SUMMARY OF EXAMPLES OF THE CANADIAN RECOMMENDED NUTRIENT INTAKE BASED ON AGE, BODY WEIGHT, AND ENERGY EXPRESSED AS DAILY RATES

Age	Sex	Weight (kg)	Energy (kcal)	Protein (g)	Vit. A (RE)	Vit. D (µg)	Vit. E (mg)	Vit. C (mg)*	Thiamin (mg)	Riboflavin (mg)	Niacin (NE)	Folate (µg)	Vit. B_{12} (µg)	Calcium (mg)	Phosphorus (mg)	Magnesium (mg)	Iron (mg)	Iodine (µg)	Zinc (mg)
Months																			
0-4	Both	6.0	600	12†	400	10	3	20	0.3	0.3	4	25	0.3	250‡	150	20	0.3§	30	2§
5-12	Both	9.0	900	12	400	10	3	20	0.4	0.5	7	40	0.4	400	200	32	7	40	3
Years																			
1	Both	11	1100	13	400	10	3	20	0.5	0.6	8	40	0.5	500	300	40	6	55	4
2-3	Both	14	1300	16	400	5	4	20	0.6	0.7	9	50	0.6	550	350	50	6	65	4
4-6	Both	18	1800	19	500	5	5	25	0.7	0.9	13	70	0.8	600	400	65	8	85	5
7-9	M	25	2200	26	700	2.5	7	25	0.9	1.1	16	90	1.0	700	500	100	8	110	7
	F	25	1900	26	700	2.5	6	25	0.8	1.0	14	90	1.0	700	500	100	8	95	7
10-12	M	34	2500	34	800	2.5	8	25	1.0	1.3	18	120	1.0	900	700	130	8	125	9
	F	36	2200	36	800	2.5	7	25	0.9	1.1	16	130	1.0	1100	800	135	8	110	9
10-12												175		1100					12
13-15	M	50	2800	49	900	2.5	9	30	1.1	1.4	20	170	1.0	1000	900	185	10	160	12
	F	48	2200	46	800	2.5	7	30	0.9	1.1	16	170	1.0	1000	850	180	13	160	9
16-18	M	62	3200	58	1000	2.5	10	40	1.3	1.6	23	220	1.0	900	1000	230	10	160	12
	F	53	2100	47	800	2.5	7	30	0.8	1.1	15	190	1.0	700	850	200	12	160	9
19-24	M	71	3000	61	1000	2.5	10	40	1.2	1.5	22	220	1.0	800	1000	240	9	160	12
	F	58	2100	50	800	2.5	7	30	0.8	1.1	15	180	1.0	700	850	200	13	160	9
25-49	M	74	2700	64	1000	2.5	9	40	1.1	1.4	19	230	1.0	800	1000	250	9	160	12
	F	59	1900	51	800	2.5	6	30	0.8¶	1.0¶	14¶	185	1.0	700	850	200	13	160	9
50-74	M	73	2300	63	1000	5	7	40	0.9	1.2	16	230	1.0	800	1000	250	9	160	12
	F	63	1800	54	800	5	6	30	0.8¶	1.0¶	14¶	195	1.0	800	850	210	8	160	9
75+	M	69	2000	59	1000	5	6	40	0.8	1.0	14	215	1.0	800	1000	230	9	160	12
	F**	64	1700	55	800	5	5	30	0.8¶	1.0¶	14¶	200	1.0	800	850	210	8	160	9
Pregnancy (additional)																			
1st Trimester			100	5	0	2.5	2	0	0.1	0.1	1	200	0.2	500	200	15	0	25	6
2nd Trimester			300	15	0	2.5	2	10	0.1	0.3	2	200	0.2	500	200	45	5	25	6
3rd Trimester			300	24	0	2.5	2	10	0.1	0.3	2	200	0.2	500	200	45	10	25	6
Lactation (additional)			450	20	400	2.5	3	25	0.2	0.4	3	100	0.2	500	200	65	0	50	6

*Smokers should increase vitamin C by 50%.
†Protein is assumed to be from breast milk and must be adjusted for infant formula.
‡Infant formula with high phosphorus should contain 375 mg calcium.
§Breast milk is assumed to be the source of the mineral.
¶Level below which intake should not fall.
**Assumes moderate (more than average) physical activity.
KEY: NE = Niacin equivalents; RE = retinol equivalents.
Modified from Health and Welfare Canada, Nutrient Recommendations; with permission of the Minister of Supply and Services Canada, 1994.

NUTRITION: ESSENTIALS
AND
DIET THERAPY

SEVENTH EDITION

NANCY J. PECKENPAUGH, M.S.Ed., R.D., C.D.E.
Dietitian in Private Practice
Lifetime Nutrition Services
Ithaca, New York

CHARLOTTE M. POLEMAN, B.S., R.D.
Community Dietitian
Broome Developmental Services
Ithaca, New York

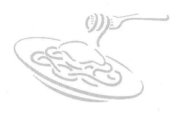

W.B. SAUNDERS COMPANY
A Division of Harcourt Brace & Company
Philadelphia   London   Toronto   Montreal   Sydney   Tokyo

W.B. Saunders Company
A Division of Harcourt Brace & Company

The Curtis Center
Independence Square West
Philadelphia, Pennsylvania 19106

Library of Congress Cataloging-in-Publication Data

Peckenpaugh, Nancy J.
    Nutrition: essentials and diet therapy. / Nancy J. Peckenpaugh,
Charlotte M. Poleman.—7th ed.
        p. cm.
    Poleman's name appears first on the earlier edition.
    Includes bibliographical references and index.
    ISBN 0–7216–5130–5
    1. Diet therapy. 2. Nutrition. I. Poleman, Charlotte M.
II. Title.
    [DNLM: 1. Nutrition—nurses' instruction. 2. Diet therapy—
nurses' instruction.   QU 145 P367n 1995]
    RM216.P67 1995   613.2—dc20
    DNLM/DLC

Nutrition: Essentials and Diet Therapy, 7th ed.   0–7216–5130–5

Printed in the United States of America.

Last digit is the print number: 9 8 7 6 5 4 3 2 1

To the nurses who have asked,
"How can you be a dietitian? Nutrition is so boring!"
and to my family and friends
who inspired and supported this endeavor.

Nancy J. Peckenpaugh

To my grandchildren:
Charlotte, Daniel, Lindsay, Sarah,
Catherine, Margaret, and Michael.

Charlotte M. Poleman

PREFACE

Every year we learn something significantly new about nutrition. Ongoing research at every level, from the biochemical to the sociocultural, expands our knowledge base in this important discipline. While this new knowledge increases our potential for improving the care we bring to our patients, it also makes the teaching and learning of nutrition more complex and difficult, particularly given the limited class time devoted to nutrition in the education of health care professionals. In writing the seventh edition of *Nutrition: Essentials and Diet Therapy,* our objective has been to provide a focused, practical approach to basic health care nutrition.

In providing better focus, we concentrate on what is most important for the health care provider to know about the nutrition basics and the application of nutrition knowledge. The previous edition was rigorously reviewed and revised toward this end:

- In order to provide a more focused examination of the nutrients, we have combined the five nutrient chapters of the previous edition into two: Chapter 3, Carbohydrate, Protein, and Fat: The Energy Macronutrients of Balanced Meals; and Chapter 5: Vitamins, Minerals, Electrolytes, and Water.
- The chapters on sports nutrition and healthy weight management have been combined to highlight their interrelationship.
- The former chapter on miscellaneous conditions has been broken up and redistributed to place the components in more relevant context.
- Application of the Health Belief Model used by health educators is included throughout the book in appropriate chapters.

To make the text more practical, we have revised the many features of the previous edition that people found most helpful and have brought some new tools for learning into the text:

- The food guide pyramid now takes a central position throughout the book, both as a guide for self-nutrition and as a tool for teaching patients about balanced diets.
- To make compliance, sociocultural, and family issues more interesting and relevant, we have introduced a special new feature at the beginning of each chapter, A Family's Perspective on Nutrition, in which the nutrition-related experiences of one extended family are described. Each episode in the family's life reflects the topic of the chapter, and reference is made to the vignette in the chapter itself to highlight certain concepts. The student learns, along with the Bernardo family, how medical nutrition therapy is central to the management of many chronic and acute health problems.
- Important notes for patient teaching have been highlighted as boxes

within the text, to provide immediate access to this important content without removing it from the context of the general discussion.

- Most of the major headings are in the form of questions, providing a better focus for the section discussions and serving as a study tool that gives immediate access to the material when it is being reviewed.
- The popular Facts and Fallacies feature has been retained to help users overcome their own as well as their patients' misconceptions about nutrition.

Discussions of important topics have been substantially updated and expanded, including those dealing with diabetes mellitus, AIDS, eating disorders, dental health, and nutritional support. The new Nutrition Screening Initiative developed by the American Academy of Family Physicians, the American Dietetic Association, and the National Council on Aging, Inc. has been included in the chapter on the older adult. A new chapter is devoted to the nursing process, including discussion of verbal and nonverbal communication strategies for effective assessment and the application of nutrition care plans.

As in previous editions, a separate instructor's manual has been made available. This helpful supplement includes answers to the text questions, suggested reading materials, sources of audiovisual aids, sample test questions, and overhead transparency masters. It also provides a guide for using the chapter-opener vignettes in classroom discussion.

Our guiding principle throughout the writing of this text is that nutrition is and increasingly will be one of the core disciplines for health care as we move into the 21st century. Not everyone takes medications, not everyone undergoes surgery or other extraordinary medical procedures, but everyone is involved in nutrition. It is the single most important factor in the care of the well and the ill client. As previously stated, our aim has been to make this body of information more accessible and useful to the people who need it most, the health care providers. We would be very interested in your views concerning how well we have met this objective and how we might better meet it in future editions. Please write to us in care of WB Saunders Company with your suggestions.

ACKNOWLEDGMENTS

We would like to pay tribute to the original author, Alberta Shackelton, who helped pioneer the advanced instruction of nutrition at Rutgers University with the first publication of this nursing textbook in 1929. The enthusiastic support of the staff at the Tompkins Day Treatment Program and their review of chapter material and assistance in providing photographs used in the text was fully appreciated. The Bernardo family case study was reviewed and modified based on the comments of Richard Cacciotti, who now runs his grandfather's Italian grocery store, and Donna Santasiero, a nurse of Italian heritage. Special recognition goes to the memory of Lynda Pryzgocki, RN, CDE, a colleague and friend who shared firsthand experience related to the importance of including the patient as a central part of the health care team. The authors further thank the dedicated staff at WB Saunders Company, especially the nursing editor Daniel Ruth for his expertise and full support of the direction taken in the seventh edition.

NANCY J. PECKENPAUGH, M.S.ED., R.D., C.D.E.
CHARLOTTE M. POLEMAN, B.S., R.D.

LIST OF REVIEWERS

Frances M. Anderson, R.N., M.S., B.S.N.
Robert Morgan Vocational Technical
Institute
Miami, Florida

Shirley Anderson
Department of Nursing
Kirkwood Community College
Cedar Rapids, Iowa

Lois Ann Dickson Caskey, M.S.N., B.S.N.
Department of Nursing
Shreveport-Bossier Regional Technical
Institute
Shreveport, Louisiana

Cheryl J. Cassis, R.N., M.S.N.
Department of Nursing
Belmont Technical College
St. Clairsville, Ohio

Patricia S. Crose, R.N., M.S.
Chairperson, Level I
St. Frances Hospital School of Nursing
Hartford, Connecticut

Sharon Fulling, M.S.N.
Assistant Dean and Director of Nursing and
PE
Mississippi County Community College
Blytheville, Arkansas

Mary P. Godwin, R.N., M.A., B.S.N., C.S.
Assistant Professor for Gerontological
Nursing
School of Nursing
Castleton State College
Castleton, Vermont

Theresa L. Hollowell, M.A., B.S., R.D.H., A.A.S.
Instructor
Nutrition Department
Kalamazoo Valley Community College
Kalamazoo, Michigan

Ruth A. Horgan, M.Ed., R.D.
Assistant Professor and Chairperson of
Dietetics Division
Laboure College
Boston, Massachusetts

Marilyn E. Hudgins, R.N., M.S.N.
LPN Instructor
George C. Wallace State Community
College
Dothan, Alabama

Patricia M. Jacobson, R.N., M.S.N.
Department of Nursing
Bullard Havens Regional Vocational
Technical School
Bridgeport, Connecticut

Cathy Kapica, Ph.D., R.D., C.H.E.
University of Pittsburgh School of Dental
Medicine
Pittsburgh, Pennsylvania
University of the Health Sciences-Chicago
Medical School
North Chicago, Illinois

Carol A. Lang, R.N., B.S.N.
Department of Nursing
L. H. Bates Technical College
Tacoma, Washington

Linda L. Love, R.N., M.A.Ed., B.S.N.
Department of Nursing
Grand Rapids Community College
Grand Rapids, Michigan

Shirley D. Miller, R.N., M.S.Ed., Ed.S., B.S.N.
LPN Instructor
Department of Nursing
Okefenokee Technical Institute
Waycross, Georgia

Carol J. Nelson, R.N., M.S.N., B.S.N.
Instructor
Department of Nursing
Spokane Community College
Spokane, Washington

Debra Phillips, R.N., M.S.N.
School of Nursing
Brunswick College
Brunswick, Georgia

Sally Roach, R.N., M.S.N.
Director of LVN Program
c/o Knapp Medical Center
Weslaco, Texas

Gayle F. Sewell, R.N., M.N., B.S.N.
Instructor
Department of Nursing
North Central Kansas Area Vocational-
Technical School and Cloud County
Community College
Beloit, Kansas

Melanie Shuran, Ph.D., R.D.
Professor and Chairperson
Department of Nutrition and Clinical
Dietetics
Finch University of Health Sciences – The
Chicago Medical School
North Chicago, Illinois

Sandra Ann Timm, B.S.
Department of Nursing
Minnesota Riverland Technical College
Rochester, Minnesota

Margaret Vogel, R.N., B.S.
Instructor
Department of Nursing
Minnesota Riverland Technical College
Rochester, Minnesota

Levia Rochella Walton, R.N., M.P.H., B.S.N.
Department of Nursing
Maui Community College
Kahului, Maui, Hawaii

CONTENTS

INTRODUCTION TO NUTRITION AND A MULTICULTURAL CASE STUDY MINISERIES

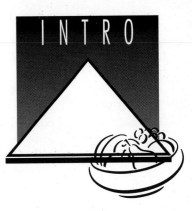

OBJECTIVES

After completing this chapter, you should be able to:
- Define terms used in the study of nutrition
- Describe basic functions of food
- Identify factors affecting health
- Describe what total health care means and how best to utilize this approach
- Discuss the importance of assessing biopsychosocial health concerns
- Discuss the attitudes, knowledge, and skills needed for effective nutrition care by the nurse or other health care professional
- Identify your personal strengths and weaknesses in nutrition knowledge and application

TERMS TO IDENTIFY

Absorption
Activities of daily living (ADL)
Biopsychosocial
Carbohydrates
Dietitian
Digestion
Fats
Food Guide Pyramid
Health

Health care team
Holistic health
Ingestion
Kilocalorie
Macronutrients
Malnutrition
Medical nutrition therapy
Minerals
Nutrient
Nutrition

Nutritional care
Nutritional status
Nutritionist
Optimal nutrition
Proteins
Prudent diet
Public health
U.S. Dietary Guidelines
Vitamins

1. **Nutrition** is the sum of the processes by which the body uses food for energy, maintenance, and growth.

2. **Malnutrition** is a state in which a prolonged lack of one or more nutrients retards physical development or causes the appearance of specific clinical conditions (e.g., anemia, goiter, rickets). Excess nutrient intake is another form of malnutrition when it leads to conditions such as obesity.

3. **Optimal nutrition** means that a person is receiving and using the essential nutrients to maintain health and well-being at the highest possible level.

4. **Nutritional status** is the condition of the body as it relates to the consumption and use of food. *Good nutritional status* refers to the intake of a balanced diet containing all the essential nutrients necessary to meet the body's requirements for energy, maintenance, and growth. This means that the body's requirements are being met. *Poor nutritional status* refers to inadequate intake (or use) of nutrients to meet the body's requirements for energy, maintenance, and growth. In nursing terms, this means that the intake is less than the body requirements. A person who is malnourished has a poor nutritional status (see section on nutritional assessment, Chapter 7).

5. A **nutrient** is a chemical substance that is present in food and needed by the body. **Proteins, carbohydrates, fats, minerals, vitamins,** and water are among the more than 50 nutrients needed by the body.

6. **Nutritional care** is the application of nutrition knowledge in the feeding of individuals.

7. A **nutritionist** is an educator as well as a counselor who usually works in a public health setting and who should have a graduate degree in nutrition.

8. A **dietitian** is concerned with the promotion of good health through proper diet and with the therapeutic use of diet in the treatment of disease. A bachelor's degree with a major in foods and nutrition or institutional management is the minimal educational requirement for a dietitian. The majority of dietitians are registered and can be identified by the initials R.D. after their name. All dietitians are nutritionists.

9. The **health care team** may be composed of various professionals, for example, physician, dietitian, nurse, pharmacist, physical and occupational therapists, speech therapist, social worker, and recreational therapist.

10. A **prudent diet** is a diet that contributes to reducing the risk for a variety of diseases, notably cardiovascular diseases, stroke, and certain types of cancer.

11. **Health** is currently recognized as being more than the absence of disease. High-level wellness means that the individual is actively engaged in moving toward fulfillment of his or her potential (O'Toole, 1992).

12. **Public health** is the field of medicine that is concerned with safeguarding and improving the health of the community as a whole. Public health nurses may work out of public health departments or private health organizations.

13. **Holistic health** is a system of preventive medicine that takes into

account the whole individual: It promotes personal responsibility for well-being and acknowledges the total influences—social, psychological, biological, and environmental—that affect health, including nutrition, exercise, and mental relaxation.

14. A **kilocalorie** (or large calorie) is a unit of measure used to express the fuel value of carbohydrates, fats, and proteins. The kilocalorie used in nutrition represents the amount of heat necessary to raise the temperature of 1 kg of water 1° C. One pound of body fat equals 3500 kilocalories.

15. **Medical nutrition therapy** (usually referred to as diet therapy) is the treatment of disease through nutritional therapy. This is the current term promoted by the American Dietetic Association.

WHAT ARE THE FUNCTIONS OF FOOD IN NUTRITION?

Food is any material, solid or liquid, that after **ingestion** (taking in food), **digestion** (the physical and chemical breaking down of food in the gastrointestinal tract), and **absorption** (absorbing food nutrients from the intestinal tract) is used to build and maintain body tissues, regulate body processes, and supply energy—also referred to as kilocalories. Any given food is a mixture of certain elements, such as minerals (calcium, phosphorus, sodium, iron, and so on), **macronutrients** (carbohydrates, fats, proteins), and water, any of which is called a nutrient.

A nutrient, therefore, is any substance that performs one or more functions in the body. Some nutrients function in more than one way. A single food might contain only one nutrient (e.g., carbohydrate in sugar) or several nutrients (e.g., carbohydrate, protein, fat, calcium, potassium, magnesium, and vitamins A, D, B_2, and B_{12} in milk). A variety of foods in the diet in the correct amounts will provide all the necessary nutrients (about 50 when the various amino acids, minerals, and vitamins are counted).

Figure 1 shows the basic functions and sources of nutrients and oxygen as represented by an analogy with a house. This analogy can also be used in patient education with children or adults who need a simple explanation. For example, without minerals and protein we could not have the solid structure of the house. Carbohydrates act like the firewood for quick and easy energy. Dietary fat can be stored as body fat (as portrayed by the coal bin) and provides a long-lasting energy source. Figure 2 shows how the macronutrients of carbohydrate, protein, and fat are represented in the **Food Guide Pyramid** (recommended intake of food to meet adequate nutritional intake while portraying the **U.S. Dietary Guidelines** of decreased fat and sugar with increased amounts of fiber) and the application to meal planning.

WHAT FACTORS AFFECT ONE'S STATE OF HEALTH?

Many factors affect one's state of health, such as proper care and functioning of all body organs, good diet, a good mental attitude, good personal hygiene and body care, genetic factors, exercise, and the environment (Table 1). It is generally agreed that one of the most important factors that affects the health of an individual, a community, or a nation is nutrition.

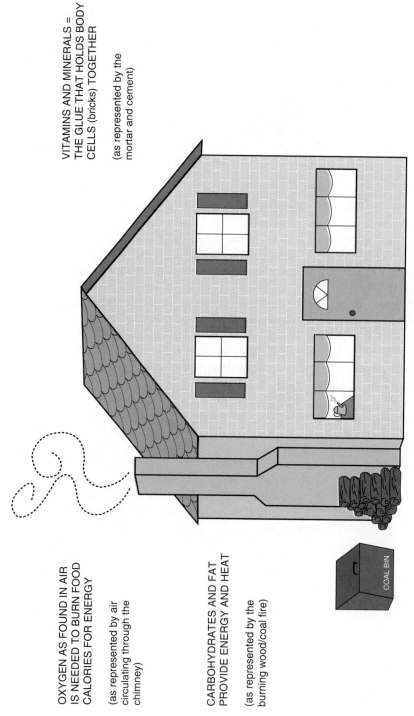

OXYGEN AS FOUND IN AIR
IS NEEDED TO BURN FOOD
CALORIES FOR ENERGY

(as represented by air
circulating through the
chimney)

CARBOHYDRATES AND FAT
PROVIDE ENERGY AND HEAT

(as represented by the
burning wood/coal fire)

STORED ENERGY = BODY FAT

(represented by the coal bin
and wood pile)

VITAMINS AND MINERALS =
THE GLUE THAT HOLDS BODY
CELLS (bricks) TOGETHER

(as represented by the
mortar and cement)

PROTEIN = BUILDING BLOCKS

(as represented by bricks)

WATER PROVIDES MOISTURE
AND PREVENTS DEHYDRATION

(as represented by the
kettle containing water)

COAL BIN

▲ FIGURE 1

Basic functions of nutrients and oxygen.

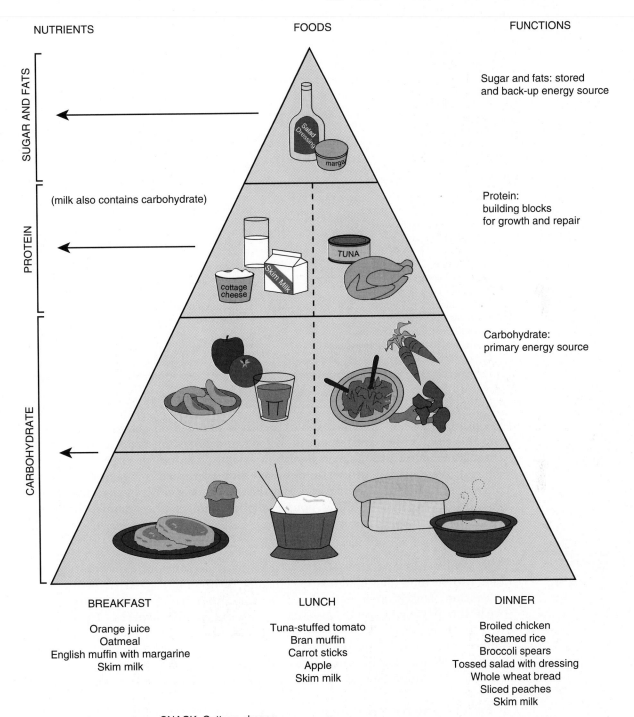

NUTRIENTS

SUGAR AND FATS

PROTEIN

CARBOHYDRATE

(milk also contains carbohydrate)

FOODS

Salad Dressing

marga

TUNA

Skim Milk

cottage cheese

FUNCTIONS

Sugar and fats: stored and back-up energy source

Protein: building blocks for growth and repair

Carbohydrate: primary energy source

BREAKFAST

Orange juice
Oatmeal
English muffin with margarine
Skim milk

LUNCH

Tuna-stuffed tomato
Bran muffin
Carrot sticks
Apple
Skim milk

DINNER

Broiled chicken
Steamed rice
Broccoli spears
Tossed salad with dressing
Whole wheat bread
Sliced peaches
Skim milk

SNACK Cottage cheese

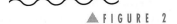

▲ F I G U R E   2

Carbohydrate, protein, and fat in one day's balanced meal plan using the Food Guide Pyramid.

▲ T A B L E   1

FACTORS THAT PROMOTE GOOD HEALTH

Good Diet
  Eating right kinds and amounts of food
  Regular meals
  Avoiding alcohol
  Drinking adequate water
Good Mental Attitude
  Positive outlook on life
  Emotional stability
  Social support group
  Stress reduction
Regular Aerobic Exercise
  Sufficient sleep and rest
Good Personal Hygiene and Habits
  Not smoking
  Good posture
  Preventive care of teeth
  Knowledge of and regular practice of self-checks for disease warnings
Regular Medical Care
  Recommended immunizations
  Needed eye and ear examinations
  Early attention to warning signs of disease

Optimal (best or most favorable) health is founded on good nutrition. Eating the right kinds and amounts of food and following good dietary habits throughout one's life mean a healthier body and mind, greater vitality and energy, greater resistance to disease, and increased longevity. The role played by food in promoting and maintaining good health is therefore a major one. Its role in fulfilling nonmetabolic social, socioeconomic, and emotional needs must be recognized as well.

HEALTH CARE DELIVERY

How Is Nutrition an Aspect of Total Health Care?

The total needs and care of the patient as a person and community member, rather than just diagnosis, continue to be emphasized in health care education. Nutrition is considered an integral part of patient care, along with the physical, social, psychiatric, and economic aspects. The patient (the term *patient* will be used throughout this book to mean client, consumer, and so on) requires adequate nutritional intake to maintain an already good nutritional state or to improve a poor one. For many patients, food is the single factor or one of several factors used to restore good health.

Patient-centered educational activities are the accepted approach in choosing learning experiences by the health professional. The result is a better understanding by the patient of medical nutrition therapy in illness and recovery as well as nutrition in everyday living. Nutrition education strategies provided throughout this textbook can later be applied to patient education. Although health may be restored without medicine, it cannot be maintained without proper nutrition.

What Are Biopsychosocial Concerns in Health Care?

Biopsychosocial concerns address the interplay of environmental (external) and internal forces. For example, the diagnosis of diabetes is primarily a biochemical or internal problem, but for the person hearing this diagnosis, it involves psychological issues of acceptance versus denial and social concerns of healthy living in an environment that is stressful and provides little opportunity for low-fat, low-sugar food choices (external problems or forces). The biochemical problem of either very high or very low blood sugar levels can also affect the ability to think (cognitive functioning) and emotions. The incidence of depression is increased with poor blood sugar control. The nurse or other health care professional who is aware of the interplay of external forces and internal forces (acceptance or denial and the ability to make appropriate personal health care decisions) will be a much more effective team member of the health care system.

What Is the Health Care Team?

The health care team comprises all the health care professionals who work with a given patient or patients and their families toward the common goal of patient health (Fig. 3). This includes the medical part of the team (physician, nurse, dietitian, physical therapist, and pharmacist), the social professionals (social worker, psychologist, occupational therapist), and other community resource personnel who play a role in facilitating good health. Since each type of health care professional has a unique perspective on needs assessment and health care planning, a team approach is most effective in eliciting positive changes in a person's well-being.

The patient should also be considered part of the health care team. The patient may arguably be the most important member of the health care team. This is especially true in managing chronic illness because of the day-to-day management decisions required by the patient in making lifestyle changes. Lifestyle changes, no matter how small, can have either a positive or a negative impact on health. It is critical that patients feel they have choices in their health care intervention; they should be considered integral to the health care team in the planning and implementation stage (see Chapter 2). The patient needs to be encouraged to contribute fully to the assessment phase and be actively involved in the planning stage. This will increase patient cooperation, leading to better compliance and improved health outcomes.

How Does the Health Care Team Coordinate Patient Services?

Each health care professional brings a unique perspective and set of skills from his or her field of knowledge. All health care professionals use a variety of patient intervention skills. Coordination of patient care is important to help ensure that appropriate and reinforcing messages are provided

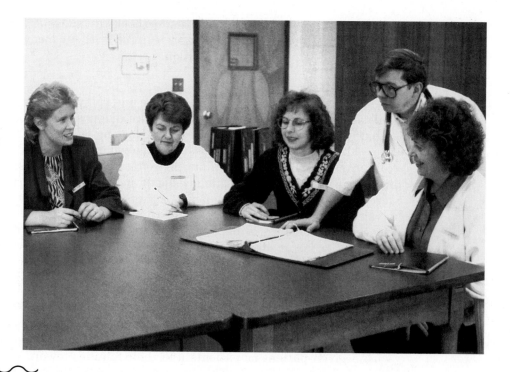

▲ FIGURE 3

The Health Care Team. (Courtesy of Broome Developmental Services, Ithaca, NY.)

by each member of the health care team. Team meetings are an effective means to coordinate patient care, but outside of institutional settings, written referrals may need to suffice. Final health care decisions often are in the realm of the physician, who should be kept informed of concerns of the health care team and their recommendations for individual patient care.

THE PHYSICIAN

Generally the person with the most broad-based knowledge related to patient health care is the medical doctor or M.D., otherwise referred to as the physician. The physician knows the patient's medical history and has a general understanding of the relationship of disease states to other health concerns. Often, however, it is in the best interest of the patient for the physician to make referrals to other complementary health services. The physician needs to be kept abreast of health services received by the patient. This may be in the form of written documentation in a hospitalized patient's chart, through standardized written correspondence from a community agency or other health care provider, or through telephone contact when there is an urgent need for the physician and the health care provider to discuss patient needs.

THE NURSE

The nurse generally has the most contact with individual patients and their families and can provide the other members of the health care team with good insight into patient needs. Ongoing assessment and monitoring of patient eating habits and health status is an important role of the nurse.

THE SOCIAL WORKER

The social worker is the health care professional who has expertise in the area of community resources, including financial, counseling, technical support, and educational services. The social worker often can help patients identify and express barriers, whether perceived or actual, that they may be facing to their goal of achieving health and wellness. Other health care professionals can best meet the patient's needs when there is feedback from the social worker. Many times the patient is not "ready" to hear health care advice because of the need to resolve and come to terms with a chronic or acute illness.

THE PHYSICAL THERAPIST

Assisting in promoting mobility and physical movement to control pain is part of the role of the physical therapist (P.T.) and physical therapy assistant (P.T.A.). A physical therapist may be involved with helping a person enhance physical capabilities that have been impaired through illness or trauma. Exercises, splints, canes, and walkers are common tools used by the physical therapist.

THE OCCUPATIONAL THERAPIST

The occupational therapist or O.T. emphasizes the remaining strengths of the individual and identifies adaptive devices that would enhance independent functioning, such as large-handled spoons and reaching devices. The O.T. works to increase the amount or types of **activities of daily living (ADL)** a patient is involved in, such as personal hygiene and eating. This is of particular importance after a person has suffered a stroke or other physical injury that impairs or prevents independent living.

THE SPEECH PATHOLOGIST

The professional to consult when assessing the seemingly simple act of swallowing is the speech pathologist. Swallowing, a series of interrelated steps, can be seriously impaired after a stroke or other neurological damage (see Chapter 11). Aspiration of food (inhaling food into the lungs) is of serious consequence and can lead to partial or full airway obstruction or pneumonia. A speech pathologist can help determine the degree of risk of aspiration and make appropriate care plans that other health care professionals can use in developing their own plans. For example, the patient may need physical therapy to position correctly for good swallowing, the occupational therapist may promote eating utensils designed for special feeding needs, and the dietitian may need to specify food of certain consistencies to facilitate effective swallowing.

THE PHARMACIST

The registered pharmacist is responsible for preparing the nutritional solutions that the physician orders. These solutions are administered through veins or enteral routes (see Chapter 14). The dietitian often makes recommendations in consultation with the physician on the solutions, so that they provide appropriate amounts of nutrients for the specific patient's needs. Having specialized knowledge about drugs and their actions, the pharmacist is able to serve as a resource person concerning drug and nutrient interactions.

THE REGISTERED DIETITIAN

The registered dietitian (R.D.) is the health care professional best qualified to interpret the science of how food is used by the body in health and disease states and how changes in the diet can improve a patient's health status. The R.D. also works with culturally diverse populations in adapting customary foods to meet ongoing health concerns and diet prescriptions. Nurses should alert a dietitian of any nutrition concerns they may have about their patients.

WHAT IS THE ROLE OF THE NURSE IN THE HEALTH OF SOCIETY?

A nurse's contact with patients in any situation provides unlimited teaching opportunities to promote better nutrition. The nurse's own dietary habits, attitudes, and state of nutrition are reflected in his or her interest and approach when helping patients understand the importance of a basic normal or modified diet. Success will more likely occur if the nurse starts with good attitudes toward the importance of nutrition. By having a good basic knowledge of nutrition and by keeping informed, the nurse can also do much to combat the misinformation forced on the public (by one or another method) by slanted advertising, food faddists, quacks, and untrained self-termed "health specialists." (Food facts and fallacies are discussed in each chapter in this text whenever appropriate.) In the community setting, the nurse has a unique opportunity to help families plan meals and is able to explain why good nutrition will promote growth and development in children and maintain good health in adults.

WHAT IS YOUR NUTRITION IQ AS YOU BEGIN THE STUDY OF NUTRITION?

Some of the following statements are true, and some are false. Read each question and then check your answer in the appropriate column before you consult the list of correct answers at the bottom of page 14. Page numbers for relevant chapter discussions are given for your convenience.

		TRUE	FALSE
1.	A daily diet for weight reduction should have adequate amounts of protein, minerals, and vitamins but should furnish less than the daily requirements for kilocalories. (p. 441)	☐	☐
2.	Margarine and butter contain the same number of kilocalories. (pp. 72, 76)	☐	☐
3.	Milk and cheese are constipating foods. (p. 271)	☐	☐
4.	One never outgrows the need for milk in the diet. (p. 460)	☐	☐
5.	A well person who eats the right kinds and amounts of foods every day does not need to take vitamin pills. (p. 97)	☐	☐
6.	Skipping meals is a good way to lose weight safely. (p. 442)	☐	☐
7.	No food can be considered "fattening" or "slenderizing." (p. 131)	☐	☐
8.	"Fast food" is unusually high in sodium and fat. (p. 34)	☐	☐
9.	Calcium supplements are the best way to increase calcium intake if one does not like milk. (p. 118)	☐	☐
10.	The risk of heart disease can be reduced by following a diet low in saturated fat, cholesterol, and sodium. (pp. 190, 204)	☐	☐
11.	White bread is the same thing as wheat bread. (p. 60)	☐	☐
12.	Olives and olive oil are low in saturated fat, and moderate amounts of each are fine for a low-cholesterol diet. (p. 75)	☐	☐
13.	Dried peas and beans are a rich source of protein, fiber, and other nutrients. (pp. 64, 70)	☐	☐
14.	One's risk of heart disease can be reduced by consuming fish from cold water regions. (p. 200)	☐	☐
15.	Pasta is a good source of complex carbohydrates. (p. 59)	☐	☐
16.	Nuts contain cholesterol. (p. 72)	☐	☐

17. A peanut butter sandwich made with whole-grain bread provides "complete protein." (p. 28) ☐ ☐

18. Fat should account for no more than 30 per cent of the total kilocalories in the daily diet. (p. 137) ☐ ☐

19. Avocados are high in fat. (p. 76) ☐ ☐

20. The best way to lose weight is to follow a diet that is low in carbohydrates. (p. 61) ☐ ☐

21. Athletes should consume twice as much protein as other people do to improve performance. (p. 434) ☐ ☐

22. Natural sweets like honey have fewer calories and less carbohydrate than sugar does. (pp. 64, 65) ☐ ☐

23. Drinking water at mealtimes may aid digestion if it is not used to wash down food. (p. 90) ☐ ☐

24. A teenager needs more milk every day than a preschooler does. (p. 389) ☐ ☐

25. Fad diets for reducing are not only ineffective for permanent weight reduction but also may be dangerous. (p. 426) ☐ ☐

26. Some foods rich in vitamin C should be eaten daily, as the body cannot store this vitamin. (p. 98) ☐ ☐

27. Orange juice loses vitamin C if exposed to air in an open container. (p. 125) ☐ ☐

28. One should eat a wide variety of foods daily to meet nutrient requirements as specified by the RDA. (pp. 132, 133) ☐ ☐

29. Vitamin E has been well proven to prevent heart disease, cancer, impotency, and circulatory problems. (pp. 109, 110) ☐ ☐

30. Beet and turnip greens contain large amounts of vitamin A. (p. 99) ☐ ☐

Number of correct answers _____
Number of incorrect answers _____
How good do you think your Nutrition Score is?

FOOD, NUTRITION, AND HEALTH IN A MULTICULTURAL CASE STUDY MINISERIES

This textbook presents a multicultural perspective with emphasis on biopsychosocial nutrition concerns. Information about all cultures will be discussed in the context of specific illnesses and diets. In addition, we will focus on the concerns of a hypothetical Italian-American family in an ongoing, miniseries approach.

The Bernardo family is not unlike the millions of other families who have immigrated to the United States in the past century. Some genetically based health problems can be traced back to our roots of heritage whether in Europe or other parts of the world. Even though we may be Americans we all share a different family heritage. Even if there is not a direct familial link, ". . . unrelated members of an ethnic group or race with common ancestry share a common gene pool and, hence, may resemble one another (biochemically and physically) more than they resemble people from other groups . . . Most chronic diseases whose etiology and pathogenesis are influenced by nutritional factors have genetic determinants. High blood pressure, obesity, hyperlipidemia, atherosclerosis, and various cancers appear to aggregate in families for genetic reasons rather than merely because of common environment" (National Research Council, 1989). While this is a land of plenty, excess food intake can cause havoc for the health of many persons.

It has been shown around the world that a change to a more Westernized diet and lifestyle, with increased kilocalories, fat, and sugar and reduced fiber and activity level resulting in obesity, increases the rate of diabetes. This has been noted with African-Americans (Auslander et al., 1992), Australian Aborigines (O'Dea, 1991), Inuits and Native Americans (Murphy et al., 1992) and Japanese who immigrated to Hawaii (Kawate et al., 1979). An interesting study showed that adult Pima Indians in Arizona reduced their near 50 per cent rate of diabetes when they returned to a more traditional lifestyle with increased activity and fibrous foods (Brody, 1991). The prevalence of diabetes in Italy is lower than it is in the United States (Bruno et al., 1992), but with increasing body weight and intake of saturated fat, persons of Italian heritage in the United States can expect to have an increased rate of diabetes compared with their counterparts in Italy.

Health care professionals need to be aware of health issues surrounding food and nutrition in a multicultural context. Health screening should assess family health history. Diabetes tends to run in families (see Chapter 9), as do lactose intolerance and food allergies (see Chapter 15), and other health concerns. Beyond the biological component, the psychosocial context of a family's lifestyle has a bearing on health care. The health care professional who is aware of these interactions can better assess family and individual needs for health care changes.

Reading about the Bernardo family's health and nutrition concerns, from their perspective, should help personalize and promote increased empathy by health care professionals. For example, what are some likely emotions of this multigenerational Italian family as they encounter common health problems in this country and attempt to follow principles of good nutrition? The impact of adolescence, pregnancy, diabetes, and weight management on diets and the concerns of the aging will be explored.

The focus on the Italian population allows an understanding of the impact of emigration on eating habits in both a positive and a negative perspective. How do Italians in Italy eat as compared with second- or third-generation Italian-Americans? How have Italian cuisine and food customs adapted to the culture of this country? What are the implications for other ethnic groups?

As a practicing health care professional, can you apply the food guides to typical Italian cuisine? Do you know how to include pizza, lasagna, or manicotti into the Food Guide Pyramid? How does olive oil fit into the Dietary Guidelines for Americans for less fat and less saturated fat? Do you know what polenta is? These and other questions about ethnic food will be explored throughout this textbook.

As you read about the Bernardo family in the coming chapters you may want to refer to this introduction to think how you would handle their unique concerns. What type of health professionals would be useful in meeting the special health-related needs of the Bernardo family? The chapter materials will give you further ideas about how you as a health care professional could help this family meet their health concerns. You might also think about other families with different cultural backgrounds and how they might be served if they faced similar problems. You may be able to share with your classmates some cultural distinctions that you have with your own family and how you would advise your classmates to make them more effective health professionals in a multicultural perspective.

STUDY QUESTIONS AND ACTIVITIES

1. Why should nutritional counseling be sought only from those with a knowledge of the science of nutrition?
2. Name three risk factors that affect one's state of health.
3. What are the functions of food in nutrition?
4. List four skills needed to apply nutrition knowledge.
5. Research ethnic cultures and foods as provided by your instructor.
6. Interview your family members to identify health problems that your parents, aunts, uncles, and grandparents have had. Do you know what countries your family ancestors came from before arriving in America?

CORRECT ANSWERS TO THE NUTRITION IQ TEST:

1. T	9. F	17. T	25. T
2. T	10. T	18. T	26. T
3. F	11. T	19. T	27. T
4. T	12. T	20. F	28. T
5. T	13. T	21. F	29. F
6. F	14. T	22. F	30. T
7. T	15. T	23. T	
8. F	16. F	24. T	

"MY FOOD AND NUTRITION EXPERIENCE DIARY"

To help make you "food- and nutrition-minded" as you study nutrition, set up a chart like the one following and jot down any food and nutrition comments, questions, or experiences you encounter. These should come from discussions with individuals outside of a classroom setting and later from your experience as you give nutritional care to patients (checking menus, setting up and serving trays, feeding patients, and so on). Assemble in a notebook (preferably), folder, or file box any available food and nutrition booklets, clippings, or other printed materials you may encounter.

Date	*Food and Nutrition Experience*	*Comments*

REFERENCES

Auslander WF, Haire-Joshu D, Houston CA, Fisher EB: Community organization to reduce the risk of non-insulin-dependent diabetes among low-income African-American women. Ethn Dis, 1992; 2(2):176–184.

Brody JE: To Preserve Their Health and Heritage, Arizona Indians Reclaim Ancient Foods. The New York Times, May 21, 1991.

Bruno G, Bargero G, Vuolo A, Pisu E, Pagano G: A population-based prevalence survey of known diabetes mellitus in northern Italy based upon multiple independent sources of ascertainment. Diabetologia, 1992; 35(9):851–856.

Kawate R, Yamakido M, Nishimoto Y, Bennett PH, Hamman RF, Knowler WC: Diabetes mellitus and its vascular complications in Japanese immigrants on the Island of Hawaii. Diabetes Care, 1979; 2:161–170.

Murphy NJ, Schraer CD, Bulkow LR, Boyko EJ, Lanier AP: Diabetes mellitus in Alaskan Yupik Eskimos and Athabascan Indians after 25 years. Diabetes Care, 1992; 15(10):1390–1392.

National Research Council, Committee on Diet and Health: Diet and Health. Washington DC, National Academy Press, 1989; pp 87 and 94.

O'Dea K: Westernization and non-insulin-dependent diabetes in Australian Aborigines. Ethn Dis, 1991; 1(2):171–187.

O'Toole M, ed.: Miller-Keane Encyclopedia & Dictionary of Medicine, Nursing, & Allied Health, 5th ed., Philadelphia, WB Saunders Co, 1992; p 649.

THE ART OF NUTRITION

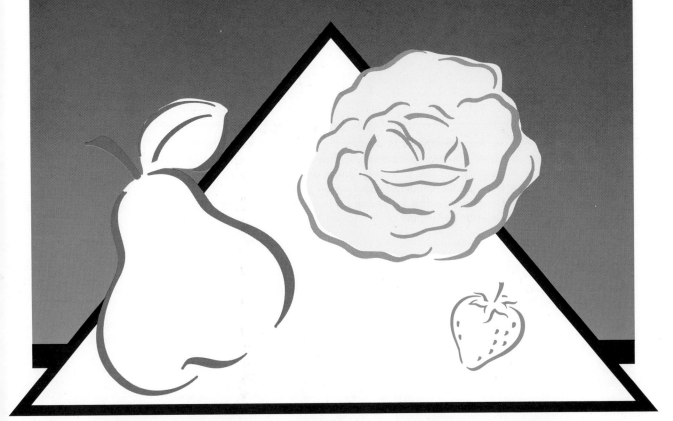

CHAPTER 1

NUTRITION IN A FAMILY MEAL ENVIRONMENT

CHAPTER TOPICS

CHAPTER INTRODUCTION
HOW FOOD AND DIETARY PATTERNS DEVELOP
CULTURAL AND SOCIETAL INFLUENCES
IMPACT OF VEGETARIANISM ON HEALTH
IMPACT OF SNACKING ON HEALTH
IMPACT OF FAST FOODS ON HEALTH
IMPACT OF ALCOHOL ON HEALTH

OBJECTIVES

After completing this chapter you should be able to:

- Identify positive and negative influences on nutritional intake and health
- Describe the role of vegetarianism on health
- Describe the impact of snacking on health
- Describe how fast foods can be included in a healthy way of eating
- Describe the impact of alcohol on health

TERMS TO IDENTIFY

Beta carotene	Goiter	Nutrient density
Cleft palate	Grazing	Recommended Dietary
Chronic disease	Learned food aversion	Allowances (RDAs)
Empty kilocalories	Legumes	Vegan
Fiber	Metabolic	Vegetarian

A FAMILY'S PERSPECTIVE ON NUTRITION

It had been good to visit family back in Italy. Rita Bernardo, affectionately referred to as Nanna by her grandchildren, thought how pleasant it had been to see her brothers and sisters again. Sitting around the noon meal, the special camaraderie of mealtime was certainly apparent. It was funny how a meal could be a treat without cake and cookies. And meat really wasn't such a necessity to have every day. Not like back here in the States. Meals were so different here. Now they were back into the fast-paced lifestyle of work, school activities, and other household routines.

She thought of her daughter-in-law Maria. How could Maria expect to feed the family well when she worked outside the home? Not like in Nanna's own day. Back in Italy, preparing meals was considered important by the women of the household. How could a family be healthy eating frozen vegetables? Growing children needed fresh foods. And eating so often in those fast food restaurants. No, she simply did not approve.

Her son Antonio was a hard worker. It wasn't his fault that he had been laid off with all those other workers at the factory. His new job didn't pay nearly enough, but it could provide for the family. They just needed to plan better. They really should eat at home more. She would speak to Maria.

Anna, thought Nanna, was looking so healthy. She couldn't understand why Maria was so concerned. Anna becoming overweight? She liked her granddaughter just the way she was. It made her look like she ate well and was healthy.

Now Joey, her grandson, here was a problem. He usually ate so well. She couldn't understand why he was so thin. He just didn't look well. But he did seem healthy, being one of the top wrestlers at his school, and he probably would make State Championships. Maybe she should say something to her son Antonio about Joey just in case. Her son would listen to her.

(This is the beginning of an on-going case study miniseries that can be found at the opening of each chapter.)

INTRODUCTION

The family used to be thought of as a mother, father, and at least two children. The concept of a family unit now includes single parent families, one child families, stepfamilies, foster care families, and families that have long-distance relationships in which children spend weekends with one parent and the school week with the other parent.

Owing to the complexities of family structures, meal planning from a health care professional's perspective is as much a science as it is an art. It can be reduced to a science through the tools of meal planning, which are the basic food groups of the Food Guide Pyramid, the Dietary Guidelines for Americans, and the **Recommended Dietary Allowances (RDAs)**— the estimated amount of nutrients needed to support health for at least 95 per cent of the population (see Chapter 6 for further discussion). The application of these guidelines in a manner conducive to a positive meal environment, however, is an art. For professionals who assist families in developing the skills necessary to attain the goal of good nutritional intake, some basic guidelines are useful.

It is helpful to begin by taking the view that family eating behaviors fall in a spectrum from ideal to poor. The ideal diet consists of a balance of high-quality, nutritionally dense foods in appropriate quantities and variety to support normal growth and repair while inhibiting the development of chronic disease. Most families probably fall somewhere in the middle between ideal and poor, but preferably closer to the ideal end of the spectrum.

POOR   IDEAL

Fortunately, the human body is quite resilient. Dietary intake of some nutrients can vary significantly without causing harm (e.g., protein, fat, and fat-soluble vitamins). However, some nutrients, such as water and water-soluble vitamins, are needed on a regular daily basis.

The concept of adequate levels of nutrients for health has been reflected in the five food groups of the Food Guide Pyramid and in the RDAs. With the advent of fortification, many deficiency diseases such as **goiter** have been overcome. (Goiter is a disease of the thyroid gland caused by lack of iodine; iodized salt helped eradicate goiter.) The focus has now shifted to setting maximum levels for prevention of **chronic disease** (any disease of long standing such as diabetes or hypertension); thus the advent of the Dietary Guidelines for Americans (see Chapter 6 for more information.)

The art of family meal planning comes through the creative solutions to the various negative influences inhibiting a family's ability to feed itself appropriately. The principles of moderation, balance, and variety should be applied.

HOW DO FOOD AND DIETARY PATTERNS DEVELOP?

Sound nutritional habits certainly begin in infancy. Ideally, the infant is exposed to a variety of foods and is fed in a manner that promotes positive meal association. The infant then becomes a child who learns to like a variety of foods that are of high quality and dense in nutrients. Since the child has been allowed to eat on the basis of his or her own hunger and satiety cues in a positive meal environment, eating takes place according to growth needs, and thus an appropriate quantity of food intake is maintained (see Chapter 17 for more detailed information on child development).

Many factors can change this ideal scenario. Some problems can be internal, such as food allergies or lactose intolerance, by which certain foods become associated with physical discomfort. Learned food aversions also fall into this classification. For example, a food that is eaten prior to the onset of an illness that is unrelated to food, such as a viral illness, becomes mistakenly connected to the illness. If this food is avoided in the future, it is appropriately termed a **learned food aversion.**

Many barriers to adequate nutrient intake are external in nature. They may be:

- economic (inadequate money to purchase food)
- physical (lack of food storage facilities or physical impairment such as **cleft palate,** a birth defect in which there is an opening in the roof of the mouth, lips or both)
- cultural (lack of exposure to a variety of food because of limited parental offerings or overemphasis on meat or high-fat and high-sugar foods)
- ecological (droughts, floods)
- emotional (television advertisements depicting non-nutritious foods as appealing)
- religious (adherence to restrictive food codes)
- political (food boycotts, forced starvation for military purposes)

Improvement in food selection patterns for bettering one's health frequently means changing habits of long standing. This is a slow, step-by-step, almost never-ending process necessitating a real desire to change, a deep conviction that change is important, and the willingness to substitute desirable food habits for undesirable ones. Persons dealing with nutritional improvement, although primarily concerned with the **metabolic** (biochemical) role of food in health, must also have some understanding of the circumstances under which dietary habits are acquired and the various meanings that food may have for different individuals. This is especially true in dealing with patients who suffer from a disorder or disease that requires drastic changes in dietary habits.

Since there appears to be no doubt that many nutritional deficiencies are caused by poor dietary habits, the establishment of correct habits early in life, and adherence to them throughout life, are of extreme importance. A good diet helps ensure good nutrition. The nurse or other health care professional has a unique opportunity to foster good food habits.

A registered dietitian is of special importance when there are complex factors that interfere with nutritional intake. Other professionals, such as the family physician (for medically related barriers), the physical therapist (for physical barriers such as cleft palate), and the social worker or mental health worker (for negative family dynamics), may need to be consulted as well. In order to make the best use of these professional resources, the nurse should first identify the patient's nutritional needs by describing the factors that are negatively influencing the family's ability to feed itself adequately. This role particularly suits the nurse, who has frequent regular contact with patients, but other health professionals may also play a part.

FACT & FALLACY

FALLACY: Children who do not "clean their plates" should not have dessert.

FACT: This commonly practiced fallacy may work in the short-term to coerce children to eat their meals, but the long-term implications outweigh any benefits. This approach implicitly conveys to children that desserts have more value than other foods, since dessert is being used as a "reward." Parents should be reminded that desserts can be nutritious, such as fresh, juicy fruit, a colorful fruit salad, or a piece of pumpkin pie or carrot cake. The "clean the plate" philosophy can also contribute to over-eating and excess weight gain. Children (and many adults) need to learn to stop eating when they are comfortably full.

WHAT ARE SOME CULTURAL AND SOCIETAL INFLUENCES ON NUTRITIONAL INTAKE?

Changing Food Habits in the United States

The traditional housewife is becoming scarce, as an estimated 53 million women work outside the home, according to the 1992 Statistical Abstract of the United States. This fact is contributing to the trend of increasing numbers of men becoming involved with food shopping and preparation (Fig. 1–1). Changing demographics also has an impact on the nutritional status of the United States as a whole, which in turn affects food choices. The number of elderly persons and households composed of single persons is growing, and there is an increased demand for more ready-to-use foods.

Americans are now eating about twice the amount of sugar that our ancestors did at the turn of the century. A big part of this increased sugar intake is through added sugar, such as high-fructose corn syrup, in the food supply (Barry, 1990). On a more positive note, several sources of data suggest a decline in meat consumption since the 1970s (Smiciklas-Wright et al, 1993). A recent Gallop Poll, commissioned in part by the American Dietetic Association (ADA), shows that more than half the people surveyed add oat bran and vitamin supplements to their diet and nearly three quarters try to reduce fats. Yet fewer than 10 per cent report eating more vegetables and fruits as recommended by most health experts (American Institute for Cancer Research, 1991).

Impact of Regional, Ethnic, and Religious Dietary Habits in Studying Nutrition and Meal Planning

A large number of ethnic groups are included in the population of the United States (Fig. 1–2). Coming as they do from all parts of the world, they have brought with them and tend to retain habits of eating and food tastes different from those Americans are familiar with. Conversely, some ethnic foods become popular with broad groups of people, such as Italian and Mexican foods. Unfortunately these foods often become "Americanized" with excess amounts of cheese and meat added. Traditional Italian and Mexican meals contain little meat and only moderate amounts of cheese.

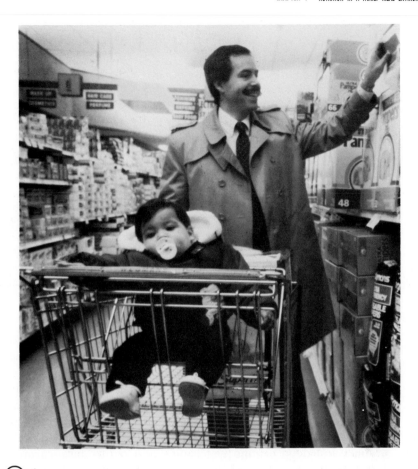

▲ FIGURE 1-1

Men are increasingly becoming involved in food shopping and meal preparation. (Courtesy of Cornell University Photography, Ithaca, NY.)

Chinese meals in China are low in fat, but Chinese restaurants in the United States often serve food high in fat, in an attempt to cater to American preferences (Hurley & Schmidt, 1993).

Unbalanced diets have been brought from some countries in which limited production has restricted the diet to a few types of foods. Persons coming from such countries need to learn better food habits in the United States and how to incorporate into their native dishes the nutrients necessary for good nutrition. More adequate diets have been brought from other countries; however, foods familiar in these countries may be rare and expensive in the United States and consequently may be omitted from the diet. If an ethnic group does give up some of its own food habits and adopts those of the new country, the poorest of the new country's nutritional habits are frequently chosen, such as a preference for excessive sweets and fats. This trend was found among second- and third-generation Mexican families

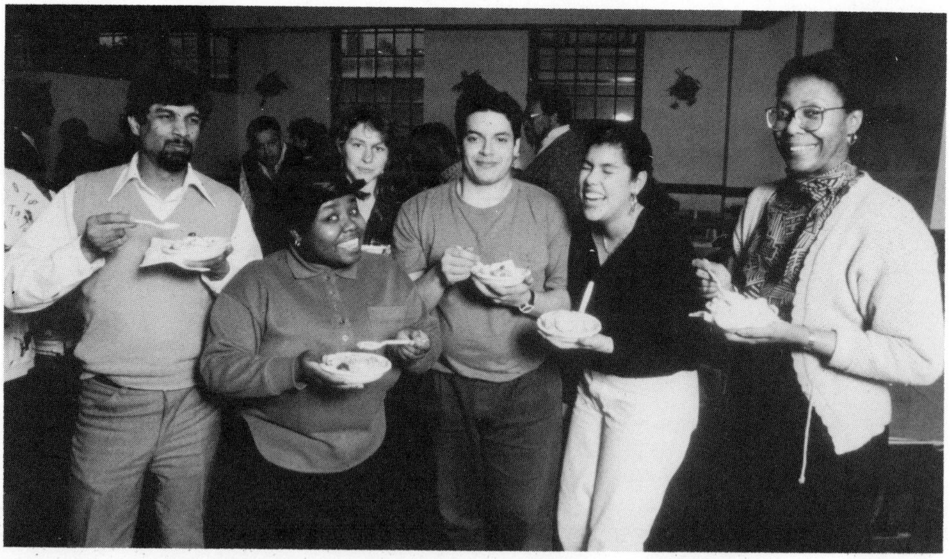

▲ FIGURE 1-2

Food as a multicultural experience in the United States (Courtesy of Cornell University Photography, Ithaca, NY.)

living in California, whose diet, as compared with the traditional diet in Mexico, showed a decrease in **beta-carotene** foods (dark green leafy vegetables and deep orange vegetables and fruits; beta-carotene turns into vitamin A in the body), in conjunction with increased sugar and fat (Romero-Gwynn et al., 1993).

If general nutrition in the United States is to be improved, educating the various ethnic groups in the best ways to supplement the good features of their native diets is an important starting point. In most cases, the answer lies in the greater use of milk, fruits, and vegetables in their cheaper forms and prepared in dishes that are accepted and enjoyed. Some assistance in planning the expenditure of food money to permit the purchase of the needed supplemental foods, as well as some help in combining these foods into dishes and meals that the family will eat, is frequently needed. The lure of foods advertised on television, which are often high in fat and sugar, also needs to be considered. It is important to acknowledge this desire to try new foods but to focus on maintaining the foundation of the diet as low-fat, low-sugar, and low-salt according to the Dietary Guidelines for all Americans.

Table 1–1 shows how the five food groups of the Food Guide Pyramid are incorporated into different types of eating patterns. A typical day's diet for any ethnic, regional, or religious group may be evaluated nutritionally by checking it against an acceptable meal plan such as the Food Guide Pyramid.

▲ T A B L E 1 - 1

ETHNIC AND REGIONAL FOOD PATTERNS ACCORDING TO THE BASIC FIVE FOOD GROUPS OF THE FOOD GUIDE PYRAMID

ETHNIC GROUP	BREAD AND CEREAL	EGGS, MEAT, FISH, POULTRY	DAIRY PRODUCTS	FRUITS AND VEGETABLES	SEASONINGS AND FATS
Italian	Northern Italy Crusty white bread Cornmeal and rice Southern Italy Pasta	Beef, chicken, eggs, fish, anchovies	Milk in coffee, cheese	Broccoli, zucchini, other squash, eggplant, artichokes, string beans, legumes, tomatoes, peppers, asparagus, fresh fruit	Olives & olive oil, balsamic vinegar, salt, pepper, garlic, capers, basil
Puerto Rican	Rice, beans, noodles, spaghetti, oatmeal, cornmeal	Dry salted codfish, meat, salt pork, sausage, chicken, beef	Hot milk in coffee	Starchy root vegetables, green bananas, plantains, legumes, tomatoes, green pepper, onion, pineapple, papaya, citrus fruits	Lard, herbs, oil, vinegar
Near Eastern	Bulgur (wheat)	Lamb, mutton, chicken, fish, eggs	Fermented milk, sour cream, yogurt, cheese	Nuts, grape leaves	Sheep's butter, olive oil
Greek	Plain wheat bread, phyllo dough	Lamb, pork, poultry, eggs, organ meats	Yogurt, cheese, butter	Onions, tomatoes, legumes, fresh fruit	Olive oil, parsley, lemon, vinegar
Mexican	Lime-treated corn tortillas	Little meat (ground beef or pork), poultry, fish	Cheese, evaporated milk as beverage for infants	Pinto beans, tomatoes, potatoes, onions, lettuce	Chili pepper, salt, garlic
Chinese	Rice, wheat, millet, corn, noodles	Little meat and no beef, fish (including raw fish) eggs of hen, duck, and pigeon, tofu and soybeans	Water buffalo milk occasionally, soybean milk, cheese	Soybeans, soybean sprouts, bamboo sprouts, soy curd cooked in lime water, radish leaves, legumes, vegetables, fruits	Sesame seeds, ginger, almonds, soy sauce, peanut oil
African American	Hot breads, pastries, cakes, cereals, white rice	Chicken, salt pork, ham, bacon, sausage	Milk and milk products (often lactase-free)	Kale, mustard, turnip greens, cabbage, hominy grits, sweet potatoes, watermelon	Molasses
Jewish	Noodles, crusty white seed rolls, rye bread, pumpernickel bread	Kosher meat (from forequarters and organs from beef, lamb, veal) Milk not eaten at same meal Fish	Milk and milk products	Vegetables— usually cooked with meat Fruits	

International research suggests that the United States might benefit by eating more like other countries, for example those described below (Broihier, 1993):

CHINESE. Studies show that the Chinese have lower blood cholesterol levels and about one-tenth the incidence of heart disease of Americans. They also have a lower cancer rate. Chinese meals focus on rice and vegetables with meat as a condiment: exactly the opposite of the typical American meal. Only 15 per cent of the Chinese diet comes from fat.

FRENCH. The French have a low risk of heart disease, second only to the Japanese. The fat content of the French diet has only recently equaled ours (since the 1980s) and their rate of heart disease may not have had time to catch up with the American rate, and thus explaining their "paradox" of high fat and low heart disease. The French, however, eat small amounts of meat and plenty of vegetables. They also eat a lot of bread, which should be the basis of any healthy diet, and tend not to eat rich desserts on a regular basis. As a rule, the French eat less shortening, oil, eggs, and sugar than Americans do.

JAPANESE. The Japanese have the lowest rate of heart disease in the world, as well as a generally low cancer risk. The Japanese diet centers around rice and vegetables but also includes lots of noodles, seaweed, fish, and soybean products including tofu.

MEDITERRANEAN REGION. Both Greeks and southern Italians have low rates of heart disease. The traditional Mediterranean diet contains lots of carbohydrate foods—vegetables, fruits, grains, and breads—along with a moderate intake of legumes and nuts. The consumption of lean red meat is usually limited to a few times per month, and fish is eaten about once a week. Milk, cheese, eggs, and sweets are eaten in small amounts. Olives and olive oil are used liberally but they are low in saturated fat and are cholesterol-free.

FACT & FALLACY

FALLACY: Italian foods are always high in fat.
FACT: In Italy little meat is eaten. Dessert is saved for special occasions only. Italian foods in this country have more meat and generally more cheese than would be used in Italy. Foods eaten in Italy meet the guidelines of the Food Guide Pyramid through the emphasis on plant foods (pasta, rice, vegetables, and legumes), moderate or small amounts of animal foods (little meat, moderate amounts of cheese), and little sugar. Olives and olive oil are low in saturated fat and their use in cooking helps prevent cardiovascular disease.

IMPACT OF VEGETARIANISM ON HEALTH

Who Follows Vegetarian Diets?

The number of vegetarians has increased rapidly over the past few decades. It is now estimated that there are 12 million Americans who consider themselves **vegetarian,** a jump of 2 million since just 10 years ago; a significant number of the new vegetarians are teenagers (Flynn, 1993). Two religious groups that forgo consumption of meat and other animal products are Seventh Day Adventists and Muslims. Others follow vegetarian diets for health, political, cultural, or economic reasons, or a combination of these.

How Do Vegetarian Diets Differ?

There are three main classifications of vegetarian diets:

1. *Lacto-ovo vegetarian.* Plant foods are supplemented with dairy products and eggs. This is probably the most common type of vegetarian diet.

NUTRITIOUS SAMPLE MENU for a VEGAN DIET

▲

BREAKFAST
Oatmeal with soy milk
Whole wheat toast with peanut butter
Orange juice
½ Grapefruit
Herbal tea

▲

LUNCH
Lentil soup
Apple slices with sesame seed butter
Whole wheat bread
Glass of soy milk

▲

SUPPER
Tofu stir fry
Fresh spinach salad
Cantalope wedges
Herbal iced tea

▲

SNACK
Walnuts
Whole wheat crackers
Glass of soy milk

Lacto comes from the word *lactose* (milk sugar) and *ovo* comes from *ovum* (egg). Lacto-ovo vegetarians often also eat fish and chicken.

2. *Lacto-vegetarian.* Dairy products are included, but eggs are not.

3. *Total vegetarian **(vegan)**.* Animal food sources (including eggs and dairy products) are completely excluded. For this reason, the diet is low or inadequate in iodine, vitamin B_{12}, iron, calcium, zinc, riboflavin, and vitamin D.

How Should One Plan a Vegetarian Diet?

The five food groups, with emphasis on a wide variety of plant foods, should be the basis of an adequate vegetarian diet (Figure 1–3 and Table 1–2). Meat is replaced with an increased intake of **legumes** (dried beans and peas), nuts, meat analogs such as soybean burgers, and nonfat or low-fat milk products.

Vegans (those persons who eliminate all animal products from the diet) must replace the nutrients found in the milk group, ideally through food alternatives (see list of vegetarian calcium sources, Table 1–3) but possibly by supplementation because of the difficulty in obtaining calcium from non-milk sources.

Because of the restrictive food code of vegetarians, it is of the utmost importance that primarily **nutrient-dense** foods (high amounts of nutrients in relation to the total kilocalories) are consumed. The use of whole grains is critical. **Empty kilocalorie** foods (foods high in kilocalories but low in nutrients) should be avoided.

Sources of Important Nutrients in Vegetarian Diets

Soybean, a legume high in protein and unsaturated fat, is particularly useful in vegetarian diets because it contains all eight essential amino acids (see Chapter 3) in abundance. Soybeans must be boiled or roasted before processing.

The addition of dairy products, with or without eggs, to a selection of legumes and whole grains, along with the use of vegetable oils that provide unsaturated fatty acids (see Chapter 3), constitutes a nutritious diet. Legumes contribute fiber as well as B vitamins and iron, and whole grains provide carbohydrates, protein, thiamine, and iron and are a good source of trace minerals. (Table 1–2 lists various non-meat food sources that contain important nutrients.)

By combining different foods in vegetarian diets, complete proteins can be formed from the available amino acids. For example, the following combinations are recommended for nutritious, meatless menu items (it should be noted that these foods do not have to be included at the same meal but do need to be included within the same day):

Whole grains plus legumes = good protein source
Legumes plus nuts or seeds = good protein source
Whole grains, legumes, nuts, or seeds plus milk products
= good protein source

Vegetarian meal planning as related to the food guide pyramid. 1-2-3-4-5 indicates the minimum number of recommended servings (see Fig. 6–1 for serving size). Group 2 (proteins) allows for a vegan approach or a lacto-ovo vegetarian approach. (From Mastrapa SC: Diet patterns for total vegetarians. Adventist Review, Aug. 1980.)

GRAINS

barley	cornmeal	rye
brown rice	millet	whole wheat
bulgur wheat	oats and oatmeal	

▲ T A B L E   1 - 2

FOOD SOURCES FOR IMPORTANT NUTRIENTS IN THE VEGETARIAN DIET

NUTRIENT	SOURCES
Calcium*	Milk and milk products, particularly cheese and yogurt; fortified soy milk; dark green leafy vegetables such as parsley, kale, spinach, and mustard, dandelion, and collard greens
Iron	Legumes, dark green leafy and other vegetables, whole-grain or enriched cereals or breads, some nuts, and dried fruits (There are many factors that may affect absorption of this nutrient)
Riboflavin (Vitamin B$_2$)	Milk, legumes, whole grains, and certain vegetables
Vitamin B$_{12}$	Milk and eggs, fortified soybean milk, and fortified soya meats
Zinc	Nuts, beans, wheat germ, and cheese

* See Table 1-3.

LEGUMES

black beans	kidney beans	peanuts
black-eyed peas	lentils	soybeans and tofu
cannelini beans	lima beans	split peas
fava beans		

NUTS AND SEEDS

almonds	pecans	sesame seeds
brazil nuts	pignoli nuts	sunflower seeds
cashews	pumpkin seeds	walnuts

▲ T A B L E   1 - 3

SOURCES OF CALCIUM IN THE VEGETARIAN DIET

FOOD SOURCE	AVERAGE CALCIUM (MG)
1 cup oysters	225
3 oz. salmon	165
3 oz. sardines	370
1 cup almonds	350
1 cup Brazil nuts	260
1 cup peanuts	105
1 cup greens	200
1 cup dried apricots	100
1 cup cranberry sauce	105
1 cup dates	130
1 tbsp blackstrap molasses	135

HOW DOES SNACKING AFFECT NUTRITION?

The traditional pattern of having only three meals daily is becoming less common with today's busy lifestyles. Many people find it more convenient to eat when they can, and snacking has become part of our culture. The term **grazing** is sometimes applied to the frequent all-day eating that many people engage in. The daily coffee break is a popular custom for people in all walks of life.

When one eats does not matter as long as there are at least three meals daily. Skipping meals in an attempt to control weight can actually have the opposite effect (see Chapter 20). Rather, it is more important to consider *what* is eaten, and *how much,* remembering the principles of moderation, balance, and variety. Three meals daily may be satisfactory for some people, but others find that the best way to receive adequate and appropriate amounts of kilocalories and nutrients is to eat more often. Snacking can be beneficial for children and adults alike, especially if appetites are small in relation to physical needs. As a general rule, snacks with low nutrient density should not replace breakfast, which is a very important meal nutritionally.

FACT & FALLACY

FALLACY: A late-night snack or meal causes weight gain.

FACT: The time when food is eaten has little impact on weight. What is more important is the total kilocalorie and fat content of meals and more frequent eating. Saving all the day's kilocalories for one late-night meal is a problem. Rather, the kilocalories should be spread out over the day, with emphasis on breakfast and at least three meals.

How Should Snacks Be Chosen?

There is no single perfect snack, but some snacks are more nutritious than others, and careful selection is necessary to avoid potential problems. Snacks should be planned according to the needs of each member of the family. An individual who nibbles food during food preparation or clean-up may find it easy to put on unwanted pounds and hard to succeed in a weight reduction program. Conversely, planned snacking can be an effective means for meeting the energy and nutrient needs of a growing or very active child or adolescent and may be an effective weight management strategy.

Many snack foods have a high fat and sugar content and do a disservice to the principles of moderation, balance, and variety. Hunger can be satisfied by foods other than candy, potato chips, and soft drinks. The traditional carrot and celery sticks or apple and banana are always wise choices, but other whole grains, fruits, and vegetables are equally appropriate snacks.

Snacks should be chosen from the five food groups. Foods such as sticky sweets, which have been found to increase susceptibility to tooth decay, should be avoided. Pizza, hamburgers, and similar fast foods are considered to be nutritious snacks but need to be planned into the day's meals to prevent overconsumption of protein, kilocalories, fat, and sodium.

HOW DO FAST FOODS AFFECT NUTRITION?

Fast food is food purchased at an outlet featuring quick service, convenience, and relatively low cost. *Fast food service* would be a more accurate term, because it is the speed and style of service, rather than the food itself, that distinguishes fast food restaurants from other eating establishments. Many families with young children eat at fast food restaurants (Figure 1–4).

What Is the Definition of Fast Foods?

It is unfortunate that fast foods are often referred to as *junk food*. This is a particularly inappropriate label now that offerings of low-fat meal choices on fast food menus have increased. The Food Guide Pyramid concept can easily be applied to fast food. To illustrate: A small cheeseburger on a bun with lettuce, tomato, and onion, plus juice, represents the five food groups;

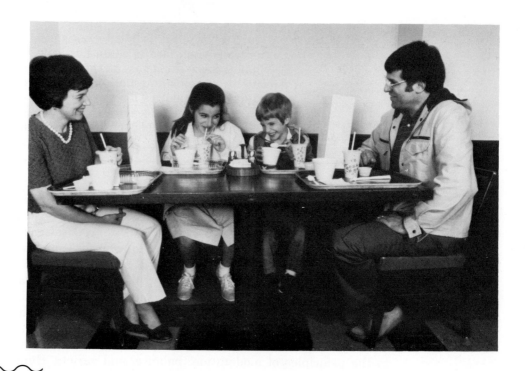

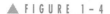

▲ FIGURE 1–4

A family eating in a fast food restaurant. (Courtesy of Cornell University Photography, Ithaca, NY.)

NUTRITIOUS MENU INCLUDING FAST FOOD

▲

BREAKFAST (AT HOME)
Toasted English muffin with peanut butter
Banana slices dipped in wheat germ
Glass of low-fat or skim milk

▲

LUNCH (CAFETERIA)
Chili con carne
Piece of cornbread
Glass of low-fat milk
Bunch of grapes (brought from home)

▲

SUPPER (FAST FOOD RESTAURANT)
Small cheeseburger
Small orange juice
Large tossed salad with 1 tbsp regular dress-
ing or free use of lemon juice or
low-kilocalorie dressing

▲

SNACK (AT HOME)
Herb-seasoned low-fat popcorn
Apple cider

a taco is composed of a shell made from grain, along with ground beef, shredded cheese, shredded lettuce, and tomato; pizza has a crust made from grain, plus tomato sauce, cheese, and various vegetable and meat toppings; a typical fried chicken dinner with mashed potato, coleslaw, a roll, and a glass of milk also represents at least four of the five food groups. Fast foods can also meet the nutrient density criteria required by the U.S. Department of Agriculture for Type A school lunches by providing one third of the RDA for selected nutrients. See Appendix 4 for a nutritional analysis of selected fast food restaurants.

What Are Some
Nutrients Found in
Fast Foods?

PROTEIN. Animal products such as fish, chicken, beef, cheese, and milk are excellent sources of protein and are available in all quick service restaurants. It is possible to fulfill 60 to 100 per cent of one's protein RDA with a single fast food meal. Other meals can be adjusted to prevent excessive intake of protein.

FAT. Some of the major components of fast foods (beef, cheese, mayonnaise, and deep-fat frying) are rich sources of fat. However, because of consumer demand, some restaurants are offering low-fat selections such as salad bars and low-fat milk. Consumers need to be aware that the salad toppings they choose might be high in fat. Lemon juice is a flavorful, low-fat topping that can be used freely.

CARBOHYDRATE AND FIBER. Complex carbohydrate is found in enriched rolls and French fries. Fast food menu items are generally low in **fiber** (the part of plant foods that resists digestion), except for salads and coleslaw. Empty kilocalories found in soft drinks and shakes can be reduced by requesting milk, juice, or water as a beverage.

CALORIES. Fast food menus include many high-kilocalorie items, but with calorie counts available, weight-conscious people can incorporate fast foods into their diets. Requests to omit high-kilocalorie toppings can be fulfilled easily. Other meals in the day can be modified to compensate for high-kilocalorie selections.

VITAMINS. Most fast food meals provide adequate amounts of thiamine, riboflavin, niacin, pyridoxine, and cobalamin. Vitamin C is found in orange juice, coleslaw, potatoes, and the increasingly available salads. Vitamin A is low in hamburger or chicken fast food meals, but Mexican-style foods and pizza provide some vitamin A from the tomato and cheese. Salads are also good sources of vitamin A if raw carrots, tomatoes, and dark green leafy vegetables are included.

MINERALS. Milkshakes and milk are high in calcium and phosphorus. Hamburgers are high in iron, and if rolls are made with enriched flour, they are also a fair source of iron. Beef and dairy products, which are used in many entrees, are good sources of zinc. Sodium can be a problem for those advised by physicians to lower their intake of that element, because many fast foods are relatively high in sodium (in the form of salt, which is sodium chloride), but again, requests for no salt can be made.

What Is Junk Food?

Many fast foods and snack type foods contain empty kilocalories (commonly called *junk food*). Empty kilocalories do provide the nutrients carbohydrate and fat, but they do not contribute any significant amounts of protein, vitamins, and minerals. Empty kilocalorie foods, such as candy, table sugar, and added fats, are appropriate when necessary for maintenance of weight, as long as the other nutrient needs are being met, or when "something is better than nothing." For other situations, the rule of moderation applies. Empty kilocalorie foods are not harmful on an occasional basis.

A useful analogy to use with children is to explain that some foods (those high in fat and sugar) help us grow outward whereas other foods (such as those in the Food Guide Pyramid) help us grow upward. Using your hands to graphically describe is very effective in getting children's attention.

Unfortunately, our society tends to overvalue many foods with empty kilocalories. Schools often reward academic achievement with candy, children of divorced parents may be given extra "treats" in attempts to lessen the guilt of the parents, and television advertisements tell us to "Go ahead, you deserve it!" Because of this reward system, many Americans have problems with overconsumption of low nutrient foods that are high in fat and sugar. It is time we put junk foods into perspective: In moderation they are fine but should never be used as a reward.

HOW DOES ALCOHOL INTERFERE WITH NUTRITIONAL STATUS?

Alcohol consumption affects health under two general, broad modes. One is the actual inhibition of food intake resulting from factors such as decreased appetite, replacement of the kilocalories in the alcohol for those in food (concern for weight control), or the use of available food money for alcohol. The other major impact is impaired absorption, reduced storage, increased metabolic needs, and impaired use of nutrients. Thiamin deficiency is often a result of excess alcohol and too little food.

WHAT IS THE ROLE OF THE NURSE OR OTHER HEALTH CARE PROFESSIONAL IN THE FAMILY MEAL ENVIRONMENT?

The nurse plays a vital role in assessing and identifying patient and family needs, while facilitating solutions in a counseling approach. Meal planning can be relatively simple when there are few or no negative forces influencing a family. The more likely scenario, however, is a combination of internal and external barriers to good nutrition, which can best be overcome through a total health care team approach. Many community services are available that can complement the skills of the health care team.

STUDY QUESTIONS AND CLASS ACTIVITIES

1. Explain what is meant by the following statement: "Good meal planning is both a science and an art."
2. How would you assist the Bernardo family, described in the opening case study, in meeting their health and nutrition needs? Describe potential nutrition problems, questions you might ask the family to

assess their nutritional intake and status, and possible intervention strategies if problems are identified. (See Chapters 2 and 7 for further ideas on nutrition assessment).

3. List nutritious snack ideas that are high (more than one third of the RDA) in one of the following nutrients: 1) vitamin A, 2) vitamin C, 3) calcium, 4) iron.

4. Plan a fast food restaurant meal that includes all of the five food groups of the Food Guide Pyramid and that is in line with the Dietary Guidelines for Americans for less fat, sugar, and salt and more fiber.

5. How would you advise a patient to overcome food dislikes or avoidances?

6. If one of the Bernardo children decided to follow a vegetarian diet, what might you suggest to ensure adequate nutritional intake?

7. Analyze food advertisements in magazines. To whom is the ad appealing? How?

8. Become familiar with the ethnic, religious, or regional diet assigned you by the instructor and summarize information about it to present to the class. Be prepared to discuss this ethnic diet in terms of the five food groups of the Food Guide Pyramid and Dietary Guidelines for Americans (see Chapter 6). What are the good points? How could the diet be improved? Each student in the class will then use the following chart to record important information about each diet presented in class.

Ethnic Dietary Habits

Regional or ethnic diet (list foods)	Characteristics and main dish	Good nutritional features	Desirable nutritional improvements

9. Students might tell about the food customs and dietary habits of their country or countries of heritage and possibly demonstrate the ethnic dishes popular in their family meals. Markets of a city, ethnic food sections of large grocery stores, and ethnic restaurants afford good opportunities for learning about foods used by families with different ethnic backgrounds. The class might prepare an Italian meal or go to lunch at an Italian restaurant to better understand the food choices of the Bernardo family.

REFERENCES

American Institute for Cancer Research, Newsletter, Issue 32, Washington DC, Summer 1991.
Barry RD: The US sugar program in the 1980's. Nat Food Rev. 1990; 13(1):55.
Broihier CA: Environmental Nutrition, April 1993; 16(4):1–4.

Hurley J, Schmidt S: Chinese food: a wok on the wild side. Nutrition Action Newsletter, Sept 1993; pp 10–12.

Flynn ME: How you can borrow from the global pantry and come up healthy. Environmental Nutrition, March 1993; 16(3):5.

Romero-Gwynn E, Gwynn D, Grivetti L, et al.: Dietary acculturation among latinos of mexican descent. Nutrition Today. July/August 1993; 6–12.

Smiciklas-Wright H, Giles LE, Wang MQ: Meat consumption of respondents to USDA's nation-wide food consumption survey. Food & Nutrition News, Jan/Feb 1993; 65(1):1.

Statistical Abstract of the United States. Washington, DC: US Department of Commerce; 1992.

THE NUTRITION CARE PROCESS AS USED BY HEALTH CARE PROFESSIONALS

CHAPTER 2

CHAPTER TOPICS

CHAPTER INTRODUCTION
THE NUTRITION CARE PLANNING PROCESS
THE HEALTH BELIEF MODEL
INTERVIEWING AND COMMUNICATION SKILLS FOR EFFECTIVE NUTRITION ASSESSMENT
NUTRITION COUNSELING TIPS FOR THE NURSE OR OTHER HEALTH CARE PROFESSIONAL

OBJECTIVES

After completing this chapter you should be able to:
- Describe the steps of the nursing process as it relates to nutrition care
- Describe the implications of the Health Belief Model for patient compliance
- Describe good communication skills
- Describe appropriate nutrition interventions for families
- Describe the role of the patient in facilitating compliance in health care and nutrition

TERMS TO IDENTIFY

Active listening
Affective
Albumin
American Heart
    Association
Change agent
Cholesterol
Cognitive

Expanded Food and
    Nutrition Education
    Program (EFNEP)
Health Belief Model
Hemoglobin
"I" versus "You"
    statements
Nonverbal communication
Nursing process

Nutrition care process
Nutrition Program for the
    Elderly
Psychomotor
Women, Infants, and
    Children (WIC)
    Supplemental
    Food Program

A FAMILY'S PERSPECTIVE ON NUTRITION

He just knew it was more bad news. Not that he could take anymore. The appointment with his doctor was in 15 minutes. Tony pushed the gas pedal to the floor. After being laid off work because of the plant shutdown, his wife informs him she's pregnant. Pregnant! There wasn't enough money to pay the bills as it was. The minimum wage job he was lucky enough to finally get just wasn't enough to make ends meet. And now he's told the doctor wants to talk with him about his lab results. Great, just great!

Donna was just preparing the file on Mr. Antonio Bernardo. A newly diagnosed case of diabetes with elevated serum cholesterol and triglycerides. And this was the first patient who she was responsible for as Dr. Shaw's new nurse. What was she going to say to Mr. Bernardo? Should she tell him he was a prime candidate for a heart attack, even though he was of Italian heritage? His risk factors clearly made him so: middle-aged, a smoker, overweight, with high cholesterol and triglycerides, a history of hypertension, and now diabetes. Where would she begin in assisting him meet his health care needs? She wished Dr. Shaw had made some time to discuss this case with her. One thing on her side, since she was of Italian heritage herself perhaps she could help reassure Mr. Bernardo. But she wasn't sure if he would have to give up his Italian foods in order to control his diabetes. She wondered if olive oil was okay for a low-cholesterol diet.

Dr. Graham Shaw was in his office thinking about Mr. Bernardo's case. Mr. Bernardo needed a variety of services and Dr. Shaw planned to review community resources with him. The first item on the agenda was breaking the news of the diagnosis of diabetes, which he knew was the last thing Tony needed to hear. He wished he had reviewed this case with his new nurse. No time now, however. He would just have to rely on the good judgment that he had sensed in Donna when he had hired her. Other needs of Mr. Bernardo included diet management; where was that dietitian's brochure? She recently had opened a private practice down the street and seemed good, especially since she was also a Certified Diabetes Educator. Oh yes, there it was—Jenny Burritt, R.D., C. D. E. Mr. Bernardo might also need to consult with a social worker with all that had happened this past year. He would suggest seeing Doris DeLong, C. S. W., as needed. It would certainly be understandable if Tony had a difficult time coping with this latest illness with all the other life stresses he was facing—the loss of a well paying job, his wife's pregnancy, coping with teenagers. And he had to help Tony realize that he must stop smoking now. Perhaps the local American Heart Association still had space in their smokers' treatment program. Dr. Shaw took a few deep breaths to relax himself before he faced the difficult situation of Mr. Bernardo.

INTRODUCTION

Imagine yourself meeting a new patient. What do you say? Where do you begin? What questions should you ask? How do you keep your patient from becoming defensive toward you? Do you present yourself as very professional and aloof or informal and witty? Perhaps a combination? What are you trying to achieve through contact with the patient? These are just some of the questions that face a new nurse or practicing health professional.

The **nutrition care process** of assessment, planning, intervention, and evaluation is the same as the **nursing process** with the omission of diagnosis. It is both a science and an art. By following the steps of the nursing process you will be a more effective health care professional. With practice and experience it will become easier, but your own unique style with patients can either help or hinder the process of nutrition and patient health care. Being very observant of **nonverbal** (facial expressions or other body language) and verbal communication from the patients you work with can guide you to become an effective **change agent** in patient compliance. As a positive change agent you are directly and indirectly involved in helping patients make changes in their lifestyle aimed toward improved health.

Generally, each step of the nursing process or nutrition care process should be followed in order. There is also a degree of integration between each step of the process, and the process is usually repeated several times during the course of patient intervention. This chapter emphasizes the importance of good communication skills in the nutrition care process of assessment, planning, intervention, and evaluation.

THE NUTRITION CARE PLANNING PROCESS

What are Assessment Strategies?

Nutrition care planning uses the same steps as the nursing process, the first of which is *assessment*. This step makes possible the identification of nutritional needs or problems. As the health care professional, you need first to establish patient rapport in order to promote a complete and accurate assessment of needs. Using a "chitchat" approach (such as discussing the weather or a local event) helps patients relax and talk more openly. You need to practice until you find an approach that is easy and comfortable for you and your patients. Being informal yet professional is a challenge for some health care professionals.

The assessment phase involves knowing the patient's or client's initial medical and nutritional status. Knowledge of any previous or current health concerns is important in determining the best course of action. One simple assessment is determining if the patient is overweight or underweight or has had a change in weight that may be indicative of a problem. Lab values such as those for **hemoglobin** (to determine iron status), **albumin** (to determine protein status), **cholesterol** and other blood fats, blood sugar, and others can help determine health needs that should be addressed in the later intervention phase. Other specific indicators for the assessment of nutritional status are covered in Chapter 7. These physical findings relate to the *bio* part of *biopsychosocial* concerns.

For effective intervention, assessment should also include the *psychosocial* issues that may be contributing to physical health concerns and may need to be addressed before realistic changes can take place in patient health care. For example, alcohol abuse or poor self-esteem may be causing negative food choices. This part of the assessment phase requires excellent communication skills to promote patient disclosure of potentially sensitive and personal lifestyle issues. The more thorough the assessment phase, the more likely that appropriate and well-focused intervention strategies can be identified and implemented. A "hit-or-miss" intervention plan is not only potentially a waste of time, energy, and money but can even be harmful to the patient.

The Health Belief Model, as discussed in a later section, complements the nursing process by assessing health values and beliefs prior to intervention. Family health history and heritage may give further useful information that can help the patient understand the need for making changes.

What are Planning Strategies?

The planning stage of the nursing process brings together all the findings of the assessment phase, starting with identifying priority health concerns, long-term health goals, and short-term objectives. Identifying small, achievable, and measurable objectives aimed at long-term goals and specified health outcomes is important for facilitating behavioral change by patients. When the health care professional is clear on goals and rationale for change, appropriate objectives and means of intervention can be determined.

Objectives are the steps needed to achieve long-term health goals. They should include measurable action verbs combined in a statement of intent or expected health outcome. For example, the action verbs *to identify, to recognize, to plan* can all be used in patient objectives. The expected time frame for achievement of the objectives is sometimes also included. Objectives for Mr. Bernardo in the case study might read as follows:

- The patient will recognize foods high in salt
- The patient will substitute low-salt foods for high-salt foods
- The patient will recognize foods high in sugar versus foods high in complex carbohydrates
- The patient will substitute complex carbohydrates for simple sugars
- The patient will identify low-fat food alternatives
- The patient will substitute low-fat alternatives for high-fat food choices

These objectives might be evaluated or measured through follow-up counseling sessions or through observation. Although objectives are aimed at short-term measurable activities or outcomes, goals should be more broad-based, such as "Patient will achieve near-normal blood pressure." It is important to write out the planning process to increase the effectiveness of the intervention, and to communicate the care plan to other members of the health care team.

The short-term objectives may need to be prioritized, starting with the most important change. A few easy changes are more likely to be implemented by the patient than are complex or too many changes at once. As objectives are met in the intervention and evaluation phases, the patient should receive positive reinforcement for these changes and then be encouraged to meet the other ones.

The evaluation plan is also determined prior to the intervention phase. Evaluation ultimately means changes in lab values or other clinical health outcomes. Educators will often dispute this point, but in the realm of limited dollars in the health care field, achieving desired health outcomes will help ensure continued funding of patient health care programs. The intervention phase can begin once the planned health outcomes are written, in the form of goals and objectives as based on the assessment phase, and the means of evaluation is determined.

What are Intervention Strategies?

Interventions are aimed at identifiable health objectives and goals; implementation of intervention strategies may involve other health care professionals. Good intervention objectives consider how health changes will be evaluated. The plans and interventions may have to be updated continually in keeping with the changing condition and needs of the patient.

Intervention approaches often begin with simple, brief reinforcing messages. In the case of Mr. Bernardo a question might be, "Have you tried the new low-fat snacks of hot pretzels or herb-seasoned popcorn? They are really delicious." A more general question might also be asked such as, "What have you done before to try to lower your fat or sugar intake?" Suggestions can then be built on the patient's earlier attempts or changes in eating habits.

Patient retention of information is enhanced by combining different modes of information dissemination. It is known that people remember best what they have heard, seen, and practiced. Therefore, verbal reinforcement of written educational material is more effective than simply giving patients a brochure. In addition, if patients are asked to attempt a change in the written educational material, learning and retention of information will be enhanced. Reviewing food labels and having patients describe the amount of sodium, sugar, or fat in the food product is another exercise that can be very effective in patient compliance. Asking patients what has been successful in the past in their attempts to improve their health is also useful. This allows reinforcement of the positive attempts or changes made in the past.

Through identifying individual or group goals and objectives, messages can be kept to a few key points. Prioritizing messages and offering sequential information needed to elicit patient health and eating changes are important. Simple concepts can later be built upon with more complex concepts. For example, decision-making skills regarding meal planning are advanced concepts and need to be stressed after there is a general understanding of the rationale for change. Messages given should offer positive reinforcement for behavior change. Scare tactics can cause inappropriate behaviors for health improvement, such as denial or tuning out the message (Gregor, 1993). Follow-up reinforcement or referral to other appropriate services can assist patients to continue developing more positive health habits.

What are Evaluation Strategies?

The final step of evaluation should be considered during the planning and intervention phases. The effectiveness of the plan in terms of the patient's progress must then be documented and evaluated by information and skills gained by the patient and by the outcomes of lab blood tests or other measures, as set forth in the specific patient goals and objectives. Examples for Mr. Bernardo might be achieving a 10 per cent weight loss, a fasting blood sugar level under 120 mg/dL, or a blood cholesterol level of 200 mg/dL. The evaluation process can help the health care professional determine if further intervention is needed.

There are many forms of evaluation. Measuring health outcomes is one important form, which might be done with ongoing, informal evaluation through observation such as at mealtimes or in other social settings, or through informal conversation such as discussion of food likes and dislikes. More formal evaluation may involve monitoring of lab values. Monitoring of growth in children and weight changes in adults is a simple but effective means of measuring nutritional status. Evaluation may also focus on knowledge gained through verbal or written questions. Before-and-after tests can evaluate the outcome of a planned intervention but should be used with caution, as many adults do not like to be "quizzed." For adults, self-quizzes may be better accepted so that no one but the patient knows the specific answers to questions.

The nutrition care plan (see Chapter 7, Fig. 7–4) should always be incorporated into the total patient care plan. This plan should be formulated by the health care team as soon as possible to establish patient-centered goals to be met before discharge. The physician will then review the plan.

In summary, the nutrition care planning process includes (1) nutrition assessment, (2) identification of nutritional needs, (3) planning how to meet nutritional needs, (4) carrying out the plan of care, (5) evaluating nutritional care, and (6) planning nutrition discharge (see Chapter 7).

WHAT IS THE HEALTH BELIEF MODEL?

The **Health Belief Model** is based on the theory that a patient makes health decisions in line with personal health values and the perceived benefits versus "costs." The cost of change, aside from the monetary aspect of health care services, relates to the social cost of eating differently from others and the psychological cost of changing food habits. For example, a person may feel that quality of life is more important than quantity of life to the point of refusing to attempt any lifestyle changes. The person's motivation to make lifestyle changes should be determined prior to the intervention phase. Providing a diet sheet of foods to avoid would be wasteful and possibly harmful psychologically if the person either is resolved not to make changes in eating habits or has so many other life concerns that meal changes take lower precedence. Rather, the intervention may more appropriately be aimed first at dealing with other life issues, such as referring to the Food Stamp program a person with inadequate food purchasing ability.

> Quality of life versus quantity of life might be addressed by asking an assessment question such as, "How do you feel about eating less cheese and butter to bring down your cholesterol level?" You might add in the case of Mr. Bernardo, "Eating less fat will also help you lose weight and thus bring down your blood sugar level. Are you willing to try low-fat cheese and to use less butter?"

By helping the person evaluate his or her health beliefs and values you may be able to promote compliance with changes in food habits. Education on the rationale of recommended lifestyle changes is critical to increasing patient compliance. In order to promote effective health changes, the benefit side of the equation needs to outweigh the cost side in the patient's perception.

The Health Belief Model as developed by Rosenstock (1982) suggests that people need to believe that (1) they are susceptible to illness, (2) the illness will have a serious impact on their lives, (3) changing their lifestyle will have a positive impact on their health, and (4) the health recommendations will provide psychological benefits.

The next section provides guidelines on interviewing and communication strategies that can be used to assess health beliefs. It is a challenge and an art to elicit true patient feelings regarding health and health practices. Many of these communication skills can be incorporated into a variety of settings, including discussions with patient family members and members of the health care team.

INTERVIEWING AND COMMUNICATION SKILLS

How are Good Communication Skills Important in Health Care?

Both the assessment phase and the intervention phase require good communication skills with patients. The planning stage also requires good written and verbal communication skills in working with other health care professionals in the coordination of patient care. Nonverbal communication is also involved. Using an authoritative manner is not as effective as using an empathetic approach when using active listening techniques. To promote patient discussion of personal health concerns, the following strategies are helpful (Fig. 2–1):

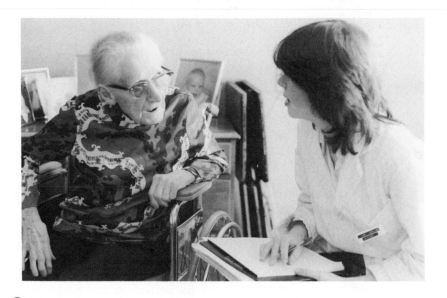

▲ F I G U R E   2 – 1

The nutrition care process begins with assessment.

- Use a warm, friendly, positive approach
- Sit in comfortable proximity, neither too close nor too far away
- Use good eye contact, with eyes intent but not staring
- Face the patient and lean forward
- Have arms unfolded and resting in a relaxed manner
- Carefully listen to what the patient is saying, using affirming responses to encourage the patient to clarify comments made
- Allow pauses in the conversation; take as long a pause as needed to consider how to best make replies—it shows that you are interested in giving correct replies

Terminology used in the intervention stage can further promote or hinder patient openness. Using overly technical medical jargon can discourage the patient's understanding and willingness to ask questions. As much as possible, the health care professional should use terms and expressions that are understood and used by the patient in everyday settings. Observing the nonverbal communication signals that the patient exhibits can assist the health care professional in determining and fine-tuning messages given based on patient needs. A patient who initially is very talkative but who becomes very quiet or begins to look at the clock is sending a powerful message. The health care professional needs to observe the verbal and nonverbal communication used by the patient and respond accordingly.

A good sense of humor can diffuse any growing tension and help redirect the message based on the patient's needs. In describing complex medical conditions you might say, "There are always fancy terms in medicine. For example, there are little doors into the body's cells that allow insulin and sugar to get in. These are called receptor sites if you do any reading on diabetes." (See Chapter 9.)

What are Some Interviewing Tips?

In the process of nutritional assessment, there are three realms that should not be overlooked in patient care: (1) **cognitive** (knowledge), (2) **affective** (attitudes), and (3) **psychomotor** or behavioral (behaviors). What is the patient's family meal environment in general? Is there adequate knowledge about good nutritional practices? Does the family value good nutrition? What constraints does the family have in gaining access to and consuming a good balanced diet? Can the patient shop and cook? Is the patient's ability to chew and digest food appropriate?

A variety of interviewing and assessment methods can be used to identify these three areas, such as diet history (see Chapter 7) and active listening–type questions (see next section). It is important to be aware that there may be misconceptions combined with accurate information. Asking patients to provide an example of a learned concept, for example, to interpret a food label, is useful in evaluating their understanding.

What is Active Listening?

Active listening is a manner of questioning and responding to a person that promotes full disclosure of opinions, feelings, emotions, and beliefs. This form of assessment can take time, but the information gathered allows for planning the most effective intervention methods. A few key questions can result in a wealth of information. Active listening is a nonjudgmental type of questioning which uses open-ended questions that elicit feelings and thoughts rather than questions that have "yes" or "no" responses. The following are examples of effective active listening questions:

GOOD INTERVIEWING QUESTIONS

How do you feel about _____?
Can you tell me what you know about _____?
Is _____ a problem for your family?
Can you tell me more about _____?

How Can "I" Versus "You" Statements Help in the Nursing Process?

"I" statements versus "You" statements complement active listening techniques. "You" statements can sound judgmental and authoritarian, which can result in a defensive reaction by the patient or client. Rephrasing "you" statements to "I" statements will enhance promotion of patient interaction and communication.

An example of a "you" statement changed to an "I" statement for Mr. Bernado is as follows: "You have a problem with fat intake" changed to "I am concerned about what appears to be a high-fat diet." (Using the term "concerned" indicates empathy. Follow this comment with an active listening questioning such as, "How do you feel about your diet?" for a very effective communication strategy.)

An "I" statement is your opinion, which makes the statement less threatening and final. Your position as an authority figure can prevent many patients from questioning statements that sound official, even if they feel that your statements are in error. A defensive reaction by the patient will essentially end your effectiveness in bringing about health changes. If patients feel that their opinions are being listened to, through the use of active listening techniques, they also will be more likely to listen to your opinions.

Does Choice Help in Patient Compliance?

Chronic illness often is best controlled or managed through ongoing support services. Developing goals and small achievable objectives is important. It is also important for the patient or client to have a feeling of choice in making health care decisions. This is often seen with acceptance of hospital food. If patients are given choices over their meal selections in the hospital, they often are more accepting of their therapeutic diet. A verbal commitment (action) from a patient can further increase the likelihood that the patient will believe in and adopt the agreed upon health change. The effectiveness of the verbal commitment will be enhanced by providing a structured choice.

Choice is important for people of all ages. Even two year olds are more likely to eat vegetables if given a structured choice such as, "Which do you want to eat tonight, carrots or broccoli?" This same principle can be applied to an adult situation, such as saying to Mr. Bernardo, "One salty food can be worked into your low-salt meal plan. Which would you prefer?" Or the choice might be between the saturated fat of cheese and that of red meat. Mr. Bernardo may be more willing to use low-fat cheese if he knows that some red meat can be included in his low—saturated fat diet.

What is the
Importance of
Honesty and Respect
in Patient Care and
Education?

It is okay to admit lack of knowledge when questioned by a patient. There is a lot to know regarding how food and nutrition affect one's health. It is much better to admit you do not know an answer than to be caught telling inaccurate information, which could forever damage your credibility as a patient educator. Instead, you might say, "That's an interesting question. Perhaps we can find the answer in this brochure."

The most important aspect of patient communication is respect. Without respect, all attempts at effective communication will be lost. For example, if you have to leave the room, tell the patient. Do not assume the patient knows you will return. If the patient makes a comment unrelated to his or her health care needs, respond anyway. Showing respect for a patient's feelings and thoughts will greatly enhance the nutrition care process.

FACT & FALLACY

FALLACY: Doctors are always the best source for nutrition information.

FACT: Most doctors receive little nutrition information in medical school, especially in the area of nutrition education. Physicians who change their own diets tend to express the most positive attitudes about nutrition and are more likely to use diet therapy in patient care (Tufts University, 1993). Physicians, other health care professionals, and even patients and their families should use the services of a registered dietitian when the need arises, even if only a phone call is made to ask a question.

COUNSELING TIPS FOR THE HEALTH CARE PROFESSIONAL IN A FAMILY MEAL ENVIRONMENT

The health care professional can help to create a harmonious mealtime—one that allows the innate satiety cues to function more effectively and also promotes the association of eating with positive feelings—by recommending the following:

- Focus on positive conversations; avoid points of potential conflict and friction
- Use candles or soft music, or both, to facilitate a quiet, relaxed atmosphere
- Eat as a family as much as possible in contrast to eating "on the run"
- Encourage young children to eat with the family but do not force them to eat; encourage the *one-taste rule* and emphasize that tastes are learned
- Serve food that looks appealing by using a combination of colors, textures, and sizes (e.g., orange carrot "coins," white chicken, crisp lettuce wedges, warm biscuits, and cold milk)
- Watch portion sizes; smaller portions are useful for small appetites and for weight control
- Provide rest and calming activities just prior to and after meals

The role of the health care professional in positively influencing family meal environments begins with an understanding of and empathy toward the various influences that have an impact on a family's ability to nourish itself appropriately. Gaining an understanding of these factors requires good interviewing skills. With the good verbal and nonverbal skills described in this chapter, the health care professional can gain knowledge of both positive and negative influences affecting families and can then make appropriate suggestions.

What are Some Common Family Nutrition Problems and Their Possible Solutions?

INADEQUATE ECONOMIC RESOURCES FOR PURCHASING FOOD

- *Refer to:*

  The Food Stamp Program

  The ***Women, Infants, and Children* (WIC) Supplemental Food Program**—a program for lower-income families that includes food coupons and nutrition education.
  Food pantries and soup kitchens
  The **Expanded Food and Nutrition Education Program (EFNEP)**—a program of the Cooperative Extension Service, for budgeting assistance

- *Use food models* to determine if excess intake in one food group (such as meat) can be reduced to allow for increase in other foods

PHYSICAL CONSTRAINTS TO OBTAINING FOOD

- *Refer to:*

  Nutrition Program for the Elderly, for meal delivery for homebound older adults
  Local grocery stores with delivery service
  Public Health Nursing for professional home-based assessment

INADEQUATE COOKING EQUIPMENT OR STORAGE FACILITIES

- *Refer to:*

  EFNEP for recipes and meal ideas

FOOD DISLIKES

- *Refer to:*

  A qualified nutritionist (or registered dietitian) for food alternatives

- *Explain* that tastes are learned; suggest the one-taste approach to facilitate acceptance

INADEQUATE TIME TO PREPARE FOOD

- *Suggest* use of nutritious but convenient food ideas:

  Vitamin A ideas: carrot sticks, apricots, cantaloupe, watermelon
  Protein ideas: cheese (low-fat or moderate amounts of natural cheese), peanut butter, eggs or egg whites

TOO MUCH SODIUM IN DIET

- *Refer to:*

  The local **American Heart Association (AHA)**—an organization promoting heart health—for recipe ideas
  A registered dietitian for individualized meal plans and behavioral change strategies

- *Suggest:*

  Use of frozen or fresh vegetables
  Use of Swiss cheese instead of high-sodium processed cheese
  Use of spices and herbs or jelly to enhance the natural flavor of food

- *Explain* that our taste for salt is both learned and unlearned
- *Explain* that salt substitutes should be used only on the advice of a medical doctor because of potential harm from the potassium content

TOO MUCH SUGAR IN THE DIET

- *Encourage* gradual sugar reduction while tastes change: use of ½ or ¾ of usual amount in baking or at the table; suggest use of fresh fruit or fruit canned in light syrup
- *Explain* that spices such as cinnamon or nutmeg can enhance the natural flavor without added sugar

TOO MUCH CHOLESTEROL, FAT, AND SATURATED FAT

- *Encourage* the use of ice water, flavored waters, iced tea, or diet soda as a replacement for soft drinks
- *Refer to:*

  American Heart Association for recipe ideas

- *Suggest* a gradual change from 4 per cent (whole milk) to 2 per cent (low-fat) to 1 per cent and ultimately to skim milk while tastes change
- *Suggest* use of less butter, margarine, mayonnaise, and oil
- *Explain* that although cholesterol is found only in animal foods, saturated fats should also be avoided; food products with ingredient labels that say *liquid oil* are better than those that say *hydrogenated oil* (see Chapter 8 for more details)

NEGATIVE EFFECTS OF COMMERCIALS ON FOOD-BUYING PRACTICES

- *Explain* that advertisements are meant to sell products; they generally are not concerned with healthy dietary habits
- *Explain to children* that many foods they see advertised help them to grow outwards, not upwards (a representation with your hands can be helpful to children)

STUDY QUESTIONS AND ACTIVITIES

1. What assessment questions should Donna, the new office nurse, ask Mr. Bernardo in the case study?
2. Why might Dr. Shaw be thinking of referral sources for Mr. Bernardo?
3. What are some good questions to ask Mr. Bernardo to determine his health belief system regarding diabetes management?
4. Should Dr. Shaw start his session with Mr. Bernardo by stating all the adverse health outcomes that can come from not taking care of his diabetes? Why or why not?

5. Should Dr. Shaw's nurse have told Mr. Bernardo his new diagnosis of diabetes on the telephone when making his appointment? Why or why not?

6. Have a class role-play with one student serving as a nurse or other health care professional attempting to use the Health Belief Model in assessing the needs of a volunteer patient. The patient should be from another ethnic background (refer to class activity in Chapter 1 regarding differences in ethnic cultures and food choices). Other class members should critique the role-play for good communication techniques and how successfully the nutrition care process was put into practice. The role-play might be repeated to cover a number of different ethnic backgrounds, including Mr. Bernardo's situation.

REFERENCES

Gregor W: Nutrition communications opportunities with patients: some guidelines for nurses. Food and Nutrition News, May/June 1993; 65(3):17.

Rosenstock IM: The health belief model and nutrition education. J Can Diet Assoc. 1982;43:184.

Tufts University: Doctors fail to make the nutritional grade. Tufts University Diet & Nutrition Letter. April 1993; 11(2):1.

THE SCIENCE AND APPLICATION OF NUTRITION

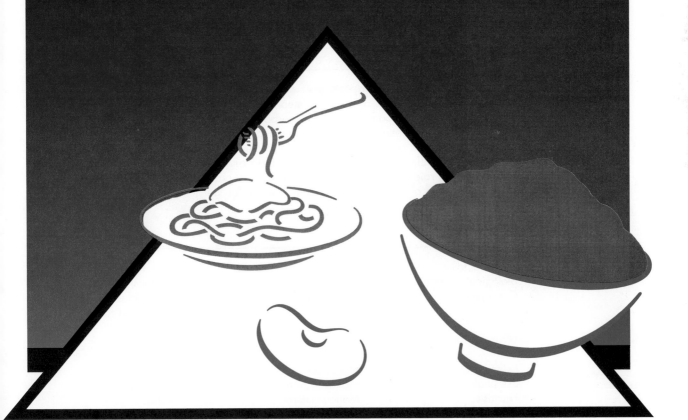

CARBOHYDRATE, PROTEIN, AND FAT: THE ENERGY MACRONUTRIENTS OF BALANCED MEALS

CHAPTER 3

OBJECTIVES

After completing this chapter, you should be able to:

- Describe the importance of balanced meals containing carbohydrate, protein, and fat
- Describe the three broad categories of carbohydrates, and their food sources and functions in promoting health and preventing disease
- Describe the food sources and functions of protein
- Describe the different types of fat found in food and their functions in health
- Describe the role of the nurse or other health care professional in promoting appropriate intake of carbohydrate, protein, and fat for the general public

TERMS TO IDENTIFY

Amino acids	Hydrogenated fat	Omega-3 fatty acid
Biological value of protein	Insoluble fiber	Photosynthesis
Cariogenic	Ketosis	Polysaccharides
Cellulose	Kwashiorkor	Polyunsaturated fat
Dietary fiber	Lactose	P:S ratio
Disaccharides	Linoleic acid	Saturated fat
Energy	Lipids	Soluble fiber
Essential amino acids	Marasmus	Sugar alcohols
Essential fatty acids	Monosaccharides	Trans fatty acid
Fructose	Monounsaturated fat	Triglycerides
Glycerol	Nitrogen balance	Unsaturated fat

Maria was tired but the kitchen was getting bare. Where was her shopping list? She found the list in her purse and started reading it over. Cornmeal, tagliatelle, fusilli, bucatini, pastini, Italian and whole-wheat bread, mozzarella, ricotta, lentils, chickpeas, fava and cannelini beans, pancetta, anchovies and anchovy paste, tuna, olive oil, unsalted butter, balsamic vinegar, capers, pignoli nuts, canned tomatoes, garlic, basil, fresh carrots, oranges, dried fruit, and a variety of frozen vegetables. Much quicker and just as good as fresh vegetables, she thought to herself. And then there were the extras for the children. Ice cream, soda pop, and baked goods. They could wait on chips this shopping trip. Now, what kind of cereal did Tony say he wanted? Something about bran. She just wanted to get home and lie down. The feeling of nausea was starting again.

INTRODUCTION

The macronutrients of food—carbohydrate, protein, and fat—are essential for life. Balanced meals contain all three macronutrients, which provide the fuel for body functioning (although of the three, protein serves this function least well). All three macronutrients contain carbon, hydrogen, and oxygen as the base. Protein foods also contain nitrogen.

The base of the diet should emphasize plant foods, which are the main source of carbohydrate, and are portrayed in the two lower levels of the Food Guide Pyramid (see Chapter 6 for more information). Grain products and legumes (dried beans and peas) also contribute significant amounts of protein and minimal amounts of fat. With emphasis on low-processed whole grains, deep orange vegetables and fruits, dark green leafy vegetables, skim or low-fat milk, and legumes, all of the nutrients needed for health can be obtained.

The main protein foods in the diet are found in the third level of the Food Guide Pyramid (Fig. 3–1). Meat, eggs, and milk all contain complete protein with all of the **essential amino acids** (the building blocks of protein that must be supplied in the diet). Since Americans typically consume two to three times the daily need for protein, meat is receiving less emphasis and is thus portrayed in smaller amounts closer to the tip of the Food Guide Pyramid. One-half cup of legumes contains as much protein as one ounce of meat. Because legumes are relatively low in fat and high in complex carbohydrate and can be eaten freely while meat should not be, there is controversy about including them in the smaller protein section of the Food Guide Pyramid.

Milk is generally promoted as a source of calcium rather than as a protein source. But for people eating less meat, skim milk or 1 per cent milk can help balance protein intake with only a trace of fat. One cup of milk has as much protein as one ounce of meat.

Fat is found in most protein foods. Exceptions are skim milk products

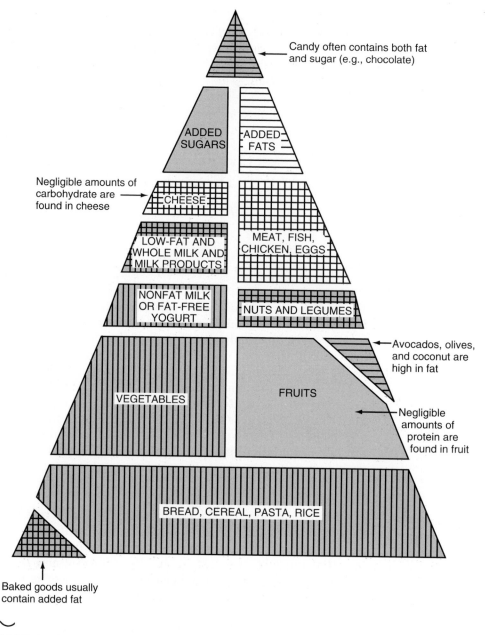

Candy often contains both fat and sugar (e.g., chocolate)

ADDED SUGARS

ADDED FATS

Negligible amounts of carbohydrate are found in cheese

CHEESE

LOW-FAT AND WHOLE MILK AND MILK PRODUCTS

MEAT, FISH, CHICKEN, EGGS

NONFAT MILK OR FAT-FREE YOGURT

NUTS AND LEGUMES

Avocados, olives, and coconut are high in fat

VEGETABLES

FRUITS

Negligible amounts of protein are found in fruit

BREAD, CEREAL, PASTA, RICE

Baked goods usually contain added fat

▲ F I G U R E   3 - 1

Carbohydrate, protein, and fat content of the Food Guide Pyramid.
KEY: Green = carbohydrate; vertical lines = protein; horizontal lines = fat.

and egg white, which are both fat-free. Legumes are also relatively low in fat and contain no cholesterol. Because the United States is primarily a nation of meat eaters, most Americans eat excessive amounts of fat. Added fats are generally not necessary for health, however.

Balanced meals contain at least one serving from each of the three lower levels of the Food Guide Pyramid. For example, a serving of grain, a vegetable or fruit, and a meat or milk source constitutes a balanced meal. In such a meal there is carbohydrate, protein, and fat, which are all helpful for proper functioning of the body.

CARBOHYDRATE—FUNCTION, SOURCES, AND RECOMMENDATIONS FOR APPROPRIATE INTAKE

What is Carbohydrate?

Carbohydrate consists of the three elements, carbon, hydrogen, and oxygen. It is formed by all green plants through a complex process known as **photosynthesis,** in which sugar is formed from carbon dioxide (CO_2) in the air and water (H_2O) in a series of reactions, with the aid of sunlight and the green plant pigment chlorophyll. Some of the sugar remains in the plant sap; the rest of the sugar units can be converted into starch and other carbohydrates, even very complex ones. The dry matter of most plants is largely carbohydrate and provides energy directly when eaten as food by humans and animals.

There are three main types of carbohydrates related to how many units of $C_6H_{12}O_6$ (C = carbon, H = hydrogen, O = oxygen) are connected.

1. Simple carbohydrates, or sugars, are single or double units ($C_6H_{12}O_6$)—also referred to as **monosaccharides** (single units) and **disaccharides** (double units).

2. Complex carbohydrates, or starch, consist of several units of sugar linked together—also referred to as **polysaccharides** (multiple units).

3. **Dietary fiber** contains complex linkages of many small units of sugar that resist digestion in the human digestive tract (Table 3–1). Fiber is further broken down into soluble and insoluble, having to do with whether it dissolves in water.

What are the Functions of Carbohydrates?

The primary function of carbohydrates is to meet the body's specific needs for **energy.** Carbohydrates are readily converted to energy. One gram of carbohydrate yields 4 kilocalories. Other functions of carbohydrate include the following:

1. It *spares* the burning of protein for energy (protein has more important functions, such as building and repair of body structures)

2. It *aids* in the more efficient and complete oxidation (burning) of fats for energy

3. As *sugar,* it produces energy quickly

4. As *starch,* it provides an economical and abundant source of energy after it is changed to glucose

5. As *lactose,* it has a certain laxative action (remains in the intestines longer and encourages desirable bacterial growth) and aids in the absorption of calcium

6. As *dietary fiber* (insoluble and indigestible), it aids in the normal functioning of the intestines. Soluble forms are believed to lower serum cholesterol levels, control blood sugar levels, and promote a healthy digestive tract (Table 3–2 and Appendix 7)

▲   **T A B L E   3 – 1**

TYPES AND SOURCES OF CARBOHYDRATES

TYPE	DESCRIPTION	SOURCES
Monosaccharides (commonly called simple sugars)		
Glucose blood sugar	The end product of all carbohydrate digestion. The form in which carbohydrates are absorbed, resulting from its being the only fuel the central nervous system can use.	Found in fruits, certain roots, corn, and honey. Also found in blood as the product of starch digestion.
Fructose fruit sugar	Gives honey its characteristic flavor. Combined with glucose in table sugar.	Found in fruit, honey, and vegetables.
Galactose	A by-product of lactose digestion.	Naturally found only in mammary glands.
Disaccharides (commonly called double sugars)		
Sucrose sugar	Composed of glucose and fructose. Commonly known as table sugar, which is made from sugar cane.	Found in sugar cane, sugar beets, molasses, maple sugar, maple syrup, many fruits and vegetables, and added to foods as table sugar.
Lactose milk sugar	Produced only by mammals. It is less soluble and less sweet than cane sugar and is digested more slowly. Composed of glucose and galactose.	Found in milk and in unfermented milk products.
Maltose malt sugar	Formed when starch is changed to sugar during digestion. Composed of two glucose molecules.	Found in malt and malt products; not free in nature.
Polysaccharides (commonly called starch, complex carbohydrates)		
Complex carbohydrate starch	The reserve store of carbohydrates in plants; changed to glucose during digestion (through intermediate steps of dextrin and maltose).	Found in grains and grain products, seeds, roots, potatoes, green bananas, and other plants.
Glycogen	The reserve store of carbohydrates in animals; changed to glucose as needed.	Stored in the liver.
Dietary fiber	Indigestible; provides bulk and stimulation for the intestines.	Found in skins and seeds of fruits, vegetables, and grains.
Dextrin	Formed from starch breakdown.	Cooked starch (toast).

What is the Role of Carbohydrate in Dental Caries?

All digestible carbohydrates are **cariogenic.** This means all forms of sugar and starch can cause tooth decay. Dietary fiber, which is not digestible, does not promote dental caries and may even be helpful in its prevention through the physical cleansing action and encouragement of saliva production. (See Chapter 19 for more information on oral and dental health.)

▲ **T A B L E   3 - 2**

FOOD SOURCES OF VARIOUS FIBER COMPONENTS

Cellulose	**Hemicellulose**	**Pectin**
Whole wheat flour	Bran	Apples
Bran	Cereals	Citrus fruits
Cabbage family	Whole grains	Strawberries
Peas and beans	**Gums**	**Lignin**
Apples	Oatmeal	Mature vegetables
Root vegetables	Dried beans	Wheat
	Brown rice	
	Barley	

FACT & FALLACY

FALLACY: It is better to eat potato chips than candy because of the low sugar content of potato chips.

FACT: Potato chips have no advantage over candy. Since they both contain carbohydrate, both contribute to dental caries. In addition, the high-fat and generally high-salt content of potato chips make them worse than pure carbohydrate foods, such as sugar, because they promote cardiovascular disease and cancer.

What are the Dietary Sources of Carbohydrate?

Carbohydrate foods are all plant foods plus milk and most milk products. Cheese, although a milk product, contains insignificant amounts of carbohydrate. Sugar increasingly is becoming a source of carbohydrate since Americans have about doubled their intake of sugar since the turn of the century. Around the world, carbohydrate foods range from an approximate 50 per cent in the American diet to a much higher proportion, as much as 80 per cent, in other countries. Knowing the carbohydrate content of foods is vital in the management of diabetes (see Chapter 9) and is also helpful in promoting an increased intake of complex carbohydrates for the general public.

GRAINS. Wheat in the form of breads, cereals, and pastas (macaroni, noodles, spaghetti) features prominently in the Western world; corn is important in the diet of native Americans as well as in the southern United States; wheat and rye are widely eaten in Europe; wheat and rice are consumed in large amounts in the Near East; and rice is important in the diet in the Far East. Italians love their pasta and have many forms such as spaghetti, macaroni, tagliatelle, fusilli, bucatini, and pastini. Polenta, which is cornmeal-based, is a favorite Italian dish.

Enriched grain products consist of grain with the bran layer and germ portion removed (Fig. 3–2). We often refer to these products as *white bread* or *white rice*. Wheat bread is often thought of as whole-grain by the public, but unless the food ingredient label includes the term "whole wheat," the bread product is probably white flour with coloring added (see Chapter 5 for more information on enrichment).

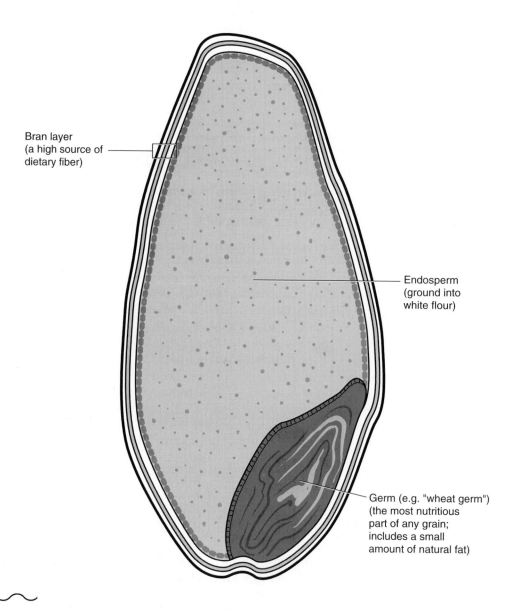

Bran layer
(a high source of
dietary fiber)

Endosperm
(ground into
white flour)

Germ (e.g. "wheat germ")
(the most nutritious
part of any grain;
includes a small
amount of natural fat)

▲ FIGURE 3-2

Anatomy of a grain. Whole grains include all three portions of the grain.

One serving of a starch contains about 15 grams of carbohydrate. Portion sizes generally equal ½ cup or the equivalent of one slice of bread. Grains that have a lot of air allow a larger volume for the same amount of carbohydrate (for example, 3 cups of popcorn). A piece of pizza that is the size of a slice of bread contains one serving of starch (about 15 grams carbohydrate). A wedge of lasagna the same diameter as a slice of bread contains the equivalent of two servings of starch (assuming there are three layers of noodles). This amount of carbohydrate is the basis of the grain/starch group of the Exchange System (see Chapter 6) as well as the Food Guide Pyramid.

There is a significant amount of protein in grains (3 grams of protein in each serving of grains), which is almost half of what 1 ounce of meat contains (1 ounce of meat contains 7 grams of protein). The protein content found in whole grains is more complete than that in white flour products, which is significant for people who want to eat less meat (see later section on protein).

There are about 2 grams of fat in each serving of whole grains because of the natural fat content of the germ portion of the grain. This quantity of fat is generally not counted. Two grams of fat is inconsequential for most persons, especially since it is a good type of fat, as found naturally in grains.

There are about 2 grams of fiber for each serving of whole grain. Wheat products contain primarily insoluble fiber. Oat products, barley, and brown rice contain primarily soluble fiber.

FACT & FALLACY

FALLACY: Starches are fattening.
FACT: Starches (complex carbohydrates) are comparable to protein in energy value with both contributing 4 kilocalories per gram. Starches play an important role for the dieter in allowing protein to be used for building purposes, thereby preventing muscle wasting. Dieters fare better through avoidance of fat, which provides 9 kilocalories per gram, being the most concentrated source of food energy. A starch food such as potato contains 80 calories per ½ cup, compared with 150 kilocalories in ½ cup of most meats (2 ounces of meat), and 500 kilocalories in only ¼ cup of oil as used in frying.

VEGETABLES. Vegetables with a high water content and low sugar content are the lowest in simple and complex carbohydrates. Examples of low-carbohydrate vegetables include the leafy green ones such as spinach, broccoli, lettuce, and cabbage. Carrots are moderately low in carbohydrate (Fig. 3–3).

Vegetables that are drier (low in water content) have more carbohydrate per volume, such as potatoes and legumes (legumes are technically a vegetable although they are sometimes counted in the meat group based on their high protein content). Legumes such as lentils, chickpeas, fava beans, cannelini beans, navy beans, and kidney beans are used regularly in Italy (Fig. 3–4).

Like the low-moisture vegetables, sweet vegetables (sweet peas, sweet corn, and sweet winter squash) are also higher in carbohydrate. These higher-carbohydrate vegetables are often referred to as *starchy vegetables* and are included in the starch group in the Exchange System (15 grams

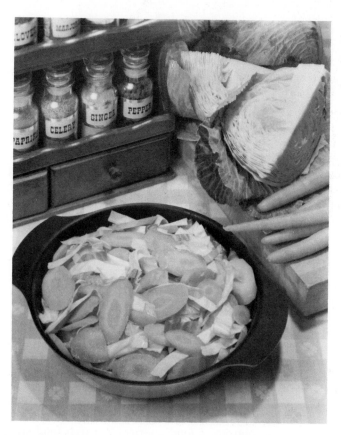

▲ F I G U R E   3 - 3

Low-calorie vegetables are those that are high in water content and relatively low in sweetness. (Courtesy of Cornell University Photography, Ithaca, NY.)

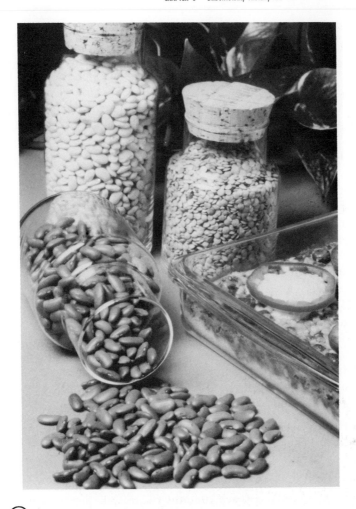

▲ F I G U R E   3 - 4

Legumes contribute significant amounts of carbohydrate to the diet, as they are a dry plant food. (Courtesy of Cornell University Photography, Ithaca, NY.)

carbohydrate per ½ cup; see Chapter 6 and Appendix 9 for more information on the Exchange System). The Food Guide Pyramid includes starchy vegetables in the vegetable group based on the nutrient content rather than the total carbohydrate content. For most vegetables, the following guidelines can be used for determining carbohydrate content. Amounts are given for cooked versions (for raw vegetables, the serving is 1 cup).

½ cup High-water, low-sweetness vegetables:	5 grams carbohydrate
½ cup Low-water (dry) vegetables:	15 grams carbohydrate
½ cup Sweet vegetables:	15 grams carbohydrate
¼ cup Dry, sweet vegetables (e.g., yams):	15 grams carbohydrate

An example you can use in patient education is, "You can almost feel the water content of green beans when you eat them and you would never say 'sweet green beans.' You also wouldn't say sweet broccoli or sweet cauliflower. These are all examples of low-calorie vegetables because they are high in water content and not considered sweet."

Vegetables contain a fair amount of protein, averaging about 2 grams per serving. There is no significant amount of fat in vegetables.

Each serving of vegetables contains about 2 grams of fiber, although legumes are much higher with about 10 grams of fiber. The fiber found in all forms of legumes, such as kidney beans, lima beans, fava beans, split peas, and lentils, is mostly of the soluble form.

FRUITS. Fruits contain a large proportion of water but are also sweet. The carbohydrate content is mostly sugar (fructose) and dietary fiber. There is the equivalent of almost 4 teaspoons of natural sugar in 1 serving of fruit. Persons with diabetes should limit fruit to one serving per meal or snack (see Chapter 9). The same principle as described above for vegetables of water content and level of sweetness can be applied to fruits. The following are some general guidelines:

1 cup High water content fruit (e.g., canteloupe):	15 grams carbohydrate
½ cup Most other fruits:	15 grams carbohydrate
¼ cup Low water content fruits (e.g., dried fruits):	15 grams carbohydrate
⅛ cup Dry, sweet fruit (e.g., raisins):	15 grams carbohydrate

Fruits have only a trace amount of protein per serving (1 gram or less). There is no significant amount of fat in fruit except for in avocados, olives, and coconuts. These fruits are found in the fat grouping of the Exchange System based on the high fat content (see Chapter 6). Most nuts are technically a type of fruit but are found in the meat group of the Food Guide Pyramid based on the high protein content. In the Exchange System, nuts are listed in the fat group because they contain more fat than protein.

Each serving of fruit contains about 2 grams of fiber. Apples and citrus fruits are high in soluble fiber.

SWEETS. Ordinary table sugar, molasses, maple syrup and sugar, corn syrup, honey, and sorghum syrup are poor sources of carbohydrates because they are concentrated, empty calories, meaning they contain carbohydrates but few vitamins or minerals. Molasses (especially blackstrap) is the one exception, as it is relatively high in some nutrients such as iron, calcium, and potassium, and it also contributes some B vitamins. Sugar can be noted on food labels as sugar, syrup, or any word that ends in -*ose* (except **cellulose,** which is a type of fiber). Fruit sugar is called **fructose,** milk sugar is **lactose,** and table sugar is sucrose. Honey is a combination of fructose and glucose (glucose is the type of sugar found in blood). One teaspoon of sugar contains 4 grams of carbohydrate.

Pure sugars have no significant amounts of protein, fat, or fiber.

MILK. There are no significant animal sources of carbohydrate except for lactose found in milk. Cheese is low in carbohydrate and is generally considered carbohydrate-free. Yogurt contains simple carbohydrate but minimal lactose, as the double sugar is converted into simple sugars. There are 12 grams of carbohydrate in 1 cup of milk or the equivalent of 3 teaspoons of lactose.

The protein content of 1 cup of milk is similar to that of 1 ounce of meat (the Exchange System uses the figures of 8 grams of protein in milk and 7 grams in meat). The various forms of milk differ mainly in the fat content. There is no significant amount of fiber in milk, as it is not a plant product.

1 cup whole milk contains the equivalent of 2 teaspoons of butter
  (10 grams fat)
1 cup 2 per cent milk contains 1 teaspoon of butter (5 grams fat)
1 cup 1 per cent milk contains ½ teaspoon butter (about 2 grams fat)
1 cup skim milk contains only a trace of butter (counted as 0 grams fat)

SUGAR SUBSTITUTES. Sugar substitutes come in two main forms: nutritive (providing a carbohydrate source) and non-nutritive (containing insignificant amounts of carbohydrate). **Sugar alcohols** are nutritive and are easy to recognize by their names, which all end in -*ol*. The main sugar alcohols are sorbitol, mannitol, and xylitol. Sugar alcohols do not contribute to dental decay but otherwise have little advantage over sugar. Saccharin, aspartame, and acesulfame-K are all non-nutritive sweeteners that are useful for the management of diabetes. See Table 9–6 for more on sugar substitutes.

What are the
Recommendations for
Carbohydrate Intake?

There is no specific requirement for carbohydrate intake. However, it is desirable to include carbohydrate in a reasonable proportion of the caloric intake (about 60 per cent of total kilocalories). The minimum amount of carbohydrate intake should be 100 g daily. This amount can prevent **ketosis** (a condition in which the end products of fat breakdown or digestion build up in the blood to dangerous levels).

The minimum number of food servings as represented in the Food Guide Pyramid (see Chapter 6) will provide about 135 grams of carbohydrate, an appropriate minimum level for most people. For someone who needs a high-calorie diet, the necessary amount of carbohydrate also goes up to reflect the ideal percentage of carbohydrate to total kilocalories.

RECOMMENDATIONS FOR SUGAR. There is controversy over how much sugar is an excess amount. For someone with diabetes mellitus or impaired glucose tolerance (see Chapter 9), the American Diabetes Association has recommended no more than 1 teaspoon of added sugar per day on a regular basis. Most Americans consume far more sugar than this, for example, one can of soda pop contains about 10 teaspoons of sugar. If adequate amounts of complex carbohydrates are consumed, simple sugars are sometimes appropriate for part of total kilocalories, if counted into the meal plan.

FACT & FALLACY

FALLACY: Juice contains less sugar than soda pop.

FACT: Juice contains as much total sugar as does soda pop. The sugar in juice is primarily fructose, whereas the sugar in soda pop is sucrose, but they both are simple sugars and will raise blood sugar for persons with impaired glucose tolerance (see Chapter 9). Juice, however, does contain vitamins and minerals, which soda pop does not.

RECOMMENDATIONS FOR FIBER. The Food Guide Pyramid, compared with earlier food guides, portrays increased amounts of fiber, with plant foods (grains, vegetables, and fruits) forming the base of the pyramid. The recommended amount of fiber (20 to 30 grams) can be met by including in the daily diet the recommended number of food servings of the Food Guide Pyramid. It is recommended that a desirable fiber intake be achieved through consumption of legumes, whole grains, vegetables, and fruits, which also provide minerals and vitamins. With any increase in fiber intake, there is also a need to increase water intake.

The increase in dietary fiber should include sources of **insoluble fiber** for the provision of bulk to the intestinal tract, which is beneficial for normal gastrointestinal functioning. Gums and pectins (classified as **soluble fiber**) should also be emphasized for other health benefits, such as the reduction of serum cholesterol levels (see Chapter 8) and blood sugar (see Chapter 9). Table 3–2 shows food sources of both types of fiber.

A method to describe the difference between soluble and insoluble fiber in patient education, such as with Mr. Bernardo in the case study, is to say, "If you put the peel of an apple in a glass of water, it will sit there day after day. That is insoluble fiber, or roughage. But if you put the white part of the apple into water, it will dissolve into little particles. This is soluble fiber, known as pectin. Soluble fiber dissolves in the digestive tract and helps to thicken and slow the movement of food through the intestinal tract, which is particularly helpful in controlling blood sugar levels. Legumes are high in soluble fiber and have the added benefit of being lower in natural sugar than fruit."

FACT & FALLACY

FALLACY: Because it is difficult to increase fiber in our diets, fiber supplements are recommended.

FACT: Except for relief from constipation, fiber supplements are not appropriate for healthy Americans. Through increased use of legumes, whole grains, and fruits and vegetables with skins and seeds, achieving appropriate levels of dietary fiber is entirely feasible. Nutritional deficiencies may result from too much fiber because certain minerals such as iron and zinc can bind with fiber and become unavailable to the body.

PROTEIN—FUNCTION, SOURCES, AND RECOMMENDATIONS FOR APPROPRIATE INTAKE

What is Protein?

Protein is the term used to describe a group of substances that are composed of many amino acids linked together. **Amino acids,** often called the building blocks of protein, are a family of molecules that are made up of carbon, hydrogen, oxygen, and nitrogen. It is the nitrogen that sets protein apart from the other macronutrients, carbohydrate and fat, and gives protein its unique function of building and repairing body tissues. Although this is protein's primary role, it can also be broken down and stripped of its nitrogen so that it can be used as an energy source.

The term **biological value** describes how well a particular protein approximates the amount and combination of amino acids in the body. A *complete* protein is said to contain all of the essential amino acids, whereas an *incomplete* protein has some of the essential amino acids but is lacking others. Generally speaking, animal sources of protein such as meat, fish, poultry, and dairy products contain complete proteins of high biological value. Incomplete yet good sources of protein foods that are lacking one or more of the essential amino acids include whole grains, legumes, corn, nuts, and seeds. Combining incomplete protein foods correctly in the diet will give the body all of the essential amino acids, which can result in adequate protein status. Therefore, vegetarians can receive adequate protein without eating meat if food choices are made wisely (see Chapter 1).

What are Amino Acids?

Twenty-two amino acids are known to be necessary for building and repairing body tissue in humans and for the formation of enzymes. Amino acids can be found in varying amounts and combinations in the food we eat, and most of them can be synthesized by the human body. However, there are nine essential amino acids that cannot be synthesized and must be obtained from the diet. These essential amino acids are:

Histidine (required for children)	Valine	Phenylalanine
Isoleucine	Lysine	Threonine
Leucine	Methionine	Tryptophan

The 13 nonessential amino acids that can be synthesized by the body in adequate amounts are:

Alanine	Cystine	Hydroxyproline
Arginine	Glutamic acid	Proline
Asparagine	Glutamine	Serine
Aspartic acid	Glycine	Tyrosine
Cysteine		

What are the Functions of Protein?

Protein is a part of all cell material and is found in muscles, organs, and glands and in all body fluids except bile and urine. Protein in the diet provides nitrogen, to be used in the synthesis of body proteins and other nitrogen-containing substances, and is involved in a variety of important metabolic functions.

1. It is essential for life, supplying material to repair or replace worn-out tissues
2. It is essential for growth, supplying material for tissue building
3. It supplies some energy (4 kilocalories/g) but is not as well equipped for this purpose as are carbohydrate and fat
4. It supplies certain essential substances for the construction and proper functioning of important body compounds (enzymes, hormones, hemoglobin, antibodies, other blood proteins, glandular secretions)

Sufficient amounts of carbohydrates and fats to provide for energy needs will prevent some of the protein needed for building and repair from being diverted for energy.

What are the Food Sources of Protein?

ANIMAL SOURCES. Animal sources include milk, cheese, yogurt, eggs, meat, fish, and poultry. Legumes and nuts, although they are from plants, provide similar amounts of protein (Fig. 3–5). Animal protein foods provide all of the essential amino acids; however, they tend to be high in fat and cholesterol. As discussed in Chapter 1, fat and cholesterol intake should be limited in the diet to prevent chronic diseases such as cardiovascular disease and possibly certain types of cancer. Therefore, animal sources of protein should be used sparingly, with an attempt to choose low-fat varieties such as skim milk, fat-free yogurt, lean meat, fish, and chicken.

One ounce of meat (¼ cup)	7 grams protein and 5 grams fat (about 2 grams fat for lean; 8 to 10 for high fat)
One cup 2 per cent milk	8 grams protein and 5 grams fat

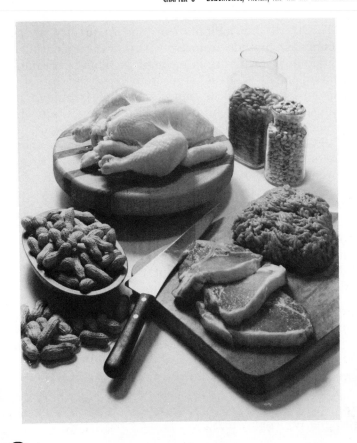

▲ FIGURE 3-5

Meat and meat alternatives for protein. (Courtesy of Cornell University Photography, Ithaca, NY.)

FACT & FALLACY

FALLACY: Skim milk is regular milk with added water.
FACT: There is no extra water added to skim milk. It tastes thinner because the fat is removed. Skim milk and powdered skim milk are as nutritious as whole milk but offer the advantage of having no cholesterol or saturated fat. Low-fat milk (1 or 2 per cent) has reduced amounts of fat but is otherwise the same as full milk. A taste for low-fat milk can be acquired through repeated trials, using 2 per cent milk as the first step toward liking skim milk.

PLANT SOURCES. Plants can (and frequently do, especially in developing countries) provide humans with all the essential amino acids, even though protein from plants is incomplete. This is accomplished by consuming different plant sources of protein over the course of the day, with emphasis on legumes, seeds, nuts, and whole grains. A vegan diet (no animal products) can help children and adults maintain or achieve desirable blood cholesterol levels. A study to this effect was undertaken with a Seventh Day Adventist population who consumed almonds, cashews, and nut butters, along with soy milk for protein sources (Resnicow et al., 1991).

The protein value of plants may also be complemented when eaten with an animal protein. This practice is common in many cultures when foods such as grilled cheese sandwiches, cereal with milk, chili containing meat and beans, and lasagna are consumed (Fig. 3–6).

Legumes are the highest source of plant protein with about 5 grams of protein per ½ cup. Whole grains contain 3 grams of protein per serving, vegetables 2 grams, and fruits about 1 gram or less.

What are the Recommendations for Protein Intake?

The protein allowance is based on the amount of protein necessary to maintain nitrogen balance (National Academy of Science, National Research Council, 1989). **Nitrogen balance** refers to a condition in which the nitro-

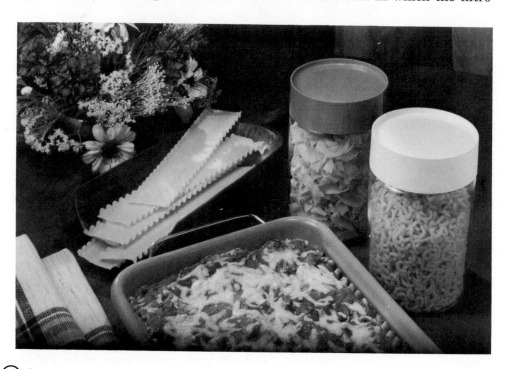

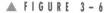

▲ F I G U R E   3 - 6

Lasagna provides protein from cheese, meat, and pasta. (Courtesy of Cornell University Photography, Ithaca, NY.)

gen consumed in the form of protein is equal to the nitrogen lost daily in the urine. At this point, intake is considered to be meeting the body's needs. The requirement is then increased to account for the mixed protein diet of the American population. The allowance is 0.8 g of protein for each kilogram of body weight. This translates into 63 g for a man weighing 79 kg and 50 g for a woman weighing 63 kg. See the inside front cover of this textbook for the RDA for protein for different ages and genders.

For infants, the allowances are based on the amount of protein provided by the quantity of milk required to ensure a satisfactory rate of growth. This is estimated to be 2.24 g/kg/day during the first month of life and falls gradually to about 1.5 g/kg/day by the sixth month of life. The protein requirement during growth is higher than that in adulthood, since nitrogen must be provided for the formation of new tissue. The allowances for children and young people are calculated from information on growth rates and body composition. The allowances decrease gradually from 1.5 g/kg/day at 6 months to 1 year to 0.8 g/kg/day by age 18 years.

During pregnancy, at least 60 g of protein daily is recommended. This is based on nitrogen retention of 16 mg/kg/day and on 50 per cent utilization of dietary protein. The dietary protein allowance for the lactating woman is about the same as that during pregnancy.

The protein requirement is increased for any condition in which the body protein is broken down, such as hemorrhage, burns, poor protein nutrition, previous surgery, wounds, and long convalescence. Protein deficiency over a long period results in muscle loss, reduced resistance to disease, skin and blood changes, slow wound healing, and a condition known as nutritional edema.

What are Problems with Inadequate Protein Intake?

The term **kwashiorkor** refers to a condition in which the individual may have an adequate caloric intake but lacks adequate dietary protein. However, protein deficiency is frequently associated with a deficiency in calories as well. When the diet is low in calories, protein is used as a source of energy, leaving little of this nutrient to build and repair tissues and maintain immune function. Such a condition is termed *protein-energy malnutrition* (also called **marasmus**) and is prevalent in most developing countries (see Chapter 22). This condition also occurs often during physiological stress (see Chapter 14).

What are Problems with Excess Protein Intake?

Excess protein is generally a problem for persons with renal insufficiency (see Chapter 10). Excess nitrogen from protein foods that must be excreted through the kidneys can place a burden on these organs. Excess protein also limits the body's ability to use calcium. And since most protein foods also contain fat, excess protein can lead to an excess intake of fat, which promotes obesity, cardiovascular disease, and cancer.

Protein intake should be about 10 to 15 per cent, up to a maximum of 20 per cent, of the total daily kilocalories. (See later section on calculating grams of protein into percentages of total kilocalories.) Figure 3–1 shows the protein content of food groups of the Food Guide Pyramid. The protein content of the recommended servings in the Food Guide Pyramid ranges from a minimum of 68 g to a maximum of 115 g of protein.

FATS—FUNCTION, SOURCES, AND RECOMMENDATIONS FOR APPROPRIATE INTAKE

What are Fat and Cholesterol?

Fats are similar to carbohydrate in that they are composed of carbon, hydrogen, and oxygen. However, they differ from carbohydrate in that they contain a greater concentration of carbon, which leads to higher energy values (at least 9 kilocalories/g versus 4 kilocalories/g for carbohydrate).

Lipids is a general term that includes all types of fats and fat-related compounds. Cholesterol is a fat-related compound that contains no kilocalories. It is found only in animal fats because it is made in the liver of animals. Fats from plant sources do not contain cholesterol.

The other main type of fat, which does contain kilocalories, is found in varying proportions in food consisting of a combination of saturated, monounsaturated, and polyunsaturated fats. If saturated acids predominate, the fat is called a **saturated fat;** if unsaturated acids predominate, the fat is called a **polyunsaturated fat.** The main **monounsaturated fat** is called oleic acid, which is found in nuts, seeds, olives, and avocados. Polyunsaturated fats are generally referred to as linoleic and linolenic acids and are found in corn oil, safflower oil, and sunflower oil (Table 3–3).

▲   T A B L E   3 - 3

FATTY ACIDS AND THEIR COMMON FOOD SOURCES

FATTY ACIDS	COMMON FOOD SOURCES
Saturated	
Lauric	Coconut, palm kernel oil
Myristic	Coconut
Palmitic	Palm oil, beef
Stearic	Cocoa butter, beef
Monounsaturated Fatty Acid	
Oleic	Olive oil, rapeseed oil, beef
Polyunsaturated Fatty Acids	
Linoleic	Corn oil, cottonseed oil, safflower oil, soybean oil, sunflower oil
Linolenic acid	Green leafy vegetables, soybean oil, soybean products (tofu)
Eicosapentaenoic acid	Mackerel, sardines, lake trout
Docosahexaenoic acid	Salmon, tuna, bluefish, halibut

In patient education, you might explain that peanuts are cholesterol-free since they grow in the ground. You can add to this by saying that cholesterol is made only in animal livers. Then you can ask in a good-natured manner, "Have you ever seen a liver in a peanut?" Most nuts can be safely eaten when a higher intake of mono-unsaturated fat is acceptable (when weight loss is not an issue).

Fats that are of a liquid consistency at room temperature are referred to as *oils,* whereas those that are solid are called *fats.* Liquid oils are composed predominantly of the **unsaturated fats;** the solid fats are the saturated forms. The most unsaturated form of fat is called **omega-3 fatty acid.** Fish from cold water areas are high in this kind of fat. Even at the cold ocean temperatures, the fat in the fish stays in semi-liquid form. Polyunsaturated fats also will stay in liquid form if placed in the refrigerator; monounsaturated fats will become viscous; and saturated fats will become so hard that you have to cut them.

The difference in degree of saturation relates to the amount of hydrogen in the fat molecule. Hydrogen atoms can be added to unsaturated liquid oils to make them more solid. For example, who wants to put corn oil on toast in the morning? By adding hydrogen the oil becomes a spread, or margarine. These are called **hydrogenated fats.** This form of fat is also now referred to as **trans fatty acid,** which may contribute to the risk of cardiovascular disease (Lichtenstein, 1993). Polyunsaturated fats have the least amount of hydrogen.

A tip for patient education to explain hydrogenation is to say, "Hydrogen is found in water (hydrogen and water). When clothes are hanging on the clothesline soaking wet, we could say they are saturated with water (or hydrogen). Thus, the more hydrogen in a fat, the more saturated it is."

Both fats and oils are composed principally of triglycerides and various fatty acids in various proportions. These differences contribute to food flavor and other properties and have health implications. **Triglycerides** consist of a base of glycerol with three fatty acids; diglycerides have two fatty acids, and monoglycerides have one.

Fats are insoluble in water. **Glycerol** is a small water-soluble carbohydrate. The addition of glycerol to fats in the body allows transport through the blood.

FACT & FALLACY

FALLACY: It is better to use butter, since we now know margarine also contributes to heart disease.

FACT: While margarine does contain trans fatty acids, which promote cardiovascular disease, butter is no better. Butter contains both saturated fat and cholesterol, increasing the risk of heart disease. Liquid or tub margarines are less hydrogenated than the harder margarines and contain less trans fatty acids. We might take the approach of Italians, who in Italy spread olive oil on their toast and avoid saturated and hydrogenated fats. (Adding a topping of basil and a very light sprinkle of parmesan makes this delicious!)

What are the Functions of Dietary Fats?

The primary function of fat is to serve as a concentrated source of heat and energy. About one third to one half of the kilocalories in the current average American diet come from fat. The body cells, with the exception of the cells of the nervous system and erythrocytes, can use fatty acids directly as a source of energy. In addition, fats perform the following functions:

1. *Furnish* essential fatty acids
2. *Spare* burning of protein for energy
3. *Add* flavor and palatability to the diet
4. *Give satiety* value to the diet (fats slow the digestive process and retard the development of hunger)
5. *Promote* absorption of fat-soluble vitamins
6. *Provide* a structural component of cell membranes, digestive secretions, and hormones
7. *Insulate* and control body temperature in the form of body fat

Animal fats and fortified margarines not only contain some of the fat-soluble vitamins (A, D, E, and K) but also aid in their absorption. They also play a role in the absorption of fatty acids. Excess fat stored in the body as adipose tissue insulates and protects organs and nerves. Fats also lubricate the intestinal tract. Fat-like substances that have important roles in the body include phospholipids (fat plus the mineral phosphorus) and sterols (ergosterol in plants and cholesterol in animal fat).

The polyunsaturated to saturated fat ratio (**P:S ratio**) can be used to determine the type of fat desirable in foods. Foods with a high P:S ratio (more polyunsaturated than saturated fat) tend to lower the body's own production of cholesterol, whereas foods with a low P:S ratio do the opposite. A P:S ratio of less than 2:1 is generally considered undesirable (see Table 3–4 for food examples, remembering that foods with a higher P:S ratio can help "balance out" those with a lower P:S ratio).

What are the Functions of Essential Fatty Acids?

Essential fatty acids are necessary for the nutritional well-being of all animals and must be supplied in the diet. The principal one for humans is called **linoleic acid** and is found in vegetable oils. Two others, arachidonic

▲ TABLE 3-4

DEGREE OF SATURATION IN COMMON FOODS, EXPRESSED AS P:S RATIO

HIGH (10:1–1:1)	MODERATE (1:2–1:10)	LOW (1:15–1:35)
Safflower oil	Tuna	Butter
Walnuts	Salmon	Hamburger, regular
Corn oil	Haddock	Cream cheese
Soybean oil	Olive oil	Coconut
Mayonnaise	Cashews	Dark chocolate
Cottonseed oil	Bacon	
Tub margarine	Chocolate cake	
Peanuts	Beef, lean	
Chicken	Egg yolk	
Whole-ground cornmeal	Lamb, lean	
Vegetable shortening	Milk chocolate	
Peanut butter	Hamburger, lean	
Avocados		

Foods are listed in the order of decreasing P:S ratio.

acid and linolenic acid, are essential, but the body generally can produce them if adequate linoleic acid is consumed.

Linolenic acid has multiple purposes, including 1) maintenance of the functioning and integrity of cellular and subcellular membranes, 2) cholesterol metabolism regulation, and 3) acting as the precursor of a group of hormone-like compounds (prostaglandins).

What are the Functions of Cholesterol?

Cholesterol has an essential role in the structure of adrenal and sex hormones and is converted to vitamin D_3 by the action of ultraviolet light on the skin. It is made and stored in the liver and also occurs in the form of a lipoprotein in the blood. Excess cholesterol intake contributes to fatty deposits in blood vessels and arteries, which in turn contributes to cardiovascular disease (see Chapter 8).

FACT & FALLACY

FALLACY: Lecithin prevents cardiovascular disease.
FACT: Lecithin is a natural fat emulsifier (helps fat mix with water) that is found in eggs, nuts, soybeans, liver, and other foods. There are claims that lecithin helps control cardiovascular disease, but there is no scientific evidence that supplements should be taken. Consuming a variety of foods will provide an adequate intake of lecithin.

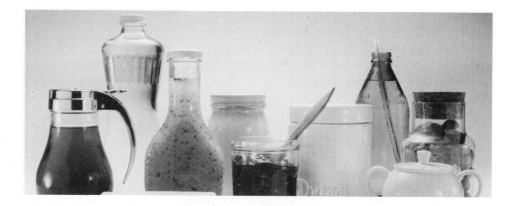

▲ FIGURE 3-7

Sources of fats and sugars in the diet. (Courtesy of the U.S. Department of Agriculture, Office of Governmental and Public Affairs.)

What are the
Common Food
Sources of Fat?

Fat is found primarily in animal foods but is also found in some plant foods such as nuts, seeds, avocados, olives, coconut, vegetable oils, shortenings, and margarines (Fig. 3–7). The plant sources of fat are all free of cholesterol and most are also low in saturated fats.

Saturated fats (e.g., stearic acid and butyric acid) typically are found in animal fat, such as milk fat, butter, and red meat. The main exceptions are coconut and palm oils: Although they are of plant origin, they are naturally high in saturated fat. Cashews and macadamia nuts are also higher in saturated fats than other nuts. (Walnuts, on the other hand, are very low in saturated fat.) Hydrogenated vegetable oils (shortening) act like saturated fats because the conversion from oil to hard shortening creates trans fatty-acids.

Unsaturated fats (mono- and polyunsaturated) are mainly of plant origin. However, fish from cold-water regions and chicken tend to be higher in unsaturated fat than in saturated fat (which is found in red meats). The texture of the fat is again the key to knowing what type the meat contains. The hard fat that needs to be trimmed from red meat is saturated; chicken fat is soft and thus lower in saturated fat; and you can't even see the fat in fish because it is in liquid form. Egg yolks contain cholesterol, but they also contain unsaturated fat as evidenced by the liquid texture even when they come straight from the refrigerator. The same is true of shellfish, in which the higher content of cholesterol is outweighed by the positive attribute of low amounts of saturated fat.

It is important to note that mineral oil is not a food fat, as it cannot be digested and used by the body. When used as a laxative, if at all, it should never be taken near mealtime.

1 teaspoon butter, margarine, mayonnaise, or oil: 5 grams fat
1 tablespoon nuts, salad dressing, or gravy: 5 grams fat
⅛ avocado: 5 grams fat
5 green olives or 3 black olives: 5 grams fat

What are Fat Substitutes?

Simplesse consists of very small particles of protein, generally of milk origin. These microparticles of protein provide a creamy consistency like fat. Simplesse is all-natural and fat-free, although it is not kilocalorie-free because it contains protein. Simplesse will increasingly be found in food products because of its acceptability. Persons with milk allergy should avoid Simplesse.

Olestra is another fat substitute that still has some unresolved problems because it is not digestible. The consequence is that excess intake can cause unpleasant gastrointestinal problems such as diarrhea.

What are the Recommendations for Intake of Fats and Cholesterol?

There are no specific requirements for fat other than the body's need for the essential fatty acids, which is usually met through a diet that contains appropriate food fats. The recommended intake of essential fatty acids for a population with a high fat intake, as is currently found in the United States, is 7 per cent of dietary calories (National Academy of Sciences, National Research Council, 1989). The Committee on Diet and Health of the Food and Nutrition Board has recently recommended that individual intakes not exceed 10 per cent of calories for either polyunsaturated or monounsaturated fats, which also contain the essential fatty acids, because there is a lack of information about the long-term consequences of a higher intake (National Academy of Sciences, National Research Council, 1989). There is also a concern that excess consumption of polyunsaturated fats increases our chances of developing cancer. A reduction in the total kilocalorie intake from fat to a maximum of 30 per cent fat, with equal distribution of polyunsaturated fats, monounsaturated fats, and saturated fats, is recommended. The Step Two diet of the National Cholesterol Education Program (NCEP) recommends lowering intake of saturated fat to 7 per cent of total kilocalories (see Chapter 8), and cholesterol intake to 200 mg or less, on average.

It is important to remember that the quantity of fat may not be as important as the quality or type of fat. For example, diets in the Mediterranean region are typically high in fat, but of the monounsaturated variety, because of the frequent use of olives and olive oil. Greenland Eskimos also have high-fat diets but consume large amounts of unsaturated fats through the use of fish. Both populations have a low incidence of cardiovascular disease.

The fat content of the recommended servings in the Food Guide Pyramid ranges from about 20 grams of fat, if skim milk, lean meat, and low-fat grain products are used, to 80 grams, if whole milk and high-fat meats are used. It is not unusual for Americans to consume 100 to 150 grams of fat per day.

HOW ARE PERCENTAGES OF THE MACRONUTRIENTS CALCULATED?

The percentage of protein as total kilocalories is calculated by first multiplying the number of grams of protein in the diet by 4 kilocalories and then dividing that number by the total caloric intake from all foods consumed in one day. For example, a 2000 kilocalorie diet containing both animal and vegetable sources of protein in the form of 3 cups milk (24 g protein), 6 slices bread (18 g protein), 3 vegetables (6 g protein), and 4 ounces meat (28 g protein) for a total of 76 grams of protein, would be calculated as follows:

$$76 \times 4 = 304 \text{ kilocalories}$$

$$304 \div 2000 \text{ calories} = 0.15 = 15\%$$

The same calculation can be used to find carbohydrate percentage (excluding fiber content, since fiber is not digestible and therefore provides no kilocalories). For calculating fat percentage, the number of grams of fat should be multiplied by 9 because fats yield 9 kilocalories per gram.

WHAT IS THE ROLE OF THE NURSE OR OTHER HEALTH CARE PROFESSIONAL IN EDUCATING THE PUBLIC ABOUT CARBOHYDRATE, PROTEIN, AND FAT INTAKE?

The goal of a nurse or other health care professional should be to educate patients about the role of carbohydrate, protein, and fat in their diets and to promote proper consumption of different sorts of foods, as based on the Food Guide Pyramid. The health care professional should use good interviewing skills in determining a patient's current dietary habits and the reasons such practices are being followed (for example, adherence to physician advice, which may have been given years ago, dental problems, health beliefs). Some patients, when given a rationale, may be receptive to dietary change whereas others may strongly resist change. The nurse should never argue or give an impression of arguing but rather indicate respect for a patient's food choices and health beliefs while also introducing new ideas about healthy diets.

Promoting consumption of complex carbohydrates and dietary fiber food sources (along with adequate fluid), and providing information on current thinking related to fiber, is an appropriate role for the health care professional. The foods portrayed at the base of the Food Guide Pyramid provide adequate carbohydrate and fiber. These foods are also low in fat and, with consideration of adequate intake of protein and calcium sources, can meet the goals of a healthy diet.

Sugar is a form of carbohydrate and thus provides the body with a fuel source, although excess sugar replaces more nutrient-dense foods and can contribute to weight problems and dental caries. A sensible, moderate approach to avoiding sugar should be used, and "scare tactics" should be avoided, to help prevent an unreasonable fear of sugar. Total rejection of sugar has led to feeding infants honey, which is linked to infant botulism. Long-term health effects of sugar substitutes, while probably safe, are not yet known, particularly as related to use during pregnancy and early childhood. The rule of moderation applies to sugar and sugar substitutes. Although a high intake of sugar cannot be supported, dental caries is the only known disease caused directly by sugar.

The health care professional can help re-educate the public about how much protein in the daily diet is really needed by the body. The amount of protein we consume can generally be safely decreased, but an assessment of usual dietary intake should be determined before automatically recommending a reduced amount. In the past, the emphasis in meal planning was to have meat as the main part of the meal with side dishes such as starch and vegetables. It is now recommended to view meat as the side dish with emphasis on vegetables and grains.

Helping individuals become aware that controlling the fat content of their diet plays a key role in the prevention and management of chronic diseases such as obesity, cardiovascular disease, and cancer is another goal of the health care professional. Beyond this awareness, individuals need to learn what foods are low in saturated fat and cholesterol; these foods should be promoted in a way that makes them practical to consume as well as appealing. Low-fat and skim milk and milk products, and meat alternatives such as legumes, for example, can be promoted simply by indicating verbally that they can be a delicious part of a meal. The health care professional should taste different low-fat dishes in order to express sincerity when promoting this concept.

Finally, the health care professional should recognize when referral to a professional nutritionist or registered dietitian is appropriate for highly motivated individuals or those at risk for obesity, cardiovascular disease, diabetes, or cancer.

STUDY QUESTIONS AND ACTIVITIES

1. What are the different kinds of carbohydrates?
2. Why is an excess of sugars and sweets in the diet generally undesirable?
3. What is the difference between soluble and insoluble fiber?
4. What are some foods on Maria's shopping list (in the case study) that would be helpful for her husband to increase his level of soluble fiber?
5. Write a day's menu, based on Maria's shopping list, that provides 20 to 30 grams of fiber.
6. What foods on Maria's shopping list are low in saturated fat?
7. How do proteins differ from carbohydrates and fats?
8. What is the difference between a complete and an incomplete protein?
9. What are some of the nutritional problems associated with an overconsumption of protein and those associated with too little protein?

10. Determine the percentage of carbohydrate, protein, and fat from the minimum number and maximum number of food servings as portrayed in the Food Guide Pyramid (1200 kilocalories and 2000 kilocalories, respectively).

11. Class activity: Students are to bring in a sample of crackers and their respective food labels. In class, students will estimate how many crackers would take up the same amount of space as a slice of bread. Compare this estimate to the food label (how many crackers does it take to equal 15 grams of carbohydrate?). Then compare fat content for the different types of crackers for one serving of starch.

12. If a food label states that one bagel contains 60 grams of carbohydrate, how many servings of grain would it contain?

REFERENCES

Lichtenstein A: Trans fatty acids, blood lipids, and cardiovascular risk: Where do we stand? Nutrition Reviews, 1993, 51(11):340.

National Academy of Sciences, National Research Council: Recommended Dietary Allowances, 10th ed. Washington DC, National Academy Press, 1989.

Resnicow K, Barone J, Engle A, et al.: Diet and serum lipids in vegan vegetarians: A model for risk reduction. J Am Diet Assoc, 1991, 91(4):447.

DIGESTION, ABSORPTION, AND METABOLISM: FOOD FOR GROWTH AND REPAIR

CHAPTER
4

OBJECTIVES

After completing this chapter, you should be able to:
- Describe the mechanical and chemical processes of digestion as related to carbohydrates, proteins, and fats
- Name the digestive enzymes and hormones and how they are involved in digestion and metabolism of carbohydrates, proteins, and fats
- Summarize the role of the mouth, stomach, and intestines in the digestive process
- Describe how absorption of nutrients takes place
- Explain the Krebs cycle
- Describe digestibility of foods as related to carbohydrates, proteins, and fats
- Describe the role of the nurse or other health care professional in aiding the digestive process

TERMS TO IDENTIFY

Absorption
Anabolism
Basal metabolism
Bile
Capillaries
Catabolism
Chyme
Cortisol
Digestion
Digestive enzymes

Duodenum
Endocrine system
Epinephrine
Estrogen
Glycogen
Growth hormone
Hormones
Hydrolysis
Ileum

Insulin
Jejunum
Krebs cycle
Metabolism
Oxidation
Peristalsis
Specific dynamic action
Thyroxine
Villi

A FAMILY'S PERSPECTIVE ON NUTRITION

Tony Bernardo sat in the dietitian's office. He was learning how balanced meals could slow down the digestion of food. This meant lowered blood sugars because food had to be digested before it could be turned into glucose. But while protein and fat were good to include with his meals, excess was also a problem. It was still confusing, but he was beginning to understand how to manage his diabetes.

He further learned that there were many aspects to how his body worked that affected his blood sugar levels. He was amazed at how complicated the body was in its use of food and controlling blood sugar. The dietitian said that when he got upset the adrenaline that was produced would raise his blood sugar. He would not only have to consider what his meals contained but would have to try to control his level of stress. He took a few deep breaths as he left her office and planned to go for a walk later.

INTRODUCTION

Good nutrition goes beyond obtaining and consuming appropriate foods in a positive meal environment. Without adequate digestion and absorption, foods cannot be used for their intended biological functions. The process of digestion and cellular nutrition can affect health more than food choices do. Health care professionals need to be aware of the digestive and metabolic impact on food use.

WHAT IS MEANT BY DIGESTION, ABSORPTION, AND METABOLISM OF FOODS?

Digestion

Digestion is the change of food from a complex to a simpler form and from an insoluble to a soluble state in the digestive tract. These changes facilitate absorption through the intestinal walls into the circulation for eventual use by the body (Fig. 4–1). The processes of digestion occur simultaneously:

1. *Physical (mechanical):* During the physical, or mechanical, process, food is broken into small particles in the mouth, then mixed with digestive juices by a churning action in the stomach, and then propelled through the digestive tract in rhythmic movements known as **peristalsis.**

2. *Chemical:* During the chemical process, enzymes in digestive juices change food nutrients into simple soluble forms that can be absorbed: carbohydrates to simple sugars, fats to fatty acids and glycerol, and protein to amino acids. This chemical breakdown is called **hydrolysis** and involves the addition of water to molecules. Water, simple sugars, salts, vitamins, and minerals require no digestion.

Each **digestive enzyme** (chemicals produced by the body to break food down in preparation for absorption in the intestinal tract) has a specific ac-

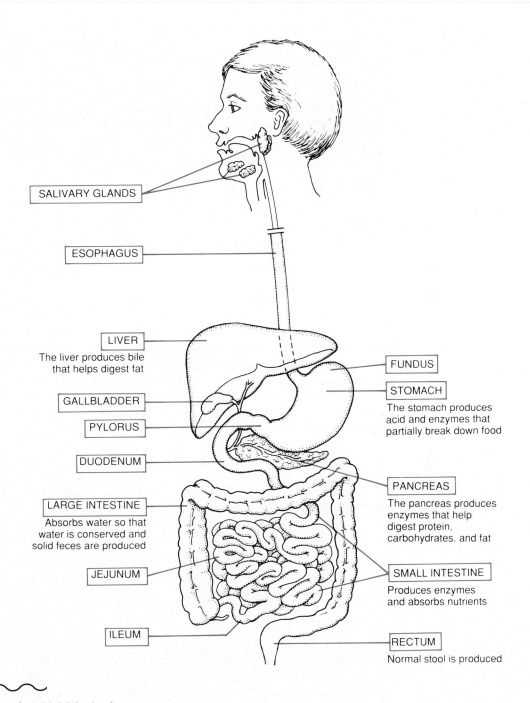

SALIVARY GLANDS

ESOPHAGUS

LIVER
The liver produces bile
that helps digest fat

FUNDUS

STOMACH
The stomach produces
acid and enzymes that
partially break down food

GALLBLADDER

PYLORUS

DUODENUM

PANCREAS
The pancreas produces
enzymes that help
digest protein.
carbohydrates. and fat

LARGE INTESTINE
Absorbs water so that
water is conserved and
solid feces are produced

SMALL INTESTINE
Produces enzymes
and absorbs nutrients

JEJUNUM

ILEUM

RECTUM
Normal stool is produced

▲ FIGURE 4-1

The digestive system.

tion and optimal conditions under which it acts. The name of each group of enzymes ends in *ase:* amylases act on starch, lipases act on fat, and proteases act on protein. Other enzymes include lactase, to digest lactose, and sucrase, to digest sucrose. Other chemical substances assist in the physical and chemical processes, such as hydrochloric acid and mucin in the gastric secretion, **bile** (which promotes the digestion of fat) excreted from the liver into the duodenum, and certain **hormones** (chemicals produced by the body that in part affect how the body uses nutrients in food).

Digestibility of food refers to the rapidity and ease of digestion as well as to its completeness. Liquid foods and thoroughly masticated solid foods are more rapidly digested than are foods left in large pieces. The well masticated food begins to leave the stomach 15 to 30 minutes after ingestion. Forms of liquid sugar such as fruit juice leave an empty stomach almost immediately.

Foods that stay in the stomach longer have a higher satiety value. Small meals move out of the stomach faster than larger ones do. Solid foods stay in the stomach longer than liquids. The amount and type of food eaten at one time also affect the rapidity of digestion. Of the three macronutrients, carbohydrates are digested and leave the stomach most rapidly (about 1 hour), proteins are digested and leave less rapidly (about 2 hours), and fats require the longest time for digestion (about 4 hours). Thus, a balanced meal stays in the stomach longer than a meal of only carbohydrate foods. Foods containing a large amount of dietary fiber are digested more slowly than are low-fiber foods.

Absorption

Absorption is the passage of soluble digested food materials through the intestinal walls into the blood, either directly or through osmosis by way of the lymph. The greater part of absorption takes place in the small intestine, lower duodenum, and upper jejunum. Tiny finger-like projections called **villi,** which contain small **capillaries** (tiny blood vessels), line the intestinal wall. The villi are in constant motion and trap the tiny nutrients, which are then taken in by the adjacent cells and transported through the circulatory and lymphatic systems to every part of the body. Microvilli are even smaller projections on the surface of the villi (Fig. 4–2).

Simple sugars, amino acids, a few fatty acids, minerals, and water-soluble vitamins reach the general circulation through the capillaries. Water is also absorbed from the large intestine. Absorbed materials are carried by the blood to various organs and tissues to be used as needed. The body is able to digest and absorb about 90 to 98 per cent of an average mixed diet.

Metabolism

Metabolism is a general term covering all physical and chemical changes that food nutrients undergo after their absorption from the gastrointestinal tract. It also covers the use of simple sugars, amino acids, fatty acids, and glycerol by the body cells. If the change is of a constructive nature, resulting in the building up of new substances, it is called **anabolism;** if it is of a destructive or oxidative nature, resulting in the release of energy, it is called **catabolism.** Energy metabolism refers to the oxidation of nutrients

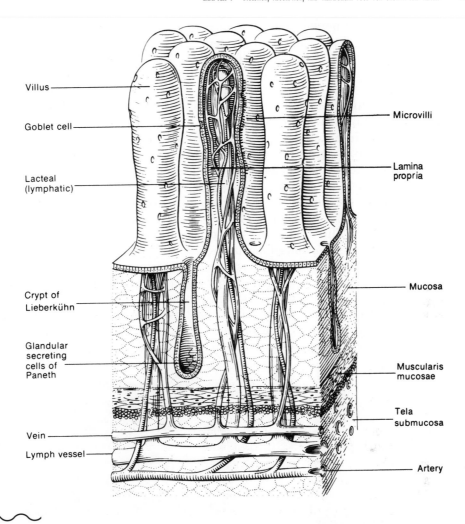

▲ FIGURE 4-2

Diagram of villi of human intestine showing their structure and blood and lymph vessels. (From Villee CA, Dethier VG: Biological Principles and Processes, 2nd ed., copyright © 1976 by Saunders College Publishing, reproduced by permission of the publisher.)

(carbohydrate, protein, and fat) within the body resulting in the release of heat and energy.

What is Basal Metabolism?

The body needs energy for the internal, involuntary activities of organs and tissues and oxidation within the tissues as well as for circulation, respiration, digestion, elimination, and maintenance of muscle tone, heartbeat, and so on. All internal activities continue 24 hours a day, while a person is asleep and awake. The amount of energy required to sustain these processes alone is known as the **basal metabolism.** The basal metabolic rate is influenced by body composition, body size, and age. The more muscle tissue a person has, the more calories are needed. The basal metabolic rate varies from person to person, but on the average it amounts to approximately 1200 to 1400 kilocalories daily for women, and 1600 to 1800 kilocalories daily for men. This minimum caloric need usually accounts for more than half the total daily energy need of a moderately active adult, and an even greater portion for a less active adult. Total energy requirements and weight maintenance are discussed in Chapter 20.

A simple and relatively accurate method of estimating basal metabolic rate is to multiply one's weight in kilograms by 0.9 for women and 1 for men, and then by 24 (which represents the number of hours in a day). This estimate is generally accurate enough, except during times of physiological stress (see Chapter 14). In large institutions, what are referred to as metabolic carts are used to measure a person's oxygen intake and carbon dioxide output. This technique can precisely measure the basal metabolic kilocalorie needs. Various measurements of oxygen use and carbon dioxide output have been used over the years to determine basal metabolic rate (Fig. 4–3).

The body also needs energy for the stimulating effect (**specific dynamic action**) that each food exerts on basal metabolism after digestion and absorption. This action raises the total energy needs about 10 per cent for a person who eats a mixed diet. Carbohydrate foods, especially, tend to raise the rate of metabolism through the process of digestion.

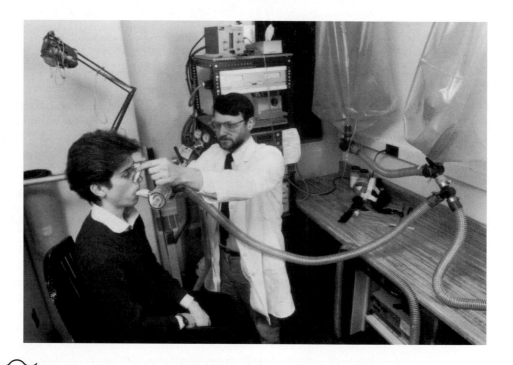

▲ FIGURE 4-3

Measuring metabolic rate. (Courtesy of Cornell University, Ithaca, NY.)

WHAT HAPPENS TO THE MACRONUTRIENTS IN THE BODY?

Carbohydrates

Carbohydrates (except for fiber) are easily digested, and the degree of absorption is high. Digestion of starch starts in the mouth and is completed in the small intestine. Glucose, which is formed from all carbohydrate eaten in food, is absorbed into the blood stream through the walls of the small intestine and is metabolized as shown in Figure 4–4.

Simple sugars such as glucose and fructose are ready for absorption in the digestive tract without digestion. Double sugars such as sucrose must be changed to simple sugars for absorption, which is a quick process. Double sugars are digested in the small intestine (see Fig. 4–4). Complex carbohydrates such as starch require two digestive steps to be changed to simple sugar (glucose) for absorption in the intestinal tract. Cooking starch facilitates digestion, as it breaks down the cell walls, which makes the action of the digestive enzymes easier. Dietary fiber is indigestible and passes through the intestinal tract virtually unchanged. Since most unprocessed plant foods contain fiber, the process of digestion is slower for them than for sugar and low-fiber plant food products such as white bread.

Proteins

The proteins in the daily diet must be broken down by digestion into their component parts, the amino acids, before the body can absorb them into the blood from the small intestine and use them. Digestion of protein is started in the stomach by enzymes in the gastric juice and is continued and completed in the small intestine by enzymes from the pancreatic and intestinal juices (see Fig. 4–4).

Fats

Fats, being insoluble in water, require special treatment in the gastrointestinal tract so that their end products can be absorbed through the intestinal wall. No digestion of fat takes place in the mouth. Only finely emulsified fats, such as those found in butter, cream, and egg yolk, can be digested in the stomach. For the most part, fats must be emulsified by bile and bile salts before they are digested in the small intestine by enzymes from the pancreatic juice. Fats are changed to glycerol and fatty acids during digestion (see Fig. 4–4).

Fatty foods are generally digested without difficulty, but they require a longer time for digestion than carbohydrates do. Softer fats are more completely digested and absorbed than harder fats. Fried foods are not necessarily indigestible but are more slowly digested. The presence of carbohydrates in the diet is necessary for the complete **oxidation** of fats (the chemical step in releasing energy from fat) in the tissues; otherwise, acetone bodies accumulate and ketosis results.

How Are Macronutrients Converted to Energy?

When the body needs energy, a series of metabolic reactions occurs called the **Krebs cycle** (see Fig. 4–5, which shows the central pathways of energy metabolism). Oxygen is necessary for the release of energy by the cells in the body. The process of combining oxygen with a molecule is called oxi-

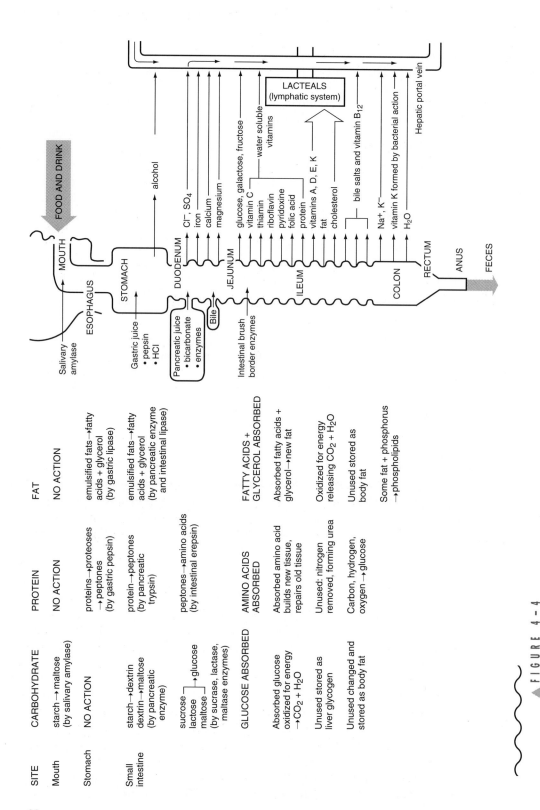

▲ FIGURE 4-4

Digestive process of carbohydrate, protein, and fat. KEY: Cl = chloride; CO_2 = carbon dioxide; HCl = hydrochloric acid; H_2O = water; K^- = potassium; Na^+ = sodium; SO_4 = sulfur. (Modified from Mahan LK, Arlin M: Krause's Food, Nutrition & Diet Therapy. 8th ed. Philadelphia, WB Saunders, 1992.)

▲ F I G U R E   4 - 5

Metabolic pathways.

dation. A person needs hemoglobin to supply oxygen to the cells, and a low level of hemoglobin means oxygen is not available for energy production, which results in a tired feeling. An increased intake of air into the body, such as that achieved with aerobic exercise, tends to raise the body's rate of metabolism through the process of oxidation (see Chapter 20).

WHAT ROLE IS PLAYED BY EACH PART OF THE DIGESTIVE TRACT?

The Mouth

The teeth provide the first mechanical function of chewing, with the cutting action with the anterior teeth (incisors) and the grinding action of the posterior teeth (molars). Chewing is important for digestion of all foods, but it is especially important for most fruits and raw vegetables because these have undigestible cellulose membranes around their nutrient portions, which must be broken before the food can be utilized.

Chewing aids the digestion of food for a simple reason. Since the digestive enzymes act only on the surface of food particles, thorough chewing increases the amount of food surface area available to these enzymes.

Another mechanical function is performed by saliva, which moistens food and prepares it for swallowing.

The chemical function of the mouth is to change cooked starch to dextrin and then to maltose by the salivary enzyme ptyalin (amylase).

FACT & FALLACY

FALLACY: Washing food down with water is a good habit.
FACT: Food must be chewed thoroughly so that it can be mixed with saliva, which aids digestion. However, a glass of water at mealtime is beneficial to the digestive process, as long as it does not take the place of mastication.

Esophagus

In general, swallowing can be divided into three stages: (1) the voluntary stage, which initiates the swallowing process, or *mechanical function;* (2) the pharyngeal stage, which is involuntary and involves the passage of food through the pharynx to the esophagus; and (3) the esophageal stage, which involves passage of food from the pharynx to the stomach through peristaltic wave contractions (Fig. 4–6).

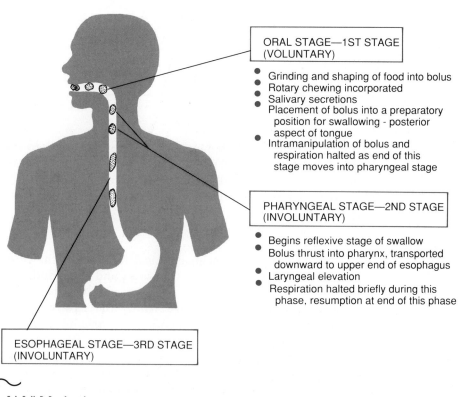

ORAL STAGE—1ST STAGE
(VOLUNTARY)

- Grinding and shaping of food into bolus
- Rotary chewing incorporated
- Salivary secretions
- Placement of bolus into a preparatory position for swallowing - posterior aspect of tongue
- Intramanipulation of bolus and respiration halted as end of this stage moves into pharyngeal stage

PHARYNGEAL STAGE—2ND STAGE
(INVOLUNTARY)

- Begins reflexive stage of swallow
- Bolus thrust into pharynx, transported downward to upper end of esophagus
- Laryngeal elevation
- Respiration halted briefly during this phase, resumption at end of this phase

ESOPHAGEAL STAGE—3RD STAGE
(INVOLUNTARY)

▲ FIGURE 4-6

The stages of swallowing. (Modified from Roeche JR: Dysphagia: An Assessment and Management Program for the Adult. Minneapolis, Sister Kenny Institute, 1980.)

Respiration is generally only minimally stopped during the act of swallowing. Poorly chewed food, however, increases the risk of obstruction of the airway, especially for persons with an impaired swallowing reflex, in whom oxygen deprivation can occur (Rogers et al., 1993).

The Stomach

The presence of food in the stomach stimulates functioning of the digestive tract. Food is kept in motion by the muscular walls of the stomach, which bring it into contact with the gastric juice secreted by stomach cells. The fundus of the stomach acts as a temporary storage place for food.

Various gastric juice enzymes work in the stomach to digest different macronutrients. Complex proteins are partially digested by pepsin (protease); milk protein is coagulated by renin and then is partially digested by pepsin. Emulsified fats are digested to fatty acids and glycerol by lipase. Hydrochloric acid aids these digestive enzymes and increases the solubility of calcium and iron. Mucus protects the lining of the stomach from the hydrochloric acid.

Once solid food is reduced to a semiliquid state **(chyme),** it is passed from the stomach to the small intestine.

FACT & FALLACY

FALLACY: Antacids promote indigestion by reducing the amount of acid secreted by the stomach.

FACT: The stomach needs the acid already secreted and reacts to the antacid by producing more acid. Indigestion could be prevented by adequately chewing food, eating more slowly, and eating less at a meal.

The Small Intestine

The small intestine is 20 feet long and is made up of the **duodenum** (the upper section), the **jejunum** (the middle section), and the **ileum** (the lower section). The food mass from a meal remains in the intestine for 3 to 8 hours, although liquids and pure carbohydrate foods pass more quickly.

Chyme mixes with the digestive juices of the small intestine, and with pancreatic juices and bile, both of which are excreted into the duodenum (bile is secreted by the liver and stored in the gallbladder). Alkaline juices from the small intestine neutralize chyme as it leaves the stomach. Bile prepares unemulsified fats for digestion. Pancreatic enzymes finish starch and fat digestion, and partially digest protein. The intestinal enzymes complete protein and carbohydrate digestion. Digested food moves with peristaltic waves through the small intestine. Unused food, waste materials, and water move to the large intestine.

The Large Intestine

The large intestine consists of the cecum, the colon, the rectum, and the anal canal. Water is drawn out of the contents of the large intestine and absorbed, and solid feces are formed. Waste, including indigestible residue, undigested food particles, meat fibers, and decomposition products, is eliminated. Because no enzymes are produced in the large intestine, no digestion takes place there.

WHAT IS THE ROLE OF THE ENDOCRINE SYSTEM ON METABOLISM AND ABSORPTION OF NUTRIENTS?

The **endocrine system** is a major control system of the body with hormones that the body produces; more than a dozen of them regulate metabolism and use of nutrients. Some hormones that have significance to nutrition and diet are as follows:

EPINEPHRINE (ALSO REFERRED TO AS ADRENALINE). This hormone is produced mainly by the adrenal glands and helps release stored sugar in the liver **(glycogen)** in response to low blood sugar or stress. Energy metabolism is increased in response to epinephrine because of the resultant increased heart rate and oxygen intake. Excess epinephrine may raise the blood sugar too high if there is insufficient insulin for the metabolism of carbohydrates (see Chapter 9).

CORTISOL. This hormone is also produced by the adrenal gland and also works in the opposite manner to insulin (see later definition of *insulin*). It is produced in increased amounts during sleep. As a result, blood sugar levels tend to run higher first thing in the morning. Steroid medications are similar to the cortisol hormone, as they tend to increase the appetite and their use is related to weight gain (see Chapter 20). They also will raise blood sugar levels.

ESTROGEN. This hormone is produced mainly in the ovaries and helps retain bone calcium, which results in a decreased risk of osteoporosis (see Chapter 21). Estrogen tends to cause blood sugar levels to rise because of its inhibiting effect on insulin. Premenstrual syndrome (PMS; see Chapter 16) may be caused in part by lowered levels of estrogen after ovulation. Without estrogen, insulin is able to lower the blood sugar level more effectively. Lowered blood sugar levels can result in the irritability, hunger, and headaches that often are associated with PMS.

GROWTH HORMONE. This hormone is produced by the pituitary gland. It raises the rate of metabolism and is associated with protein anabolism, which produces a positive nitrogen balance. It is also referred to as diabetogenic because it works against insulin in muscle tissue (Ganong, 1991). Adolescents have an increased need for insulin because of increased levels of growth hormone.

INSULIN. This hormone is produced in the pancreas and allows carbohydrates to be metabolized for energy by facilitating the entry of blood sugar (glucose) into the cells where the Krebs cycle takes place. Insulin also affects the metabolism of fat. Excess insulin in the body leads to fat deposition (Sharkey, 1990). Insulin deficiency decreases the body's ability to metabolize carbohydrates and fats, and contributes to weight loss.

THYROXINE. This is one of the hormones produced in the thyroid that raises the rate of metabolism. A high level of thyroxine will increase the metabolic rate in part because it increases oxygen consumption. The thyroid hormones also help regulate lipid (fat) metabolism and increase the absorption of carbohydrates from the intestine (Ganong, 1991). Iodine binds to thyroxine, so measuring the amount of protein-bound iodine found in a blood sample is one technique to measure the basal metabolic rate. The more iodine found bound to thyroxine, the more active the thyroid gland, therefore, the greater the metabolic rate.

WHAT IS THE ROLE OF THE NURSE OR OTHER HEALTH PROFESSIONAL IN AIDING THE DIGESTIVE PROCESS?

The nurse or other health care professional in an institutional setting can indirectly promote the digestive process by providing a relaxed and unhurried atmosphere where patients can feel at ease to thoroughly chew their food. Direct intervention might include emphasizing the importance of thorough chewing.

The health care professional should be aware of possible issues of digestion in patients, such as swallowing problems and intestinal or gastric surgery, and should be alert to signs of malabsorption such as chronic diarrhea and unexplained weight loss. Patients with these types of problems should be referred to a registered dietitian with the approval of the attending physician. Digestive or intestinal problems, such as chronic constipation, may also be improved by following a dietitian's suggestions. See Chapter 11 for more information on gastrointestinal diseases and disorders.

STUDY QUESTIONS

1. What is the purpose of digestion?
2. What is absorption? In what part of the body does it take place?
3. In what form are all carbohydrates absorbed? All fats? All proteins?
4. Why did the dietitian recommend balanced meals which include protein and fat for Mr. Bernardo?
5. What other hormone besides epinephrine might affect Mr. Bernardo's blood sugar levels?
6. Why might taking baking soda for indigestion retard digestion in the stomach?
7. How is energy produced by the Krebs cycle made available for use by the body?
8. Name the enzymes involved in the digestion of maltose and fructose.

PRACTICAL APPLICATION

Trace the digestion of a meal composed of a ham sandwich on whole wheat bread, a glass of low-fat milk, and a fresh apple. Describe the mechanical and chemical processes that occur and name the enzymes that are involved.

REFERENCES

Ganong WF: Review of Medical Physiology. Norwalk, CT, Appleton & Lange, 1991; pp 302, 378–379.

Rogers BT, et al.: Hypoxemia during oral feeding of children with severe cerebral palsy. Dev Med Child Neurol. 1993; 35:3–10.

Sharkey BJ: Physiology of Fitness, 3rd ed. Champaign, IL, Human Kinetics Books, 1990, p 32.

CHAPTER 5

VITAMINS, MINERALS, ELECTROLYTES, AND WATER

CHAPTER TOPICS

CHAPTER INTRODUCTION
FOODS VERSUS SUPPLEMENTS AS SOURCES OF VITAMINS AND MINERALS
THE ROLE OF VITAMINS IN NUTRITION
FAT-SOLUBLE AND WATER-SOLUBLE VITAMINS: DEFICIENCIES, TOXICITIES, FOOD SOURCES
MAJOR MINERALS AND TRACE MINERALS: DEFICIENCIES, TOXICITIES, FOOD SOURCES
FOOD PREPARATION FOR PRESERVATION OF VITAMINS AND MINERALS
FOOD FORTIFICATION
ELECTROLYTES, THEIR ROLES, AND PROBLEMS WITH IMBALANCES
FUNCTION AND FOOD SOURCES OF WATER
THE ROLE OF THE NURSE OR OTHER HEALTH CARE PROFESSIONAL IN PROMOTING GOOD
    INTAKE OF VITAMINS AND MINERALS

OBJECTIVES

After completing this chapter you should be able to:
- Describe the main difference between the fat-soluble and water-soluble vitamins
- Recognize at least one function of each of the vitamins and minerals that have established RDAs
- List foods high in the various vitamins and minerals
- Describe the role of electrolytes and where they are found in food
- Describe the importance of water and how to include appropriate amounts in the diet
- Describe how the nurse or other health professional can most appropriately promote intake of vitamins, minerals, electrolytes, and water

TERMS TO IDENTIFY

Acid-base balance	Elemental	Iron overload
Anemia	Enrichment	Neuropathy
Arthralgias	Fat-soluble vitamins	Pellagra
Beriberi	Fortification	Pernicious anemia
Cardiomyopathy	Heme iron	Precursor
Carotene	Hemoglobin	Prothrombin
Celiac sprue	Hypocalcemia	Rebound scurvy
Cirrhosis	Hypoparathyroidism	Retinol equivalent (RE)
Cretinism	Hyperosmotic diarrhea	Rickets
Crohn's disease	International unit (IU)	Sickle cell disease
DNA	Intrinsic factor	Tetany

A FAMILY'S PERSPECTIVE ON NUTRITION

Joey Bernardo sat in chemistry class. They were studying the periodic table. Potassium, sodium. Interesting, he thought. His dad was supposed to be eating less sodium. As a family they had begun to read food labels. He wondered if this was the same thing. And potassium. He recalled his dad saying he needed to eat more leafy green vegetables for potassium instead of the orange juice and bananas he used to have. This was to help control his blood sugar while still getting the potassium he needed. And there were other terms in this periodic chart that sounded like vitamins—magnesium, chromium, selenium. He didn't think he would be learning about nutrition in chemistry class . . .

INTRODUCTION

As we become knowledgeable about our vitamin and mineral needs, it is helpful to keep their history in perspective. Initially, food was recognized as the important element in health. One of the first major discoveries about the role of vitamins was that the use of lemons and limes protected against the dreaded scurvy that plagued ocean voyagers. Prior to this revelation, sailors often developed this severe vitamin C deficiency, which resulted in internal bleeding and death.

It was not until this century that vitamins were chemically identified. This author had the rare opportunity of talking personally with a retired scientist who recalled being one of the first people asked to chemically isolate vitamin C during the 1920s. He and his colleagues laughed at the foolishness of this idea. We may no longer laugh about the importance of vitamins, but we cannot expect that in one person's lifetime, all has been learned about the body's need for vitamins.

Minerals, the seeming equivalent of vitamins in the consumer's eye, are elemental inorganic substances that have some similarities to vitamins but also have many differences. The most notable difference is that minerals are **elemental,** meaning that they do not break down. This characteristic of minerals prevents their destruction by heat and air, to which vitamins are susceptible. The elements found in the chemical periodic table are minerals. In the saying, "Ashes to ashes and dust to dust," the ashes are the minerals found in the body.

The roles and functions of vitamins and minerals in health are complex, and a body of knowledge is accumulating. Excess of one vitamin or mineral can compete with another; for example, zinc competes with copper, and vitamin E can inhibit the activity of vitamin K. The most prudent approach for achieving an optimal vitamin and mineral nutritional status is by a varied diet, with emphasis on whole grains, legumes, dark green leafy vegetables, orange vegetables and fruits, meat, and milk. Vitamin and mineral supplements, which generally are unnecessary, should not exceed 100 per cent of the RDA (see RDA table inside the front cover). Exceptions to this guideline should be made only with a warranted medical condition and the advice of a physician.

Health care professionals are in a unique position of being able to influence positively a patient's nutrient intake. This chapter is aimed at increasing appreciation for the micronutrients our bodies require and recognition of the food sources to obtain them.

SHOULD VITAMINS AND MINERALS COME FROM FOOD SOURCES OR FROM SUPPLEMENTS?

As already implied, the vitamin pill industry has had a short history. It should therefore be apparent that there is likely a great deal more to learn about the human body's need for nutrients and how best to supply them. As of now, food sources of vitamins and minerals are superior to those offered through vitamin pill technology. Food offers more nutritional value than do pills, as it provides the macronutrients carbohydrate, protein, and fat. Vitamin and mineral supplements are no substitute for a balanced, varied diet, and with such a diet, pills are generally unnecessary and costly. Only individuals with conditions that increase vitamin and mineral needs or impair the absorption and utilization of these essential nutrients should worry about supplements. A physician or registered dietitian can best determine this need.

Reliance on food sources for vitamins and minerals (Tables 5–1 through 5–4) offers little risk of ingesting toxic amounts and is therefore safer. In persons requiring medications, excess ingestion of vitamins and minerals may be harmful (see Table 7–9). Many individuals do not realize that substances that are essential at one level can be harmful at higher doses. There are no long-term studies that establish the safety of large doses of vitamins (Community Nutrition Institute, 1993). "The lack of controlled trials prevents us from defining the lowest human neurotoxic dose of any vitamin. Large differences in individual susceptibility to vitamin neurotoxicity probably exist, and ordinary vitamin doses may harm occasional patients with genetic disorders" (Snodgrass, 1992). Foods may also offer as yet undiscovered nutrients important for health. It would be much better if people took the 2.7 billion dollars that the FDA estimates is spent on vitamin and mineral supplements, and bought vegetables, fruits, and whole grains instead.

Set off by the box is the statement on vitamin and mineral supplementation that was prepared by the American Dietetic Association, the American Institute of Nutrition, the American Society for Clinical Nutrition, and the National Council Against Health Fraud representing registered dietitians, nutrition research scientists, and physicians. The American Medical Association's (AMA) Council on Scientific Affairs has reviewed the joint statement and finds it consistent with AMA policy.

STATEMENT ON VITAMIN AND MINERAL SUPPLEMENTS

Healthy children and adults should obtain adequate nutrient intakes from dietary sources. Meeting nutrient needs by choosing a variety of foods in moderation, rather than by supplementation, reduces the potential risk for both nutrient deficiencies and nutrient excesses. Individual recommendations regarding supplements and diets should come from physicians and registered dietitians.

Supplement usage may be indicated in some circumstances, including:

- Women with excessive menstrual bleeding may need to take iron supplements.
- Women who are pregnant or breast-feeding need more of certain nutrients, especially iron, folic acid, and calcium.
- People with very low calorie intakes frequently consume diets that do not meet all their needs for all nutrients.
- Some vegetarians may not be receiving adequate calcium, iron, zinc, and vitamin B_{12}.
- Newborns are commonly given, under the direction of a physician, a single dose of vitamin K to prevent abnormal bleeding.
- Certain disorders or diseases and some medications may interfere with nutrient intake, digestion, metabolism, or excretion and thus change requirements.

From the American Dietetic Association, et al.: Statement on vitamin and mineral supplements. Nutrition Today 22 (3), © by Williams & Wilkins, 1987. By permission of the American Dietetic Association.

WHAT IS THE ROLE OF VITAMINS IN NUTRITION?

Vitamins are present in foods and are needed by the body in only minute amounts, but proper growth and development and optimal health are impossible without them. Some vitamins may be synthesized in the body, but for the most part, they must be supplied in the daily diet of normal healthy persons. Early attention to the clear-cut manifestations of diseases caused by vitamin deficiencies (Fig. 5–1), seldom seen now, obscured for a time the very important function of vitamins in the prevention of nutritional deficiencies, as is the focus today.

Vitamins, although organic in nature, do not provide energy. But they do help in the metabolism of the macronutrients. In this role vitamins are thought to act as catalysts.

Vitamins are classified as *body regulators* because of the following functions:

1. They regulate the synthesis of many body compounds (bones, skin, glands, nerves, brain, and blood).

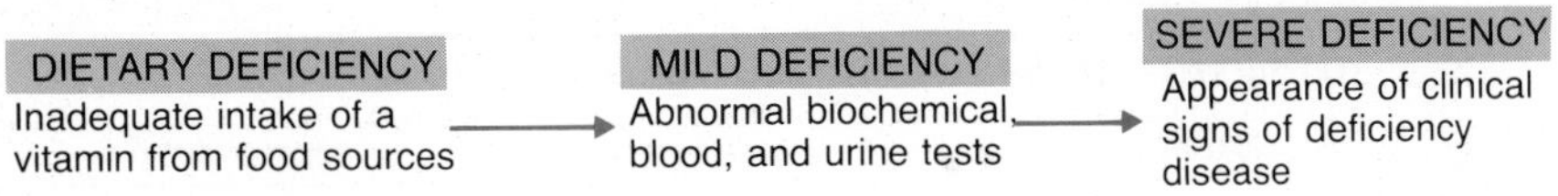

DIETARY DEFICIENCY	MILD DEFICIENCY	SEVERE DEFICIENCY
Inadequate intake of a vitamin from food sources	Abnormal biochemical, blood, and urine tests	Appearance of clinical signs of deficiency disease

▲ FIGURE 5-1

The progression of the development of vitamin deficiencies.

2. They participate in the metabolism of protein, carbohydrates, and fats.

3. They prevent nutritional deficiency diseases and allow for optimal health at all ages.

WHAT IS THE DIFFERENCE BETWEEN FAT-SOLUBLE AND WATER-SOLUBLE VITAMINS?

Generally, vitamins are classified into two groups: fat-soluble (vitamins A, D, E, and K) and water-soluble (B-complex vitamins and vitamin C). Water-soluble vitamins are not stored in any significant amounts in the body, which means that they need to be included in the diet on a daily basis. In contrast are the **fat-soluble vitamins,** which are stored in body fat and can reach toxic levels. Deficiencies of fat-soluble vitamins in healthy individuals are less likely to occur than deficiencies of water-soluble vitamins.

The absorption of fat-soluble vitamins is enhanced by dietary fat (Table 5–5). Individuals afflicted with malabsorption of fat would be at higher risk for development of fat-soluble vitamin deficiencies. Fat-soluble vitamins are generally more stable than water-soluble vitamins and are less prone to destruction by heat, air, and light.

The following section reviews some of the basic distinctions of the various vitamins (see also Tables 5–1 through 5–4). The RDAs for fat-soluble vitamins are given in the table inside the front cover. Figure 5–2 shows the vitamin and mineral content of foods in the Food Guide Pyramid.

FAT-SOLUBLE VITAMINS

FUNCTIONS	GOOD SOURCES	SYMPTOMS OF DEFICIENCY	SYMPTOMS OF TOXICITY
Vitamin A (Nomenclature: Preformed—retinol, retinal, retinoic acid; Precursor—carotene)			
Maintenance of epi-thelial cells and mucous membranes Constituent of visual purple, important for night vision Necessary for normal growth, development, and reproduction Necessary for adequate immune response	Preformed vitamin A: liver Carotene (dark green leafy): Spinach Broccoli Kale Swiss chard Turnip greens Collard greens Carotene (deep orange): Carrots Sweet potatoes Orange winter squash Pumpkin Tomatoes Apricots Watermelon Cantaloupe	Nyctalopia (night blindness) Keratinized skin (rough, dry skin) Dry mucous membranes Xerophthalmia (an eye disease)	Appetite loss Hair loss Dry skin Bone and joint pain Enlarged liver and spleen Fetal malformations Headache Weakness Vomiting Irritability Hydrocephalus (children) Brittle nails Gingivitis Cheilosis Ascites
Vitamin E (Nomenclature: Tocopherol)			
Prevents oxidative de-struction of vitamin A in the intestine Protects red blood cells from rupture (hemolysis) Helps maintain normal cell membranes by reducing the oxidation of polyunsaturated fatty acids	Wheat germ Vegetable oils Legumes Nuts Whole grains Fish Green leafy vegetables	Breakdown of red blood cells	Decreased thyroid hormone level Modest increases in triglycerides
Vitamin K (Nomenclature: Menadione [vitamin K_3], Phylloquinone [vitamin K_1])			
Necessary for formation of prothrombin and other factors necessary for blood clotting	Dark green leafy vegetables Cauliflower Soybean oil Green tea Synthesis of intestinal bacteria	Hemorrhage	No toxicity known
Vitamin D (Nomenclature: Ergocalciferol [vitamin D_2], cholecalciferol [vitamin D_3]; Precursors—Ergosterol [plants], 7-dehydrocholesterol [in skin]			
Aids in absorption of calcium and phosphorus Regulates blood levels of calcium Promotes bone and teeth mineralization	Fortified milk Fish with bones (e.g., salmon, sardines)	Rickets (children) Osteomalacia (adults)	Calcification of soft tissues Hypercalcemia Renal stones Appetite and weight loss Nausea and fatigue Growth failure in children

Data from the National Research Council: Diet and Health, Washington, DC, National Academy Press, 1989; Mahan KL, Arlin M: Krause's Food, Nutrition & Diet Therapy, 8th ed., Philadelphia, WB Saunders, 1992; and Davis J, Sherer K: Applied Nutrition and Diet Therapy for Nurses, 2nd ed., Philadelphia, WB Saunders, 1994.

WATER-SOLUBLE VITAMINS

FUNCTIONS	GOOD SOURCES	SYMPTOMS OF DEFICIENCY	SYMPTOMS OF TOXICITY
	Vitamin B$_1$ (Nomenclature: Thiamine)		
Plays a role in carbohydrate metabolism Helps the nervous system, heart, muscles, and tissue to function properly Promotes a good appetite and good functioning of the digestive tract	Whole grains Wheat germ Enriched white flour products Organ meats Pork Legumes Brewer's yeast	Polyneuritis Beriberi Fatigue Depression Poor appetite Poor functioning of intestinal tract Nervous instability Edema Spastic muscle contractions Wernicke's encephalopathy Korsakoff's psychosis	No toxicity known
	Vitamin B$_2$ (Nomenclature: Riboflavin [formerly vitamin G])		

Essential for certain enzyme systems that aid in the metabolism of carbohydrate, protein, and fat	Milk and milk products
	Eggs
	Green leafy vegetables
	Organ meats
	  Liver
	  Kidney
	  Heart
	Dry yeast
	Peanuts
	Peanut butter
	Whole grains
		Tongue inflammation
		Scaling and burning skin
		Sensitive eyes
		Angular stomatitis and cheilosis
		Cataracts
			No toxicity known in humans

	Vitamin B$_3$ (Nomenclature: Niacin, nicotinic acid)		
Part of two important enzymes that regulate energy metabolism Promotes good physical and mental health and helps maintain the health of the skin, tongue, and digestive system	Meats and organ meats Whole grain flour products Enriched white flour products Legumes Brewer's yeast	Pellagra (rare) with skin and mouth manifestations Gastrointestinal disturbances Photosensitive dermatitis Depressive psychosis	Flushing caused by vasodilation Nausea and vomiting Abnormal glucose metabolism Abnormal plasma uric acid levels Abnormal liver function tests Gastric ulceration Anaphylaxis (swelling, pain, fever, or asthmatic symptoms caused by physical sensitivity) Circulatory collapse
	Vitamin B$_6$ (Nomenclature: Pyridoxine, pyridoxal, pyridoxamine)		
Important in metabolism of protein and amino acids, carbohydrate, and fat Essential for proper growth and maintenance of body functions	Liver and red meats Whole grains Potatoes Green vegetables Corn	Not fully established but believed to lead to convulsions, peripheral neuropathy, secondary pellagra, possible depression, oral lesions	Sensory nerve damage Numbness of extremities Ataxia Bone pain Muscle weakness
	Vitamin B$_{12}$ (Nomenclature: Cobalamin)		
Aids in hemoglobin synthesis	Foods of animal origin Meats	Pernicious (megaloblastic) anemia	No toxicity known

Table continued on following page

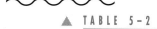

▲ T A B L E   5 – 2

WATER-SOLUBLE VITAMINS *Continued*

FUNCTIONS	GOOD SOURCES	SYMPTOMS OF DEFICIENCY	SYMPTOMS OF TOXICITY
	Vitamin B$_{12}$ (Nomenclature: Cobalamin) *Continued*		
Essential for normal functioning of all cells, especially nervous system, bone marrow, and gastrointestinal tract Important in energy metabolism, especially folic acid metabolism	Organ meats Dry milk and milk products Whole egg and egg yolk Not found in significant amounts in plant sources	Subacute combined degeneration of the spinal cord Various psychiatric disorders May cause anorexia	
	Folacin (Nomenclature: Folic acid)		
Functions in the formation of red blood cells and in normal functioning of gastrointestinal tract Aids in metabolism of protein	Glandular meats Yeast Dark green leafy vegetables Legumes Whole grains	Impaired cell division Alterations of protein synthesis with possible neural tube defect Various psychiatric disorders Megaloblastic anemia Supplements mask the symptoms of pernicious anemia but not the neurological manifestations	No toxicity known
	Choline		
A constituent of several compounds necessary for certain aspects of nerve function and lipid metabolism	Synthesized from methionine (an amino acid)	Occurs only when protein intake (methylamine) is low	No toxicity known in humans
	Pantothenic Acid		
Essential part of complex enzymes involved in fatty acid metabolism	Animal products Liver Eggs Whole grains Legumes White potatoes Sweet potatoes	Nutritional melalgia (burning foot syndrome) Headache Fatigue Poor muscle coordination Nausea Cramps	Possible diarrhea
	Biotin (Nomenclature: Once known as vitamin H)		
Essential for activity of many enzyme systems Plays a central role in fatty acid synthesis and in the metabolism of carbohydrates and protein	Liver Meats Milk Soy flour Brewer's yeast Egg yolk (raw egg white destroys biotin) Bacteria in the intestinal tract also produce biotin	Rare, but includes certain types of anemia, depression, insomnia, muscle pain, dermatitis	No toxicity known in humans

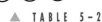

▲ TABLE 5-2

WATER-SOLUBLE VITAMINS *Continued*

FUNCTIONS	GOOD SOURCES	SYMPTOMS OF DEFICIENCY	SYMPTOMS OF TOXICITY
	Vitamin C (Nomenclature: Ascorbic acid, dehydroascorbic acid)		
Helps protect the body against infections and in wound healing and recovery from operations Is important for tooth dentin, bones, cartilage, connective tissue, and blood vessels	Citrus fruits Tomatoes Strawberries Cantaloupe Currants Green leafy vegetables Green peppers Broccoli Cabbage Potatoes	Anemia Swollen and bleeding gums Loose teeth Ruptures of small blood vessels (bruises) Scurvy (rebound scurvy can occur when large doses, or megadoses, are suddenly stopped)	Urinary stones Diarrhea Hypoglycemia Interferes with tests for fecal and urinary occult blood Will provide a false positive test for glucosuria

Data from the National Research Council: Diet and Health, Washington, DC, National Academy Press, 1989; Mahan KL, Arlin M: Krause's Food, Nutrition & Diet Therapy, 8th ed., Philadelphia, WB Saunders, 1992; and Davis J, Sherer K: Applied Nutrition and Diet Therapy for Nurses, 2nd ed., Philadelphia, WB Saunders, 1994.

Fat-Soluble Vitamins

VITAMIN A. Vitamin A can be obtained in two forms: in the **precursor** form of *carotene,* which is found in abundance in dark green leafy vegetables and deep orange vegetables and fruits, and is converted into vitamin A in the liver; or as preformed vitamin A, also called *retinol,* which is found in animal products such as liver, milk fat, and egg yolks. Preformed vitamin A is the type often found in vitamin supplements. It can reach toxic proportions, primarily because it is stored in the liver, whereas the **carotene** found in plant products cannot. However, it should be noted that

Text continued on page 108

FACT & FALLACY

FALLACY: Because vitamin A is suspected to lower the risk of cancer, all people should take a supplement to ensure adequate intake.

FACT: Although a correlation has been shown between increased vitamin A intake and a lower incidence of cancer, the research is based on food intake. Thus, it may be the vitamin A specifically in these foods or some other nutrient yet to be identified that helps prevent cancer. In addition, it is known that excess vitamin A from supplements is toxic and, even in small amounts, can cause severe problems in a growing fetus if taken during pregnancy. Thus, the best and safest approach is to choose adequate dietary sources such as the deep orange and dark green leafy vegetables and deep orange fruits (see Table 5-1).

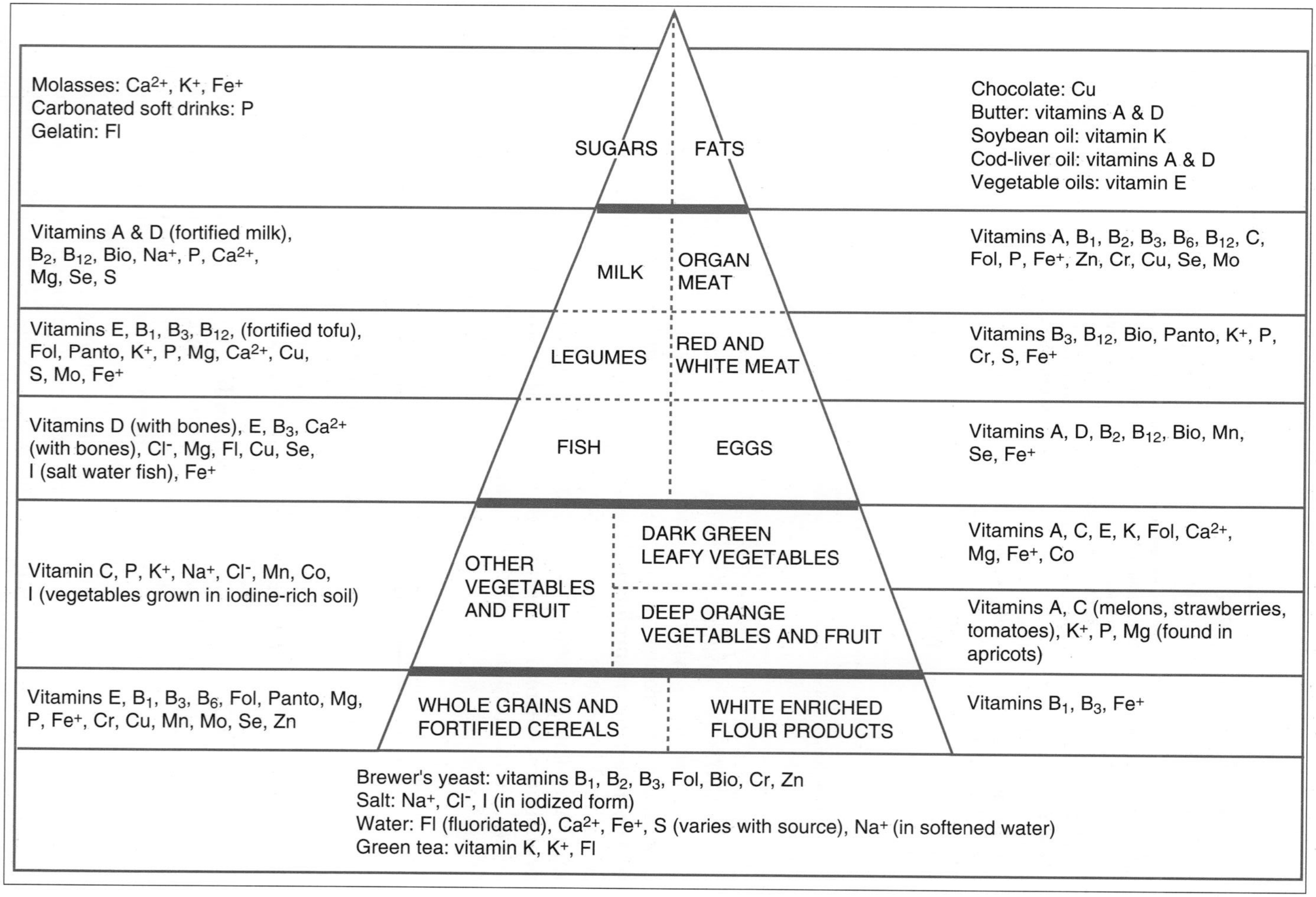

Chocolate: Cu
Butter: vitamins A & D
Soybean oil: vitamin K
Cod-liver oil: vitamins A & D
Vegetable oils: vitamin E

FATS / SUGARS
Vitamins A, B_1, B_2, B_3, B_6, B_{12}, C, Fol, P, Fe^+, Zn, Cr, Cu, Se, Mo

ORGAN MEAT / MILK
Vitamins B_3, B_{12}, Bio, Panto, K^+, P, Cr, S, Fe^+

RED AND WHITE MEAT / LEGUMES
Vitamins A, D, B_2, B_{12}, Bio, Mn, Se, Fe^+

EGGS / FISH
Vitamins A, C, E, K, Fol, Ca^{2+}, Mg, Fe^+, Co

DARK GREEN LEAFY VEGETABLES / OTHER VEGETABLES AND FRUIT

DEEP ORANGE VEGETABLES AND FRUIT
Vitamins A, C (melons, strawberries, tomatoes), K^+, P, Mg (found in apricots)

WHITE ENRICHED FLOUR PRODUCTS / WHOLE GRAINS AND FORTIFIED CEREALS
Vitamins B_1, B_3, Fe^+

Molasses: Ca^{2+}, K^+, Fe^+
Carbonated soft drinks: P
Gelatin: Fl

Vitamins A & D (fortified milk), B_2, B_{12}, Bio, Na^+, P, Ca^{2+}, Mg, Se, S

Vitamins E, B_1, B_3, B_{12}, (fortified tofu), Fol, Panto, K^+, P, Mg, Ca^{2+}, Cu, S, Mo, Fe^+

Vitamins D (with bones), E, B_3, Ca^{2+} (with bones), Cl^-, Mg, Fl, Cu, Se, I (salt water fish), Fe^+

Vitamin C, P, K^+, Na^+, Cl^-, Mn, Co, I (vegetables grown in iodine-rich soil)

Vitamins E, B_1, B_3, B_6, Fol, Panto, Mg, P, Fe^+, Cr, Cu, Mn, Mo, Se, Zn

Brewer's yeast: vitamins B_1, B_2, B_3, Fol, Bio, Cr, Zn
Salt: Na^+, Cl^-, I (in iodized form)
Water: Fl (fluoridated), Ca^{2+}, Fe^+, S (varies with source), Na^+ (in softened water)
Green tea: vitamin K, K^+, Fl

▲ FIGURE 5-2

Vitamin and mineral content of the Food Guide Pyramid (listed in the following order: fat-soluble vitamins, water-soluble vitamins, major minerals, and trace minerals). KEY: Bio = biotin; Ca^{2+} = calcium; Cl^- = chloride; Co = cobalt; Cr = chromium; Cu = copper; Fe^+ = iron; Fl = fluorine; Fol = folate; I = Iodine; K^+ = potassium; Mg = magnesium; Mn = manganese; Mo = molybdenum; Na^+ = sodium; P = phosphorus; Panto = pantothenic acid; S = sulfur; Se = selenium; Zn = zinc.

▲ T A B L E   5 - 3

MAJOR MINERALS (MACRONUTRIENTS)

FUNCTIONS	SOURCES	DEFICIENCY SYMPTOMS	TOXICITY SYMPTOMS
	Mineral and Elemental Symbol: Calcium (Ca^{2+})		
Helps muscles to contract and relax, thereby helping to regulate heartbeat Plays a role in the normal functioning of the nervous system Aids in blood coagulation and the functioning of some enzymes Helps build strong bones and teeth May help prevent hypertension	Primarily found in milk and milk products; also found in dark green leafy vegetables, tofu and other soy products, sardines, salmon with bones, and hard water	Poor bone growth and tooth development, leading to stunted growth and increased risk of dental caries, rickets (bowing of legs) in children, osteomalacia (soft bones) and osteoporosis (brittle bones) in adults, poor blood clotting, and possible hypertension	Kidney stones in predisposed individuals
	Mineral and Elemental Symbol: Chloride (Cl^-)		
Involved in the maintenance of fluid and acid-base balance Provides an acid medium, in the form of hydrochloric acid, for activation of gastric enzymes	Major source is table salt (sodium chloride); also found in fish and vegetables	Disturbances in acid-base balance, with possible growth retardation, psychomotor defects, and memory loss	No toxicity known
	Mineral and Elemental Symbol: Magnesium (Mg^{2+})		
Helps build strong bones and teeth Activates many enzymes Participates in protein synthesis and lipid metabolism Helps regulate heartbeat	Raw dark green vegetables, nuts and soybeans, whole grains and wheat bran, bananas and apricots, seafoods, coffee, tea, cocoa, and hard water	Rare, but in disease states may lead to central nervous system problems (confusion, apathy, hallucinations, poor memory) and neuromuscular problems (muscle weakness, cramps, tremor, cardiac arrhythmia)	Increased calcium excretion
	Mineral and Elemental Symbol: Phosphorus (P)		
Helps build strong bones and teeth Present in the nuclei of all cells Helps in the oxidation of fats and carbohydrates (energy metabolism) Aids in maintaining the body's acid-base balance	Milk and milk products, eggs, meats, legumes, whole grains, soft drinks (used to make the "fizz")	Rare, but with malabsorption can cause anorexia, weakness, stiff joints, and fragile bones	Hypocalcemic tetany (muscle spasms)

Table continued on following page

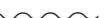

▲ TABLE 5-3

MAJOR MINERALS (MACRONUTRIENTS) *Continued*

FUNCTIONS	SOURCES	DEFICIENCY SYMPTOMS	TOXICITY SYMPTOMS
	Mineral and Elemental Symbol: Potassium (K⁺)		
Plays a key role in fluid and acid-base balance	Apricots, bananas, oranges, grapefruit, raisins, green beans, broccoli, carrots, greens, potatoes, meats, milk and milk products, peanut butter, legumes, molasses, coffee, tea, and cocoa	May cause impaired growth, hypertension, bone fragility, central nervous system changes, renal hypertrophy, diminished heart rate, and death	Hyperkalemia (excess potassium in the blood) with cardiac function disturbances
Transmits nerve impulses and helps control muscle contractions and promotes regular heartbeat			
Needed for enzyme reactions			
	Mineral and Elemental Symbol: Sodium (Na⁺)		
Plays a key role in the maintenance of acid-base balance	Salt (sodium chloride) is the major dietary source; minor sources occur naturally in foods such as milk and milk products and several vegetables	Hyponatremia (too little sodium in the blood)	May cause hypertension, which can lead to cardiovascular diseases and renal (kidney) disease; in the form of salt tablets, can cause gastric irritation
Transmits nerve impulses and helps control muscle contractions			
Regulates cell membrane permeability			
	Mineral and Elemental Symbol: Sulfur (S)		
Part of three amino acids, and the B vitamins thiamine and biotin	Protein-rich foods (meat, eggs, milk)	None documented in humans	Unlikely to cause significant symptoms
Plays a role in oxidation-reduction reactions			

Data from the National Research Council: Diet and Health, Washington, DC, National Academy Press, 1989; Mahan KL, Arlin M: Krause's Food, Nutrition & Diet Therapy, 8th ed., Philadelphia, WB Saunders, 1992; and Davis J, Sherer K: Applied Nutrition and Diet Therapy for Nurses, 2nd ed., Philadelphia, WB Saunders, 1994.

FACT & FALLACY

FALLACY: Hair analysis is an excellent way to determine nutritional status.

FACT: Although hair analysis has some value in assessing nutritional status, it is too limited in scope because various nutrients are stored in different parts of the body. Blood test results are more significant. Height and weight are also important indicators of nutritional status.

TRACE MINERALS (MICRONUTRIENTS)

FUNCTIONS	SOURCES	DEFICIENCY SYMPTOMS	TOXICITY SYMPTOMS
	Mineral and Elemental Symbol: Chromium (Cr^{3+})		
Activates several enzymes Enhances the removal of glucose from the blood	Liver and other meats, whole grains, cheese, legumes, and brewer's yeast	Weight loss, abnormalities of the central nervous system, and possible aggravation of diabetes mellitus	Liver damage and lung cancer caused by industrial exposure
	Mineral and Elemental Symbol: Cobalt (Co^{2+})		
An essential component of vitamin B_{12} Activates enzymes	Figs, cabbage, beet greens, spinach, lettuce, watercress	Pernicious anemia	Polycythemia (excess number of red corpuscles in blood) Hyperplasia of bone marrow Increased blood volume
	Mineral and Elemental Symbol: Copper (Cu^{2+})		
Aids in the production and survival of red blood cells Part of many enzymes involved in respiration Plays a role in normal lipid metabolism	Shellfish—especially oysters—liver, nuts and seeds, raisins, whole grains, chocolate, and legumes	Anemia, central nervous system problems, abnormal electrocardiograms, bone fragility, impaired immune response; may be a factor in failure to thrive in premature infants	In Wilson's disease, copper accumulation causes neuron and liver cell damage
	Mineral and Elemental Symbol: Fluorine (F^-)		
Helps the formation of solid bones and teeth, thereby reducing incidence of dental caries (see Chapter 19) and may help prevent osteoporosis	Fluoridated water (and foods cooked in fluoridated water), fish, tea, gelatin	Increased susceptibility to dental caries	Fluorosis and mottling of teeth
	Mineral and Elemental Symbol: Iodine (I^-)		
Helps regulate energy metabolism as a part of thyroid hormones Essential for normal cell functioning, helping to keep skin, hair, and nails healthy	Primarily from iodized salt, also found in saltwater fish, seaweed products, vegetables grown in iodine-rich soils	Goiter, cretinism in infants born to iodine-deficient mothers, with accompanying mental retardation and diffuse central nervous system abnormalities	Little toxic effect in individuals with normal thyroid gland functioning Goiter may also occur in toxic states
	Mineral and Elemental Symbol: Iron (Fe^{3+})		
Essential to the formation of hemoglobin, which is important for tissue respiration and ultimately growth and development Part of several enzymes and proteins in the body	Heme sources: organ meats—especially liver, red meats, and other meats Nonheme sources: iron-fortified cereals, dark green leafy vegetables, legumes, whole grains, blackstrap molasses, dried fruit, and foods cooked in iron pans	Iron-deficiency anemia and possible alterations that impair behavior	Idiopathic hemochromatosis, which can lead to cirrhosis, diabetes mellitus, and cardiomyopathy

Table continued on following page

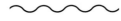

▲ **T A B L E   5 – 4**

TRACE MINERALS (MICRONUTRIENTS)   *Continued*

FUNCTIONS	SOURCES	DEFICIENCY SYMPTOMS	TOXICITY SYMPTOMS
	Mineral and Elemental Symbol: Manganese (Mn^{2+})		
Needed for normal bone structure, re-production, normal functioning of cells and the central nervous system A component of some enzymes	Nuts, whole grains, vegetables and fruits, coffee, tea, cocoa, and egg yolks	None observed in humans	Parkinson-like symp-toms have been noted in miners
	Mineral and Elemental Symbol: Molybdenum (Mo)		
A component of three enzymes Important for normal cell function	Organ meats, legumes, whole grains, dark green vegetables	Vomiting, tachypnea (fast breathing), tachycardia, coma, hypermethioninemia in premature infants (methionine is an amino acid)	No toxicity known
	Mineral and Elemental Symbol: Selenium (Se)		
Part of an enzyme sys-tem Acts as an antioxidant with vitamin E to protect the cell from oxygen	Protein-rich foods (meat, eggs, milk), whole grains, sea-food, liver and other meats, egg yolks, and garlic	Keshan's disease (a human cardiomyo-pathy) and Kashin-Beck disease (an endemic human osteoarthropathy)	Physical defects of the fingernails and toe-nails and hair loss Nausea Abdominal pain Diarrhea Peripheral neuropathy Fatigue Irritability
	Mineral and Elemental Symbol: Zinc (Zn^{2+})		
Plays a role in protein synthesis Essential for normal growth and sexual development, wound healing, immune function, cell divi-sion and differentia-tion, and smell acuity	Whole grains, wheat germ, crabmeat, oysters, liver and other meats, brew-er's yeast	Depressed immune function, poor growth, dwarfism, impaired skeletal growth and delayed sexual maturation, acrodermatitis	Severe anemia, nau-sea, vomiting, ab-dominal cramps, diarrhea, fever, hypocupremia (low blood serum cop-per), malaise, fatigue Impaired immunity also found in toxic states Renal damage

Data from the National Research Council: Diet and Health, Washington, DC, National Academy Press, 1989; Mahan KL, Arlin M: Krause's Food, Nutrition & Diet Therapy, 8th ed., Philadelphia, WB Saunders, 1992; and Davis J, Sherer K: Applied Nutrition and Diet Therapy for Nurses, 2nd ed., Philadelphia, WB Saunders, 1994.

carotene is stored in the adipose tissue, and an excess is known to cause a yellowing of the skin, an innocuous but undesirable effect. This skin color-ing can be reversed by a decreased intake of foods high in carotene (see Table 5–1 and Fig. 5–2).

Deficiency of vitamin A has long been known to increase the risk of infec-tion and is associated with blindness in many countries (see Chapter 22). It

▲ TABLE 5-5

SOME NUTRIENT INTERACTIONS WITH VITAMINS AND MINERALS

NUTRIENT	INHIBITING NUTRIENT	ENHANCING NUTRIENT
	Vitamins	
Vitamin A (carotene)	Excess vitamin E, deficiency of protein, iron, and zinc	Dietary fat
Vitamin D		Dietary fat
Vitamin E		Dietary fat
Vitamin K	Excess vitamin E	Dietary fat
Vitamin B_1	Tannins (as found in coffee)	
Vitamin B_2	Excess vitamin B_1	
Vitamin B_3	Deficiency of vitamin B_6	
Vitamin B_6	Excess choline and leucine	Deficiency of vitamin C
Vitamin B_{12}	Excess vitamin C, deficiency of vitamin B_6	
Folacin	Thiamine hastens decomposition in supplements	
Choline	Excess inositol	
Vitamin C	Deficiency of vitamin B_6	
	Minerals	
Calcium	Excess sodium, protein, phosphorus, oxalates	Vitamin D, lactose, and certain amino acids
Phosphorus	Excess iron	
Magnesium	Excess sodium, calcium, vitamin D, phosphate, protein, and alcohol	
Iron	Excess manganese	Vitamin C, copper, cobalt
Zinc	Excess iron, copper, tin, folic acid, tannins, and possibly calcium	Possible fluoride role
Copper	Excess zinc, molybdenum, and vitamin C	Possible fluoride role Estrogen increases copper serum levels
Molybdenum	Excess sulfur	

is now known that a good intake of vitamin A helps with growth, the formation of sperm, and fetal growth starting in the embryonic stage (Ross, 1991).

WHAT IS THE DIFFERENCE BETWEEN IU AND RE FOR VITAMIN A?

Retinol equivalents (REs) and **international units (IUs)** are two different methods of describing the amount of vitamin A in foods. The use of IU indicates that both preformed vitamin A and carotenoids are measured; this is still a common method used in food composition tables and in diet planning. Because the biological activities of carotenoids and vitamin A are different, however, REs began to be used. Simply said, numbers used in the IU system are about five times those expressed in the RE system.

VITAMIN D. Active research on the prevention of **rickets** (bowing of the legs caused by the increasing weight on the soft bones of growing children who do not receive enough vitamin D) began during World War I, although rickets in children had been recognized for centuries (Fig. 5–3). After vitamin D was chemically isolated in 1935, it was eventually added to milk (to the relief of many children who had previously taken cod liver oil to prevent rickets). Milk was an appropriate food to fortify with vitamin D, since this vitamin greatly enhances the absorption of calcium, of which milk is the best source.

Sunlight also contributes to vitamin D status by converting a vitamin D precursor in the skin to an active form. This conversion varies according to the length and intensity of exposure and the color of the skin. Institutionalized elderly people are at high risk for vitamin D deficiency because of negligible exposure to the sun. However, excessive sun exposure is related to the development of skin cancer; thus, although a little is good, too much is harmful. A vitamin D supplement in addition to a calcium supplement may help reverse the cycle of bone loss and fracture in very old women (Chapuy, 1992). Patients with renal (kidney) disease may also require supplementation because of impaired metabolism (see Chapter 10).

VITAMIN E. Initially, vitamin E was recognized as essential for reproduction in rats. Since the role of this vitamin is still not well defined, it has

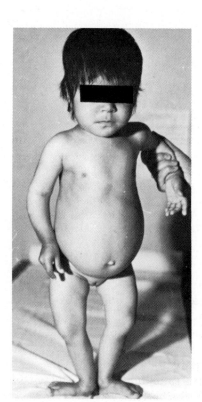

▲ FIGURE 5-3

Rickets in young child. Chest and lower extremities are deformed. (From Harrison HE, Harrison HC: Disorders of Calcium and Phosphate Metabolism in Childhood and Adolescence. Philadelphia: WB Saunders, 1979, p. 153.)

become the target of many unscientific claims. Vitamin E acts as an antioxidant and therefore may serve a role in preventing cell damage from oxidation. Although known toxic effects from excess ingestion of vitamin E are limited primarily to premature infants, persons receiving anticoagulant medications may have complications associated with megadoses of vitamin E because it inhibits the clotting action of vitamin K (National Research Council, 1989). At this time, there is not enough medical justification for the use of large doses of vitamin E, particularly since it is widely distributed in common foods.

VITAMIN K.   Vitamin K was first recognized as an antihemorrhagic factor. Because vitamin K is essential for the formation of **prothrombin** (a clotting factor), defective coagulation of the blood is the main symptom of vitamin K deficiency. In addition to dietary sources (see Table 5–1), vitamin K is synthesized by bacteria in the jejunum and ileum.

Vitamin K deficiency is most likely to occur in individuals receiving antibiotics over an extended period who are not able to absorb fat and who have a low intake of foods containing vitamin K. Infants are also at risk because of their inability to adequately colonize the vitamin K–synthesizing bacteria. Vitamin K injections are recommended for newborn infants, and infant formulas are now routinely supplemented with this vitamin. Persons receiving antibiotic therapy should be considered for vitamin K supplementation (Suttie, 1992). Persons who take coumarin to reduce the risk of blood clot formation need to use caution with foods high in vitamin K because this vitamin can counteract the effect of coumarin.

WATER-SOLUBLE VITAMINS

The Vitamin B Complex

The term *vitamin B complex* refers to all water-soluble vitamins except ascorbic acid (vitamin C). Vitamin B_1 was the first of this group to be discovered and was found to prevent **beriberi** (a condition involving inflammation of the nerves). With further study, vitamin B proved to be not a single substance but a combination of substances, each one of which was given a letter or a descriptive term, or later a chemical designation as its chemical nature became known.

Several factors in the vitamin B complex are recognized today. The RDAs have been established for six: thiamine (vitamin B_1), riboflavin (vitamin B_2, formerly vitamin G), niacin (nicotinic acid), vitamins B_6 and B_{12}, and folacin (see table on the inside front cover). Important functions in the body have been assigned to biotin, choline, and pantothenic acid, but no definite daily allowances have been established, although estimated safe and adequate intakes are now given.

A lack of B-complex vitamins is one of the widespread forms of malnutrition. Because of the similar distribution of the B vitamins in foods, a deficiency of several factors is observed more often than is a deficiency of a single factor. The interrelationship of many of these vitamins in life processes means that signs of dietary deficiency are often similar when the diet lacks any one of several factors (Fig. 5–4). Many physiological and pathological stresses influence the need for the B vitamins, but generally an adequate diet will meet these needs.

THIAMINE (VITAMIN B$_1$). The requirement for thiamine is small but important, and is based on the kilocalorie requirement. Thiamine is needed in increased amounts during pregnancy and lactation, but these levels are easy to achieve through an increased intake of food. In excess, as with in-

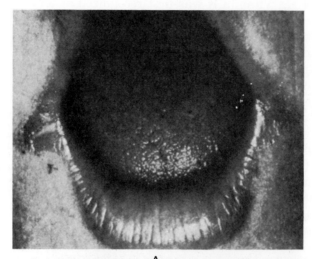

A

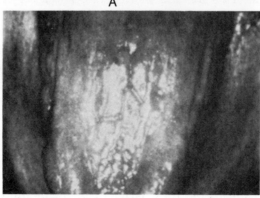

B

▲ FIGURE 5 – 4

Vitamin B deficiencies. *A,* Angular cheilosis due to vitamin B complex deficiency. *B,* Depapillation of the tongue from the same cause. (From Schneider HA, et al: Nutritional Support of Medical Practice. Hagerstown, MD, Harper & Row Publishers, Inc., 1977.)

travenously administered thiamine, fatal reactions can occur (Snodgrass, 1992). Thiamine:

- plays a role in carbohydrate metabolism
- promotes good appetite and good functioning of the digestive tract
- helps the nervous system, heart, and muscles function properly

Many foods contain thiamine. It is found in whole-grain and enriched flour and bread, meats (especially organ meats), fish, and poultry. Pork contains three times as much thiamine as other meats do. Dry beans and peas and peanuts contain thiamine, and small amounts can be found in milk and eggs. Brewer's yeast and wheat germ are also sources of thiamine.

RIBOFLAVIN (VITAMIN B$_2$). The requirement for riboflavin is also related to kilocalorie needs. Riboflavin:

- is essential for certain enzyme systems that aid in the metabolism of carbohydrates, proteins, and fats
- is important for healthy eyes, skin, lips, and tongue

Riboflavin is found in milk, cheese, eggs, green leafy vegetables, organ meats (liver, kidney, and heart), dry yeast, peanuts, and peanut butter. Without an adequate consumption of milk, riboflavin intake is likely to be impaired.

NIACIN (NICOTINIC ACID OR VITAMIN B$_3$). Niacin requirements are related to kilocalorie intake. Niacin:

- functions as part of two important enzymes that regulate energy metabolism
- promotes good physical and mental health
- helps maintain the health of the skin, tongue, and digestive system

Good food sources include organ meats (kidney, liver, and heart), other meats, poultry, fish, whole-grain and enriched cereal products, meat drippings, and brewer's yeast. Niacin can also be synthesized in the body from tryptophan (an amino acid) in protein. Precursors of niacin can be found in milk and eggs. Niacin deficiency can result in **pellagra,** a syndrome of various skin, digestive, and mental disturbances.

VITAMIN B$_6$. Three interrelated substances—pyridoxine (from plants), pyridoxal, and pyridoxamine (from animal products)—are collectively known as vitamin B$_6$. The need for vitamin B$_6$ increases in conjunction with high-protein diets, pregnancy, certain tuberculosis therapies, certain medications, and some contraceptives. Vitamin B:

- functions primarily in protein and amino acid metabolism
- is important in energy metabolism
- may be of importance in red blood cell regeneration and normal nervous system functioning

Excess pyridoxine can be related to neuropathy (Berger et al., 1992). Women who take 500 to 5000 mg vitamin B_6 per day to treat PMS (premenstrual syndrome, see Chapter 16) have shown peripheral **neuropathy** (problems of the peripheral nervous system, commonly found in persons with diabetes) within 1 to 3 years. The use of vitamin B_6 at doses less than 100 milligrams per day appears safe for adults. Pyridoxine has also been suggested to treat Down's syndrome and autism but not enough data exist at this time to suggest a safe amount in a therapeutic range for children (Bernstein, 1990). Renal patients who are deficient in this nutrient should receive supplementation (Wilkens and Brouns Schiro, 1992).

FACT & FALLACY

FALLACY: Women experiencing premenstrual syndrome (PMS) should be advised to take a vitamin B_6 supplement.

FACT: There is no scientific evidence to support this hypothesis. Women who are insistent on this approach would be better off increasing their vitamin B_6 intake through the use of whole grains, such as wheat germ, or legumes. A balanced diet, evenly spaced throughout the day to help maintain blood glucose levels, would also be advisable. Individuals who are still insistent on the use of a vitamin supplement should be strongly advised not to exceed 100 per cent of the RDA (1.6 mg), since larger doses are potentially harmful or even toxic.

VITAMIN B_{12} (COBALAMIN). Cobalt, a mineral, is an essential part of vitamin B_{12}. **Pernicious anemia** (a form of anemia that can lead to permanent neurological impairment and death) is caused by a lack of **intrinsic factor,** a glycoprotein secreted in the stomach that attaches to vitamin B_{12} to aid its absorption. Vitamin B_{12}:

- is essential for normal functioning of all cells, particularly those of the bone marrow, the nervous system, and the gastrointestinal tract
- is important in energy metabolism, especially folic acid metabolism

Vitamin B_{12} is found bound to protein in foods of animal origin. There is relatively little in vegetables, which is why strict vegetarians (vegans) may need a vitamin B_{12} supplement. Kidneys and liver are high in vitamin B_{12}, with only moderate amounts found in other meats. Milk, most cheeses, shellfish, most fish, whole egg, and egg yolk are all additional sources of vitamin B_{12}.

FOLATE. The active form of folate is folic acid, which is formed from folate by vitamin C. There are many forms of this water-soluble vitamin. Folate:

- is important in the formation of red blood cells
- helps in normal gastrointestinal functioning
- aids in the metabolism of protein and **DNA** (deoxyribonucleic acid, a basic structure of genes and therefore found in all cells)

At high-risk for folate deficiency are premature, low birth-weight infants. A subcommittee of the American Society for Clinical Nutrition recommends daily parenteral folate intake of 56 mg/kg body weight/day for preterm infants. Other high-risk groups that may benefit from a folate supplement, as recommended by the National Academy of Sciences, include pregnant women who smoke, use specific medications, abuse alcohol, lack the ability to purchase folate-dense foods, are adolescents, or are carrying multiple fetuses. The recommended amount of supplementation is 300 mg (Bailey, 1992). In normal, healthy adults, supplemental folate can be considered nontoxic, but very large doses (100 times the RDA) may precipitate convulsions in epileptic patients. Vitamin B_{12} status should be assessed before initiating folate therapy (Bailey, 1992).

Folate can be found in a wide variety of foods of animal and plant origin, particularly glandular meats, yeast, dark green leafy vegetables, dried beans, whole grains, peanuts, walnuts, and lentils. Ideally, raw, fresh, dark green leafy vegetables such as spinach or broccoli should be consumed, since folate may be destroyed in cooking and lost in cooking water.

CHOLINE. Choline is a constituent of several compounds that are necessary for certain aspects of nerve function and lipid metabolism. No RDA has been established and no disease related to choline deficiency has been demonstrated in humans. Mixed diets are estimated to provide adults with 400 to 900 mg of choline daily, and such diets are evidently adequate. In addition, the body can synthesize choline from methionine (an amino acid).

PANTOTHENIC ACID. Pantothenic acid is an essential constituent of complex enzymes involved in fatty acid metabolism and synthesis of certain products. It is widely distributed in foods, occurring abundantly in animal sources, whole-grain cereals, and legumes. The estimated safe and adequate intake is 4 to 7 mg daily; the higher level is suggested for pregnant and lactating women. Dietary deficiencies are unlikely, but marginal deficiencies may exist in generally malnourished individuals, along with deficiency of other B-complex vitamins. The usual dietary intake is between 5 and 20 mg daily.

BIOTIN. Biotin is essential for the activity of many enzyme systems. It is widely distributed in nature and is bound to protein in foods and tissues. It plays a central role in synthesis of fatty acid and participates in several metabolic reactions. The estimated safe, adequate intake is 100 to 200 μg daily for adults.

Vitamin C

Vitamin C (ascorbic acid) performs a variety of functions. Higher levels may be necessary during conditions of stress, with certain medications, or in persons who smoke. Inadequate vitamin C intake may eventually lead to swollen and bleeding gums, loose teeth, and ruptures of small blood vessels (Fig. 5–5), which are early forerunners of scorbutus, also known as scurvy. However, these increased needs can easily be met with an extra serving of a food high in vitamin C. Vitamin C:

- aids in the formation and maintenance of the intracellular cement substance of body tissues
- is important for tooth dentin, bones, cartilage, connective tissue, and blood vessels
- is thought to help protect the body against infections
- helps in wound healing and recovery following operations
- participates in the formation of red blood cells in the bone marrow
- is involved in changing folate to folic acid
- increases the absorption of iron

Fruits and vegetables are the main sources of vitamin C. They contain more of the vitamin when they are fresh or frozen. Foremost among them are citrus fruits, tomatoes, strawberries, cantaloupes, and some of the green leafy vegetables. Additional sources of vitamin C are green peppers, broccoli, raw greens, cabbage, and newly harvested potatoes.

Vitamin C is generally not toxic in high doses. However, some individuals are at risk of toxicity. These include about one-eighth of the men with a heritage of African, Asian, Sephardic Jewish, and Mediterranean basin ori-

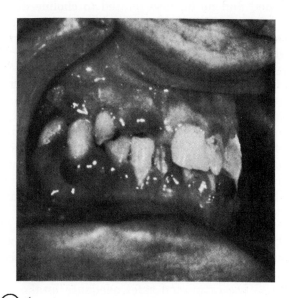

▲ FIGURE 5-5

Scorbutic gingivitis. (From Nizel AE, Papas AS: Nutrition in Clinical Dentistry, 3rd ed. Philadelphia, WB Saunders, 1989.)

gin who were born with glucose-6-phosphate dehydrogenase deficiency. In these individuals, megadoses of vitamin C will instantly affect red blood cells and can lead to death within hours. In addition, megadoses of vitamin C can precipitate an acute sickle cell crisis in all those with **sickle cell disease** (a disease in which the red blood cells take on a sickle shape). And since megadoses of vitamin C cause **hyperosmotic diarrhea** (when excess substances attract water in the intestinal tract through the process of osmosis, resulting in watery stools), persons with pre-existing diarrhea, such as 60 per cent of AIDS patients, can go into hypovolemic shock. Oxalate kidney stones, oxalate deposits in the heart and other body tissues, urinary tract irritation, and potentially problematical increased iron absorption can occur (Herbert, 1993). **Rebound scurvy** may occur if the body has become accustomed to high blood plasma levels of vitamin C and the dose is then discontinued. A gradual decrease from high doses is recommended. Much more research is needed on the safety of high doses of vitamin C as well as of other vitamins. A more prudent approach at the present time is to obtain vitamin C and other vitamins and minerals from food sources to help avoid toxicity problems.

FACT & FALLACY

FALLACY: People who have colds should take megadoses of vitamin C (1 g/day).

FACT: Although minor lessening of cold symptoms may occur, the risks of large doses of vitamin C outweigh any possible benefits. Since the RDA for vitamin C is less than 100 mg/day, a 1-gram dose is more than ten times the RDA. This quantity can result in rebound scurvy when the dosage is stopped. If the vitamin C supplement is in chewable pill form, dental decay is promoted because the acidity of vitamin C is very destructive to dental enamel.

HOW DO MINERALS FUNCTION IN NUTRITION?

Minerals have building functions and regulating functions. As building material, the following minerals enter into the formation of:

- *Bony tissue:* Calcium and phosphorus in bones and teeth, and fluoride in teeth
- *Soft body tissue* (muscles, nerves, glands): All salts, especially phosphorus, potassium, sulfur, and chloride
- *Hair, nails, skin:* Sulfur
- *Blood:* All salts, especially iron for hemoglobin and copper for red blood cells
- *Glandular secretions:* Chlorine in gastric juice, sodium in intestinal juice, iodine in thyroxine, manganese in endocrine secretions, and zinc in enzymes

As regulators, the following minerals play a role in:

- *Fluid pressure:* All salts, especially sodium and potassium
- *Muscle contraction and relaxation:* Calcium, potassium, sodium, phosphorus, and chlorine
- *Nerve responses:* All salts, with a balance between calcium and sodium
- *Blood clotting:* Calcium
- *Oxidation in tissues and blood:* Iron, iodine
- *Acid-base balance:* Balance between acid compounds—chlorine, sulfur, and phosphorus—and base compounds—calcium, sodium, potassium, and magnesium

HOW ARE MINERALS CLASSIFIED?

Minerals are usually classified into two groups: major minerals and trace minerals. The major minerals (also referred to as macrominerals) are those present in amounts greater than 5 grams in the human body. The trace minerals (also referred to as microminerals) are found in the human body in amounts less than 5 grams. See Tables 5–3 and 5–4 for lists of the major and trace minerals, their functions and sources, and symptoms of deficiency and toxicity. The RDA for minerals can be found inside the front cover.

Major Minerals

CALCIUM. As calcium phosphate, calcium is the major mineral constituent of the body. Ninety-nine per cent of calcium is found in bones (giving rigidity) and teeth, with the remainder in the blood, other body fluids, and soft tissues. Vitamin D is required for proper absorption and utilization of dietary calcium. Inadequate calcium in the diet leads to poor bone growth and tooth development, stunted growth, rickets in children (Fig. 5–3), osteomalacia and osteoporosis in adults, thin and fragile bones, and poor blood clotting.

> An interesting experiment and useful teaching technique is to soak a chicken bone in vinegar, which leaches the calcium from the bone. This activity clearly demonstrates how calcium lends rigidity to the bone, as without it bone becomes extremely soft and pliable.

In conjunction with the other minerals, calcium:

- promotes bone growth and strength
- helps muscles to contract and relax normally
- takes part in the normal functioning of the nervous system
- facilitates passage of materials into and out of cells

- aids in blood coagulation
- helps in the functioning of some enzymes

Milk, the best source for calcium, is also a major contributor of protein, vitamin D, riboflavin, potassium, and magnesium. For this reason, milk intake is vital for health. Calcium supplements cannot replace the nutritive value of milk. For persons who are weight-conscious or trying to control their fat intake, low-fat or skim milk can be used. For individuals who cannot tolerate milk, there are alternatives such as low-lactose milk and soy milk. Figure 5–2 shows where calcium foods are found in the Food Guide Pyramid. Although dark green leafy vegetables are high in calcium, the calcium in chard, beet greens, spinach, and rhubarb generally is not available to the body. This is because an insoluble salt forms with the oxalic acid found in these foods. It is important to note that protein intake may affect calcium needs by increasing the acidity of urine. Vegetarians, with their lower meat and protein intake, generally have a less acidic urine, which is believed to help the body retain calcium (Mickelsen and Marsh, 1989).

FACT & FALLACY

FALLACY: Butter and eggs are high in calcium because they are dairy products.

   FACT: Butter comes from milk fat and does not contain significant amounts of calcium. (Margarine, which contains milk solids, has more calcium than butter does.) Eggs do not have any significant amounts of calcium either.

CHLORIDE.   Chloride is an electrolyte and it:

- provides an acidic medium for activation of gastric (stomach) enzymes
- aids in maintaining osmotic pressure

Its major dietary source is table salt (sodium chloride), and it is also found in the chlorinated water used in urban settings.

MAGNESIUM.   Deficiency of magnesium is rare because normal kidney functioning helps maintain appropriate levels of magnesium in the body. Magnesium deficiency in diabetes does occur as a result of frequent urination and the use of diuretics (American Diabetes Association, 1992). Conversely, renal insufficiency and reduced renal function in general in the elderly population increase the risk for toxicity symptoms as a result of excessive intake. Antacids, laxatives, or other drugs containing magnesium should be used cautiously in such individuals. Along with the other minerals, magnesium:

- is a component of bones and teeth
- is vital for the metabolism of adenosine triphosphate (ATP)
- plays a role in metabolic processes and muscle contractions

The major food sources of magnesium are those containing chlorophyll (magnesium is a part of the chlorophyll molecule), such as the dark green leafy vegetables. It is also found in high quantities in nuts, whole grains, seafoods, coffee, tea, cocoa, and hard (versus soft) water.

PHOSPHORUS. The amount of phosphorus in the body is second only to the amount of calcium. The largest amount of phosphorus is found with calcium in the bones; the remainder is in soft tissues and fluids. A wide variation in the ratio of calcium to phosphorus is tolerated in the adult diet that includes adequate vitamin D. A ratio of 1.5:1 is recommended in early infancy to prevent tetany caused by **hypocalcemia** (low blood levels of calcium). Phosphorus:

- is involved in bone and tooth structure
- is present in the nuclei of all cells
- helps in oxidation of carbohydrates and fats
- helps enzymes act in energy metabolism

Rich sources of phosphorus include milk, meat, eggs, cheese, dried beans, nuts, and whole-grain cereals. A diet adequate in protein and calcium will provide sufficient phosphorus for body needs.

POTASSIUM. Potassium is an electrolyte. Serum potassium fluctuations can be fatal because potassium affects the heartbeat. This is one reason that taking potassium supplements (as found in salt substitutes [potassium chloride]) should be based on physician recommendation. It is imperative that individuals who are taking potassium-depleting diuretics receive additional potassium, preferably through food and again on the advice of a physician. Potassium:

- aids in the regulation of nerve impulses and muscle contractions
- is necessary for enzyme reactions intracellularly as well as for the synthesis of proteins

There is no RDA for potassium; however, the recommended intake is about 1500 to 6000 mg, which is easily met by food sources. Foods high in potassium include citrus fruits, bananas, tomatoes, potatoes, meat, milk, legumes, and dark green leafy vegetables.

SODIUM. Sodium is an electrolyte and is involved in:

- transmission of nerve impulses
- controlling muscle contractions
- regulating permeability of the cell membrane

Sodium is naturally found in low levels in food, although rather significant levels are found in some foods such as milk and certain vegetables. The major dietary sources are table salt (sodium chloride) and foods that have added salt, such as processed meats, convenience foods, and canned vegetables and soups (canned fruit is low in sodium). One teaspoon of salt contains about 2000 mg of sodium.

There is no RDA for sodium, but the recommended range for healthy individuals is between 2000 and 4000 mg, a level lower than that generally consumed. The recommended intake of 2400 mg of sodium per day for the general public appears on the new food labels. See Chapter 8 for a more detailed discussion of sodium as related to heart disease.

SULFUR. Sulfur is a component of skin, hair, nails, cartilage, and some organ tissue. It is a component of all body proteins, along with thiamine and biotin. No deficiency of sulfur has been documented in humans.

Meat, eggs, poultry, and milk are all important food sources of sulfur. No RDA has been established, but diets adequate in protein provide liberal amounts of sulfur.

Trace Minerals

IRON. Populations at risk for iron deficiency include infants older than 6 months, young children through the preschool years, adolescents, menstruating women, and pregnant women. These individuals need carefully planned diets to meet iron needs. Supplements may be necessary during pregnancy.

More than one half of the 4 to 5 grams of iron in the body is in hemoglobin. **Hemoglobin** facilitates tissue respiration by carrying oxygen from the lungs to the tissue cells and by carrying the carbon dioxide formed in oxidation away from cells. Copper, protein, vitamin B_{12}, and folate are necessary for hemoglobin synthesis. Tests for levels of hemoglobin indicate whether **anemia** (a condition of reduced oxygen delivery to the body cells) is present.

Excess iron inhibits absorption of zinc (see Table 5–5) but true toxicity from food sources has been documented only from long-term ingestion of home brewed alcohol made in iron stills. However, toxic overdoses from iron supplements do occur in the United States. **Iron overload** (idiopathic hemochromatosis), which was once considered a rare genetic disease, has recently been estimated to occur heterozygously in about 1 in 10 individuals and homozygously in 2 to 3 of 1000 individuals in northern Europe, North America, and Australia. Various complications of iron overload, such as **cirrhosis** (a disease of the liver), diabetes mellitus, skin pigmentation, **arthralgias** (joint pain), and **cardiomyopathy** (a heart condition), can be averted by early detection (Skikne and Cook, 1987) and avoidance of excess iron intake.

It is important to recognize that iron comes in two forms: heme, found in meat, and nonheme, found in plant products. **Heme iron**—which is found in high quantities in red meat and organ meats such as liver, kidney, and heart—is absorbed extremely well by the body. In contrast, nonheme iron found in plant foods such as blackstrap molasses, whole grains, iron-fortified cereals and enriched breads, dark green leafy vegetables, dried fruit, and legumes is poorly absorbed unless vitamin C foods or meat are consumed at the same meal. For example, orange juice or coleslaw, with its high vitamin C content, would enhance the iron absorption from a peanut butter sandwich or other nonheme iron source. The use of iron cooking pans is also known to increase the iron content of food greatly; the amount of increase is related to the length of cooking time and acidity of the food.

IODINE. Iodized salt and ocean or saltwater fish are the most common sources of iodine. Inadequate iodine intake leads to goiter (Fig. 5–6). **Cretinism,** or mental retardation, was once a relatively common phenomenon in infants born to mothers who had iodine deficiency during pregnancy. Such a deficiency generally is no longer a concern, however. Iodine:

- is a constituent of the thyroid hormones thyroxine and thyroglobulin
- helps regulate energy metabolism through the thyroid hormones.

SELENIUM. The RDA for selenium was first set in 1989 (see table on the inside front cover). The selenium requirement for adults appears to be related to body weight. The best food sources of selenium include whole grains, seafood, kidneys, and liver. Selenium:

- functions as part of an enzyme system
- acts as an antioxidant with vitamin E to protect the cells

Selenium toxicity and deficiency have been noted mainly as a result of soil selenium content. Hair loss and toxic defects in fingernails and toenails have been found in regions of the United States where there is a high content of selenium in the soil.

ZINC. Zinc is a component of more than 50 enzymes. Although zinc is stored primarily in bone, it is poorly mobilized, and therefore regular di-

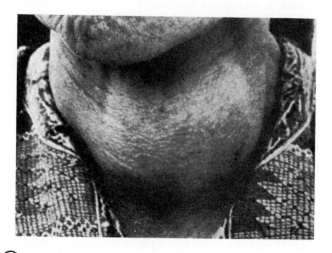

▲ FIGURE 5–6

Goiter. (From Nizel AE: Nutrition in Preventive Dentistry: Science and Practice, 2nd ed. Philadelphia, WB Saunders Co., 1981, p. 248.)

etary intake is crucial. Individuals with malabsorption, such as those with chronic diarrhea, chronic pancreatitis, **celiac sprue** (a condition involving the intestinal tract that is caused by an allergy to gluten found in certain grains, see Chapters 11 and 15), **Crohn's disease** (an inflammatory disease of the intestinal tract, see Chapter 11), and the short bowel syndrome, are at particular risk for zinc deficiency. Zinc absorption is also impaired by excessive intake of iron, copper, tin, folic acid, and possibly calcium. Persons who have polyuria from uncontrolled diabetes (see Chapter 9) or who take diuretics may be predisposed to loss of zinc in the urine. Zinc:

- is essential for normal growth
- promotes wound healing
- is involved in immunity
- promotes cell division and differentiation, mainly because of its role in protein synthesis
- influences taste sensitivity
- can also reduce the risk of retinal degeneration of the eye among older adults (Flynn, 1993)

Food sources high in zinc include high-protein foods, especially oysters and liver. Legumes, leafy green vegetables, and whole grains are also high in zinc.

OTHER TRACE MINERALS

The following minerals do not have established RDAs at present but are essential to the body. Human requirements for these minerals are not known, but estimated safe and adequate intakes have been suggested until further data are available (Table 5–6).

CHROMIUM. This mineral activates several enzymes. It plays a role in carbohydrate metabolism as a component of glucose tolerance factor, which enhances the removal of glucose from the blood. Good sources of chromium

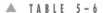

▲ TABLE 5-6

TRACE MINERALS: ESTIMATED SAFE AND ADEQUATE DAILY DIETARY INTAKES

CATEGORY	AGE (Years)	COPPER (mg)	MANGANESE (mg)	FLUORIDE (mg)	CHROMIUM (µg)	MOLYBDENUM (µg)
Infants	0–0.5	0.4–0.6	0.3–0.6	0.1–0.5	10–40	15–30
	0.5–1	0.6–0.7	0.6–1.0	0.2–1.0	20–60	20–40
Children and	1–3	0.7–1.0	1.0–1.5	0.5–1.5	20–80	25–50
adolescents	4–6	1.0–1.5	1.5–2.0	1.0–2.5	30–120	30–75
	7–10	1.0–2.0	2.0–3.0	1.5–2.5	50–200	50–150
	11+	1.5–2.5	2.0–5.0	1.5–2.5	50–200	75–250
Adults		1.5–3.0	2.0–5.0	1.5–4.0	50–200	75–250

From National Academy of Sciences, National Research Council: Recommended Dietary Allowances, 10th ed. Washington, DC, National Academy of Sciences, National Academy Press, 1989.

include brewer's yeast, liver, whole-grain cereals, meat, and cheese. Most of the chromium is removed from grains during the processing of white flour products and is not returned during the enrichment process.

COBALT. This mineral is an essential component of vitamin B_{12}. Inadequate intake of cobalt results in pernicious anemia.

COPPER. This mineral aids in the absorption of iron from the intestinal tract and in the production and survival of red blood cells and is an essential part of many enzymes. There is also evidence that copper helps prevent heart disease.

Foods rich in copper include legumes, liver, kidney, nuts, seeds, whole grains, and raisins. Chocolate is also high in copper, but the high fat content rules out its being regularly included in a healthy diet.

FLUORIDE. This mineral helps in the formation of solid bones and teeth. It also helps reduce the incidence of dental caries (see Chapter 19). There is some evidence that it aids calcium in bone formation. The Food and Nutrition Board recommends fluoridation of public water supplies if natural fluoride levels are low. The American Dental Association recommends fluoride supplements until about age 13 years or until the adult teeth are fully formed. Like other trace minerals, fluoride is toxic when consumed in excessive amounts.

MANGANESE. This mineral is essential for normal bone structure, normal reproduction, and normal functioning of the central nervous system. It is a component of some enzymes. The best sources of manganese are nuts and whole grains. A manganese intake of 2 to 5 mg/day is recommended by the Food and Nutrition Board for adolescents and adults of both sexes (National Research Council, 1989).

MOLYBDENUM. This essential mineral is a component of an enzyme (xanthine oxidase). The best sources of molybdenum include organ meats, some cereals, and legumes.

NICKEL, TIN, VANADIUM, AND SILICON. Findings produced in experimental animal feeding suggest that these elements are essential, but the implications for human nutrition are unknown.

ARE THERE ANY HARMFUL MINERALS?

Arsenic is probably the best known of the harmful minerals. In addition, mercury and lead need to be avoided. For this reason, some fish products need to be used sparingly because of their mercury content, and bone meal supplements, which tend to be high in lead, should be avoided. Other potential lead-contaminant sources are wine decanters with the lead crystal (it is advised to avoid storage of wine in decanters), ceramic dishes with a lead glaze, food left in opened cans that have lead solder, household water pipes that are either made from lead (older homes) or have lead in the solder (running the tap water 1 to 2 minutes prior to use each morning is advised), lead paint (now illegal in the United States but still found in older homes), lead-based fuel including its fumes, and dirt and dust contaminated with lead residue. Young children are particularly susceptible to lead poisoning, in part because of an increased risk of exposure from playing in dirt contaminated with lead (one reason that washing hands before eating is so important) and from eating peeling lead paint, which has a sweet taste. As previously noted, all minerals in excess are generally harmful.

HOW CAN VITAMINS AND MINERALS BE PRESERVED IN FOOD PREPARATION?

The following is a list of food handling practices that will enhance vitamin and mineral retention:

1. Store vegetables properly to avoid wilting and drying out, which cause loss of vitamins A and C.
2. Cook vegetables whole as often as possible. Cutting and peeling release oxidative enzymes and increase surfaces from which water-soluble vitamins and minerals leach out.
3. Use cooking water and canned food juices to conserve soluble nutrients, or, preferably, steam fresh or frozen vegetables to lessen the leaching of water-soluble vitamins and minerals.
4. Avoid use of baking soda in cooking vegetables, as it is destructive to thiamine and ascorbic acid. Avoid long cooking for the same reason. Cooling meat drippings before use allows easy removal of solidified fats without sacrificing thiamine and niacin.
5. Store fats covered and preferably refrigerated to prevent them from becoming rancid, which destroys vitamin A.
6. Keep milk in glass containers away from light, which is destructive to riboflavin, or put in opaque containers. Waxed cardboard containers for milk prevent destruction of riboflavin by light.
7. Keep fruit juices covered and cold to prevent oxygen from destroying ascorbic acid.
8. While cooking foods containing ascorbic acid, do not stir, as oxygen destroys vitamin C.
9. Cook vegetables quickly in a covered container until just fork-tender. Store leftovers covered.

WHAT IS FOOD FORTIFICATION?

The war among cereal brands ("How many bowls of your cereal does it take to equal one of ours?") is an example of food fortification, which differs from **enrichment**, a method to replace known nutrients lost in processing such as the B vitamins and iron in white flour products. In contrast, **fortification** means "to make stronger; to fortify" and involves either adding nutrients in higher amounts than naturally occur or adding nutrients that are generally not present, for example, adding calcium to orange juice. Food fortification does play an important role in the promotion of the health of our society. Examples are iodized salt, which helped eradicate goiter, and iron-fortified cereal and infant formula, which help prevent iron deficiency anemia. However, fortified foods can be used inappropriately.

The food industry generally has a profit motive rather than society's health as its basis for food fortification. Advertisements that promote fortified food as the best alternative can mislead the public. To use the preceding example, calcium-fortified orange juice is not a replacement for milk, since milk offers many other nutrients. Also, since we know that overconsumption of vitamins and minerals can be harmful, if not toxic, indiscriminate use of and reliance on fortified foods is not a healthful practice, particularly if those foods are used as a replacement for a balanced, varied diet.

WHAT ARE ELECTROLYTES?

An electrolyte is a compound that, when dissolved in water, separates into charged particles (ions) capable of conducting an electrical current. Within the body, electrolytes play an essential role in maintaining fluid and **acid-base balance** (a state of equilibrium in the body between acidity and alkalinity of body fluids, Fig. 5–7). Diet, however, is considered to play only a small role in maintaining an appropriate acid-base balance.

The chief electrolyte ions are sodium, potassium, calcium, magnesium, chloride, and phosphate. All body fluids contain electrolytes. The chief electrolytes outside the cell (extracellular) are sodium and chloride. Potassium, magnesium, and phosphate are found in large amounts inside the cell (intracellular).

Changes in the electrolyte composition of body fluids create electrical charges, which, in turn, are responsible for electrochemical reactions such as transmission of nerve impulses, contraction of muscles, and glandular cell secretions. Shifts in the electrolyte balance that cause either an excess or a deficiency of electrolytes may occur as the result of various disease conditions. Alterations in electrolyte balance can cause death. Thus, careful monitoring of the blood levels of electrolytes is necessary, especially during times of illness.

Correction of malnutrition, as with the initiation of nutrition support, can cause shifts in electrolyte balance. The refeeding syndrome (see Chapter 14

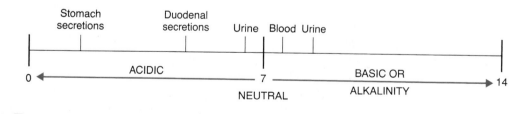

▲ FIGURE 5-7

The pH of various body fluids.

for details) is related to electrolyte shifts from outside the cells to inside (extracellular to intracellular movement). Serum phosphorus levels (extracellular), for example, can become low as phosphorus moves back into the cell.

Low levels of magnesium in the blood can be caused by alcoholism, malabsorption, hyperthyroidism, use of steroids, and massive blood transfusions. High levels can be caused by renal failure, heavy use of laxatives and antacids, dialysis or total parenteral nutrition (TPN, see Chapter 14), and inadequate amounts of the hormone aldosterone.

Low levels of calcium in the blood can lead to **tetany,** a condition of muscle twitchings, cramps, and convulsions (O'Toole, 1992). The condition is not likely caused by inadequate calcium intake but rather by **hypoparathyroidism** (reduced function of the parathyroid gland), some bone diseases, certain kidney diseases, and low serum protein. High levels of calcium can be caused by excessive vitamin D intake, hyperparathyroidism, cancer, or prolonged excessive milk intake (Davis and Sherer, 1994).

WATER

Water is the principal constituent of the body. One half to three quarters of body weight is water. Most water is in cells (intracellular), and the remainder is in blood, lymph, various secretions and excretions, and around cells (extracellular). The water requirement for adults is 1 mL per kilocalorie, and for infants is 1.5 mL per kilocalorie. Fluid balance is essential, and intake must balance output. Fluid requirements are closely related to salt requirements; intake of increased amounts of water is needed under conditions of extreme heat or excessive sweating. Water is absorbed in the small intestine and colon with digested food. Since it is not stored, daily intake is necessary. Water requirements are increased for infants receiving high-protein formulas; comatose patients; those with fever, polyuria, or diarrhea; or those on high-protein diets. Water is normally lost through urine, in expired air, in feces, and through the skin. Water:

- helps every organ to function properly
- aids digestion, absorption, circulation, and excretion
- functions as a solvent for body constituents and as a medium for all chemical changes in the body
- carries nutrients to and waste products from cells as part of the blood
- participates in the regulation of body temperature
- is involved with the lubrication of the moving parts of the body

Water can be found in varying quantities in foods (foods contain from 10 to 98 per cent water); it is formed in the body's metabolic processes, and is an end product of oxidation. The average diet with milk (87 per cent water) contains about 1000 mL water daily. With the addition of 1 quart of water (4 cups), the recommended 2000 mL of water can be met. Beverages containing caffeine or alcohol should not be counted as fluid because these substances promote diuresis and do not contribute to the body's need for fluid.

WHAT IS THE ROLE OF THE NURSE OR OTHER HEALTH CARE PROFESSIONAL IN EDUCATING THE PUBLIC ON VITAMINS AND MINERALS?

The nurse or other health care professional needs to be aware of how positive nutritional messages about food can be conveyed in informal settings, such as while a patient is eating a meal. Emphasis should be on positive messages such as, "That cantaloupe looks really good. Did you know that one half of a cantaloupe has all the vitamin A and vitamin C that you need for the day?" or "No milk? Can I get you something else in the dairy group—pudding, yogurt, cheese?" These types of messages reinforce good nutritional practices.

It is a disservice to consumers to speak of minerals as if they alone can cure some of humankind's ills. Claims such as "Calcium prevents osteoporosis," "Selenium prevents cancer," or "Zinc promotes sexual performance" have an element of truth but are simplistic messages at best. Rather, a better approach would be to take facts, put them in their proper perspective, and apply them to the relevant food sources. For example, a nurse might say, "Milk and milk products help prevent osteoporosis," "Whole grains may be helpful for cancer prevention," or "Wheat germ and legumes help promote sexual maturation." This approach will promote good nutritional status without placing undue emphasis on one mineral over another. This is particularly important in our "pill-popping society" in which interactions of one mineral with another or excess intake can lead to toxicity or other problems.

The health care professional should also assess supplement usage. Are excessive amounts being taken, particularly of the fat-soluble vitamins? For persons concerned with their vitamin needs, a quick comparison of their diet to the foods in the Food Guide Pyramid can decrease their fears of vitamin deficiency. People need to be reminded that nature supplies us with our needed vitamins, minerals, and other nutrients through foods; the vitamin pill industry is a profit-oriented one that does not have the experience of Mother Nature. It may be helpful to point out that an excess of one vitamin or mineral (in supplement form) can have a negative impact on the body's use of other vitamins or minerals. Also, it cannot be stressed enough that if a person chooses to take a supplement it should not exceed 100 per cent of the RDA. Referral to a medical doctor or a registered dietitian is appropriate for high-risk individuals (persons with an impaired ability to excrete excess vitamins, such as persons with renal disease, elderly individuals, pregnant women, or young children).

STUDY QUESTIONS AND ACTIVITIES

1. Why do minerals not break down when cooked, as some vitamins do?
2. Why must some foods containing vitamins be eaten daily? Which vitamins can be stored by the body? Which ones cannot be stored?

3. What is meant by the vitamin B complex? What foods need to be included in the diet to ensure an adequate amount of the B-complex vitamins?

4. List the foods in the Food Guide Pyramid, with the correct servings, that will help meet your vitamin and mineral requirements. Could the foods from Maria Bernardo's food shopping list (Chapter 3 case study) meet the RDA for vitamins and minerals?

5. List menu items that include legumes. Locate Italian cookbooks to determine how the Bernardo family might eat the legumes noted in the family shopping list from Chapter 3.

6. Calculate the calcium content of your diet. How could you meet the RDA for calcium without relying on supplements?

7. Name several procedures in food care, preparation, and cooking that will help retain the water-soluble vitamins and minerals.

8. Role-play in class, portraying each of three negative characteristics (lack of knowledge, food dislikes, or inadequate food habits), singly or in combination, in order to practice strategies to encourage adequate intake of foods high in vitamin A.

REFERENCES

American Diabetes Association: Magnesium supplementation in the treatment of diabetes. Diabetes Care. 1992; 15:1065–1067.

American Dietetic Association, American Institute of Nutrition, American Society for Clinical Nutrition, and the National Council Against Health Fraud: Statement on vitamin and mineral supplements. Nutrition Today. June 1987; 22(3):28.

Bailey LB: Evaluation of a new Recommended Dietary Allowance for folate. J Am Diet Assoc. 1992; 92(4):466–467.

Berger AR, Schaumburg HH, Schroeder C, et al.: Dose response, coasting, and differential fiber vulnerability in human toxic neuropathy: a prospective study of pyridoxine neurotoxicity. Neurology. 1992; 42(7):1367–1370.

Bernstein AL: Vitamin B6 in clinical neurology. Ann NY Acad Sci. 1990; 585:250–260.

Chapuy MC, Arlot ME, Duboeuf F, et al.: Vitamin D3 and calcium to prevent hip fractures in elderly women. N Engl J Med. 1992; 327:1637–1642.

Community Nutrition Institute, Nutrition Week. May 21, 1993; XXIII, (19), p. 3.

Davis JR, Sherer K: Applied Nutrition and Diet Therapy for Nurses, 2nd ed. Philadelphia, WB Saunders Co., 1994; p. 227.

Flynn ME: Environmental Nutrition, March 1993; 16(3), p. 5.

Herbert V: Viewpoint: Does mega-C do more good than harm, or more harm than good? Nutrition Today. Jan/Feb, 1993; pp 28–32.

Mickelsen O, Marsh AG: Calcium requirement and diet. Nutrition Today. Jan/Feb, 1989; p. 31.

National Research Council: Recommended Dietary Allowances, 10th ed. Washington, DC, National Academy of Sciences, National Academy Press, 1989.

O'Toole M, ed: Miller-Keane Encyclopedia & Dictionary of Medicine, Nursing, & Allied Health, 5th ed. Philadelphia, WB Saunders Co, 1992.

Ross AC: Vitamin A: current understanding of the mechanisms of action. Nutrition Today, Jan/Feb, 1991; p. 6.

Skikne BS, Cook JD: Screening test for iron overload. Am J Clin Nutr. 1987; 46(5):840.

Snodgrass SR: Vitamin neurotoxicity. Mol Neurobiol. 1992; 6(1):41–73.

Suttie JW: Vitamin K and human nutrition. J Am Diet Assoc. 1992; 92(5):585–589.

Wilkens KG, Brouns Schiro K, eds: Suggested Guidelines for Nutrition Care of Renal Patients, 2nd ed. Chicago, The American Dietetic Association, 1992, p. 49.

GUIDES FOR GOOD FOOD CHOICES

CHAPTER

6

OBJECTIVES

After completing this chapter you should be able to:
■ Recognize and differentiate between the various food guides available
■ Evaluate a daily diet for moderation, variety, and balance
■ Explain the significance of nutrition labeling

TERMS TO IDENTIFY

Daily Reference Values
  (DRVs)
Nutrition Labeling

Recommended Dietary
  Allowances (RDAs)

Reference Daily Intakes
  (RDIs)

A FAMILY'S PERSPECTIVE ON NUTRITION

Anna Bernardo was sitting in health class. The teacher was talking about the Food Guide Pyramid. He was saying that this food plan could help her lose weight by emphasizing less fat. He also said that the risk of heart disease could be lowered by eating this way. Anna wondered if her dad's dietitian had talked to him about the guide. She knew that he was worried about heart disease with his high cholesterol level.

INTRODUCTION

The definition of healthy eating has changed over the years. In the 1940s, there were seven recommended food groups, and butter was one of them. In the 1920s, even sugar was considered a food group. It's no wonder that many older Americans find the new guidelines confusing. In the 1950s, the time the baby-boomer generation was being born, the Basic Four Food Groups classification (meat, grains, dairy, and vegetables and fruits) was developed by the U.S. Department of Agriculture (USDA) to replace the older concept of seven food groups. In 1990, the USDA replaced the Basic Four with the Food Guide Pyramid (Fig. 6–1), only to be met with an uproar from the meat and dairy industries because consumption of less meat and milk was being advocated by their position in the smaller portion of the pyramid. The dried bean and lentil industry was not pleased either because legumes were placed in the upper portion of the pyramid rather than at the base. Nutritionists also agree that legumes are a healthy substitute for meat and should be recommended for more use, not less (Smith, 1992). Nevertheless, the Food Guide Pyramid best represents healthy eating in the 1990s and is here to stay until at least the 21st century.

Ever since World War II, the formulation of national and international food and nutrition policies has been based on the Recommended Dietary Allowances (RDAs). In the last decade, the USDA, the U.S. Department of Health and Human Services, the American Medical Association, the American Institute of Cancer Research, and governments of other countries including Canada have developed guidelines in which moderation, variety, and balance are the focus. The Food Guide Pyramid and the new food labels meet these goals.

Health professionals should understand how to use the new food labels, the Food Guide Pyramid, and other guides such as the RDAs to educate the general public in sound nutrition practices. These guidelines can also be used to evaluate your own dietary habits.

WHAT IS MEANT BY MODERATION, VARIETY, AND BALANCE?

Moderation means that any food can be worked into a healthy way of eating. There are no good foods and bad foods. Foods that are higher in fat and sugar should be eaten in smaller amounts or less frequently than foods that are nutrient-dense. Variety refers to eating a number of different foods within each of the food groups of the Food Guide Pyramid—not just the

▲ What is the Food Guide Pyramid?

The Food Guide Pyramid is an outline of what to eat each day. It lets you choose a healthful diet that's right for you. The Food Guide Pyramid is based on the Dietary Guidelines for Americans, nutrition advice for healthy Americans ages 2 years and over. You can use the Food Guide Pyramid to make your daily food choices.

The Pyramid calls for eating a variety of foods to get the nutrients you need while eating the right amount of calories to maintain a healthy weight.

Food Guide Pyramid
A Guide to Daily Food Choices

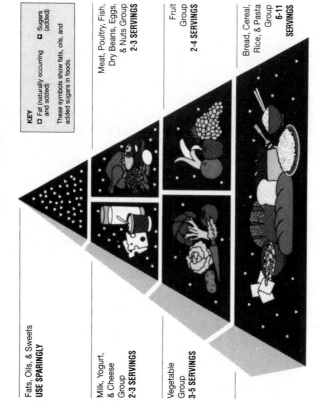

KEY
□ Fat (naturally occurring and added) ■ Sugars (added)

These symbols show fats, oils, and added sugars in foods.

Fats, Oils, & Sweets
USE SPARINGLY

Milk, Yogurt, & Cheese Group
2-3 SERVINGS

Meat, Poultry, Fish, Dry Beans, Eggs, & Nuts Group
2-3 SERVINGS

Vegetable Group
3-5 SERVINGS

Fruit Group
2-4 SERVINGS

Bread, Cereal, Rice, & Pasta Group
6-11 SERVINGS

The Food Guide Pyramid emphasizes foods from the five food groups shown in the lower three levels of the Pyramid. Each of these food groups provides some, but not all, of the nutrients you need. No one food group is more important than another—for good health, you need them all.

▲ What Counts As One Serving?

Here are some serving size examples for each food group. If you eat a larger portion, count it as more than one serving.

Be sure to eat at least the lowest number of servings from the five food groups each day.

Bread, Cereal, Rice, and Pasta Group (6-11 servings)
- 1 slice of bread
- 1 ounce of ready-to-eat cereal (check labels: 1 ounce = ¼ cup to 2 cups, depending on cereal)
- ½ cup of cooked cereal, rice, or pasta
- ½ hamburger roll, bagel, english muffin
- 3 – 4 plain crackers (small)

Vegetable Group (3-5 servings)
- 1 cup of raw leafy vegetables
- ½ cup of other vegetables, cooked or chopped raw
- ¾ cup of vegetable juice

Fruit Group (2-4 servings)
- 1 medium apple, banana, orange, nectarine, peach
- ½ cup of chopped, cooked, or canned fruit
- ¾ cup of fruit juice

Milk, Yogurt, and Cheese Group (2-3 servings)
- 1 cup of milk or yogurt
- 1½ ounces of natural cheese
- 2 ounces of process cheese

Meat, Poultry, Fish, Dry Beans, Eggs, and Nuts Group (2-3 servings)
- 2 – 3 ounces of cooked lean meat, poultry, or fish
- (1 ounce of meat = ½ cup of cooked dry beans, 1 egg or 2 tablespoons of peanut butter)

From The New York State Dietetic Association [NYSDA], Albany, NY, 1992.]

▲ FIGURE 6 - 1

The Food Guide Pyramid. (From The New York State Dietetic Association [NYSDA], Albany, NY, 1992.)

same two or three types of vegetables, for example. Balance refers to the amount of macronutrients as well as the micronutrients in the diet. Selecting foods from each of the three lower levels of the Food Guide Pyramid will allow for a balanced diet (see Fig. 6–1).

WHAT ARE THE RECOMMENDED DIETARY ALLOWANCES (RDAs)?

"RDAs are the levels of intake of essential nutrients that, on the basis of scientific knowledge, are judged by the Food and Nutrition Board to be adequate to meet the known nutrient needs of practically all healthy persons" (National Research Council, 1989). The RDA guide is revised at regular intervals, and the tenth edition was published in 1989. It is shown inside the front cover of this text. Intakes amounting to less than the lower end of the range of the RDAs are likely to lead to deficiency. Intakes amounting to more than the upper limit may give rise to toxic effects, especially involving trace elements. Recommended Dietary Allowances should not be confused with *requirements* for a specific individual because requirements vary considerably. Most authorities believe that two thirds of the RDA will meet the nutrient needs of healthy individuals. However, problems such as premature birth, inherited metabolic disorders, infections, chronic diseases, and the use of medications may require special dietary modifications. These special circumstances are not addressed in the RDAs.

The *allowance* refers to the amount of nutrient that must be consumed to ensure that the requirements of most people are met. Recommendations for dietary intake must make allowance for the portion of the ingested nutrient that is not absorbed or digested. The allowance is set above the average requirement and varies from nutrient to nutrient (National Research Council, 1989). For some nutrients, there is limited information about the variability of individual requirements, and judgments must be made. Thus the *R* in RDAs stands for *recommended,* not required.

The allowances for energy are treated differently from the allowances for specific nutrients. Recommended energy allowances for groups of people represent the average needs of individuals, whereas recommended allowances for nutrients are high enough to meet the upper level of requirement among individuals within the groups. Energy needs vary from person to person depending on physical activity and the characteristics of the individual, including age, sex, body size and composition, and genetic factors. Therefore, the average energy needs for each age and sex group should be used only as a guideline (National Research Council, 1989).

WHAT ARE DAILY REFERENCE VALUES?

Daily Reference Values (DRVs) is a term developed for the new food labels. This term includes **Reference Daily Intakes (RDIs),** which are essentially equivalent to the old U.S. RDAs (the highest level of RDAs as listed on the old-style food labels). The main difference between U.S. RDAs and RDIs is that RDIs now reflect the *average* amounts of the updated 1989 RDAs. RDIs can be found on the new food labels for vitamins A and C and the minerals calcium and iron (Fig. 6–2). The vitamins thiamine and

The New Food Label at a Glance

The new food label will carry an up-to-date, easier-to-use nutrition information guide, to be required on almost all packaged foods (compared to about 60 percent of products up till now). The guide will serve as a key to help in planning a healthy diet.*

Serving sizes are now more consistent across product lines, are stated in both household and metric measures, and reflect the amounts people actually eat.

The **list of nutrients** covers those most important to the health of today's consumers, most of whom need to worry about getting too much of certain nutrients (fat, for example), rather than too few vitamins or minerals, as in the past.

The label of larger packages may now tell the number of calories per gram of fat, carbohydrate, and protein.

New title signals that the label contains the newly required information.

Calories from fat are now shown on the label to help consumers meet dietary guidelines that recommend people get no more than 30 percent of the calories in their overall diet from fat.

% Daily Value shows how a food fits into the overall daily diet.

Daily Values are also something new. Some are maximums, as with fat (65 grams or less); others are minimums, as with carbohydrate (300 grams or more). The daily values for a 2,000- and 2,500-calorie diet must be listed on the label of larger packages.

Nutrition Facts

Serving Size 1 cup (228g)
Servings Per Container 2

Amount Per Serving

Calories 260   Calories from Fat 120

	% Daily Value*
Total Fat 13g	**20**%
Saturated Fat 5g	**25**%
Cholesterol 30mg	**10**%
Sodium 660mg	**28**%
Total Carbohydrate 31g	**10**%
Dietary Fiber 0g	**0**%
Sugars 5g	
Protein 5g	

Vitamin A 4%	•	Vitamin C 2%
Calcium 15%	•	Iron 4%

* Percent Daily Values are based on a 2,000 calorie diet. Your daily values may be higher or lower depending on your calorie needs:

		Calories:	2,000	2,500
Total Fat	Less than		65g	80g
Sat Fat	Less than		20g	25g
Cholesterol	Less than		300mg	300mg
Sodium	Less than		2,400mg	2,400mg
Total Carbohydrate			300g	375g
Dietary Fiber			25g	30g

Calories per gram:
Fat 9 • Carbohydrate 4 • Protein 4

* This label is only a sample. Exact specifications are in the final rules.
Source: Food and Drug Administration, 1994

▲ F I G U R E   6 – 2

The new food label: a tool to healthier diets. (From Food Insight, Jan/Feb 1993, IFIC.)

riboflavin were removed from the new food labels, as they are generally included in adequate amounts in the current food supply.

Daily Reference Values also include the recommended amounts of fat, saturated fat, total carbohydrate, and dietary fiber based on preset kilocalorie levels of 2000 and 2500. Recommendations for fat and carbohydrate are based on percentages of total kilocalories, so for persons requiring different levels of kilocalorie intake, these recommended amounts will change. A registered dietitian can calculate the recommended nutrient intakes for individual patients who have different kilocalorie and nutrient needs.

The reference quantity for sodium intake on the new food labels is 2400 mg per day. This amount will meet required sodium needs in all healthy Americans without providing an excess. Medical conditions may necessitate a smaller or larger intake of sodium. Cholesterol is another DRV not based on kilocalorie intake (300 mg).

WHY WERE FOOD LABELS CHANGED?

Mandatory **nutrition labeling** went into effect in 1994 with the goal of helping consumers adhere to the Dietary Guidelines (see following section). The change is aimed at reducing the prevalence and complications of chronic illnesses such as heart disease, hypertension, and diabetes (see Chapters 8 and 9).

The new labels are also designed to increase consumer confidence and ability to make wise food choices. Older food labeling made it difficult for consumers to see the total picture; for example, formerly food manufacturers were allowed to label a food "low cholesterol" without indicating that the food was high in fat. Health claims on food labels now must follow strict guidelines so that consumers cannot be as easily misled in their attempt to choose healthier foods. The health claims that can be made on food labels under the new law are as follows:

1. Fiber: Foods high in fiber may reduce the risk of cancer and heart disease.
2. Fat: A low-fat diet may reduce the risk of cancer and heart disease.
3. Sodium: A low-sodium diet may help prevent high blood pressure.
4. Calcium: Foods high in calcium may help prevent osteoporosis.

Current food labels have more uniform and expected serving sizes. Older food labels were able to use nutrition analysis based on unrealistically small portions.

Ingredients are listed in order of quantity in a product. If sugar is listed as the first ingredient, the amount of sugar in the product is greater than the amount of any of the other ingredients. In the past, food companies could "hide" the amount of sugar a product contained by using smaller amounts of several different forms of sugar. Now the total amount of sugar in a food is listed.

Daily Reference Values are found on the new food labels based on the reference kilocalories of 2000 and 2500 per day and are calculated as follows:

- Fat is based on 30 per cent of kilocalories
- Saturated fat is based on 10 per cent of kilocalories
- Carbohydrate is based on 60 per cent of kilocalories
- Fiber is based on 11.5 grams of fiber per 1000 kilocalories

Foods exempt from nutrition labeling include those sold in restaurants, cafeterias, and airplanes, unless a health claim is made. Coffee, tea, spices, and foods produced by small businesses or packaged in small containers are not required to carry a nutrition label (Dairy Council Digest, 1993).

How Does Nutrition Labeling Aid the Consumer?

Nutrition labeling is a valuable tool in learning to apply nutrition information in a practical way. A health-conscious shopper uses the percentages shown on the label to determine how well each serving of the food fulfills recommended nutritional requirements (Fig. 6–3). For example, if one serving of a food contains 25 per cent of the RDA of a particular nutrient, it means that each serving is good for one fourth of a person's recommended daily requirement for that vitamin, mineral, or amount of fat.

If consumers use the food labels while making food purchases, they will be promoting their health through the inclusion of adequate nutrient intake (protein, carbohydrate, vitamins, and minerals) while reducing their risk of chronic illness through a reduction of fat, salt, and sugar and an increase in fiber. Food labels used in conjunction with the Food Guide Pyramid can be a highly effective and ultimately simple means to promote health.

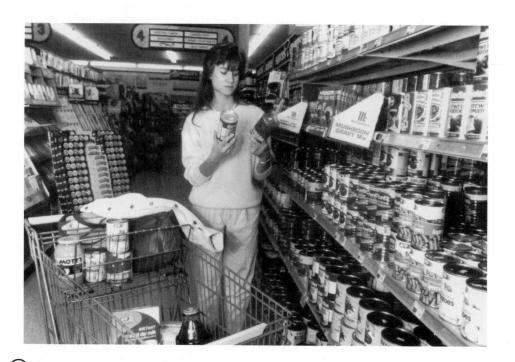

▲ FIGURE 6-3

A health-conscious shopper using food labels. (Courtesy of Cornell University Photography, Ithaca, NY.)

In 1980, the Public Health Service of the Department of Health and Human Services, together with the U.S. Department of Agriculture, published the first edition of *Dietary Guidelines for Americans*. This report, revised in 1985, includes seven recommendations that address the relationship between diet and chronic diseases. The wording of these guidelines was subsequently modified in 1990 to reflect a more positive tone. Table 6–1 gives suggestions on how often foods should be consumed in order to meet the Dietary Guidelines. Table 6–2 shows the evaluation of an adequate diet for an adult. The seven Dietary Guidelines follow.

EAT A VARIETY OF FOODS

The greater the variety of foods in the diet, the less likely that either a deficiency or an excess of any single nutrient will occur. Variety also reduces the likelihood of exposure to excessive amounts of contaminants in any single food item.

One way to assure variety, and with it a well-balanced diet, is to select foods each day from each of the five major groups of the Food Guide Pyramid (see Fig. 6–1).

MAINTAIN HEALTHY WEIGHT

If weight loss is necessary, it should be undertaken at a maximum rate of 1 to 2 pounds per week until the goal is reached. The process of losing weight successfully depends on good eating habits, which include eating slowly, preparing smaller portions, and avoiding second helpings. It is also important to increase physical activity. Emphasis should be on foods with high nutrient density that are low in fat and sugar. Alcohol should be avoided because of its low nutrient density.

CHOOSE A DIET LOW IN FAT, SATURATED FAT, AND CHOLESTEROL

To avoid consumption of too much fat, especially saturated fat and cholesterol, lean meat, fish, poultry, and legumes are recommended as protein

---

FACT & FALLACY

FALLACY: Eggs are high in cholesterol and should be avoided.
FACT: The egg is one of nature's most nutritious foods; it has a low to moderate fat content and provides a good source of vitamins A, D, and B_{12} and iron. Even though eggs contain about 250 mg of cholesterol, researchers now suggest that the amount of total and saturated fat in the diet is more important in lowering serum cholesterol than the amount of cholesterol. Up to four whole eggs per week is considered appropriate. Egg whites are fat-free and thus cholesterol-free.

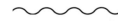

▲ T A B L E 6 - 1

FREQUENCY OF USE OF FOODS FOR IMPLEMENTING DIETARY GUIDELINES

FOOD GROUPS	CHOOSE MORE OFTEN	CHOOSE LESS OFTEN	MAJOR CONTRIBUTIONS
Fats	Corn, cottonseed, olive, sesame, soybean, safflower, sunflower, peanut, canola oils Mayonnaise or salad dressing (made from above oils) Avocado Olives	Butter, lard Margarine made from hydrogenated or saturated fats Coconut or palm oil Hydrogenated vegetable shortening Bacon Meat fat/drippings, gravy, sauces	Vitamin A, calories, essential fatty acids
Soups	Lightly salted soups with fat skimmed Cream-style soups (with low-fat milk) Reduced sodium soups	Commercially prepared soups and mixes	Fluid, calories (may contain a variety of vitamins, minerals, and protein, dependent upon type)
Sweets and desserts	Desserts that have been sweetened lightly and/or contain only moderate fat, such as puddings made from skim milk, angel food cake, fruit-based desserts	Desserts high in sugar and/or fats, such as candy, pastries, cakes, pies, whole-milk puddings, cookies	Calories (fats, carbohydrates)
Beverages	Water Unsweetened soft drinks Decaffeinated drinks	Sweetened beverages Caffeine-containing beverages Alcoholic beverages	Fluid, calories (unless sugar substitute is used)
Milk and milk products	Low-fat or skim milk Low-fat cheeses Low-fat yogurt	Whole milk Whole-milk cheeses Whole-milk yogurt Ice cream	Calories, calcium, protein, phosphorus, vitamins A and D, riboflavin
Vegetables, including starchy vegetables	Fresh, frozen, or canned; potatoes—baked or boiled Include one dark green or deep orange vegetable daily	Deep-fat fried vegetables, chips Pickled vegetables Highly salted vegetables or juices	Calories, vitamins A and C, dietary fiber, potassium, zinc, cobalt, folic acid

sources. Eggs and organ meats, such as liver, should be eaten in moderation. Low-fat or non-fat milk is encouraged. The maximum amount of fat in the diet should be 30 per cent of total daily kilocalories. Of this amount, an equal breakdown of saturated, monounsaturated, and polyunsaturated fats (10 per cent each) is recommended for the general public.

CHOOSE A DIET WITH PLENTY OF VEGETABLES, FRUITS, AND GRAIN PRODUCTS

Eating complex carbohydrates (starches) is recommended. This can be achieved by selecting foods that are good sources of fiber. For most Ameri-

▲ T A B L E   6 - 1

FREQUENCY OF USE OF FOODS FOR IMPLEMENTING DIETARY GUIDELINES *Continued*

FOOD GROUPS	CHOOSE MORE OFTEN	CHOOSE LESS OFTEN	MAJOR CONTRIBUTIONS
Fruits	Unsweetened fruits or juices Include one citrus fruit/juice or one tomato/juice daily	Sweetened fruits or juices Coconut Avocado	Calories, dietary fiber, vitamins A and C
Breads, starches, and cereals	Whole grain breads or cereals Enriched breads or cereals Muffins, bagels, tortillas Enriched pasta, rice, grits, or noodles	Snack chips or crackers Sweetened cereals Pancakes, doughnuts, biscuits	Calories, B-complex vitamins, magnesium, copper, iron, dietary fiber
Meats or substitutes	Lean meats, fish, shellfish, poultry without skin Low-fat cheeses (such as cottage cheese and part skimmed mozzarella) Peanut butter Soybeans, tofu Dry beans and peas	Fried or fatty meats/fish Fried poultry or poultry with skin High-fat cheeses (such as cheddar and processed cheeses) Eggs—limit to three per week Nuts	Calories, protein, iron, zinc, copper, B-complex vitamins
Miscellaneous	Herbs, spices, flavorings	Salt and salt/spice combinations	Sodium

Modified from Manual of Clinical Dietetics developed by The Chicago Dietetic Association and The South Suburban Dietetic Association of the American Dietetic Association, Chicago, 1988.

cans, a moderate increase in dietary fiber is desirable, although it is not clear exactly how much and what type of fiber we need in our daily diet. There is no need to take fiber supplements unless medically indicated. The use of whole grains and legumes along with the recommended amounts of vegetables and fruits will provide adequate fiber (20 to 30 g daily). Dark green leafy and orange vegetables and most orange fruits will provide more β-carotene, which is believed to lower cancer risk. Vitamin C is also associated with reduced cancer risk and is found in vegetables and fruits.

USE SUGARS ONLY IN MODERATION

To avoid excessive consumption of sugar, it is recommended that less-refined sugars, as well as foods containing these sugars, be used. Fresh fruits or fruits canned without sugar or those in light syrup rather than heavy syrup should be selected. Food labels now indicate sugar content. Sugar in most recipes can be reduced by one third or more, and spices such as cinnamon, nutmeg, ginger, and vanilla can enhance the impression of sweetness.

▲ T A B L E   6 – 2
EVALUATION OF THE FOUNDATION OF AN ADEQUATE DIET FOR AN ADULT

FOOD	AVERAGE SERVING						MINERALS		VITAMINS				
	Household Measure	Weight (g)	KILO-CALORIES	PROTEIN (g)	FAT (g)	CARBO-HYDRATE (g)	Calcium (mg)	Iron (mg)	A (RE)	Ascorbic Acid (mg)	Thiamine (mg)	Riboflavin (mg)	Niacin (mg)
Milk (whole or equivalent)	1 pt	488	300	16	16	22	582	0.2	152	4	0.18	0.8	0.4
Meat group													
Eggs	1	50	80	6	6	1	28	1	78	0	0.04	0.15	trace
Meat, poultry, fish[1]	3 oz (cooked)	85	322	19	26	0	9	2	trace	—	0.09	0.19	4.6
Vegetable and fruit group													
Vegetables:													
Deep green or orange[2]	1 salad or cooked	50 raw or cooked	23	0.9	trace	5	20	0.5	2644	9	0.03	0.06	0.3
Other cooked[3]	½ cup	85	52	2.5	trace	13	19	1.1	54	4.8	0.04	0.26	0.4
Potato, peeled and boiled	1 medium	122	90	3	trace	20	8	0.7	trace	22	0.12	0.05	1.6
Fruits:													
Citrus[4]	1 serving	125	50	0.3	trace	13.5	23	0.4	28	50	0.07	0.03	0.31
Other (fresh and canned)[5]	1 serving	135	99	0.4	trace	25	8	0.6	23	6	0.03	0.04	0.36

Bread and cereal group												
Cereal (whole-grain and enriched)[6]	½ cup cooked	25 (dry)	80	2.2	1	16	6	0.65	379	4.5	0.20	0.18	1.5
Bread (whole grain and enriched)	3 slices 1 whole wheat 2 white	78	170	7	3	40	90	2	trace	trace	0.29	0.15	2.4
Totals[7]			1266	57.3	52	180.5	793	9.61	3358[8]	100.3	1.09[9]	1.9	11.9[10,11]
Recommended Daily Dietary Allowances*													
Man (age 25–50 years: wt, 174 lb; ht, 70 inches)			2900	63			800	10	1000 RE	60	1.5	1.7	19
Woman (age 25–50 years: wt, 138 lb; ht, 63 inches)			2000	50			800	15	800 RE	60	1.1	1.3	15

Data from Nutritive Value of Foods, Home and Garden Bulletin No. 72, US Department of Agriculture, 1986.

[1] Evaluation based on figures for cooked (lean and fat) beef, lamb, and veal.
[2] Evaluation based on lettuce, cooked carrots, green beans, winter squash, and broccoli.
[3] Evaluation based on average for cooked peas and beets.
[4] Evaluation based on Florida oranges and white and pink grapefruit—whole and juice.
[5] Evaluation based on canned peaches, applesauce, raw pears, apples, and bananas.
[6] Evaluation based on oatmeal and corn flakes.
[7] With the addition of more of the same foods, or other foods, to meet calorie requirement, the totals will be increased.
[8] With the use of liver, this figure will be markedly increased.
[9] With the use of pork, legumes, and liver, this figure will be markedly increased.
[10] The average diet in the United States, which contains a generous amount of protein, provides enough tryptophan to increase the niacin value by about one third.
[11] These figures are expressed as niacin equivalents, which include dietary sources of the preformed vitamin and the precursor, tryptophan.
* Recommended Dietary Allowances, 10th ed. National Research Council, Washington, DC, 1989.

USE SALT AND SODIUM ONLY IN MODERATION

Fresh fruits, vegetables, meats, and unprocessed grains are generally low in sodium. Most convenience foods contain added sodium compounds, and "fast foods" are often high in sodium. Consumption of salted potato chips, pretzels, nuts, and popcorn; condiments such as soy sauce, steak sauce, and garlic salt; cheese; pickled foods; and cured meats and cold cuts should be limited. It is important to read food labels carefully to determine the amounts of sodium in processed foods and snack items. The recommended daily amount as listed on the new food labels is 2400 mg per day.

To avoid too much sodium, only a small amount of salt should be used in cooking, and only a little salt, if any, should be added at the table. In most recipes, the salt content can be reduced by one half or eliminated entirely. It is good to experiment with spices and herbs for seasoning instead of salt and to learn to enjoy the flavor of foods without salt. Salt substitutes containing potassium should be used only upon the advice of a physician, as excess potassium can be harmful for some persons.

IF YOU DRINK ALCOHOLIC BEVERAGES, DO SO IN MODERATION

Alcoholic beverages tend to be high in kilocalories and low in nutrients. For persons who drink alcohol, a maximum of 1 to 2 drinks per day is recommended. Vitamin and mineral deficiencies occur commonly in heavy drinkers, in part because of poor intake but also because alcohol alters the absorption and use of some essential nutrients such as fat and water-soluble vitamins.

FACT & FALLACY

FALLACY: Following the *Dietary Guidelines for Americans* will guarantee well-being.

FACT: Even though good eating habits are basic to good health and vitality, it is important to remember that lifestyle, heredity, and environment also play important roles. Moderate exercise, for example, is a primary factor in controlling hypertension, weight, osteoporosis, and other chronic health conditions.

HOW DO THE RDAs AND THE DIETARY GUIDELINES RELATE TO THE FOOD GUIDE PYRAMID?

The U.S. Department of Agriculture's Food Guide Pyramid, which was released in the 1990s, portrays the Dietary Guidelines by emphasizing maximum amounts of foods (see inside back cover). The RDAs can also be applied to the five food group system of the pyramid. Nutritional adequacy can be met by meeting the RDAs through the minimum number of recommended food servings in the Food Guide Pyramid (see Fig. 6–1). Choosing a wide assortment of foods from the two lower levels of the pyramid (foods that are high in carbohydrate and fiber and low in fat), moderate amounts of foods from the third level (the protein foods, which generally contribute fat as well), and minimal amounts from the upper tip of the pyramid (added fats and sugars) is advised. Selecting foods in this manner will allow adherence to the Dietary Guidelines while meeting the RDAs. Other countries have similar guides that vary with cultural food habits and the availability of foods. Canada's new food guide is represented as a rainbow and is shown inside the back cover (reprinted with permission of the Minister of Supply and Services, Canada). The *Guide To Good Eating* by the National Dairy Council uses the five food groups and can be used in conjunction with the Food Guide Pyramid (Fig. 6–4).

How Do the Pyramid Groups Supply Needed Nutrients?

As shown in Figures 3–1 and 5–2, all of the needed nutrients can be found in the lower three levels of the Food Guide Pyramid. Complete analytical data regarding food supply and human needs are available for key nutrients (see Appendix 5 for food composition tables).

Foods within the five food groups can also be identified for their macronutrient and vitamin and mineral content. For example, animal products in the milk and meat groups (third level of the pyramid) have more protein and fat than foods found in the fruit, vegetable, bread, and grain groups. Foods in the second level (vegetables and fruits) provide the main source of vitamins A, C, and folic acid, while the foods in the base of the pyramid are the main source of carbohydrate and the B vitamins.

FACT & FALLACY

FALLACY: Children instinctively know how to make food choices to stay healthy.

FACT: Children need the guidance of adults in selecting foods. Many chronic diseases such as cancer, heart disease, and high blood pressure may start developing in childhood as a result of poor food choices. Using the Food Guide Pyramid to teach children to eat more plant foods is appropriate.

WHAT IS THE EXCHANGE SYSTEM AND HOW DOES IT COMPARE WITH THE FOOD GUIDE PYRAMID?

The Exchange System, developed by the American Dietetic Association and the American Diabetes Association, is a food guide aimed at managing diabetes and weight (see Chapter 9 for more information and Appendix 9 for the complete Exchange System). The Exchange System groups foods according to the amounts of the macronutrients carbohydrate, protein, and fat that they contain. The Food Guide Pyramid puts less emphasis on amounts of carbohydrate and fat in foods.

The Exchange System counts cheese in the meat group based on the similar protein content but in recognition of the higher fat content. Cheese is not included in the milk group because skim or 1 per cent milk is recommended there. Cheese is also low in carbohydrate, making it more similar to meat. The Food Guide Pyramid does not distinguish the fat or carbohydrate content of milk versus that of cheese.

GUIDE TO GOOD EATING

Every day eat different foods from each food group.

MILK
Group
2-4 servings

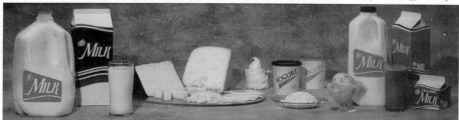

MEAT
Group
2-3 servings

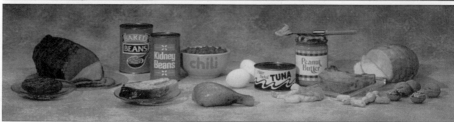

VEGETABLE
Group
3-5 servings

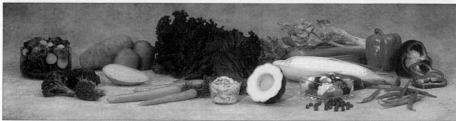

FRUIT
Group
2-4 servings

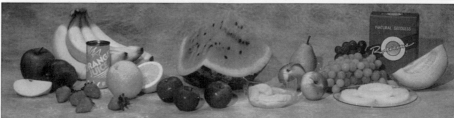

GRAIN
Group
6-11 servings

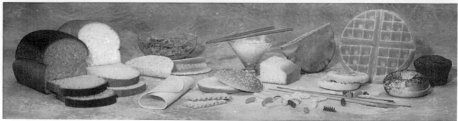

The Guide to Good Eating can be used in conjunction with the Food Guide Pyramid

▲ FIGURE 6-4

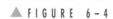

Guide to good eating. (From the National Dairy Council, Rosemont, IL, 1992.)

GUIDE TO GOOD EATING

Anyone can eat for good health.
Just follow these 2 simple steps:

1. **Eat foods from all Five Food Groups every day.**
Each food group provides you with different nutrients.

2. **Eat _different_ foods from each food group every day.**
Some foods in a food group are better sources of a nutrient than others. By eating several foods from each food group, you increase your chance of getting all the nutrients you need.

Every day eat:	Suggested Serving Sizes				
MILK Group _for calcium_ **2-4 servings**	Milk 1 cup	Yogurt 1 cup	Cheese 1½ – 2 oz	Cottage cheese ½ cup	Ice cream, ice milk, frozen yogurt ½ cup
MEAT Group _for iron_ **2-3 servings**	Cooked, lean meat 2-3 oz	Cooked, lean poultry, fish 2-3 oz	Egg 1	Peanut butter 2 tbsp	Cooked, dried peas, dried beans ½ cup
VEGETABLE Group _for vitamin A_ **3-5 servings**	Juice ¾ cup	Raw vegetable ½ cup	Raw leafy vegetable 1 cup	Cooked vegetable ½ cup	Potato 1 medium
FRUIT Group _for vitamin C_ **2-4 servings**	Juice ¾ cup	Raw, canned, or cooked fruit ½ cup	Apple, banana, orange, pear 1 medium	Grapefruit ½	Cantaloupe ¼
GRAIN Group _for fiber_ **6-11 servings**	Bread 1 slice	English muffin, hamburger bun ½	Ready-to-eat cereal 1 oz	Pasta, rice, grits, cooked cereal ½ cup	Tortilla, roll, muffin 1

Some foods don't have enough nutrients to fit in any of the Five Food Groups.
These foods are called "Others." These foods are okay to eat in moderation.
They should not replace foods from the Five Food Groups.

"OTHERS" _Category_

Fats and oils, sweets, salty snacks, alcohol, other beverages, and condiments

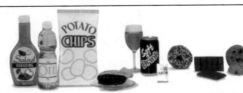

0001N ② 1993, Copyright © 1992, 6th Edition, NATIONAL DAIRY COUNCIL®, Rosemont, IL 60018-5616. All rights reserved. Printed in U.S.A.

 RECYCLED PAPERS RECYCLABLE PAPER   AGRI-TEK

▲ FIGURE 6-4   _Continued_

The Exchange System counts legumes in the starch/bread group based on the comparable carbohydrate content (⅓ cup of legumes contains about 15 grams carbohydrate and 80 kilocalories—equivalent to a serving of starch). Because of the high protein content of legumes (about 5 grams per ½ cup serving), the Food Guide Pyramid includes legumes in the meat group.

Carbohydrate content of the fruit group is not considered in the Food Guide Pyramid. It counts one whole banana as a serving, whereas the Exchange System counts only one half of a banana as a serving. The Exchange System calculates 15 grams of carbohydrate for one serving of fruit.

The Exchange System counts a fat serving as 5 grams of fat, which is equivalent to 1 teaspoon of added fat. The Food Guide Pyramid does not specifically state portion sizes for fats.

WHAT IS THE ROLE OF THE NURSE OR OTHER HEALTH PROFESSIONAL IN THE USE OF FOOD GUIDES?

The nurse or other health professional should be aware of nutritional inadequacies or excesses as represented in the Food Guide Pyramid. For persons who require a higher kilocalorie intake, the addition of more foods from the base of the Food Guide Pyramid (whole grains, vegetables, and fruits) would be the wisest choice. Many patients will require dietary modification for various conditions, such as cardiovascular disease, which requires a lower sodium intake. Foods needed for long-term health, however, should still fall within the parameters of the Food Guide Pyramid. In the case of limiting sodium intake, it would be appropriate for a nurse to advise reading labels for sodium content. Emphasis should be placed on the fact that food groups should not be omitted in an attempt to limit sodium. Problems with patient adherence to the goals of nutrition or multiple therapeutic diets beyond normal nutrition should be documented and referral made to a registered dietitian.

STUDY QUESTIONS AND ACTIVITIES

1. How do the Dietary Guidelines for Americans fit into the Food Guide Pyramid?

2. Why should the RDAs not be used to evaluate the adequacy of an individual's diet?

3. Name some of the factors that affect an individual's nutrient requirements.

4. How are the RDAs intended to be used?

5. On the table of RDAs printed on the inside front cover of this text, underline in red pencil the figures that indicate the requirements for calories and each of the nutrients for a person of your age and jot them down on the chart below. You will be referring to these figures throughout the course.

My RDA:

Kcalories _____		Vitamin B$_6$ _____ mg	
Protein _____ gm		Folate _____ gm	
Vitamin A _____ IU		Vitamin B$_{12}$ _____ μg	
Vitamin D _____ IU		Calcium _____ mg	
Vitamin E _____ IU		Phosphorus _____ mg	
Vitamin C _____ mg		Magnesium _____ mg	
Vitamin K _____ μg		Iron _____ mg	
Thiamine _____ mg		Zinc_____ mg	
Riboflavin _____ mg		Iodine _____ μg	
Niacin _____ mg		Selenium _____ μg	

6. Bring some sample nutrition labels to class to discuss how you would use the percentage values on the label in planning a day's menu for yourself.

7. Categorize the foods in Maria Bernardo's shopping list from Chapter 3 according to the five food groups of the Food Guide Pyramid. Plan a day's menu using the maximum recommended number of servings for a total intake of about 2000 kilocalories.

8. This menu was eaten by Anna Bernardo, Maria's teenaged daughter:

Breakfast:	Lunch:	Dinner:
Banana	Hot dog on roll	Cheeseburger
Corn flakes	Mustard and relish	French fries
Whole milk	Chocolate chip cookies	Coleslaw
Sugar	Coke	Milkshake
Toast, butter, and jelly		

Judge the meals according to the Food Guide Pyramid.
List the foods and amounts lacking for Anna.
Is Anna likely to lose weight eating this way? Why or why not?
What suggestions would you make?

WHAT HAS HAPPENED TO YOUR FOOD HABITS AND NUTRITIONAL ATTITUDES AS YOU HAVE STUDIED ABOUT NUTRIENTS AND FOODS FOR GOOD NUTRITION?

Now is a good time for you to check your food habits.

1. Keep a record of your food intake (at meals and between meals) for 1 week.

2. Score your diet for each day, using the accompanying Food Selection Score Card, and determine your average score for the week. Repeat this activity later in the semester and compare the scores to see if you have made an improvement in your eating habits.

3. Analyze and comment on your last food selection score in the space provided.

FOOD GROUPS	PERFECT SCORE	MY SCORE	COMMENTS
Milk group			
Meat group			
Vegetable group			
Fruit group			
Bread and cereal group			
Water			
	100		

▲　FOOD SELECTION SCORE CARD

Score your diet for each day and determine your average score for the week. If your final score is between 85 and 100, your food selection standard has been good. A score of 75 to 85 indicates a fair standard. A score lower than 75 indicates a low standard.

MAXIMUM SCORE FOR EACH FOOD GROUP	CREDITS	COLUMNS FOR DAILY CHECK
20	Milk Group: Milk (including foods prepared with low-fat milk, part skim cheese and yogurt) Adults: 1 glass, 10; 1½ glasses, 15; 2 glasses, 20 Children: 1 glass, 5; 1½ glasses, 10; 2 glasses, 15; 4 glasses, 20*	
25	Meat Group: Eggs, meat, cheese, fish, poultry, dry peas, dry beans, and nuts 1 serving of any one of above, 10 1 serving of any two of above, 20	
35	Vegetable and Fruit Group: Vegetables: 1 serving, 5; 2 servings, 10; 3 servings, 15 Potatoes may be included as one of the preceding servings If dark green or orange vegetable is included, extra credit, 5 Fruits: 1 serving, 5; 2 servings, 10 If citrus fruit, raw vegetable, or canned tomatoes are included, extra credit, 5†	
15	Bread and Cereal Group: Bread—dark whole grain, enriched or restored Cereals—dark whole grain, enriched or restored 2 servings of either, 10; 4 servings of either, 15	
5	Water (total liquid including milk, decaffeinated coffee and tea, or other beverage): Adults: 6 glasses, 2½; 8 glasses, 5 Children: 4 glasses, 2; 6 glasses, 5	
100	Final Score	

* Count ½ cup milk in creamy soups, puddings, cream pies.
† Count ½ serving vegetables in soups or fruit in salad.
Deductions from final score: Each meal omitted, 10; excessive consumption of soft drinks, 10.

What improvements have you made in your food selection habits thus far?

What further improvements do you think are desirable to make?

What thought have you given to the principles of meal planning as you have selected the necessary foods for your various meals?

Note to Instructor: It is suggested that each student keep and score a week's food intake at least once more (preferably twice) before the end of the course.

4. Why are good food habits important? How are they formed? How can they be improved?

5. What are five good food habits for *you* to acquire and follow daily?

REFERENCES

New Food Labeling Regulations. Dairy Council Digest. May/June 1993; 64(3).

National Research Council: Recommended Dietary Allowances, 10th ed. Washington, DC, National Academy of Sciences, National Academy Press, 1989.

Smith SM: Basic Four Is No More: USDA's Food Pyramid Debuts—Again. Environmental Nutrition, June 1992.

US Department of Agriculture, US Department of Health and Human Services. Nutrition and Your Health: Dietary Guidelines for Americans, 3rd ed. Home and Garden Bull. N. 232. Washington DC, Government Printing Office, 1990.

CHRONIC AND ACUTE ILLNESS

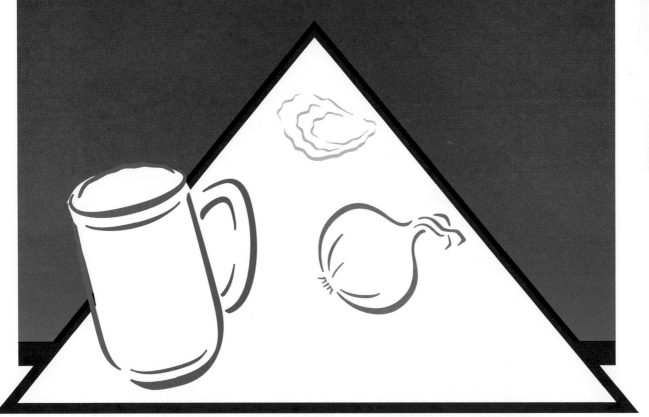

NUTRITION IN THE INSTITUTIONAL SETTING: THE INTERPLAY BETWEEN CHRONIC AND ACUTE ILLNESS

CHAPTER 7

OBJECTIVES

After completing this chapter you should be able to:
- Describe strategies used to modify the normal diet during illness
- Discuss meal service considerations in institutional settings
- Identify patient risk factors for poor nutritional status
- Recognize potential drug and nutrient interactions
- Discuss nutrition discharge planning

TERMS TO IDENTIFY

Addison's disease
Albumin
Anthropometry
Ascites
Atherosclerosis
Custodial approach
Diabetes
Diuretics
Diverticulitis
Dumping syndrome
Elbow breadth
Gastrostomy
Gluten
Gluten-sensitive enteropathy
Glycosuria

Gout
Hepatitis
Hyperglycemia
Hyperlipoproteinemia
Hypoglycemia
Ketogenic diet
Megaloblastic anemia
Mid-arm circumference
Nephrosis
Neuroleptic drugs
Osteomalacia
Pernicious anemia
Phenylalanine
Phenylketonuria (PKU)
Polyneuritis

Protein-energy malnutrition
Purines
Reactive hypoglycemia
Renal disease
Restorative approach
Tetany
Therapeutic diet
Total parenteral nutrition
Toxemia—pregnancy-
   induced hypertension
Triceps skin fold
Tube feeding
Uremia
Wilson's disease
Xerophthalmia

A FAMILY'S PERSPECTIVE ON NUTRITION

Maria awoke in the hospital to the sound of babies crying. She and her baby would be fine, she told herself. She wished she were home, with Tony. How were Anna and Joey managing without her? Even though Nanna Bernardo could drive her mad at times, she was very glad she was there with the children. She hoped the doctor came soon to tell her how she and the baby were doing. She hoped she hadn't lost any more weight. She was only 12 weeks pregnant but it seemed like forever. Constant nausea. Constant vomiting. Just when she thought she was getting better, the nausea would begin again. Like waves, it would overcome her and she would not be able to keep even water down. How could she possibly have lost 20 pounds? At her height of 5'5" she wasn't underweight at 165 pounds but she knew she shouldn't be losing weight while she was pregnant. Oh, if someone would bring her a piece of dry toast, maybe she could keep it down now, before the next wave of nausea began. The breakfast meal was taking so long to come this morning. She shouldn't have let her son Joey eat those crackers the dietitian had left for her. The dietitian had been so helpful arranging between-meal snacks and visiting daily to see how she was eating. It was nice to know someone was watching out for her in this place. But even the dietitian couldn't keep the nausea away.

INTRODUCTION

In the previous two sections, the relationship of good nutrition to health was discussed in terms of the following:

1. Nutrients: their functions, recommended dietary allowances, food sources, and use by the body
2. Foods: nutritional contributions, selection and care, and daily requirements
3. The application of basic nutritional principles to family feeding
4. The nutrition care planning process

This section deals further with the nutritional care process in an institutional setting. The purpose of this chapter is to alert the health care professional to the many different types of therapeutic diets. Specific guidelines should be provided by a registered dietitian. The nurse can assist the patient best by reinforcing the importance of therapeutic diets. Food can make an important contribution to recovery from illness and is a fundamental aspect of total care. Good nutritional status should be maintained and poor nutritional status must be improved during treatment of illness or injury. The diet is no less important than other therapies and medications. Although the correct diet is important in any situation, it carries special importance in diseases of long duration and for anyone in a stressed condition. More specific dietary intervention guidelines can be found in other chapters throughout this textbook. You may also want to refer to a diet manual such as the one used by your local hospital.

WHAT IS THE ROLE OF THERAPEUTIC NUTRITION?

Therapeutic nutrition is simply the role of food and nutrition in the treatment of various diseases and disorders. Also referred to as medical nutrition therapy or a **therapeutic diet,** it involves the modification or adaptation of the normal or basic diet according to the needs of the individual.

Medical nutrition therapy may be necessary for one or more of the following reasons:

1. To maintain or improve nutritional status
2. To improve clinical or subclinical nutritional deficiencies
3. To maintain, decrease, or increase body weight
4. To rest certain organs of the body
5. To eliminate particular food constituents to which the individual may be allergic
6. To adjust the composition of the normal diet to meet the ability of the body to adjust, metabolize, and excrete certain nutrients and other substances

HOSPITAL DIETS

What is Meant by a Basic Hospital Diet?

For reasons of economy, efficiency, convenience, and uniformity of service, a basic routine diet is a necessity in the many hospitals and other types of institutions that care for the sick. Such a routine diet must be nutritionally adequate to maintain good nutrition or improve nutritional status. The Food Guide Pyramid continues to be the basis for any therapeutic diet.

The basic routine diet, variously referred to from hospital to hospital as the *house, general, regular, standard, full diet,* or *diet as tolerated (DAT)* is served to patients who do not require a therapeutic diet. Many factors affect the choice of foods to be served on this basic diet. For example, the type of hospital (e.g., private or state), budget, food preferences of patients, adaptability to large-quantity preparation, and so forth are taken into consideration with institutional menus.

The consistency of the basic diet may be modified in progressive steps from a liquid diet to a regular diet. Liquid diets are often ordered on a patient's admission to the hospital or after surgery. The most restrictive form of liquid diets is the clear liquid diet, which generally includes gelatin, some fruit juices, and fat-free broth. As a patient becomes able to handle milk products, there may be a transition to a full liquid diet including cream-based soups and ice cream. The next transition may be to the soft diet, which is moderately low in roughage and fatty foods.

Table 7–1 lists information about each of the basic hospital diets. There are some differences from hospital to hospital in the foods allowed in each category, as well as in the number of kinds of diets. When a patient is admitted to the hospital, the type of diet will be selected by the physician, but often with input from a staff dietitian. In some hospitals, the dietitians are responsible for ordering hospital diets. Diets may be changed if and when the patient's condition makes it desirable. The nursing staff often identifies and communicates needed changes in the patient's diet.

The method of feeding and the time for feeding may also vary. For example, tube or intravenous feedings may be desirable to meet an individual's needs. Sometimes hourly feedings or several small meals a day are preferred to three meals daily (see section below on meal service considerations). Providing several small meals per day would be recommended for Maria Bernardo in the opening chapter case study. If you were the nurse working with Mrs. Bernardo, you would be expected to alert the staff dietitian to her nausea and vomiting. Any further nutritional problems Mrs. Bernardo has should also be brought to the attention of the dietitian.

How are Hospital Diets Modified for Therapeutic Purposes?

The basic diet becomes therapeutic when it is modified in the following ways:

1. The energy value (kilocalories) may be increased or decreased.
2. Fiber (bulk, roughage) may be increased or decreased.
3. Specific nutrients (one or more) may be increased or decreased.
4. Specific foods or types of foods (such as allergens for persons with allergies, fried foods, or gas-forming foods) may be increased or decreased.
5. Any one of these modified diets may be further altered to become a soft or liquid diet.
6. Condiments and any specific foods that are not tolerated by the individual may be eliminated from the diet.

Tables 7–2 and 7–3 give sample menus for therapeutic diets and how the food groups of the Food Guide Pyramid are included in the modified menus.

How are Therapeutic Diets Named and Described?

Therapeutic diets are named in terms of the diet modification, not the name of the disease (except in the case of the diabetic diet) or its symptoms or the name of the person or persons who may have originated or modified the diet. This makes possible a universal understanding of terms and also reduces the number of therapeutic diets.

Adaptations are sometimes classified as *qualitative* when they are in types of foods or consistency and *quantitative* when they consist of increases or decreases of certain nutrients or calories. It is desirable that every therapeutic diet be planned for the particular patient for whom it is ordered. It is the ultimate responsibility of the staff dietitians to assess the appropriateness of diets ordered by physicians and to document in the patient's chart any further recommendations for modifications to the physician's diet order.

The diet prescription is ideally written in terms of energy requirements based on the individual's weight and activity, and in terms of requirements for protein, fat, carbohydrate, minerals, vitamins, and fiber, with regard for the increased or decreased needs for each because of the patient's illness. This prescription is translated into foods and meals by the dietitian for hospital meal planning. If the patient needs to adhere to the diet after hospital discharge, the dietitian then instructs the patient regarding the diet. The

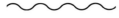

▲ **TABLE 7-1**

PROGRESSIVE BASIC HOSPITAL DIETS

	CLEAR LIQUID DIET	FULL LIQUID DIET	SOFT DIET*	REGULAR, HOUSE, GENERAL, OR FULL DIET
Characteristics	Temporary diet of clear liquids without residue. Nonstimulating, non-gas-forming, nonirritating. 400–500 kilocalories	Foods liquid at room temperature or liquefying at body temperature	Normal diet modified in consistency to have limited fiber. Liquids and semisolid food; easily digested	Practically all foods. Simple, easy-to-digest foods, simply prepared, palatably seasoned; a wide variety of foods and various methods of preparation; individual intolerances, food habits, ethnic values, and food preferences considered
Adequacy	Inadequate; deficient in protein, minerals, vitamins, and kilocalories	Can be adequate with careful planning; adequacy depends on liquids used. If used longer than 48 hours, high-protein, high-calorie supplements to be considered	Entirely adequate liberal diet	Adequate and well balanced
Use	Acute illness and infections. Postoperatively. Temporary food intolerance. To relieve thirst. To reduce colonic fecal matter. 1- to 2-hour feeding intervals. Prior to certain tests	Transition between clear liquid and soft diets. Postoperatively. Acute gastritis and infections. Febrile conditions. Intolerance for solid food. 2- to 4-hour feeding intervals	Between full liquid and light or regular diet. Between acute illness and convalescence. Acute infections. Chewing difficulties. Gastrointestinal disorders. Three meals with or without between-meal feedings	For uniformity and convenience in serving hospital patients. Ambulatory patients. Bed patients not requiring therapeutic diets
Foods	Water, tea, coffee, coffee substitutes. Fat-free broth. Carbonated beverages. Synthetic fruit juices. Ginger ale. Plain gelatin. Sugar. No milk or fats. Orange juice may cause distention	All liquids on clear liquid diet plus: All forms of milk. Soups, strained. Fruit and vegetable juices. Eggnog. Plain ice cream and sherbets. Junket and plain gelatin dishes	All liquids. Fine and strained cereals. Cooked tender and puréed vegetables. Cooked fruits without skin and seeds. Ripe bananas. Ground or tender meat, fish, and poultry	All foods from the Food Guide Pyramid

▲ **T A B L E   7 - 1**   *Continued*

PROGRESSIVE BASIC HOSPITAL DIETS

CLEAR LIQUID DIET	FULL LIQUID DIET	SOFT DIET*	REGULAR, HOUSE, GENERAL, OR FULL DIET
Salt, plain hard candy, fruit ices, all fruit juices without pulp	Soft custard Cereal gruels	Eggs and mild cheeses Plain cake and puddings Moderately seasoned foods	
	Puréed meat and meat substitutes only; for use in soups only Butter, cream, margarine, sugar, honey, hard candy, syrup; salt, pepper, cinnamon, nutmeg, and flavorings; puréed vegetables for use in soups only	Enriched white, refined whole wheat bread (no seeds)	

Modification

CLEAR LIQUID DIET	FULL LIQUID DIET	SOFT DIET*	REGULAR, HOUSE, GENERAL, OR FULL DIET
Liberal clear liquid diet includes fruit juices, egg white, whole egg, thin gruels	Consistency for tube feedings: foods that will pass through tube easily	Low residue—no fiber or tough connective tissue; traditional bland—no chemical, thermal, physical stimulants, cold soft—tonsillectomy; mechanical or "dental" soft—requiring no mastication (diced, chopped, mashed foods in place of puréed); light or convalescent diet—intermediate between soft and regular	For a light or convalescent diet, fried foods, rich pastries, foods rich in fats, coarse vegetables, possibly raw fruits and vegetables, and gas-forming vegetables may be omitted

* Because of trend toward more liberal interpretation of diets and foods, in some hospitals the soft diet may be combined with the light diet, with cooked low-fiber vegetables allowed in place of purées.

importance of the diet and guidance on how to follow the meal plan at home is reviewed with the patient by the dietitian. The dietitian also communicates with the nurses on staff so that they can reinforce the meal plan with the patient and the patient's family.

What are Examples of Therapeutic Diets and Indications for Use?

MODIFICATIONS IN CONSISTENCY

Other than liquid, soft, or regular diets, the following additional modified diets are used: mechanical soft (for any patient with chewing problems), **tube feeding** (provision of a liquid supplement through a tube placed in

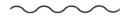

▲ T A B L E 7 - 2

MENU MODIFICATION OF FOOD GROUPS OF THE FOOD GUIDE PYRAMID FOR THERAPEUTIC DIETS

FOOD GROUP	REGULAR	SOFT	LIBERAL BLAND	SODIUM RESTRICTED	LOW-FAT	KILOCALORIE RESTRICTED
Breads and cereals	All breads and cereals allowed	All breads and cereals allowed Modify in consistency as needed (milk toast, rice pudding, and so on)	Allowed as tolerated	Avoid instant hot cereals, breads with salted toppings, salted crackers Salt-free products may be used, depending on level of sodium restriction	Avoid products with added fat	Avoid products with added fat
Fruits and vegetables	All fruits and vegetables allowed	Use juices, soft, canned, or cooked vegetables and fruits; chop and mash as needed	Allowed as tolerated	Avoid dried fruits with sodium preservatives Avoid high-sodium vegetables and juices	Avoid vegetables in cream or cheese sauces	Avoid vegetables in cream or cheese sauces, fruits packed in syrup Limit to amounts prescribed in diet
Milk	All milk and dairy products allowed	All milk and dairy products allowed	Allowed as tolerated	Milk may be limited depending on level of sodium restriction	Use skim milk and low-fat cheeses	Use skim milk and low-fat cheeses unless calorie level allows use of higher fat products
Meat	All meat and alternates allowed	Use soft, tender, or ground meats plain or in casseroles and soups	Avoid spicy meats and high-fat meats if not well tolerated	Avoid all processed and cured meats	Use lean meats	Use lean meats, limit to amounts prescribed in diet
Fats, sugars and miscellaneous	Condiments and seasonings as desired Fats, sugar, and alcohol in moderation	Condiments and seasonings as desired Fats, sugar, and alcohol in moderation	*Omit:* Black pepper, chili powder, alcohol, and caffeine-containing beverages	Avoid salt and salt seasonings, salted snack foods, commercially canned soups	Limit use of fats and oils	Limit use of fats, oils, alcohol, and foods high in sugar

the nose, see Chapter 14), bland diet, restricted-residue diet, and high-residue or high-fiber diet.

MECHANICAL SOFT DIET. This type of diet is used for the individual who has difficulty in chewing because of lack of dentures or teeth or because of inflammation of the oral cavity. Severe dental decay may cause pain upon chewing.

TUBE FEEDING. This type of feeding is used for patients with an esophageal obstruction or severe burns or those who have undergone gastric surgery or who, for some other reason, have an inability to chew or

▲ **TABLE 7-3**

SAMPLE MENUS FOR THERAPEUTIC DIETS

MEAL	REGULAR	SOFT	LIBERAL BLAND	SODIUM RESTRICTED	LOW-FAT	KILOCALORIE RESTRICTED
Breakfast	Orange juice Corn flakes Poached egg Buttered toast Milk Coffee Sugar Salt, pepper	Orange juice Cream of wheat Poached egg Buttered toast Milk Coffee Sugar Salt, pepper	Orange juice Corn flakes Poached egg Buttered toast Milk Sugar Salt	Orange juice Shredded wheat cereal Poached egg Buttered toast Milk Coffee Sugar Salt substitute Pepper	Orange juice Corn flakes Poached egg Toast 1 tsp butter Skim milk Coffee Sugar Salt, pepper	Orange juice Corn flakes Poached egg Toast 1 tsp butter Skim milk Coffee Sugar substitute Salt, pepper
Lunch	Vegetable soup Crackers Turkey sandwich Fresh fruit salad Vanilla pudding Milk Tea Sugar Salt, pepper	Vegetable soup Crackers Ground turkey sandwich Canned fruit salad Vanilla pudding Milk Tea Sugar Salt, pepper	Vegetable soup Crackers Turkey sandwich Fresh fruit salad Vanilla pudding Milk Salt	Salt-free vegetable soup Salt-free crackers Turkey sandwich on bread Fresh fruit salad Lemon sherbet Milk Tea Sugar Salt substitute Pepper	Vegetable soup Crackers Turkey sandwich (use white meat) Fresh fruit salad Lemon sherbet Skim milk Tea Sugar Salt, pepper	Vegetable soup Crackers Turkey sandwich (use white meat) Fresh fruit salad Skim milk Tea Sugar substitute Salt, pepper
Dinner	Tossed salad with dressing Baked chicken Baked potato Buttered carrots Peach slices Dinner roll Brownie Milk Tea Sugar Salt, pepper Butter	Tomato juice Baked ground chicken Baked potato Buttered carrots Peach slices Dinner roll Brownie (no nuts) Milk Tea Sugar Salt, pepper Butter	Tossed salad with dressing Baked chicken Baked potato Buttered carrots Peach slices Dinner roll Brownie Milk Salt Butter	Tossed salad with salt-free dressing Baked chicken Baked potato Buttered salt-free carrots Peach slices Dinner roll Milk Tea Sugar Salt substitute Pepper Butter	Tossed salad with low-calorie dressing Baked chicken (no skin) Baked potato Carrots Peach slices Dinner roll Skim milk Tea Sugar Salt, pepper 1 tsp butter	Tossed salad with low-calorie dressing Baked chicken (no skin) Baked potato Carrots Peach slices (packed in water) Dinner roll Skim milk Tea Sugar substitute Salt, pepper 1 tsp butter

Low-fat milk is recommended but not required unless indicated. Margarine may be preferable to butter owing to its being cholesterol-free.

swallow without aspirating. It is also sometimes necessary for patients with anorexia nervosa (see Chapter 15). Tube feeding is appropriate only when the gastrointestinal system is functioning. The site of placement needs to be considered as well. For example, a **gastrostomy** (a surgical opening into the stomach) feeding site may be indicated in the case of esophageal obstruction.

RESTRICTED-RESIDUE DIET. This diet may be used for patients after gastrointestinal surgery, or for those with gastritis, Crohn's disease, severe diarrhea, ulcerative colitis, **diverticulitis** (an inflammatory condition of the intestines, see Chapter 11), typhoid fever, or partial intestinal obstructions.

HIGH-RESIDUE OR HIGH-FIBER DIET. This type of diet may be prescribed for atonic constipation (intestinal stasis) or for diverticulosis. It is also being promoted for the prevention or therapy of gastric ulcers, cancer of the colon, hypercholesterolemia, **diabetes** (a condition of elevated blood sugar, see Chapter 9), and obesity. An intake of about 20 to 30 grams of fiber per day is recommended (see Chapter 3 for the average fiber content of the Food Guide Pyramid; Chapter 6 describes how to read food labels for fiber content).

MODIFICATIONS IN CARBOHYDRATE, PROTEIN, AND FAT

The diabetic diet; the low-calorie diet; the high-protein, high-fat, low-carbohydrate diet; and the **ketogenic diet** (a diet high in fat and low in carbohydrate, see Chapter 18) are all examples of diets that control carbohydrate, protein, and fat intake.

DIABETIC DIET. This diet is carefully calculated for each patient to minimize the occurrence of **hyperglycemia** (elevated blood sugar), **hypoglycemia** (low blood sugar), and **glycosuria** (sugar in the urine, see Chapter 9) and to attain or maintain ideal body weight and promote good health. Diabetic diets are ordered as a kilocalorie level followed by the acronym ADA, which stands for American Diabetes Association. For example, the diet might read 1200 ADA or 2000 ADA.

LOW-KILOCALORIE DIET. This diet is used to achieve weight loss in individuals with cardiovascular and **renal diseases** (diseases of the kidney, see Chapter 10), diabetes, hypertension, gallbladder disease, **gout** (a disease of the joints, see Chapter 21), or hypothyroidism, and for severely ill patients who cannot tolerate large amounts of food. See Chapter 20 for more guidelines on weight loss.

HIGH-PROTEIN, LOW SIMPLE-CARBOHYDRATE DIET. This diet is used for patients with **reactive hypoglycemia** (a condition related to inappropriate insulin secretion, see Chapter 9) and includes six small meals. Emphasis is on complex carbohydrates with protein at each meal.

HIGH-FAT DIET. This diet may be indicated for purposes of weight gain. The type of fat ideally should be monounsaturated fat, to help prevent cardiovascular disease.

KETOGENIC DIET. In some cases, a ketogenic diet is used to control a type of epilepsy. This diet is high in fat; protein and carbohydrate are controlled.

MODIFICATIONS IN FAT

Fat-modified diets include the restricted-fat diet, the fat-controlled low-cholesterol diet, and the dietary management of **hyperlipoproteinemia** (elevated lipids in the blood, see Chapter 8).

RESTRICTED-FAT DIET. Fat is restricted for patients with diseases of the liver, gallbladder, or pancreas, in which disturbances of digestion and absorption of fat may occur. Generally 40 to 50 grams of fat per day is an adequate and realistic restriction.

FAT-CONTROLLED LOW-CHOLESTEROL DIET. This diet is used in individuals with elevated blood cholesterol levels and for those with **atherosclerosis** (a form of heart disease with plaque buildup inside blood vessels and arteries, see Chapter 8).

DIETARY MANAGEMENT OF HYPERLIPOPROTEINEMIA. This diet is important for lowering the risk of cardiovascular disease. The diet is individualized based on specific serum lab values for the various blood lipids (cholesterol, high-density lipoprotein cholesterol, low-density lipoprotein cholesterol, and triglycerides, see Chapter 8).

MODIFICATIONS IN PROTEIN

Protein-modified diets include the restricted-protein, gluten-free, restricted-phenylalanine, restricted-purine, low-tyramine, and high-protein diets.

RESTRICTED-PROTEIN DIET. This diet is used for patients in hepatic coma or with chronic **uremia** (a condition of severe kidney disease, see Chapter 10), renal disease, or liver disease.

GLUTEN-FREE DIET. Gluten is the protein found in grains. Individuals with celiac disease (often referred to as nontropical sprue in children, also known as **gluten-sensitive enteropathy,** see Chapter 11) have gluten intolerance and must be on a gluten-free diet. Foods omitted are those that contain even trace amounts of wheat, oats, rye, barley, and triticale (a hybrid grain).

RESTRICTED-PHENYLALANINE DIET. This diet is used in confirmed cases of **phenylketonuria (PKU)** (an inborn error of metabolism, see Chapter 18), in which **phenylalanines** (a type of amino acid) cannot be processed by the body. All babies have a PKU test at birth.

RESTRICTED-PURINE DIET. A decrease in **purines** (a form of protein) may be useful in lowering the blood uric acid level in gout.

LOW-TYRAMINE DIET. This diet is designed to restrict foods containing tyramine and related compounds. It is used for patients who are taking medications known as monoamine oxidase (MAO) inhibitors for clinical depression. The diet helps to prevent adverse reactions such as palpitation, severe headache, and hypertension. Table 7–4 lists foods excluded on a low-tyramine diet.

HIGH-PROTEIN DIET. A high-protein diet is used to correct a protein inadequacy for any reason such as pre- and postoperative nutritional

▲ T A B L E   7 - 4

FOODS EXCLUDED ON A LOW-TYRAMINE DIET

Aged cheese—All cheeses except cottage, cream, and other unripened cheeses
Fermented sausage—Bologna, salami, pepperoni, and liver sausage
Pickled herring and salted dried fish
Broad beans and pods—Lima and Italian beans, lentils, snow peas, dried beans and peas, and
    soybeans
Fruits—Bananas, avocados, canned figs, and raisins
Cultured dairy products—Buttermilk, yogurt, and sour cream
Chocolate and products made with chocolate
Caffeine—Coffee, tea, and cola drinks
Beer and ale
Wines (especially Chianti)
Yeast extracts
Licorice
Soy sauce and any food product that is made with soy sauce

needs, high fever, burns, injuries, increased metabolism, **nephrosis** (a form of kidney disease found in children that may or may not be treated with a high-protein diet), chronic nephritis (unless there is nitrogen retention), **pernicious anemia** (a form of megaloblastic anemia characterized by lack of vitamin B_{12}, a vitamin found in animal protein foods such as meat and milk), ulcerative colitis, **hepatitis** (inflammation of the liver, see Chapter 11), celiac disease and cystic fibrosis, tuberculosis and other wasting diseases, wounds, or nutritional anemia. A low serum **albumin** level (a lab value that indicates protein status) may indicate a need for a high-protein diet.

MODIFICATIONS IN CARBOHYDRATE

Both the lactose-free diet and the **dumping syndrome** (see definition following) diet are based on modifications in carbohydrate intake.

LACTOSE-FREE DIET. Patients who have a total or partial inability to metabolize this milk sugar must avoid lactose in their diet.

DUMPING-SYNDROME DIET. Patients who have had a partial gastrectomy or gastric bypass surgery may require this special diet. This diet is low in concentrated sweets and limits fluids at mealtimes to avoid "dumping" of the stomach contents into the small intestines, which results in diarrhea. It is generally a temporary diet until normal stomach function returns after surgery.

MODIFICATIONS IN MINERALS AND ELECTROLYTES

In these diets, minerals and electrolytes may be increased or restricted depending on lab values. Common modifications include alterations of sodium, potassium, calcium, phosphorus, and iron.

INCREASED-SODIUM DIETS. These diets may be useful in **Addison's disease** (in which the body loses excess salt). Four thousand to 6000 mg sodium is a high level that is easily included in a day's diet.

RESTRICTED-SODIUM DIETS. These diets are very common and are prescribed for patients with congestive heart failure, hypertension, renal disease with edema, cirrhosis of the liver with **ascites** (a buildup of abdominal fluid often associated with liver disease), and possibly for **toxemia,** also referred to as **pregnancy-induced hypertension** (see Chapter 16 for further discussion). The level of sodium restriction most often ranges between 2000 and 3000 mg sodium per day. More restrictive sodium levels, such as 1000 mg, are generally reserved for congestive heart failure.

RESTRICTED-POTASSIUM DIET. If potassium is not excreted from the body properly, a restricted diet may be necessary. This commonly occurs in renal disease (see Table 10–3 for food items low in potassium).

INCREASED-POTASSIUM DIETS. Persons on potassium-depleting medications, such as diuretics, need to have a high-potassium diet. Table 7–5 lists high-potassium foods.

RESTRICTED-COPPER DIET. **Wilson's disease** (in which the body stores excess amounts of copper), oliguria, and anuria (see Chapter 10) all

~~~~~~~~~

▲   **TABLE 7 - 5**

FOODS HIGH IN POTASSIUM

VERY HIGH POTASSIUM SOURCES (>300 mg potassium)
Milk, 1 c
Yogurt, 1 c
Apricots, 3 whole or 6 halves
Banana, 1 small
Broccoli, 1 stalk or 1 c cooked
Canteloupe, 1 quarter
Carrots, 1 c cooked
Potatoes, ½ c
Spinach, ½ c cooked
Turnips, 1 c cooked
Winter squash, ½ baked
Legumes (dried beans & peas), ½ c cooked

MODERATELY HIGH POTASSIUM SOURCES (>200 mg potassium)
Grapefruit, 1 whole
Oranges, 1 whole or 4 oz juice
Green beans, 1 c
Tomato, 1 whole or ½ c juice
Peanut butter, 2 tbsp
Molasses, 1 tsp blackstrap or 4 tsp "green label"

call for a restriction of copper intake. High-copper foods such as shellfish, liver, legumes, and whole grains should be avoided (see Table 5–4 and Fig. 5–2).

HIGH-CALCIUM AND HIGH-PHOSPHORUS DIET. An increase in calcium and phosphorus intake is desirable in a person with rickets, **osteomalacia** (a condition in which the bones become soft), **tetany** (a condition that comprises muscle spasms generally related to low blood levels of calcium), dental caries due to poor calcification of teeth, and acute lead poisoning.

HIGH-IRON DIET. Nutritional or hemorrhagic anemia calls for a high intake of dietary iron. Only iron-deficient forms of anemia are treated with iron.

HIGH-VITAMIN DIET. If a specific vitamin deficiency is diagnosed, an increased intake of vitamins may be necessary. An increase in vitamin A is necessary to combat night blindness and **xerophthalmia** (an eye disease); increased intake of vitamin D is recommended for rickets and osteomalacia; increased vitamin K is needed in persons receiving long-term antibiotics who have fat malabsorption; increased thiamine (vitamin B_1) is necessary to avoid beriberi and **polyneuritis** (inflammation of nerves); increased niacin (vitamin B_3) is needed to combat pellagra; and increased ascorbic acid (vitamin C) may improve wound healing and fight scurvy.

WHAT ARE SOME COMMON TEST DIETS?

A variety of diets have been established to aid in the assessment of certain disorders or as part of diagnostic tests. The following are among the most common.

- **Fecal Fat Determination Diet:** It is necessary to measure fecal fat for one step in the diagnosis of cystic fibrosis or malabsorption syndromes. The test diet includes a minimum of 100 g of fat per day for 2 to 3 days prior to the test.
- **Glucose Tolerance Test Diet:** Unless contraindicated, the patient scheduled for a glucose tolerance test (used to aid in the diagnosis of diabetes mellitus) will have a high-carbohydrate diet (300 g for 3 days) prior to the test. This test is also used in the diagnosis of reactive hypoglycemia.
- **Meat-free Test Diet:** Meat, poultry, and fish contain hemoglobin, myoglobin, and enzymes that may give a false positive result in tests for gastrointestinal bleeding. Therefore, patients scheduled for these tests must sometimes eat a meat-free diet for as many as 4 days before the tests.
- **Calcium Test Diet:** This test determines urinary calcium excretion, as for the diagnosis of hypercalciuria. A diet of 1000 mg calcium is necessary and may be supplied with a combination of dietary and supplemental intake. Three cups of milk or its equivalent will provide almost 1000 mg calcium.

WHAT ARE IMPORTANT CONSIDERATIONS IN MEAL SERVICE?

Attractive food service plays an important role in stimulating the appetite and enjoyment of food. A good appetite is necessary to ensure adequate nutritional intake. Mealtime is often the major event of the day for the patient, and every effort must be made to prepare the room and the patient to receive the meal. Some patients will eat better if arrangements can be made for the use of china dishware. Holidays are often a time of sadness for patients in an institutional setting. Using colorful napkins and tray decorations at these times can stimulate the appetite.

The patient's attitude toward food may reflect a more general attitude toward illness, as it may be the one area about which they feel free to vent negative feelings. The nurse needs to listen to what the patient is really saying. Any complaints of meal service should be taken seriously, especially if there is a poor intake of food. A request for a staff dietitian consultation is appropriate when the complaints are severe enough that the patient is at nutritional risk. Food from home can be calculated into the diet when a cooperative plan is made. Caution needs to be made to ensure food poisoning does not result. Poor food handling at home or failure to keep hot foods hot while they are being transported to the hospital can cause food poisoning (see Chapter 22).

What are Some Suggestions for Assisting a Patient During Mealtimes?

The patient's room should be adjusted for adequate but not glaring light and a comfortable temperature. If the patient wears glasses, make sure that they are on and are clean. If the patient is blind, the foods should be described before eating begins. Medication for pain or nausea is sometimes indicated for improved meal intake.

It is important that you, as the person assisting the patient, be relaxed and seated in a comfortable position. You should engage in pleasant neutral conversation, avoiding discussion of the patient's illness, or any criticism of the meal or the patient. This is a good time to teach the patient. Explain the reasons for the various foods offered, especially if the patient does not understand the diet well.

If the patient must be fed, you should alternate one food with another and offer liquids frequently. Offer liquids also whenever they are requested. Open containers, cut meat, and apply condiments if necessary to ensure an adequate intake. If the patient cannot eat a meal or a portion of the meal for valid reasons, such as the meat being too tough, offer to get substitute food (providing the patient's condition warrants it).

How Can the Hospital Diet be Modified for the Patient Who Cannot Eat Enough at Mealtimes?

A referral to a staff dietitian should be made for a patient who is losing weight or not gaining weight adequately. The person may be a candidate for:

- between-meal nourishments such as sandwiches, puddings, or milkshakes
- addition of high kilocalorie items on meal trays such as extra margarine, mayonnaise, gravy, or desserts
- liquid nutritional supplements with meal trays or between meals
- tube feedings or **total parenteral nutrition** (the provision of a special liquid nutrition mixture through an artery, see Chapter 14).

WHAT IS LONG-TERM CARE?

Long-term care consists of a whole group of medical and psychosocial activities and services designed to keep a person as independent as possible for as long as possible. Acute care is undertaken in a hospital setting, whereas long-term care is provided in a variety of settings. Currently, long-term care generally involves placement in a nursing home. As the cost of health care continues to rise, the setting increasingly is in the home. Services brought to the patient such as meals, home-health aide assistance, and public health nursing can help maintain a person's independence.

What are the Differences Between the Custodial and Restorative Approaches of Long-term Care?

The **custodial approach** or perspective is characterized by staff performing *for* the resident, resulting in a lack of progress on the part of the patient. In respect to nutrition, the resident who is wheelchair-bound may not be allowed independence in wheeling to the dining room, or may be fed instead of assisted, even though encouragement, adaptive feeding utensils, and transfer to a regular chair may promote independence. The **restorative approach** is characterized by allowing the resident to do things for himself or herself, such as ambulating independently to the dining area and self-feeding. The focus is on consumption of a balanced meal, appropriate food consistency, and where and how the meal is consumed. The dining atmosphere, quality of food, and the service provided are all conducive to rehabilitation.

TEAMWORK: THE OPTIMAL DELIVERY OF NUTRITION CARE IN AN INSTITUTIONAL SETTING

The institutional setting is the ideal place for implementation of the total health care team philosophy. Most, if not all, of the respective health care professionals are available for consultation by each team member. Recommendations for input by the various health care professionals should be documented in the patient charts and personal or verbal contact made. This form of communication will help ensure that patients receive the best care possible and do not accidentally "slip through the cracks." The nurse is in the ideal position to make sure all necessary health care professionals are consulted. There may be regular team meetings to help ensure effective coordination of patient care.

Various activities or interventions are needed to carry out plans to meet patient-centered nutritional goals. They include diet prescription, any necessary modification of food consistency, nutritional supplements, nutritional support, assistance and encouragement at mealtime, counseling, and advice about meeting the individual's nutritional needs after discharge. Implementation includes ongoing monitoring of laboratory data, weight records, and food and fluid intake.

Each member of the health care team has an opportunity to aid in implementing the nutrition care plan, whether it be in the form of encouraging the patient to eat, providing adaptive eating equipment, or providing encouragement to exercise and socialize.

HOW IS NUTRITIONAL STATUS ASSESSED?

As soon as the patient arrives at the institution, members of the health team proceed to gather pertinent and accurate information. Professionally standardized techniques are used in assessing three main areas: (1) dietary history, (2) anthropometry, and (3) biochemical and clinical data. The patient is weighed and several body measurements, including height, are taken. The nurse inquires about food intolerances and allergies. If family members are present, they may also contribute to the assessment by revealing the individual's past health and eating habits. The social worker writes the social history, which the dietitian uses in gathering dietary information. The physician's report of the physical examination; results of blood, urine, and skin tests; anthropometric measurements; and the diet history are equally important in assessing nutritional status, which is the first step in nutritional care planning. The data obtained are recorded and analyzed so that the professional can identify those individuals who may need prompt nutritional support and those who may need only a modified diet and counseling. Very often a person looks well nourished but through proper assessment is found to be in a high-risk state. Table 7–6 gives indicators of good and poor nutritional status.

Dietary History

There are many factors that influence a person's nutritional status, and they should be taken into account in a dietary history. Asking what types of foods the individual eats and how often—over at least a 24-hour period or ideally for an average of 3 to 7 days—will help the dietitian determine if the patient is in the habit of consuming the basic five food groups regularly. Appetite and weight changes may be significant and should be analyzed. There may also be a recent change in eating habits as a result of illness. Recent versus usual dietary intake should be noted. It is important to note if the patient has unintentionally lost more than 10 pounds within the last 6 months, but especially if there has been a more rapid weight loss. Chewing and swallowing difficulties can hamper the individual's intake of food and may thus be detrimental to nutritional status. A sore mouth and ill-fitting dentures are potential problems to be noted in the dietary history. Medications and illnesses, especially those involving the gastrointestinal tract, are noted because they may affect the appetite or nutrient utilization, or both. Elimination practices may indicate the need for additional roughage and liquids.

Cultural and religious food habits, food preferences, the impact of food and drug interactions, meal patterns, and lifestyle cannot be overlooked in planning nutritional care for an individual. The psychological significance of food needs to be considered. Food may have been used as a reward or withheld during punishment, which can affect why a person chooses specific foods to eat or to avoid. The fact that food tastes and habits cannot be changed overnight, or in some cases, ever, must be understood by the health care professional. Minor modification of the diet may be the best goal in some situations.

No nutrition care plan, including the therapeutic diet, will be effective if the meals are not eaten. The patient's own acceptance of the plan is as important a factor in recovery (or more important in some cases) as medication or physical treatment. Timing of medications in relation to mealtimes may need to be considered in order to promote better nutritional intake. Scheduling of tests in consideration of mealtime is also important. The

▲ TABLE 7-6

PHYSICAL SIGNS INDICATIVE OR SUGGESTIVE OF MALNUTRITION

	NORMAL APPEARANCE	SIGNS ASSOCIATED WITH MALNUTRITION	POSSIBLE DISORDER OR NUTRIENT DEFICIENCY	POSSIBLE NON-NUTRITIONAL PROBLEM
Hair	Shiny; firm; not easily plucked	Lack of natural shine; dull and dry Thin and sparse Dyspigmented Flag sign Easily plucked (no pain)	Kwashiorkor and, less commonly, marasmus	Excessive bleaching of hair Alopecia
Face	Skin color uniform; smooth, healthy appearance; not swollen	Nasolabial seborrhea (scaling of skin around nostrils) Swollen face (moon face) Paleness	Riboflavin Kwashiorkor	Acne vulgaris
Eyes	Bright, clear, shiny; no sores at corners of eyelids; membranes a healthy pink and moist; no prominent blood vessels or mound of tissue or sclera	Pale conjunctiva Bitot's spots Conjunctival xerosis (dryness) Corneal xerosis (dullness) Keratomalacia (softening of cornea) Redness and fissuring of eyelid corners Corneal arcus (white ring around eye) Xanthelasma (small yellowish lumps around eyes)	Anemia (e.g., iron) Vitamin A Riboflavin, pyridoxine Hyperlipidemia	Bloodshot eyes from exposure to weather, lack of sleep, smoke or alcohol
Lips	Smooth, not chapped or swollen	Angular cheilosis (white or pink lesions at corners of mouth)	Riboflavin	Excessive salivation from improper fitting dentures
Tongue	Deep red in appearance; not swollen or smooth	Magenta tongue (purplish) Filiform papillae atrophy or hypertrophy —red tongue	Riboflavin Folic acid Niacin	Leukoplakia
Teeth	No cavities; no pain; bright	Mottled enamel Caries (cavities) Missing teeth	Fluorosis Excessive sugar	Malocclusion Periodontal disease Health habits
Gums	Healthy; red; do not bleed; not swollen	Spongy, bleeding Receding gums	Vitamin C	Periodontal disease
Glands	Face not swollen	Thyroid enlargement (front of neck swollen) Parotid enlargement (cheeks become swollen)	Iodine Starvation Bulimia	Allergic or inflammatory enlargement of thyroid

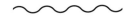

TABLE 7-6 *Continued*

PHYSICAL SIGNS INDICATIVE OR SUGGESTIVE OF MALNUTRITION

	NORMAL APPEARANCE	SIGNS ASSOCIATED WITH MALNUTRITION	POSSIBLE DISORDER OR NUTRIENT DEFICIENCY	POSSIBLE NON-NUTRITIONAL PROBLEM
Nervous system	Psychological stability; normal reflexes	Psychomotor changes	Kwashiorkor	
		Mental confusion	Thiamine	
		Sensory loss		
		Motor weakness		
		Loss of position sense		
		Loss of vibration		
		Loss of ankle and knee jerks	Thiamine	
		Burning and tingling of hands and feet (paresthesia)		
		Dementia	Niacin, vitamin B_{12}	

From Mahan CK, Arlin M: Krause's Food, Nutrition and Diet Therapy, 8th ed. Philadelphia, WB Saunders, 1992; p. 304.

nurse can be very helpful in arranging logistics of patient care while ensuring that the patient has adequate time and opportunity to eat meals. Some attention to food preferences, as much as is possible with the necessary dietary restrictions and limited hospital personnel facilities, needs to be made. Attention to the appearance and service of the food and the attitude of the person who serves it also contribute to the acceptance of the diet and the success of treatment.

Anthropometry

The science that deals with body measurements, such as size, weight, and proportions, is called **anthropometry.** It is especially useful in screening hospitalized patients who may have varying degrees of **protein-energy malnutrition** (kwashiorkor and marasmus are two forms, see Chapter 3). This condition is most likely to develop when the patient is under the stress of an acute illness or major surgery, at which time the desire or ability to eat is impaired. Risk of infection and complications may easily develop. It has been estimated that 50% or more of hospitalized patients suffer from malnutrition (Rombeau, 1993). This has been referred to as the "skeleton in the closet," as malnourished hospitalized patients have often gone unrecognized in the past. The nurse is in the ideal position to note patient dietary intake and changes in anthropometric or biochemical data in order to alert the physician or clinical dietitian to the need for more aggressive nutritional support.

WHO SHOULD BE ASSESSING ANTHROPOMETRY?

The nurse is in the best position to monitor patient weight status. It is especially important to regularly monitor weights of children (Fig. 7–1), and any undesirable changes should be reported to the staff dietitian. Monitor-

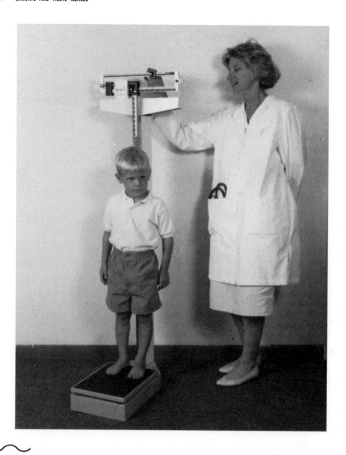

▲ F I G U R E   7 - 1

Monitoring patient weight. (From Jarvis C: Physical Examination and Health Assessment. Philadelphia, WB Saunders Co., 1992, p. 186.

ing of weight should be done at least on a weekly basis. High-risk patients can benefit from daily weight monitoring in order to aggressively treat weight problems. Bed scales are sometimes available for weight monitoring (Fig. 7–2).

The dietitian is the professional trained in anthropometry; he or she takes measurements of elbow breadth, skin-fold thickness, and mid-upper arm circumference to help determine the extent of the body's fat and protein stores in relation to body frame size and height. A discussion of various anthropometric measurements follows.

TRICEPS SKIN FOLD.　**Triceps skin fold** is an index of the body's fat or energy stores. A low skin-fold thickness measurement may indicate malnutrition. Figure 7–3 shows how the measurement is taken. This technique is used for both men and women. The most common site for

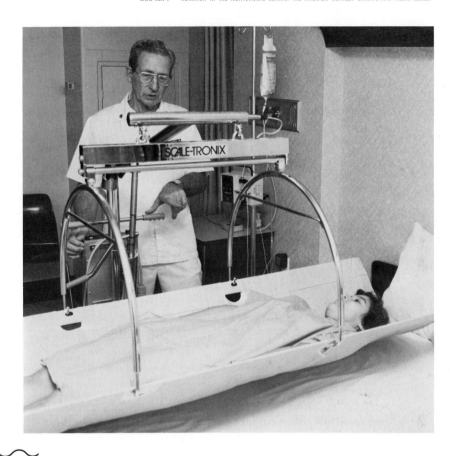

▲ F I G U R E   7 - 2

Bed scales will provide accurate weight for the patient unable to stand or get out of
bed. (Courtesy of the Faxton Hospital, Utica, NY.)

measuring skin-fold thickness is the posterior side of the upper arm at the
midpoint. Accuracy and consistency of measurement are paramount.

MID-ARM CIRCUMFERENCE.   Mid-arm circumference indicates
the level of the body's protein stores, which are found mainly in the
muscles. The nondominant arm is flexed at a 90-degree angle, and the
circumference is measured with a nonstretchable measuring tape after
the midpoint of the upper arm is determined (see Fig. 7–3).

ELBOW BREADTH.   Elbow breadth determines body frame size. It is
a reliable measurement that changes little with age and is not affected
by body fat stores. The elbow breadth measurement is helpful in determining desirable weight ranges, since body frame size reflects factors that
influence weight, such as bone thickness, muscularity, and length of trunk
in relation to total height. Calipers are applied to either side of the two

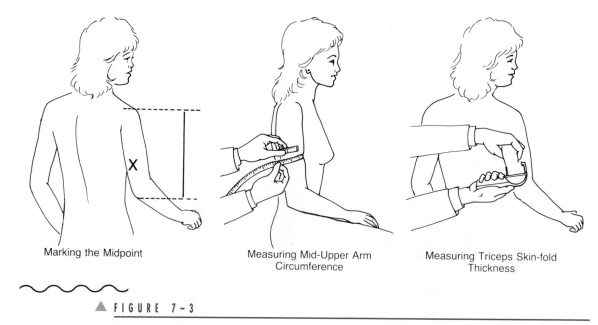

Marking the Midpoint   Measuring Mid-Upper Arm   Measuring Triceps Skin-fold
                                    Circumference   Thickness

▲ FIGURE 7-3

Measuring mid-upper arm circumference and triceps skin-fold thickness (the same procedure is used for men).

prominent bones of the elbow while the forearm is bent upward at a 90-degree angle. The fingers are straight and the inside of the wrist is turned toward the body. See Appendix 14 for frame size measurements.

BODY WEIGHT. This measurement is often expressed as relative weight, desirable weight, or as a percentage of usual weight. Any assessment of body weight can be misleading if the patient is retaining fluid or is dehydrated. Weight loss is best expressed in terms of percentage of weight change:

$$\text{Usual weight} - \text{present weight} \div \text{usual weight} \times 100$$

or

$$\text{Loss of weight in kilograms} \div \text{usual weight in kilograms} \times 100$$

Anthropometric measurements are not as precise as biochemical methods for assessing nutritional status, but they are inexpensive, noninvasive, and easily obtained. According to some clinical researchers, accurate body composition measurements are more difficult to obtain for obese people than for thin people because of the compression factor involving the use of the calipers. Measurements are more likely to be accurate if the subject is thin (Forbes and Griffiths, 1988). However, anthropometric measurements are very useful because they can help justify the use of special nutritional support when a patient is shown to be at risk for development of protein-energy malnutrition.

Biochemical and
Clinical Data

Several lab tests of the blood, urine, and skin are used in assessing nutritional status. Protein-energy malnutrition in its various forms can be detected by monitoring the blood serum levels of albumin, transferrin, and lymphocytes. These elements are all associated with body protein status. A person's level of immunity is discovered with skin antigen tests.

A nitrogen balance study can also be helpful in determining nutritional status. A negative nitrogen balance signifies that the body is using some of its protein reserves for energy. Nitrogen balance is determined from the urinary urea nitrogen content of a 24-hour urine collection. Clinical dietitians can calculate nitrogen balance with this information and determine patient protein needs to promote healing or preserve lean muscle mass.

Certain vitamin and mineral deficiencies may also be detected with lab tests when the tests are evaluated in conjunction with physical findings and dietary assessment of usual intake.

A summary of the nutrition assessment process is shown in Table 7–7. A nutrition assessment form is found in Figure 7–4.

HOW IS THE NUTRITION CARE PLAN IMPLEMENTED AND EVALUATED?

To carry out plans to meet patient-centered nutritional goals, various activities or interventions are needed. These activities include the diet prescription, any necessary modification of food consistency, nutritional supplements, nutritional support, assistance and encouragement at mealtime, and nutrition counseling in preparation for discharge.

▲   TABLE 7-7

SUMMARY OF THE NUTRITIONAL ASSESSMENT PROCESS

AREA OF SCREENING	METHOD	INFORMATION GATHERED
Diet history	Patient family interview	Food preferences and intolerances; taste, appetite, and recent weight changes; desired weight and usual weight; estimation of typical kilocalorie and nutrient intake
Clinical	Physical examination	Indicators of malnutrition: appearance of hair, skin, oral cavity, fingernails, presence of edema
	Radiography	Skeletal condition
	Anthropometry	Level of protein and fat reserves in the body, body frame size, weight, and height
Biochemical	Laboratory tests of blood and urine	Composition of blood to compare with normal ranges for hemoglobin, albumin, transferrin, total plasma protein, and so on; nitrogen content in 24-hour urinary output
	Skin tests	Immunity to certain diseases, response to antigens; possible identification of vitamin and mineral deficiencies

Name _____ Date of Birth _____ Male/Female

Diet Prescription _____ Diagnosis _____

Activity Level _____ Appetite _____

Medications   Meal Pattern

                                              B   L   S

Food Preferences: Food Intolerances/Dislikes:

_____

Clinical Data: Skin Condition _____ Edema _____

Impairments: Eyesight _____ Hearing _____ Speech _____ Taste _____

               Chewing and Swallowing Ability _____

Present Weight _____ Usual Weight _____ Desired Weight Range _____

Elbow Breadth _____ Midarm Circumference _____ Triceps Skin Fold_____

Height _____

Meal Observation: Percentage of food consumed _____ Fluid intake _____ ml

               Type of assistance needed _____

               Affective response to food _____

Biochemical Data:

Serum laboratory values: _____

_____

▲ FIGURE 7-4

Sample nutrition assessment and care plan.

Urinalysis: _____

Skin Tests: _____

Evaluation and Recommendation:

Problem/Need	Intervention	By Whom	Goal	Response/Date

By: _____ Title: _____

Date: _____

▲ FIGURE 7-4 *Continued*

Evaluation is achieved through observation of the individual's condition and acceptance of dietary changes. Weight status and improvements in lab values must also be evaluated. New methods for achieving a nutritional goal can then be tried and evaluated. Progress should be written in the medical record. Figure 7–4 shows a sample nutrition assessment and planning form that may be used.

FOOD AND DRUG INTERACTIONS

Why are Food and Drug Interactions Considered in the Nutritional Care Planning Process?

The health care team must be aware of the many factors that can adversely affect a person's nutritional status, including the effects of drugs on nutrient absorption, excretion, and metabolism, especially when long-term and multiple-drug therapy is necessary (Table 7–8). Children, elderly persons, chronically ill persons, and those with a marginal or inadequate nutrient intake are most susceptible to drug-induced nutritional deficiencies. A good nutritional status and a nutritious diet can reduce this risk. A proper diet can also reduce the risk of any altered effectiveness of drugs. The success of a patient's treatment often depends on the effectiveness of medications. The registered dietitian can provide specific dietary instructions to the patient as to when to take medications in relation to meals and which foods, if any, must be avoided. The staff pharmacist may also need to be consulted for multiple medication regimens.

▲ **TABLE 7-8**

DRUG-NUTRIENT INTERACTIONS*

DRUGS	VITAMINS/MINERALS DEPLETED	SUGGESTED FOODS TO EAT	FOODS TO AVOID
Analgesics			
Aspirin	Folic Acid	Yeast, wheat germ, whole grains, enriched breads, corn, cornmeal, egg yolk, legumes, nuts, organ meats, lean pork, almonds, milk and dairy products, leafy vegetables, oysters	Crackers, jellies, syrups, other processed high-carbohydrate foods
	Iron	Liver, fortified cocoa, lentils, lean roast beef, nuts, molasses, apricots, enriched breads and cereals, dark green leafy vegetables, pork	
	Vitamin C	Black currants, broccoli, Brussels sprouts, raw green cabbage, cauliflower, leafy green vegetables, paprika, pimentos, strawberries, citrus fruits	
Antacids			
Aluminum hydroxide (Amphojel)	Phosphorus, thiamine	Poultry, fish, meats, enriched breads, cereals, nuts, legumes, milk and milk products	Alcoholic beverages
Bicarbonate (Tums)	Iron, thiamine	Same as Analgesics	Alcoholic beverages; for sodium bicarbonate, anything high in sodium
Antibiotics			
Penicillins	Iron, potassium	Same as Analgesics; banana, citrus, and other high-potassium foods	*Note:* Avoid foods high in iron for at least 2 hours after taking any antibiotic
Tetracyclines	Vitamin C; B vitamins	Same as Analgesics	Do not take with food or any dairy products
Neomycins	Vitamin B$_{12}$	Liver, kidney, milk, muscle meats, fish	Alcoholic beverages
	Vitamin A and D, iron	Fish-liver oils, leafy green vegetables, apricots, beet tops, butter, deep orange vegetables, cheese, egg yolk, deep orange fruits (peaches, mangos, papayas), milk	

▲ **T A B L E   7 - 8**

DRUG–NUTRIENT INTERACTIONS* *Continued*

DRUGS	VITAMINS/MINERALS DEPLETED	SUGGESTED FOODS TO EAT	FOODS TO AVOID
Anticoagulants			
Coumadin, Dicumarol			Alcoholic beverages, caffeine, fried or boiled onions, leafy green vegetables, liver
Antidiabetic Drugs			
			Excessive sugar, alcohol
Antihypertensive Drugs			
	Vitamin K	Leafy vegetables	Excessive imported licorice
Digitalis			
Cardiovascular	Vitamin K, potassium	Same as Antihypertensive Drugs; foods high in potassium (see Diuretics)	Foods high in sodium, high-fiber foods, prune juice, herbal teas
	Magnesium	Nuts, legumes, whole grains, leafy vegetables, water	
Diuretics			
Potassium-wasting	Potassium	Apricots, molasses, dates, bananas, milk, nuts, bamboo shoots, prunes, mushrooms, grapefruit, oranges	Alcoholic beverages
Triamterene (potassium-sparing)	Folic acid	Same as Analgesics	Foods high in potassium
Gantrisin			
(Anti-infective)	Folic acid, vitamin K, other B vitamins	Same as Analgesics	Alcoholic beverages
Laxatives			
Mineral oil (not currently recommended as a laxative but included because of its depletion effect on nutrients)	Vitamin A	Same as Antibiotics	Fried greasy foods, fatty foods
	Vitamin D	Yeast, milk and milk products, fish-liver oils, salmon, sardines, egg yolk, butter	
	Vitamin K	See Antihypertensive Drugs	

(Table continued on following page)

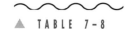

▲ T A B L E   7 - 8

DRUG–NUTRIENT INTERACTIONS*   *Continued*

DRUGS	VITAMINS/MINERALS DEPLETED	SUGGESTED FOODS TO EAT	FOODS TO AVOID
	Calcium	Milk, cheese, ice cream, leafy green vegetables, Brazil nuts, legumes, clams, oysters, tofu, whole grains, water	
Phenolphthalein	Phosphorus; vitamins A, D, and K	Same as Antacids and Laxatives	
Dioctyl sodium sulfo-succinate (stool softener)	Vitamin A	Same as Antacids and Laxatives	
Bisacodyl	Potassium	Same as Diuretics	Fried, greasy food, fatty foods, do not take *with* milk and milk products
Levodopa	Vitamin C, Vitamin B$_{12}$	Same as most foods under Analgesics; note those to avoid	Coffee, dry skim milk, beans, oatmeal, wheat germ, beef liver, pork, tuna, sweet potatoes, peas, bacon, avocado, malted milk, cheese, wine
Oral Contraceptives			
Estrogen-containing	Thiamine, folic acid, riboflavin	See Analgesics (folic acid)	
	Vitamin B$_6$	Wheat germ, corn, soybeans, liver, meat, whole grains, peanuts	
	Vitamin B$_{12}$	See Antibiotics, Analgesics	
Thyroxine			
			Excessive soy-protein products, kale, cabbage, carrots, cauliflower, spinach, pears, peaches, Brussels sprouts, turnips
Tranquilizers			
Barbiturates	Folic acid	See Analgesics	Alcoholic beverages

* Perhaps vitamins or minerals in foods will be adversely affected by prescribed drugs. Check with the physician—a vitamin/mineral supplement may be necessary.

From Resource Kit for Modified Diets—Nutrition Education Materials published by the American Dietetic Association, Chicago, Illinois.

How Do Drugs Affect Nutrient Absorption?

Drugs may affect absorption of nutrients by damaging the intestinal mucosa, by binding with nutrients, or by decreasing the availability of bile acid, which would inhibit the absorption of the fat-soluble vitamins. Folate absorption is decreased by the use of the anti-inflammatory agent sulfasalazine, but rather than the use of folate supplements, a varied and adequate diet should be encouraged.

How Do Food and Nutrients Affect Drug Action?

Food and some beverages, such as coffee or cola drinks, as well as specific nutrients can adversely affect drug action. For example, natural licorice in large quantities can complicate treatment in patients receiving antihypertensive agents because licorice can cause sodium retention, which could result in edema and hypertension.

How Do Food and Vitamin Supplements Affect Drug Action?

Some patients benefit from nutritional supplements, but the health professional needs to be aware of potential interaction with medications (Table 7–9). Large amounts of vitamin K in a supplement, for example, can reduce the effectiveness of anticoagulants. Tetracycline should not be administered at the same time as a mineral supplement, since the absorption of the minerals would be inhibited.

How Do Drugs Affect Nutrient Excretion?

Certain drugs such as **diuretics** (medications that cause fluid loss) can deplete potassium (e.g., furosemide, thiazide). A sodium-restricted diet and potassium-rich foods are often prescribed. Potassium-depleting medications often induce hyperglycemia with a resultant need to follow a diabetic diet. When a diuretic and digitalis are given together, two conditions may result—hypokalemia and hypomagnesemia—and digitalis toxicity must be guarded against. It must be remembered, however, that other diuretics such as spironolactone are potassium-conserving, in which case extra dietary potassium is not necessary and may even create a problem.

How Do Drugs Affect Nutrient Metabolism?

Certain drugs bind with enzymes and affect the metabolism of some nutrients. For example, long-term ingestion of pyrimethamine, an antimalarial drug, will likely produce **megaloblastic anemia** (a form of anemia often associated with lack of vitamin B_{12}, or folic acid or folacin), because it antagonizes folacin. Phenobarbital and phenytoin, which are used in the treatment of epilepsy, can increase bone demineralization. Ingestion of adequate dietary vitamin D should be encouraged to promote the absorption of calcium.

Can Drugs Cause Weight Gain and Electrolyte Imbalance?

Weight gain associated with the use of medications such as steroidal, antihypertensive, and anti-inflammatory agents occurs frequently because of sodium or water retention. A sodium-restricted diet may be prescribed along with a diuretic for treating the edema due to sodium retention. Potassium-rich foods may also be necessary to prevent electrolyte imbalance (see Table 7–5). All **neuroleptic drugs** (drugs used in psychiatric illness because of their tranquilizing effect) have an effect on appetite, which may result in weight gain.

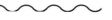

▲ TABLE 7-9

DRUGS THAT INTERACT WITH VITAMINS AND MINERALS

	CLINICAL CONSEQUENCES	NURSING CONSIDERATIONS
Anticoagulants interact with		
Vitamin C	Large doses of ascorbic acid—3 g or more—may inhibit absorption of warfarin (Coumadin, Panwarfin, Sofarin), lowering plasma levels of the drug. That in turn can reduce the drug's anticoagulant effect.	If prothrombin time decreases in patients taking warfarin and vitamin C, the vitamin may have to be discontinued or the vitamin dose lowered.
Vitamin E	Very large doses of vitamin E—1200 IU a day—may increase warfarin's anticoagulant effects and the risk of bleeding.	Advise patients taking warfarin to avoid vitamin E supplements, unless a doctor prescribes them.
Vitamin K	If patients taking warfarin or dicumarol increase their intake of green, leafy vegetables or other foods rich in vitamin K, prothrombin time may decrease. A diet that's low in the vitamin, on the other hand, may prolong PT and increase the risk of hemorrhage.	Caution patients on anticoagulant therapy not to significantly increase or decrease their intake of foods rich in vitamin K, particularly spinach, kale, cabbage, cauliflower, and liver.
Anticonvulsants interact with		
Folic acid	Prolonged use of phenytoin (Dilantin), phenobarbital, or primidone (Myidone, Mysoline) may cause folic acid deficiency, bringing on megaloblastic anemia, depression, apathy, and, on rare occasions, dementia. However, folate supplements may interfere with the drugs' effects, increasing the risk of seizures.	Check serum and RBC folic acid levels periodically. If folate supplements are needed to correct anemia, the daily dose should not exceed 1 mg. The doctor may increase the anticonvulsant dosage accordingly.
Vitamin D	Long-term therapy with phenytoin (Dilantin) or phenobarbital can cause vitamin D deficiency by inactivating the vitamin in the liver and increasing its biliary excretion.	Because vitamin D deficiency inhibits calcium absorption, serum calcium levels should be monitored. Also watch for signs and symptoms of osteomalacia: increased serum alkaline phosphatase, bone pain in the back, thighs, shoulders, and ribs, and muscle weakness in the legs. Patients on phenytoin or phenobarbital should take 400 to 800 IU of vitamin D daily and maintain a diet rich in calcium.

▲ TABLE 7-9

DRUGS THAT INTERACT WITH VITAMINS AND MINERALS   *Continued*

	CLINICAL CONSEQUENCES	NURSING CONSIDERATIONS
Antipsychotics interact with		
Vitamin B$_2$	Chlorpromazine (Thoradol, Thor-Prom, Thorazine), fluphenazine (Permitil, Prolixin), and thioridazine (Mellaril) may cause a mild vitamin B$_2$ deficiency by interfering with the vitamin's metabolism.	Encourage a diet rich in B vitamins, including milk, cheese, and green, leafy vegetables. Watch for early signs of B$_2$ deficiency, including sore, burning lips, tongue, and mouth; photophobia; and blurred vision. Administer vitamin B$_2$ supplements, as ordered, if a deficit develops. Severe depletion can bring on angular stomatitis—cracks at the corners of the mouth—and seborrheic dermatitis in the nasolabial folds.
Bile acid sequestrants interact with		
Beta carotene	The cholesterol-lowering agents cholestyramine (Questran) and colestipol (Colestid) can cause deficiencies in beta carotene, a vitamin A precursor, and other fat-soluble vitamins, by binding bile acids, which in turn interferes with the bile-dependent absorption of fat-soluble vitamins.	Patients may need beta carotene supplements if signs and symptoms of a vitamin A deficiency—night blindness, and dry, scaly, rough skin—develop.
Iron	Patients taking the cholesterol-lowering agents cholestyramine and colestipol may not respond to iron supplements because the drugs bind to iron in the gastrointestinal tract, inhibiting its absorption.	Advise patients to take iron supplements at least 1 hour before or 4 to 6 hours after taking cholestyramine or colestipol.
Cephalosporins interact with		
Vitamin K	Cefamandole (Mandol), cefotetan (Cefotan), cefoperazone (Cefobid), and moxalactam (Moxam) can cause vitamin K deficiency and subsequent bleeding by destroying the intestinal flora that make the vitamin.	Monitor prothrombin time. If bleeding occurs, stop the drug and administer vitamin K IM, as ordered. Elderly patients and those with malnutrition, renal impairment, or hepatic impairment are at high risk for bleeding and may require prophylactic vitamin K.

(Table continued on following page)

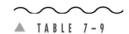

▲ T A B L E   7 - 9

DRUGS THAT INTERACT WITH VITAMINS AND MINERALS *Continued*

	CLINICAL CONSEQUENCES	NURSING CONSIDERATIONS
Chloramphenicol (Chloromycetin) interacts with		
Vitamin B$_{12}$	Patients who take this antibiotic and parenteral B$_{12}$ (cyanocobalamin) for pernicious anemia may not respond to the vitamin because the drug inhibits maturation of RBC precursors in the bone marrow.	Monitor reticulocyte count closely. If it doesn't improve during vitamin B$_{12}$ therapy, the doctor may have to switch to another antibiotic.
Iron	Patients with iron-deficiency anemia may not respond to iron supplements if they're taking chloramphenicol.	If the patient cannot be switched to another antibiotic, higher doses of iron may be needed.
Cisplatin (Platinol) interacts with		
Magnesium	This antineoplastic agent can cause magnesium deficiency by increasing the urinary excretion of the mineral.	Monitor serum Mg levels, and watch for signs and symptoms of a deficiency—muscle spasms, depression, premature ventricular beats, and tachycardia. Encourage a Mg-rich diet including nuts, fish, whole-grain breads and cereals, and green, leafy vegetables. If cisplatin-induced nausea makes that impossible, Mg supplements—the usual daily dose is 350 mg—may be needed.
Digoxin (Lanoxin, Lanoxicaps) interacts with		
Magnesium	By increasing urinary excretion of watch magnesium, digoxin can cause Mg deficiency, which in turn increases the drug's toxicity.	Monitor serum Mg levels and for signs of a deficiency. Instruct patients on digoxin to avoid alcohol, which increases Mg excretion.
Diuretics interact with		
Vitamin B$_1$	Loop diuretics such as furosemide (Lasix) can cause a B$_1$ deficiency by increasing urinary excretion of the vitamin.	Patients may need vitamin B$_1$ supplements if signs of a deficiency develop; monitor blood vitamin levels for a therapeutic response. A mild deficit can cause confusion, muscle weakness and tenderness, fatigue, and depression. More severe depletion causes paralysis and edema in the legs and congestive heart failure.

▲ TABLE 7-9

DRUGS THAT INTERACT WITH VITAMINS AND MINERALS   *Continued*

CLINICAL CONSEQUENCES	NURSING CONSIDERATIONS
Isoniazid (INH, Laniazid, others) interacts with	
Vitamin B$_6$ — Patients taking this drug may develop vitamin B$_6$ deficiency because it blocks the vitamin's conversion to its active form and increases its urinary excretion.	Monitor closely for convulsions and peripheral neuropathy, a particular risk for diabetics and alcoholics. Administer 25 mg/day of vitamin B$_6$, as ordered, as prophylaxis.
Isotretinoin (Accutane) interacts with	
Vitamin A — Combining isotretinoin—used to treat severe cystic acne—and vitamin A supplements can cause vitamin A and drug toxicity. Both the drug and the vitamin are members of the retinoid family, so the combination increases the risk of retinoid overload.	Advise patients taking the drug to avoid vitamin A and multivitamin supplements. Report signs and symptoms of retinoid toxicity: headache, nausea, vomiting, elevated liver enzymes, hair loss, hepatomegaly, and dry, fissured skin.
Levodopa (Larodopa, Dopar) interacts with	
Vitamin B$_6$ — B$_6$ supplements can diminish the therapeutic effects of this anti-Parkinsonian drug by accelerating its metabolic breakdown, reducing the amount that reaches the brain.	Advise patients on levodopa not to take vitamin B$_6$ supplements. Patients who take Sinemet, a combination of carbidopa and levodopa that isn't affected by the vitamin, may take the supplements.
Lithium (Eskalith, Lithane, others) interacts with	
Sodium — The risk of lithium toxicity increases when a patient goes on a low-sodium regimen, while a sudden increase in salt may blunt drug action.	Advise patients on lithium to maintain their normal sodium intake. If restrictions are required, watch for and report early signs of lithium toxicity—nausea, abdominal pain, diarrhea, vomiting, sedation, and mild tremor. More severe reactions include extreme thirst, frequent urination, an enlarged thyroid gland, hypotension, and seizures.
Methotrexate (Folex, Mexate, others) interacts with	
Folic acid — The drug can cause folic acid depletion, leading to megaloblastic anemia.	Monitor patients for evidence of megaloblastic anemia: pallor, irritability, dyspnea, glossitis, low RBC count, and increased mean corpuscular volume (MCV). Patients on long-term therapy with large doses of methotrexate will probably need leucovorin (Wellcovorin), an activated form of folic acid.

(Table continued on following page)

▲ T A B L E 7 - 9

DRUGS THAT INTERACT WITH VITAMINS AND MINERALS   *Continued*

	CLINICAL CONSEQUENCES	NURSING CONSIDERATIONS
Pentamidine (Pentam 300, NebuPent) interacts with		
Folic acid	The drug, taken by HIV-positive patients for the prevention and treatment of *Pneumocystis carinii* pneumonia (PCP), can cause folic acid deficiency and subsequent megaloblastic anemia.	Monitor patients for signs of megaloblastic anemia. Patients may need folic acid supplements if they're on long-term pentamidine therapy.
Pyrimethamine (Daraprim) interacts with		
Folic acid	This anti-parasitic agent, which is used to treat toxoplasmosis, can cause folic acid deficiency and subsequent megaloblastic anemia.	Monitor patients for megaloblastic anemia. The doctor may order 3 to 9 mg IM of leucovorin daily to be administered with pyrimethamine as prophylaxis.
Trimethoprim (Proloprim, Trimpex, and contained in Bactrim and Septra) interacts with		
Folic acid	Prolonged use of trimethoprim, an antibiotic used to treat PCP and urinary tract infection, may cause mild folate depletion by blocking an enzyme that activates folic acid.	The drug is contraindicated in patients with folic-acid deficiency anemia. Patients on long-term trimethoprim therapy should receive folate supplements.
Verapamil (Calan, Isoptin) interacts with		
Calcium	Calcium supplements may reduce the drug's therapeutic effect.	If the patient must take IV or oral calcium, monitor closely for elevated BP and arrhythmias.

From Cerrato PL, Vitamins and Minerals. RN, June 1993, pp. 29–32. © Medical Economics Publishing, Montvale, NJ. Reprinted by permission.

What are Some Dietary Suggestions to Aid in the Relief of Drug Side Effects?

LOSS OF APPETITE

1. Question the patient regarding factors contributing to appetite loss.
2. If early satiety occurs, offer small, frequent, attractive meals or snacks.
3. Enhance flavors by using seasonings. Requests can be made from the dietary department for small containers of spices to be kept at the patient's bedside.
4. Encourage weakened patients to select easy-to-chew menu items.
5. Consider liquid nutrition supplements until the appetite returns.

TASTE/SMELL DYSFUNCTION

1. Offer sugarless gum or candy, water, or lemon juice as mouth rinses.
2. Encourage good oral hygiene before and after meals.

DRY OR SORE MOUTH

1. Avoid dry, acidic, spicy, or salty foods. Moisten foods in liquids (milk, gravy).

2. Offer moist, soft foods such as custards, casseroles, or mashed potatoes.

3. Suggest that the patient lick or suck ice chips. Add cold foods such as ice cream or sherbet to menu selections.

4. Offer warm water rinses or saliva substitutes.

5. Stress good oral hygiene. Lack of saliva production can quickly induce severe dental caries.

APPETITE STIMULATION OR WEIGHT GAIN

1. Encourage a slow rate of eating with increased chewing.

2. Encourage low-calorie foods to abate hunger.

3. Encourage adequate fiber intake, which may help induce satiety (a sense of fullness).

NAUSEA

1. Respect patients' food preferences. If a food item does not sound appealing to a patient, it should not be forced. Often what patients think will agree with their system is well tolerated.

2. Provide small or even half portions with between-meal nourishments.

3. Cold foods may be better tolerated than hot foods.

4. Emphasize low-fat foods, which will leave the stomach earlier than greasy foods.

5. Monitor for weight loss to determine if more aggressive nutritional support is warranted.

6. Collaborate with the physician to prescribe antiemetics ½ hour before meals.

DIARRHEA

1. Focus on fluid and electrolyte replacement by providing potassium-rich fruit juices and sodium through broths or other foods. Pedialyte is often used with children. Sports drinks such as Gatorade may be appropriate for adults.

2. A clear liquid diet may be necessary for 24 hours or longer to provide bowel rest. Low-residue, lactose-free liquid supplements may be tolerated and needed for extended bowel rest.

3. Return to normal diet gradually, being careful of high-roughage foods.

FLATULENCE (GASTROINTESTINAL GAS)

1. Evaluate possible causes of ingested air such as eating fast, chewing gum, or drinking through a straw.

2. Avoid vegetables and fruits known to cause gas such as beans, cabbage, cauliflower, and broccoli. Consider offering an enzyme product known as "Beano" to help digestion and thereby reduce gas production.

3. Evaluate for lactose intolerance and provide a low-lactose diet as warranted.

CONSTIPATION

1. Evaluate if prolonged reliance on chemical laxatives has led to poor bowel reflexes.

2. Evaluate the diet for fiber and water content.

3. Encourage adequate intake of fiber or other non-laxative bulking agents and water. Promote regular exercise. (Smith, 1993).

WHAT IS DISCHARGE PLANNING?

The last step in the nutrition care planning process, called discharge planning, begins as soon as the patient is admitted to the health care facility. By the time the patient is ready to leave, needs have already been assessed

Name: _____ Age: _____ Birthdate: _____

Weight: _____ Height: _____

Diagnosis: _____

_____

Diet: _____

Meal Pattern: _____

Appetite: _____

Approximate Caloric Intake: _____

Food Preferences

Beverage: _____

Meat & Meat Sub: _____

Vegetables: _____

Fruit: _____

Other: _____

Allergies: _____ Dislikes: _____

Recommendations (Include special needs in relation to weight, medications, present illness)

_____

_____

Signature _____

Date _____

▲ FIGURE 7-5

Sample nutrition discharge summary form.

and nutritional status evaluated, and changes have been made in the nutrition care plan in response to the patient's progress. Before developing a final meal plan, input is gained from the patient so that goals are mutually
determined. This helps in promoting dietary compliance after discharge.
Recommendations should also be in line with the needs of other family
members. Dietary instruction should include counseling on weight control,
diet in relation to the patient's medications and physical condition, and a
review of the foods allowed and avoided on a modified dietary regime. It
needs to be stressed to the patient that one dietary instruction may not be
sufficient for long-term dietary modification. Identification of an ongoing
support system for change should be made whether it is referral to an outpatient dietitian or other community program. Figure 7–5 shows a sample
nutrition discharge summary form.

STUDY QUESTIONS AND ACTIVITIES

1. Name six ways the basic normal diet is modified for therapeutic
   purposes.
2. Name six considerations to remember in meal service. How would
   you as a nurse talk with Mrs. Bernardo from the case study during
   mealtimes? What would you need to avoid saying in order to promote a pleasant meal environment and a good dietary intake?
3. What are some possible effects of her hospital admission on Mrs.
   Bernardo's family?
4. List some characteristics of good and poor nutritional status that may
   be noted in the clinical area of assessment.
5. Why should food and drug interactions be considered in the assessment process?
6. Complete a nutrition assessment and care plan form on Maria
   Bernardo, as described in the opening case study, using Figure
   7–4. Comment on ways the various health care team members
   could be involved in nutrition care of the patient in the institution.
7. List appropriate reasons to request a dietary consultation by a dietitian for a patient.
8. Calculate the percentage of weight change for an individual who
   currently weighs 110 pounds and whose usual weight is 130
   pounds.
9. If a man who is 5'10" has an elbow breadth of 2.5 inches, what is
   his body frame size? (Refer to Appendix 14.)
10. How is protein-energy malnutrition detected in a hospital patient?
11. If a patient is placed on a low-protein diet, what groups of the Food
    Guide Pyramid will be affected? What advice could be given to fol-
    low a low-protein diet without jeopardizing nutritional intake?

REFERENCES

Forbes G, Griffiths H: Arm muscle plus bone area: Anthropometry and CAT scan compared. Am J Clin Nutr 1988; 47:929.

Perket S, Swartz A: Back to the Table. Program presented in Utica, NY, June 6, 1988.

Rombeau JL, Caldwell MD: Clinical Nutrition: Parenteral Nutrition, 2nd ed. Philadelphia, WB Saunders, 1993; p. 285.

Smith CH: In Powers and Moore's Food Medication Interactions, 8th ed., edited by Pronsky ZM. Published and distributed by Food-Medication Interactions, Pottstown, PA, 1993; pp. 15–18.

CARDIOVASCULAR DISEASE

OBJECTIVES

After completing this chapter, you should be able to:
- Identify risk factors related to the development of cardiovascular disease
- Describe dietary prevention and treatment of cardiovascular disease and hypertension
- Describe the rationale for lowering saturated fat to prevent cardiovascular disease
- Identify foods appropriate for a low-cholesterol/low–saturated fat diet
- List foods low in sodium
- Describe the role of the nurse or other health care professional in the prevention and
  management of cardiovascular disease

TERMS TO IDENTIFY

Antioxidants	Edema	Myocardial infarction (MI)
Arteriosclerosis	Endocardium	Myocardium
Cardiovascular disease (CVD)	Hypercholesterolemia	National Cholesterol Education Program (NCEP)
Cerebrovascular accident (CVA)	Hypertension	
	Lipids	
Congestive heart failure (CHF)	Lipoprotein	Pericardium
	Morbidity	Sodium
Coronary thrombosis	Mortality	Trans fatty acids

A FAMILY'S PERSPECTIVE ON NUTRITION

Well, here he was. At least he was only in the hospital lab, Tony Bernardo thought to himself. What a way to start the day. And he was starving after that 12-hour fast. But Dr. Shaw said it was important to know his lipids. Lipids, what did the doctor say they were? Something about good cholesterol and bad cholesterol. But wasn't all cholesterol bad? Eventually he would understand what was happening inside his body.

INTRODUCTION

If you are like most people, you probably do not worry about heart disease. In a national survey of women, only 4% cited heart disease as the most serious health problem facing them even though it is currently the deadliest disease for women in general (Environmental Nutrition, 1993). **Cardiovascular disease (CVD),** or more simply heart disease, kills more people than all forms of cancer combined and has been the leading cause of death since the 1950s (American Heart Association, 1991). Although the words *sugar, additives,* and *preservatives* cause alarm in many individuals, it is only now that Americans are coming to appreciate that the fat content of their diets plays a leading role in the development, or prevention, of CVD. The good news is that there has been progress in preventing the **mortality** (death) and **morbidity** (effects of disease) of heart disease. The proportion of Americans with high cholesterol has dropped from 26 to 20 per cent since 1978, according to the National Center for Health Statistics (Food Insight, 1993).

It remains a major challenge, however, to alter the eating habits of the public. The aim is to reduce fat intake, particularly saturated fat and cholesterol. Part of the challenge is to convince the public that low-fat eating can be enjoyable. To this end, the renowned chef Julia Child has joined forces with the American Dietetic Association to promote the concept that "healthy food can be tasty" and "tasty food can be healthy." Reducing fat intake is generally easier than most people realize. And small changes in eating habits can have a significant impact on **lipids** (different fats in the blood).

Although it is true that some individuals are not prone to CVD, the general population will benefit from dietary changes that lower the total fat content—specifically cholesterol and saturated fat—and reduce sodium. However, individual guidance should complement the general guidelines to allow for specific needs, for example, in frail, elderly persons or terminally ill patients who may need to rely on high-fat foods for adequate kilocalorie intake. For everyone, attempts to lower the risk of CVD should not take precedence over sound nutritional intake. Meat, milk, and cheese are still important to one's diet; however, through moderation and emphasis on low-fat and low-sodium alternatives, a healthy balance can result. Figure 8–1 shows the Eating Plan Tips of the American Heart Association

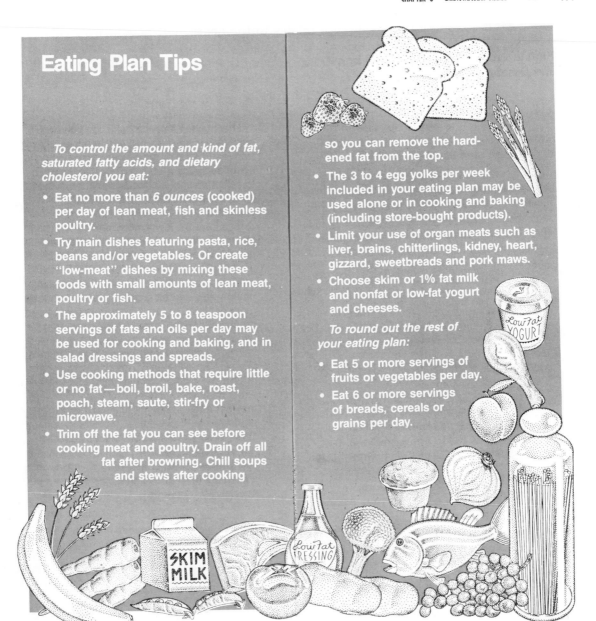

Eating Plan Tips

To control the amount and kind of fat, saturated fatty acids, and dietary cholesterol you eat:

- Eat no more than *6 ounces* (cooked) per day of lean meat, fish and skinless poultry.

- Try main dishes featuring pasta, rice, beans and/or vegetables. Or create "low-meat" dishes by mixing these foods with small amounts of lean meat, poultry or fish.

- The approximately 5 to 8 teaspoon servings of fats and oils per day may be used for cooking and baking, and in salad dressings and spreads.

- Use cooking methods that require little or no fat—boil, broil, bake, roast, poach, steam, saute, stir-fry or microwave.

- Trim off the fat you can see before cooking meat and poultry. Drain off all fat after browning. Chill soups and stews after cooking so you can remove the hardened fat from the top.

- The 3 to 4 egg yolks per week included in your eating plan may be used alone or in cooking and baking (including store-bought products).

- Limit your use of organ meats such as liver, brains, chitterlings, kidney, heart, gizzard, sweetbreads and pork maws.

- Choose skim or 1% fat milk and nonfat or low-fat yogurt and cheeses.

To round out the rest of your eating plan:

- Eat 5 or more servings of fruits or vegetables per day.

- Eat 6 or more servings of breads, cereals or grains per day.

▲ F I G U R E   8 - 1

The American Heart Association Diet: An eating plan for healthy Americans. (From the American Heart Association, National Center, Dallas, Texas, Copyright 1991; used with permission.)

WHAT ARE THE TYPES AND CAUSES OF CARDIOVASCULAR DISEASE?

Cardiovascular disease relates to the heart and the entire vascular system. Thus, **hypertension** (high blood pressure), **cerebrovascular accident** (**CVA** or, more commonly, stroke), and **arteriosclerosis** (hardening of the arteries) are all examples of cardiovascular disease. In diseases of the heart, one or several parts may be damaged. The affected part may be the muscle (**myocardium**), the outer covering (**pericardium**), the lining (**endocardium**), the blood vessels, or the valves.

What Is Atherosclerosis?

Atherosclerosis is a complex disease of the arteries; it is a form of arteriosclerosis. The passageways through the arteries become roughened and clogged with fatty deposits so that blood cannot flow freely, like clogged sink pipes that are full of grease. (Fig. 8–2). Atherosclerosis is thought to be a cause of heart attack (**coronary thrombosis** or **myocardial infarction [MI],** or plain "coronary") and CVA.

WHAT ARE RISK FACTORS FOR CARDIOVASCULAR DISEASE?

New guidelines were developed by the Adult Treatment Panel (ATP) of the National Cholesterol Education Program (NCEP). These risk factors include:

1. Elevated total blood cholesterol at or above 240 mg/dL
2. Increased low-density lipoprotein cholesterol at or above 160 mg/dL
3. Male gender, 45 years or older
4. Female gender, 55 years or older or with premature menopause and no estrogen replacement therapy
5. Decreased high-density lipoprotein cholesterol less than 35 mg/dL
6. Hypertension
7. Cigarette smoking
8. Diabetes mellitus
9. Family history of premature coronary heart disease (Schaefer, 1993)

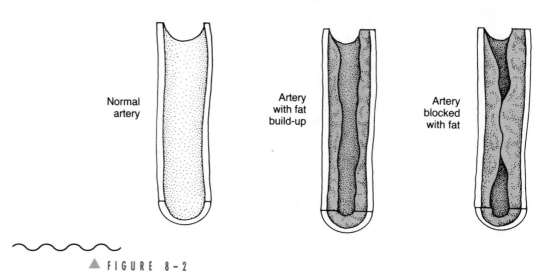

Normal artery

Artery with fat build-up

Artery blocked with fat

▲ FIGURE 8-2

The atherosclerosis process. (From Mahan LK, Arlin M: Krause's Food, Nutrition & Diet Therapy, 8th ed. Philadelphia, WB Saunders, 1992; p. 360.)

FACT & FALLACY

FALLACY: My grandfather lived to be 100 and ate eggs and bacon daily; therefore I do not have to worry about heart disease.

FACT: For individuals who subscribe to the preceding idea, it needs to be pointed out that one's heredity also comes from the grandmother's side of the family as well as from both parents. Upon careful questioning, it is often found that there is some form of CVD in the family's history, even if it is not heart disease specifically. There may also be other risk factors that did not apply previously, such as cigarette smoking or diabetes. In addition, Grandpa was probably more involved in physical activities. Many people believe this type of fallacy. However, the fact is that the mortality and morbidity from CVD is extremely high. It is the number one killer in the United States.

What Are Safe Blood Cholesterol Levels?

Although controversy exists in the medical community regarding safe and ideal blood values for total cholesterol and low-density lipoprotein cholesterol, there is growing recognition that lower levels are best. The levels set by the **National Cholesterol Education Program (NCEP)** coordinating committee indicate that total cholesterol should be less than 200 mg/dL; levels between 200 and 239 mg/dL are defined as borderline high blood cholesterol and those greater than 240 mg/dL as high-risk levels. The NCEP also indicates that low-density lipoprotein cholesterol should be less than 130 mg/dL, with borderline levels being 130 to 159 mg/dL and high-risk levels being those greater than 160 mg/dL (NCEP, 1990). Table 8–1 shows high-risk cholesterol values based on age and gender.

What Are Lipoproteins and the Different Forms?

High-density lipoprotein (HDL), low-density lipoprotein (LDL), and very–low-density lipoprotein (VLDL) are all forms of cholesterol found in the blood. **Lipids** is a term used to describe all forms of fat found in the blood. Chylomicrons are another form of lipoprotein. VLDL is the main carrier of triglycerides synthesized in the body. It is believed that HDL, which has more protein than does LDL or VLDL, allows more cholesterol to be taken from the body's cells, resulting in greater transport and removal of cholesterol through the liver. HDLs have been termed the "good" lipoproteins or fats, and in fact researchers have found that individuals with more HDLs have less heart disease. An easy way to remember the role of HDL is to think *H* for *housecleaner,* as a high level of HDL seems to keep blood vessels and arteries clean. Fortunately, recommended dietary changes to reduce serum cholesterol generally raise HDLs while lowering LDLs (Table 8–2). It is likely that Mr. Bernardo in the opening case study has elevated

▲ TABLE 8-1

PLASMA CHOLESTEROL CONCENTRATIONS ASSOCIATED WITH INCREASED RISK OF CARDIOVASCULAR DISEASE*

Age yr	TOTAL CHOLESTEROL, mg/dL		LDL CHOLESTEROL, mg/dL		HDL CHOLESTEROL,† mg/dL
	Moderate Risk	High Risk	Moderate Risk	High Risk	Increased Risk
Men					
0–14	173	190	106	120	38
15–19	165	183	109	123	30
20–29	194	216	128	148	30
30–39	218	244	149	171	29
40–49	231	254	160	180	29
≥50	230	258	166	188	29
Women					
0–14	170	174	113	126	36
15–19	173	195	115	135	35
20–29	184	208	127	148	35
30–39	202	220	143	163	35
40–49	223	246	155	177	34
≥50	252	281	170	195	36

* Values are adopted from the 75th percentile (moderate-risk) and 90th percentile (high-risk) values obtained by the Lipid Research Clinics.

† The HDL cholesterol values for the lower fifth percentile were taken from the Lipid Research Clinics.

KEY: LDL = low-density lipoproteins; HDL = high-density lipoproteins. From Hoeg JM et al. An approach to the management of hyperlipoproteinemia. JAMA 1986; 255(4):514–519. Copyright 1986, American Medical Association.

From Hoeg JM et al. An approach to the management of hyperlipoproteinemia. JAMA 1986; 255(4):514–519. Copyright 1986, American Medical Association.

cholesterol, LDL, and triglyceride values and a low HDL. This lipid pattern is commonly found in persons with diabetes mellitus (see Chapter 9). Weight loss should have a dramatic impact on his lipid values, if indeed they follow this pattern.

HOW IS CARDIOVASCULAR DISEASE PREVENTED AND TREATED BY DIET CHANGES?

The American Heart Association (AHA) advises that the nature of coronary heart disease is such that prevention is the primary means by which a reduction in morbidity and mortality will be accomplished. Therefore, it appears prudent to follow a diet aimed at lowering serum lipid concentrations. Many persons in the United States and the world have consumed diets similar to those recommended by the National Cholesterol Education Program (NCEP's Step One Diet) for many years (Table 8–3).

Studies have shown that there is a low incidence of coronary disease in populations who habitually subsist on a low-fat and low-cholesterol diet or on a diet that is low in saturated fats and cholesterol. For example, it might be pointed out to Mr. Bernardo that Italians in Italy have a low incidence of heart disease. This is felt to be related to a low intake of saturated

▲ **TABLE 8-2**

PREVENTIVE NUTRITION GUIDELINES IN CORONARY HEART DISEASE

Dietary Component	SOURCE OF RECOMMENDATION*			
	AHA	**Dietary Goals**	**Dietary Guidelines**	**ISCHDR**
Calories	Adjust to reach or maintain ideal body weight	Maintain ideal body weight	Avoid overweight; if overweight, lower caloric intake and increase exercise	Achieve and maintain optimal weight with exercise and food intake
Total fat calories	30%	30%	Avoid too much fat	Less than 30%; de-emphasize red meats, dairy products, baked goods; choose lower fat content poultry
Saturated fat calories	10%	10%	Avoid too much saturated fat	Less than 8%
Polyunsaturated fat calories	Up to 10%	10%	No specific level ↑ or ↓	Up to 10%
Monounsaturate fat calories	Remainder of ingested fat	10%	No specific level ↑ or ↓	10%
Cholesterol	About 300 mg	300 mg	No specific level ↑ or ↓	Less than 250 mg/day, lower egg yolk consumption
Carbohydrate (CHO)	Replace fat calories; emphasize complex CHO—10%	Complex CHO—48% calories;; refined CHO—10%	Eat foods with adequate starch and fiber	50% of calories; reduce sugar intake; provide whole-grain cereals, fruits, vegetables, and legumes to ensure adequate micronutrients
Salt	Avoid excess salt	5 g	Avoid too much salt	Less than 4 g/day
Dietary variety	No specific recommendation	No specific recommendation	Eat a variety of foods	Encouraged
Alcohol	No specific recommendation	No specific recommendation	If you drink alcohol, do so in moderation	Described as empty calories that are an obstacle to obesity control

* AHA = American Heart Association; Dietary Goals = Senate Select Committee on Nutrition and Human Needs: Eating in America. Dietary Goals for the United States; Dietary Guidelines = U.S. Department of Agriculture and Department of Health, Education and Welfare: Nutrition and Your Health: Dietary Guidelines for Americans; ISCHDR = Inter-Society Commission for Heart Disease Resources.

From Posner BM, DeRusso PA, Norquist SL, et al. Preventive nutrition intervention in coronary heart disease: Risk assessment and formulating dietary goals. J Am Diet Assoc 1986; 86(10): 1396.

fat even though total fat intake is high because of the use of olives and olive oil. To be maximally effective in the prevention of atherosclerosis, a diet that reduces serum lipids will need to be consumed throughout life. It should be palatable, effective, economically feasible, and nutritionally adequate to allow for long-term use.

There is some question as to whether the AHA's recommendation that fat intake equal 30 per cent of total kilocalories is strict enough (Table 8–4) shows amounts of fat to equal 30 per cent at a variety of kilocalorie levels and how to calculate amounts of fat for different percentages). Dr. Dean Ornish is one person who believes in the old Pritikin plan, which follows the theory that a stricter fat intake of less than 10 per cent of total kilocalories can actually reverse the plaquing process (Ornish, 1990). A total fat intake of 10 per cent of 2000 kilocalories, for example, equals 22 grams of fat, the equivalent of about ½ cup of gourmet ice cream! If a person is interested and motivated, this stricter recommendation for fat intake can be followed in a healthy way, but it is certainly a challenge in our society, which con-

▲ T A B L E   8 – 3

RECOMMENDED DIET MODIFICATIONS TO LOWER BLOOD CHOLESTEROL: THE STEP ONE DIET

FOOD GROUP	CHOOSE	DECREASE
Fish, chicken, turkey, and lean meats	Fish; white-meat poultry without skin; lean cuts of beef, lamb, pork or veal; shellfish	Fatty cuts of beef, lamb, pork; spare ribs; organ meats; regular cold cuts; sausage; hot dogs; bacon; sardines; roe
Skim and low-fat milk, cheese, yogurt, and dairy substitutes	Skim or 1% fat milk (liquid, powdered, evaporated); buttermilk; substitute 1 cup skim milk alone or with up to 1 cup nonfat dry-milk powder added instead of whole milk (for consistency in cooking);	Whole milk (4% fat): regular, evaporated, condensed; cream; half and half; 2% milk; imitation milk products; most nondairy creamers; whipped toppings
	For acceptable whipped topping: combine 1/3 cup ice water, 1 tbsp lemon juice, 3/4 tsp vanilla, and 1/3 cup nonfat dry-milk powder; beat 10 minutes or until stiff; add 2 tbsp sugar	
	Nonfat (0% fat) or low-fat yogurt	Whole-milk yogurt
	Low-fat cottage cheese (1% or 2% fat)	Whole-milk cottage cheese (4% fat)
	Low-fat cheeses, farmer, or pot cheeses (all of these should be labeled no more than 2–6 g fat/oz)	All-natural cheeses (e.g., blue, Roquefort, Camembert, Cheddar, Swiss)
		Low-fat or "diet" cream cheese, low-fat or "diet" sour cream
		Cream cheese, sour cream
	Sherbet, sorbet	Ice cream
Eggs	Egg whites (2 whites = 1 whole egg in recipes), or mix together 1 egg white, 2 tsp nonfat milk powder, and 2 tsp acceptable oil*; cholesterol-free egg substitutes	Egg yolks
Fruits and vegetables	Fresh, frozen, canned, or dried fruits and vegetables	Vegetables prepared in butter, cream, or other sauces
Breads and cereals	Homemade baked goods using unsaturated oils sparingly, angel food cake, low-fat crackers, low-fat cookies	Commercial baked goods: pies, cakes, doughnuts, croissants, pastries, muffins, biscuits, high-fat cookies
	Rice, pasta, barley, bulgur, legumes	Egg noodles
	Whole-grain breads and cereals (oatmeal, whole wheat, rye, bran, multigrain, etc.)	Breads in which eggs are a major ingredient, cereals with coconut oil or palm oil or palm kernel oil
Fats and oils	Acceptable unsaturated vegetable oils*	Butter, coconut oil, palm oil, palm kernel oil, bacon fat, hydrogenated vegetable shortening
	Margarine or shortening made from one of the acceptable unsaturated oils	
	Reduced-fat margarine	
	Mayonnaise, salad dressings made with acceptable unsaturated oils	Dressings made with egg yolk
	Low-fat dressings	
	Seeds and nuts, nonhydrogenated, old-fashioned-style peanut butter (100% peanuts)	Coconut, hydrogenated peanut butter

* Acceptable oils include canola, corn, cottonseed, olive, safflower, sesame, soybean, and sunflower.
From National Cholesterol Education Program Expert Panel. Report on detection, evaluation, and treatment of high blood cholesterol in adults. *Arch Intern Med*. 1988; 148:36.

sumes so many high-fat foods. Based on the success of Dr. Ornish's approach, the first comprehensive health insurance reimbursement based on preventive care was approved in 1993 by Mutual of Omaha. It is expected that other insurance companies will follow this trend toward preventive health services.

▲ TABLE 8-4

RECOMMENDED TOTAL FAT FOR VARIOUS
KILOCALORIE LEVELS

KILOCALORIE LEVEL	TOTAL RECOMMENDED FAT (30%)
1200 kilocalories	40 g fat
1500 kilocalories	50 g fat
1800 kilocalories	60 g fat
2100 kilocalories	70 g fat
2400 kilocalories	80 g fat
2700 kilocalories	90 g fat
3000 kilocalories	100 g fat

To calculate percentage of fat of total kilocalories:

1. Multiply total kilocalories by percentage of fat (0.30 used above), which yields the number of kilocalories to be contributed by fat.
2. Divide the number of kilocalories of fat by 9 to determine the total grams of fat.

To calculate the percentage of total kilocalories of a given amount of fat:

1. Multiply grams of fat by 9 to equal kilocalories contributed by fat.
2. Divide kilocalories from fat by total kilocalories to determine the percentage.

An easier way to calculate the recommended number of grams of fat is to divide the total kilocalories by 30. For example:

$$\frac{1800 \text{ kilocalories}}{30} = 60 \text{ gm of fat}$$

Use the exchange list system (see Chapters 6 and 9) for an easy method to calculate fat content from a given menu. Foods not listed in the exchange list will generally be listed in a food composition table from which fat content can be determined (see Appendix 5).

WHAT ARE THE AMERICAN HEART ASSOCIATION DIETARY GUIDELINES?

1. Total fat intake should be less than 30 per cent of total kilocalories (Table 8-4 shows total recommended fat for various kilocalorie levels).

2. Saturated fatty acid intake should be less than 10 per cent of total kilocalories.

3. Polyunsaturated fatty acid intake should be no more than 10 per cent of total kilocalories.

4. Monounsaturated fatty acids make up the rest of total fat intake, about 10 to 15 per cent of total kilocalories.

5. Cholesterol intake should be no more than 300 mg per day.

6. Sodium intake should be no more than 3000 mg (3 g) per day (AHA, 1991).

What Advice Is Appropriate for Children's Needs?

Since atherosclerosis, or the accumulation of plaque in the arteries, begins in childhood, it is believed that adult nutrition guidelines may be helpful for healthy children older than 2 years of age (National Cholesterol Education Program, 1991). Because of a child's growth needs, however, as well as a need to develop positive associations with eating, a punitive, overly restrictive diet is not in a child's best interest. Parents may be advised to limit fatty foods but to do so with an attitude of moderation, not total elimination. Parents can place positive emphasis on low-fat foods such as fruits, vegetables, low-fat milk products, and low-fat, whole-grain products and thereby help promote a healthy attitude toward eating. If a low-fat diet is undertaken with too much zeal, a child may experience undesirable weight loss or stunting of growth. An increased intake of monounsaturated fats would be appropriate in such situations. Foods such as peanut butter, olives, avocados, and most nuts (if the child is old enough to avoid choking) can provide adequate kilocalorie intake without increasing saturated fats.

How Can Dietary Intake of Cholesterol-Rich Food and Fat Be Controlled?

1. Eat no more than three or four egg yolks a week, including eggs used in cooking.

2. Moderate the use of shrimp and limit organ meats.

3. Use fish, skinless chicken and turkey, and veal in most of the meat meals for the week; use moderate-sized portions (3 oz meat equals the size of a deck of cards) of beef, lamb, pork, and ham less frequently. Substitute low-fat protein foods such as legumes for meat occasionally (e.g., red beans and rice or tofu and vegetable stir-fry).

4. Choose lean cuts of meat, trim visible fat, and discard the fat that cooks out of the meat. Removing the skin from a piece of chicken eliminates about 1 teaspoon of fat.

5. Avoid deep-fat frying and use an oil that is low in saturated fats (corn, safflower, sunflower, peanut, or canola) when frying is done.

6. Restrict the use of fatty luncheon and variety meats such as sausage and salami.

7. Instead of butter and cooking fats that are solid or completely hydrogenated, emphasize liquid vegetable oils, such as olive oil or sesame seed oil, and soft or liquid margarines. Cooking with other liquids such as wine, water, broth, or fruit juice will help reduce the fat content of meals.

8. Instead of whole milk and cheeses made from whole milk and cream, use skim milk and skim or part-skim milk cheeses.

9. Use more plant foods in place of animal foods. For example, fill up on whole-grain breads and vegetables rather than meat. Think of meat as a side dish rather than as the main dish.

10. When shopping, look for food labels with less than 15 grams of fat for a meal and less than 2 grams of fat for a snack. The level of saturated fat should be no more than one third of the total amount of fat. An acceptable level of sodium per meal is 800 mg; snack foods should have less than 200 mg sodium per serving.

Where Is
Cholesterol Found?

There are two main sources of cholesterol. One is the body's natural production of cholesterol in the liver, in the gastrointestinal tract, and in almost all body cells that have a nucleus. This natural cholesterol production is affected by diet. Saturated fats tend to increase the production of cholesterol, and unsaturated fats tend to have the opposite effect. Intake of cholesterol in the diet has little impact on the body's own natural cholesterol production.

The second source of cholesterol is the foods we eat. It is important to remember that cholesterol is found only in animal products and specifically in animal fat. Skim milk and egg whites, although both animal products, have no measurable fat and therefore no significant amount of cholesterol. Plant fats such as peanut butter do not contain any cholesterol. It now appears that reducing saturated fat in the diet is more important than reducing cholesterol intake.

Where Are Saturated
Fats Found?

Saturated fat is more challenging to identify. Saturated fat is found in animal fat and in some vegetable fats (see Chapter 3). Although coconut and palm oils are naturally saturated, there are many other manufactured saturated fats. These saturated fats are made so that the vegetable oil remains hard at room temperature. In other words, vegetable oil is turned into a solid fat. This is achieved by adding extra hydrogen to the oils, and these oils are referred to as hydrogenated fats or **trans fatty acids.** Reading food labels will tell you what kind of fat was used—whether it was animal fat or vegetable oil and if the vegetable oil was left in its liquid state or was hydrogenated (saturated). You can determine if the vegetable oil used is saturated (palm oil and coconut oil), polyunsaturated (liquid corn, safflower, or sunflower oil), or monounsaturated (peanut oil, olive oil, canola oil, and the form of fat found in avocados). The new food labels state total fat grams and amounts of saturated fat per serving of food.

An easy way to determine if a fat is saturated is by its texture. If it is hard at cold temperatures it contains saturated fats. For example, if you take butter out of the refrigerator it is so hard you cannot even cut it. Fat on red meat is saturated, which you can tell as you cut it off. But you have never cut a layer of fat off fish because the fat found in fish is primarily unsaturated (in liquid form). The same applies to chicken, in which the fat is soft; in other words, chicken has less saturated fat than red meat does.

What Is the Role of
Unsaturated Fats in
the Prevention and
Control of CVD?

As discussed in Chapter 3, polyunsaturated fats are known to reduce the body's own natural production of cholesterol. Foods with a high P:S ratio (the amount of polyunsaturated versus saturated fat) are helpful in preventing and controlling CVD (see Table 3–4).

Monounsaturated fats have long been considered neutral in their influence on CVD. However, there is growing evidence that monounsaturated fats such as olive oil are helpful in the prevention and control of CVD. However, both polyunsaturated and monounsaturated fats should not be considered "free foods," as excess total fat may contribute to the development of CVD through the promotion of obesity.

The general recommendation is to consume equal amounts (10 per cent each of total kilocalories) of saturated, monounsaturated, and polyunsaturated fats, composing a total of 30 per cent of fat in the diet. For individuals with elevated total cholesterol and LDL cholesterol who do not respond to this dietary pattern, even less saturated fat and more monounsaturated fat should be consumed, as noted in the Step One and Step Two Diets of the NCEP (Table 8–3 and Fig. 8–3).

What Are Omega-3 Fatty Acids?

The most unsaturated form of fat found in foods is referred to as omega-3 fatty acids. This form of fat is prevalent in cold-water fish and other foods such as dark-green leafy vegetables. Given the example earlier of saturated fats becoming hard in cold temperatures, can you imagine what would happen to fish that live in cold water if their body fat was primarily of the saturated form? Mother Nature made fish living in cold water regions with unsaturated fats that can stay soft at cold temperatures.

Omega-3 fats are known to reduce blood levels of triglycerides and thus are recommended in the control of cardiovascular disease. These fats also reduce the inflammation process of the body and tend to reduce clotting time of the blood. It was found that men who ate as little as 30 g (1 oz) of fish daily reduced their risk of CVD by two and a half times (Kromhout et al., 1985).

FACT & FALLACY

FALLACY: Fish oil capsules should be recommended for management of CVD.

FACT: Fish from the cold northern oceans contain more omega-3 fatty acids than do fish from temperate southern seas. Since Greenland Eskimos, who have a low incidence of atherosclerosis, have a high intake of omega-3 type of fat through consumption of almost 1 pound of fish daily, this is an area of promise. However, since the optimal dose of these omega-3 fatty acids has not been established, recommending the widespread use of these fatty acid concentrates should be discouraged (Kris-Etherton, 1990). In addition, it is not known if it is EPA (a form of omega-3 fatty acids) or other substances in the fish that are the reason for the lower incidence of cardiovascular disease among the Greenland Eskimos. Advice to eat more tuna fish would be well accepted and appropriate.

Nutrient	Recommended intake	
	Step One diet	*Step Two diet*
total fat	Less than 30% of total calories	
saturated fatty acids	Less than 10% of total calories	Less than 7% of total calories
polyunsaturated fatty acids	up to 10% of total calories	
monounsaturated fatty acids	10% to 15% of total calories	
carbohydrates	50% to 60% of total calories	
protein	10% to 20% of total calories	
cholesterol	Less than 300 mg/day	Less than 200 mg/day
total calories	to achieve and maintain desirable weight	

▲ FIGURE 8-3

Dietary therapy for high blood cholesterol recommendations of the Adult Treatment Panel of the National Cholesterol Education Program. (From Ernst ND, et al.: The National Cholesterol Education Program: Implications for dietetic practitioners from the Adult Treatment Panel Recommendations. Copyright the American Dietetic Association. Reprinted by permission of the Journal of the American Dietetic Association. 1988; 88(11):1405.)

What Is the Connection Between CVD and Fiber?

There is growing evidence that dietary fiber may play a role in preventing and controlling CVD. As noted in Chapter 3, the water-soluble fibers— pectins from fruits, gums from legumes, and the water-soluble fiber in oat grain—appear to be effective in reducing serum cholesterol levels. The benefits of soluble fiber are so impressive that daily consumption has been advised, whether it comes from oat bran, brown rice, legumes, barley, or other sources (See Appendix 7 for fiber content of foods).

ONE DAY SAMPLE MENU
for a STEP ONE DIET
(approximately 2000 kilocalories)

▲

BREAKFAST
6 oz grapefruit juice
½ c strawberries
½ c oatmeal
1 slice whole-wheat toast
1 tsp tub margarine
8 oz skim milk
Coffee
2 tsp sugar or jelly

▲

LUNCH
Turkey sandwich:
3 oz turkey (no skin)
2 slices bread
1 tsp mayonnaise
½ c cole slaw with low-calorie dressing
Small orange
Tea with lemon and honey

▲

AFTERNOON SNACK
8 oz skim milk

▲

SUPPER
3 oz lean roast beef
1 c pasta
½ c mixed vegetables
2 tsp oil
½ c broccoli
½ c tossed salad with 1 tbsp Italian dressing
8 oz skim milk

▲

EVENING SNACK
1 oz low-salt pretzels

Modified from Kris-Etherton PM: Cardiovascular Disease: Nutrition for Prevention and Treatment. Chicago, The American Dietetic Association, © 1990. Used by permission.

If you were a health care professional working with Mr. Bernardo you might ask him if his heritage is Italian, as his name suggests. This would allow you to discuss how the inclusion of legumes in the typical diet of Italy may contribute to a lessened risk of heart disease. Then ask Mr. Bernardo if he feels he could emphasize dried beans more in his diet.

What Are Anti-Oxidants and What Is Their Role in CVD?

The main **antioxidants** are vitamins C, E, and beta-carotene (the precursor to vitamin A). These nutrients are believed to help prevent harm from oxygen in the blood vessels, thereby reducing the plaquing process on artery walls. Foods containing these antioxidants are known to reduce CVD (see Chapter 5).

Can Excess Iron in the Diet Cause CVD?

A study in Finland suggests that elevated serum iron levels (specifically ferritin levels) increase the risk of a myocardial infarct in men (Salonen, 1992). The hypothesis has been raised that women are at decreased risk of heart disease because of menstruation and loss of iron with blood flow. Women after menopause do have an increased rate of heart disease. The role of iron in heart disease is still, however, in the theory stage. As iron-deficiency anemia is a health problem, caution should be exercised. Individuals at risk of high serum iron levels, such as those with hemochromatosis (see Chapter 5) should be advised to avoid iron. For the general public, avoidance of iron is not yet recommended.

WHAT IS THE ROLE OF EXERCISE IN THE MANAGEMENT OF CARDIOVASCULAR DISEASE?

Exercise is a well-known component of weight control, and since obesity is a risk factor associated with the development of CVD, it should be an integral approach in both the prevention and the treatment of CVD. However, exercise as appropriately determined by a physician should be practiced, particularly for the person at high risk for CVD.

In addition, regular aerobic exercise (any exercise that makes a person take in more air, such as a brisk walk) is associated with increased levels of HDL cholesterol and decreased levels of LDL cholesterol, and it has been recommended that patients with low HDL levels (see Table 8–1) be encouraged to exercise. Again, aerobic exercise should be appropriate for the person's condition, and consultation with a physician is always prudent.

WHAT IS THE ROLE OF DRUG THERAPY IN THE MANAGEMENT OF CARDIOVASCULAR DISEASE?

Drug therapy has a place in the management of CVD. However, as all drugs have potential negative side effects, diet control should be the first step in CVD management. For those individuals with familial (hereditary) **hypercholesterolemia** (high blood cholesterol levels) that does not respond to dietary intervention, there are several medications that may be prescribed in addition to dietary modifications. Niacin (at levels high enough to be considered a drug even though it is a vitamin) is the drug of choice. If there are contraindications to the use of niacin (e.g., diabetes mellitus, peptic ulcer disease, or symptomatic gout), a bile acid sequestrant, such as Questran, or another drug, such as gemfibrozil, clofibrate, probucol, or neomycin sulfate, may be prescribed. The level of elevated lipids also dictates the drug of choice, as some medications lower total cholesterol and LDL cholesterol while others lower triglycerides or elevate HDL cholesterol.

FACT & FALLACY

FALLACY: Niacin therapy, through over-the-counter vitamin supplements, should be recommended to all persons with elevated cholesterol levels.

FACT: The amount of niacin shown to be effective in lowering cholesterol levels is large enough for it to be considered a drug. Drugs need to be monitored by a physician, since there can be adverse side effects. In the case of niacin, it may be contraindicated for persons with diabetes mellitus and other disorders. Dietary control through food modification is the first and safer approach before drugs are advised.

WHAT IS HYPERTENSION AND WHAT IS ITS ROLE IN CVD

Hypertension is an elevation of the blood pressure to greater than normal levels, which is generally considered to be more than 140/90 mm Hg (the top number is the systolic pressure and the bottom number is the diastolic pressure), with the diastolic pressure being the more significant number. Hypertension is often associated with CVD, diabetes, and renal disease. It is one of the most important risk factors associated with the development of CVD. The underlying insulin resistance with hyperinsulinemia (see Chapter 9) of diabetes found in adults is generally felt to increase sodium retention. Thus diabetes and hypertension are often found together, as in the case of Mr. Bernardo as described in Chapter 2.

WHAT DIETARY TREATMENTS ARE USED FOR THE CONTROL OF HYPERTENSION?

Since obesity is a predisposing factor in hypertension, a low-kilocalorie diet is often prescribed to reduce weight. Sodium restriction is often recommended. Further adjustments in protein and fluids as well as sodium intake are made if there is kidney involvement. Sodium restriction improves the effectiveness of diuretic therapy. If potassium-depleting diuretics are taken, patients are advised to increase their potassium intake to replenish what is lost in the increased urine volume. Bananas and orange juice are frequently recommended for their potassium content, but there are many foods high in potassium. Most fresh vegetables (especially dark green leafy ones), fruits, legumes, milk, and fresh meats are good sources of potassium and add only a small amount of sodium to the diet. Physicians should be consulted before using a potassium substitute for salt.

Salt is often linked to hypertension simply because the **sodium** in salt causes the body to accumulate fluid. Any excess fluid puts greater pressure on the walls of the blood vessels, creating higher blood pressure. For many people with high blood pressure, reducing salt in the diet will often bring it within normal range.

Excess alcohol may also raise blood pressure. A moderate intake of alcohol is generally considered safe unless there are contraindications to its use. A low saturated fat intake may also lower blood pressure.

What Are the Purposes and Indications for Sodium-Controlled Diets?

There are several reasons for restricting sodium intake (see Chapter 5 to review information on sodium). The indications for restricting sodium intake include:

1. Hypertension: to relieve elevated or high blood pressure
2. **Congestive heart failure (CHF)** (a condition in which the heart cannot pump blood adequately)
3. To aid the body in eliminating sodium and fluids (to prevent **edema,** a condition of fluid build-up)
4. Renal disorders with edema
5. Adrenocorticotropic hormone and cortisone therapy
6. Cirrhosis of the liver with ascites (a disease often caused by alcoholism but also from other causes)
7. To meet the Dietary Guidelines for Americans of 2400 mg of sodium per day

What Is a Sodium-Restricted Diet?

A sodium-restricted diet is a normal adequate diet with a modified sodium content, from a very low amount of 250 mg to 3000 mg.

An average diet prepared in the kitchen with some commercially prepared foods, foods salted during cooking, and some salt added at the table provides about 3000 to 7000 mg of sodium daily. (These numbers should not be confused with salt intake—sodium composes 40 per cent of salt. One teaspoon of salt contains about 2000 mg of sodium.) For therapeutic purposes, sodium intake may vary from 250 mg daily to 2000 mg or more. Diets in which sodium is limited were formerly called low-salt diets, when salt was omitted only in the preparation of food, and salt-free diets, when it was not allowed either in cooking or at the table. Such diets are now named in terms of the level of sodium restriction, the most usual being the 2000 to 4000 mg sodium diet (mild restriction), the 1000 mg sodium diet (moderate), and the 500 mg sodium diet (strict). Table 8–5 shows the differences among sodium-restricted diets for different sodium levels. See Chapter 5 for more information on sodium.

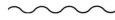

▲ **TABLE 8-5**

SODIUM RESTRICTED DIETS

FOODS	2–4 g SODIUM	1 g SODIUM	500 mg SODIUM
Milk	3 c milk or yogurt, no processed cheese; natural cheese (1 oz) can replace 1 c milk; free use of low-sodium cheese	2 c milk or yogurt; up to 1 oz natural cheese can be substituted for 1 c milk; free use of low-sodium cheese	Use low-sodium products in limited amounts
Meat and meat substitutes	Limited use of processed meats; free use of fresh meat	No processed meat; use salt-free canned tuna; limited use of regular peanut butter; free use of low-sodium peanut butter	Limited portions of fresh meat; no eggs or fish; use low-sodium peanut butter
Breads and cereals	Avoid breads and crackers with salt topping; regular bread may be used in normal amounts; free use of low-sodium bread and cereal products; avoid canned soups and vegetables and cereals with added salt	Up to 2 slices regular bread may be used or 1 serving regular processed cereal; free use of low-sodium breads and cereals	Limited use of low-sodium products
Vegetables and fruits	All fresh, frozen, and dried; all canned fruit but limited use of canned vegetables; free use of low-sodium canned vegetables; no salted products such as potato chips or french fries	Use only low-sodium canned vegetables; limited use of naturally high-sodium vegetables (beets, carrots, celery, spinach); free use of all others	No naturally high-sodium vegetables (beets, carrots, celery, spinach); no dried fruit; limited use of all others
Condiments			
Sweets			
Brown sugar	Free use	Free use	Limited use
Table sugar	Free use	Free use	Limited use
Honey	Free use	Free use	Limited use
Jams and jellies	Free use	Free use	Limited use
Maple syrup	Free use	Free use	Limited use
Molasses	Free use	Free use	Limited use
Sauces			
Catsup	Limited use	Use low-sodium	Use low-sodium limited
Mayonnaise	Limited use	Use low-sodium	Use low-sodium limited
Mustard	Limited use	Use low-sodium	Use low-sodium limited
Soy sauce	Limited use	Use low-sodium	Use low-sodium limited
Worcestershire sauce	Limited use	Not allowed	Not allowed
Butter/margarine	Limited use	Use low-sodium	Use low-sodium, limited
Other			
Cooking oil	Free use	Free use	Free use
Vinegar	Free use	Free use	Free use
Spices			
Natural	Free use	Free use	Free use
Salt-based	Limited use	Not allowed	Not allowed
Lemon	Free use	Free use	Free use
Horseradish	Free use	Limited use	Not allowed
Salt	Very limited use (few sprinkles)	Use salt substitute (physician approval)	Use salt substitute (physician approval)

Although the initial elimination of salt from the diet is very difficult for a person used to its taste, the taste for salt can be unlearned. Use of spices, herbs, lemon juice, or vinegar can help enhance the taste appeal of food while the preference for salt is changing.

Is Calcium Related to Hypertension?

There is growing evidence that adequate calcium nutritional status plays a role in the control of hypertension. However, the situation appears to be more complex with other nutrients, such as sodium, potassium, and magnesium. Milk contains calcium, potassium, and magnesium. Vegetarians generally have lower blood pressure, and one explanation is that the lower protein and sodium content of their diets allows more efficient use of dietary calcium. Weight control, sodium restriction, avoidance of excess protein, and adequate intake of calcium and potassium food sources (milk, fruit, and vegetables) all contribute to the control of hypertension (Zemel, 1988).

WHAT IS THE ROLE OF THE NURSE OR OTHER HEALTH CARE PROFESSIONAL IN THE PREVENTION AND CONTROL OF CARDIOVASCULAR DISEASE?

The nurse and other health care professionals are important team members in the fight against CVD. There is a large body of evidence to reinforce the belief that nutritional changes can lower the risk of CVD. For instance, each 1 per cent reduction in blood cholesterol levels results in a 2 per cent reduction in CVD mortality for individuals with elevated cholesterol levels (Kris-Etherton, 1990). Yet many individuals either are not aware of how to make appropriate dietary changes to help prevent CVD or believe that the cost of change is greater than the results accrued. The nurse has the opportunity through direct patient contact to assess the reasons that various individuals may not be following the general CVD reduction guidelines.

A health care professional can assess whether lack of knowledge is the reason for poor dietary compliance by saying, "You probably have heard about cholesterol and saturated fat in television commercials, but are you aware of which foods contain high amounts?" Or, a negative attitude or belief may be the reason for not making dietary changes. To assess this, a good question would be, "How do you feel about all the talk concerning cholesterol?"

Through positive reinforcement of steps taken, no matter how small, and referral to appropriate services, the nurse and other health care professionals can play a key role in reducing this society's primary health risk. Figure 8–4 shows when referral to a registered dietitian is recommended by the National Cholesterol Education Program.

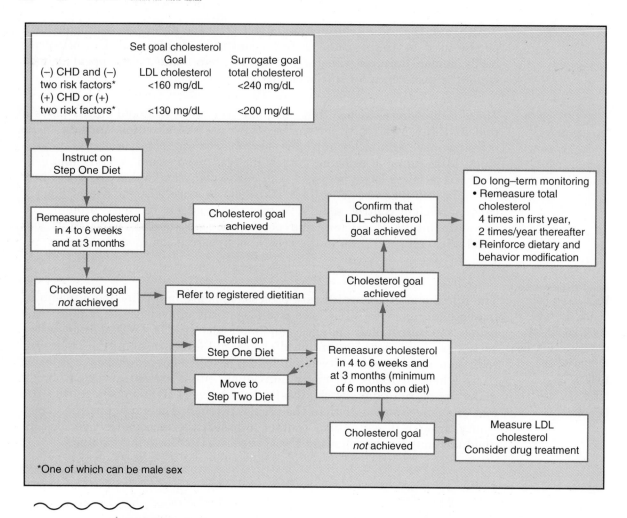

▲ FIGURE 8-4

Classification and treatment decisions for LDL-cholesterol levels. (From National Cholesterol Education Program Expert Panel. Report on detection, evaluation, and treatment of high blood cholesterol
in adults. Arch Intern Med 1988; 148:36.)

STUDY QUESTIONS AND ACTIVITIES

1. List the known risk factors of Mr. Bernardo for cardiovascular disease.
2. Interview family members regarding personal family history of CVD
   and hypertension. Use Figure 8–5 to determine your personal risk
   factors for heart disease.
3. Collect samples of vegetable oils, including at least one saturated
   fat and one polyunsaturated fat, and refrigerate all of them. Compare textures to determine the degree of solidity.

4. Taste-test low-sodium food products. Compare these foods with different seasonings, such as spices, herbs, lemon, and jelly.
5. Have the class list 20 everyday foods and then read food labels of these foods to determine fat and sodium content.
6. Have each student evaluate his or her family's sodium intake.
7. Class role-play: one volunteer to serve as Mr. Bernardo; another to serve as a health care professional describing the different types of blood fats and food fats and how they interact. The health care professional should assess Mr. Bernardo's health belief values toward cardiovascular disease and offer options for dietary changes to decrease his risk of CVD.
8. If your client has been placed on a low-fat diet, what could you recommend he take for lunch to his construction worksite? What could you recommend for a dessert?
9. Collect some family recipes and bring them to class. Assess whether these recipes contribute to heart disease because they are high in saturated fat or sodium, or both. What recipe modifications could be made to lower the fat and sodium content if needed?

H   E   A   R   T

Everyone plays the game of health whether he wants to or not. What is your score? Add up the numbers in each category that most nearly describe you.

	1	2	3	4	6
Heredity	No known history of heart disease	One relative with heart disease over 60 years	Two relatives with heart disease over 60 years	One relative with heart disease under 60 years	Two relatives with heart disease under 60 years
	1	2	3	5	6
Exercise	Intensive exercise, work and recreation	Moderate exercise, work and recreation	Sedentary work & intensive recreational exercise	Sedentary work & moderate recreational exercise	Sedentary work & light recreational exercise
	1	2	3	4	6
Age	10–20	21–30	31–40	41–50	51–65
	0	1	2	4	6
Lb	More than 5 lb below standard weight	± 5 lb standard weight	6–20 lb overweight	21–35 lb overweight	36–50 lb overweight
	0	1	2	4	6
Tobacco	Nonuser	Cigar or pipe	10 cigarettes or fewer per day	20 cigarettes or more per day	30 cigarettes or more per day
	1	2	3	4	5
Habits of eating Fat	0% No animal or solid fats	10% Very little animal or solid fats	20% Little animal or solid fats	30% Much animal or solid fats	40% Very much animal or solid fats

Your risk of heart attack:
  4–9 Very remote   16–20 Average   26–30 Dangerous
10–15 Below average   21–25 Moderate   31–35 Urgent danger — reduce score!
Other conditions — such as stress, high blood pressure, and increased blood cholesterol — detract from health and should be evaluated by your physician.

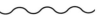

▲ FIGURE 8-5

Risk factors in heart disease. (Courtesy of the School of Public Health, Loma Linda University, Loma Linda, CA.)

10. What advice might you give Mr. Bernardo to help his family prevent the development of cardiovascular disease?

REFERENCES

American Heart Association: The American Heart Association Diet, An Eating Plan for Healthy Americans, 1991.

Environmental Nutrition, The Newsletter of Diet, Nutrition and Health. September 1993; 16(9):3.

Food Insight, Current Topics in Food Safety and Nutrition. July/Aug 1993; p. 8.

Kris-Etherton PM, ed.: Cardiovascular Disease: Nutrition For Prevention and Treatment. The American Dietetic Association, 1990.

Kromhout D, Bosschieter EB, Conlander L: The inverse relation between fish consumption and 20-year mortality from coronary heart disease. N Engl J Med 1985; 312:1205.

National Cholesterol Education Program: Report of the Expert Panel on Population Strategies for Blood Cholesterol Reduction. NIH publication No. 90-3046, US Dept. of Health and Human Services, 1990; p. 7–9.

National Cholesterol Education Program: Report of the Expert Panel on Blood Cholesterol Levels in Children and Adolescents. NIH publication No. 91-2732, US Dept. of Health and Human Services, 1991; pp 1–2.

Ornish D: Dr. Dean Ornish's Program for Reversing Heart Disease. New York, Ballantine Books, 1990.

Salonen JT, Nyyssonen K, Korpela H, et al.: High stored iron levels are associated with excess risk of myocardial infarction in Eastern Finnish men. Circulation 1992; 86:803–811.

Schaefer EJ: new recommendations for the diagnosis and treatment of plasma lipid abnormalities. Nutrition Reviews. 1993; 51(8):246.

Zemel MB: Calcium utilization: Effect of varying level and source of dietary protein. Am J Clin Nutr 1988; 48(3):880.

CHAPTER 9

DIABETES MELLITUS

OBJECTIVES

After completing this chapter, you should be able to:
- Describe the different types of diabetes mellitus
- Describe the symptoms and clinical findings of diabetes mellitus
- Relate the nutritional management of diabetes mellitus to the Dietary Guidelines for
    Americans and the Food Guide Pyramid
- Explain differences in nutritional management of the different forms of diabetes
- Describe the importance of self monitoring of blood glucose
- Explain the role and special concerns of exercise in diabetes management
- Describe the role of health care professionals in facilitating the nutritional aspects of
    diabetes management

TERMS TO IDENTIFY

Autonomic neuropathy
Beta cells
Carbohydrate counting
Counter-regulatory
    hormones
Diabetes management
Diabetes mellitus
Diabetic coma
Diabetic retinopathy
15:15 rule
Food exchange lists
Gastroparesis
Gestational diabetes
    mellitus (GDM)

Glucagon
Glucose
Glycemic index
Glycogenolysis
Glycosuria
Hemoglobin A_{1C}
    (Hgb A_{1C})
Honeymoon period
Hormones
Hyperglycemia
Hyperglycemic hyperos-
    molar nonketotic coma
    (HHNK)
Hyperinsulinemia

Hypertriglyceridemia
Hypoglycemic
    unawareness
Insulin-dependent dia-
    betes mellitus (IDDM)
Insulin resistance
Insulin shock
Islets of Langerhans
Ketoacidosis
Ketonuria
Non–insulin-dependent
    diabetes mellitus
    (NIDDM)

Oral hypoglycemic
    agents
Pancreas
Peripheral neuropathy
Podiatrist
Polydipsia
Polyphagia
Polyuria
Postprandial
Reactive hypoglycemia
Receptor sites
Renal threshold
Self monitoring of blood
    glucose (SMBG)

A FAMILY'S PERSPECTIVE ON NUTRITION

Tony pricked his finger. This actually wasn't so bad, he told himself. It had increasingly become a part of the routine. Check his blood sugar in the morning and at least one other occasion at various times of the day. And his almost daily walks really did help keep his blood sugar under control while helping him to lose weight and feel a bit more positive.

Maria's being in the hospital, however, seemed to affect his blood sugar levels at times. Sometimes it seemed like it was related to eating in the hospital cafeteria. But at other times it seemed like it was related to stress. Such as when he found out that Maria's morning sickness was really serious. His blood sugar went over 200 mg/dL that night!

And a diabetic way of eating really wasn't so bad. It certainly was easier than he thought it was going to be. It would even be a good way of eating for the rest of the family. Less fat, less sugar, less salt, more fiber, and balanced meals. Once you got in the swing of eating a more natural way, the way his ancestors had eaten in their native Italy, it was actually even enjoyable. It was really like the way he and Maria had eaten on their recent trip to Italy. Smaller portions of meat, more reasonable portions of pasta, not like in American restaurants. Fewer desserts and sweets. Fruit at the end of the meal. He especially liked stewed dried fruit with a small chunk of parmesan cheese as his dessert. His dietitian had shown him how to safely work dried fruit and cheese into a healthy way of eating. But he was curious to know how his blood sugar was going to be affected after eating just a small piece of cake for his upcoming birthday. . . .

He certainly felt better these days. He had more energy, and the realization that he could live a longer life to see his new baby grow up made changing his eating and exercise habits worth it.

INTRODUCTION

Diabetes mellitus, commonly referred to by the public as "having sugar," is a serious metabolic disorder related to the utilization of carbohydrate and its end product **glucose** (blood sugar). The metabolism of protein and fat is affected as well. Diabetes affects approximately 13 million individuals in the United States, of whom the majority have **non–insulin-dependent diabetes mellitus,** otherwise referred to as **NIDDM** (see following section for a description). Of the 1 in 20 Americans who have diabetes, only about half know they have it. Mortality statistics of diabetes are greatly underrated since most people with diabetes die from related causes such as heart disease.

The Food Guide Pyramid and the Dietary Guidelines for Americans, appropriate for the general public, are specific management strategies for the control of diabetes. Maintenance of desirable body weight, emphasis on complex carbohydrates and fiber, and avoidance of sugar, fat, and sodium all help the person with diabetes live a full and productive life.

The changing demographics of this country will increase the number of persons with diabetes because of an increased proportion of elderly persons and of persons of color in the population: Both groups are at high risk for diabetes. There is also a growing recognition that a higher than normal blood sugar level that is not actually diabetes is linked to heart disease. All health care professionals, especially nurses, should become thoroughly versed in the management of diabetes. Very few people know that diabetes is related to heart disease, stroke, kidney disease, hypertension, blindness, and circulation problems. Health care professionals can play a vital role in educating the public about diabetes.

WHAT ARE THE BASIC FACTS ABOUT DIABETES MELLITUS?

Etiology

One form of diabetes mellitus can result from a destruction of the beta cells in the pancreas, causing a complete lack of insulin production (**insulin-dependent diabetes mellitus [IDDM]**). This form of diabetes was previously referred to as juvenile-onset because the peak age of onset is during puberty. It was also formerly called Type I diabetes. The other main form of diabetes, formerly called Type II, is related to insulin resistance at the cell level with varying amounts of insulin production: high, normal, or low. **Insulin resistance** means that the body cells resist the action of insulin. The resistance occurs at the **receptor sites** (doors of entry) of the cells. Insulin is used inefficiently, causing elevated blood sugar levels (**hyperglycemia**) (Fig. 9–1). This form of diabetes is non–insulin-dependent diabetes mellitus (NIDDM), otherwise called adult-onset because it usually does not develop until after age 40. Figure 9–2 shows the differences between IDDM and NIDDM.

Heredity is a risk factor for the development of diabetes. It is generally believed that IDDM is an autoimmune disease in which a stress such as a virus causes the body's natural immune system to attack the beta cells where insulin is produced. Persons with IDDM tend to have few relatives with diabetes but do have the genetic predisposition for its development. Higher rates of IDDM are generally found among people with family heritage from northern latitudes. One exception to this is Sardinia, Italy, which has the second highest rate of IDDM behind Finland (Muntoni and Songini, 1992).

Heredity plays a critical role in the development of NIDDM. The propensity to insulin resistance is inherited and is exacerbated by obesity and excess saturated fat intake. Individuals with insulin resistance often produce two to three times more insulin than is normally expected. Persons with NIDDM generally have many family members with a history of diabetes, high blood pressure, heart disease, and obesity. The genetic predisposition and incidence of NIDDM increase in people with heritage from regions nearer the equator, with the highest prevalence being among persons of African, Native American, Asian, Pacific Island, and Southern European heritage. Persons of northern European heritage tend to have a lower incidence of NIDDM.

There is a great deal of evidence that links a more westernized lifestyle (low-fiber and high-fat and high-sugar diet with low levels of physical activity) with the development of NIDDM. But the genetic predisposition toward diabetes must be present before diet and obesity can cause diabetes.

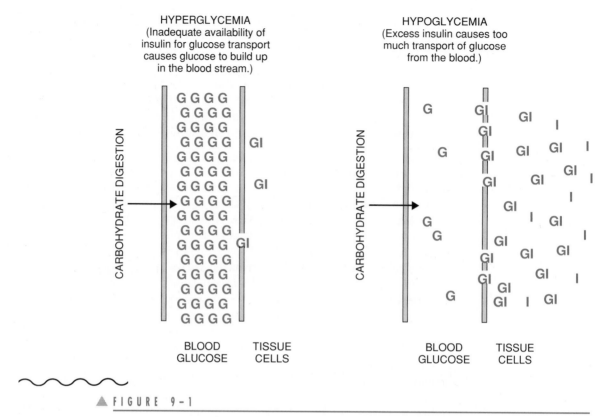

Hyperglycemia and hypoglycemia as a result of inadequate or excess levels of available insulin.
Normal glucose levels are in the range of 70/80 to 120/140. KEY: G = glucose; I = insulin.

Classifications

By the year 2000 we are likely to have many new classifications for diabetes. This is because there are different levels of inadequate insulin production and insulin resistance. Treatment goals will also likely be modified
as we learn more about diabetes. The current major forms of diabetes are
as follows:

INSULIN-DEPENDENT DIABETES MELLITUS

Because insulin production is minimal or completely lacking in IDDM, insulin is required in daily injections (Table 9–1; it should be noted that individual differences are found in the timing of insulin peak action. Human
insulin has a shorter peak action time than beef and pork insulin). Without
insulin, ketoacidosis sets in quickly and makes a person very ill. **Ketoacidosis** is an acidic state caused by a rapid breakdown of body fat. The onset
of this type of diabetes is usually sudden and severe. The person with
IDDM has most, if not all, of the clinical signs and symptoms that will be
discussed in following sections. Control is accomplished only through insulin injection with structured meals and exercise. During the first year af-

	INSULIN-DEPENDENT	NON–INSULIN-DEPENDENT
GENDER:	Males and females.	Increased rate among females.
ETHNICITY:	Increased rates among persons with Northern European heritage.	Increased rates among persons with heritage from equatorial countries (highest rates found with Native American, Hispanic, African American, Asian, Pacific Islander, Mediterranean).
AGE OF ONSET:	Generally under 30 years with peak onset prior to puberty.	Generally over 40 years, although the genetic predisposition is inherited and onset may be seen at younger ages.
WEIGHT:	Usually normal or underweight; unintentional weight loss often precedes diagnosis.	Usually overweight but may be of normal weight.
TREATMENT:	Insulin injections necessary to prevent death. Food and exercise have to be balanced with insulin injections.	Weight loss is usually the first goal. Reduction of sugar and fat, and increase of fiber (soluble) helpful. Oral hypoglycemic agents or insulin or both may be necessary for good blood sugar management but are not necessary to prevent imminent death. Exercise important.
BETA CELL* FUNCTIONING:	Totally absent (no insulin is produced) after the "honeymoon period": residual insulin is produced for about 1 year after diagnosis.	Excess insulin production usually evident (hyperinsulinemia) but due to insulin resistance at the cell level, there is relative insulin insufficiency. Insulin production may also be normal or below normal.

* Beta cells are found in the pancreas.

Pancreas: no insulin production, leads to weight loss

Pancreas: excess insulin production to compensate for insulin resistance at the cell level

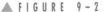

▲ FIGURE 9-2

Differences between insulin-dependent diabetes mellitus (Type I) and non–insulin-dependent diabetes mellitus (Type II).

▲ TABLE 9-1

TYPES OF INSULIN

TYPE OF INSULIN	PEAK ACTION (HOURS)	DURATION OF ACTION (HOURS)
Rapid-acting (Regular, Semilente)	3–4	6–8
Intermediate (Lente, NPH, globin)	9	24
Slow acting (PZI, Ultralente)	20	36

ter diagnosis of IDDM there may be a temporary period of insulin production before the beta cells completely exhaust their insulin production. This is referred to as the **honeymoon period.**

Since onset typically begins in childhood, management issues become complex. The complete lack of natural insulin production makes balancing of food and exercise with insulin injection a challenge. Regular blood sugar monitoring is required to prevent and compensate for high and low blood sugar readings. There is great stress on the family to care for a child with diabetes. Sibling relationships can suffer. Diabetes summer camp programs in which acceptance of the disease and control strategies are emphasized can be very helpful for families.

Approximately 5 to 10 per cent of all cases of diabetes are IDDM.

NON-INSULIN-DEPENDENT DIABETES MELLITUS

Insulin resistance at receptor sites is the underlying mechanism in NIDDM. Elevated production of insulin occurs, leading to excess insulin in the blood, known as **hyperinsulinemia.** The onset of this type of diabetes is slow and gradual. Hyperglycemia is usually evident, but ketoacidosis is frequently not a problem at the time of diagnosis, as it is with IDDM. NIDDM is more stable and can usually be controlled with diet and exercise alone. If there is an inadequate amount of insulin for the body's needs, oral hypoglycemic drug therapy (Table 9–2) or insulin, or both, may be required. Weight reduction in obese individuals is essential to successful treatment. Even though a person with NIDDM does not require insulin for survival, insulin may be needed for good control of blood glucose. A person in this situation would be described as having "non–insulin-dependent diabetes requiring insulin." (This distinction is confusing to many physicians as well!) Thus a person with NIDDM requiring insulin may be able to decrease or discontinue insulin treatment eventually with good dietary and exercise management. Reduction of stressors such as infection, burns, and surgery is also important for blood glucose management without insulin.

▲ TABLE 9-2

ORAL HYPOGLYCEMIC AGENTS

HYPOGLYCEMIC AGENT	DURATION OF ACTION
First-Generation	
Tolbutamide (Orinase)	6-10 hours
Chlorpropamide (Diabinese)	Up to 60 hours
Tolazamide (Tolinase)	12-18 hours
Acetohexamide (Dymelor)	12-20 hours
Second-Generation	
Glyburide (Diabeta and Micronase)	12-24 hours
Glipizide (Glucotrol)	10-16 hours
Gliclazide (Diamicron)	10-20 hours

Modified from Krall LP, Beaser RS: Joslin Diabetes Manual, 12th ed. Philadelphia, Lea & Febiger, 1989; pp. 390-392.

Most persons with diabetes have NIDDM, and most of these persons are overweight.

GESTATIONAL DIABETES

Gestational diabetes mellitus (GDM) is a temporary form of diabetes that occurs during pregnancy. A woman who has diabetes before pregnancy is not said to have GDM. The woman who has IDDM prior to conception will have increased needs for insulin during the latter stages of pregnancy.

In NIDDM, the primary goal is weight loss for the majority of patients, but this is not an appropriate goal for the woman with gestational diabetes because of the growth needs of the developing fetus. Diet control focuses on slow but steady weight gain, avoidance of concentrated sugar sources, and frequent small, balanced meals. A prescribed kilocalorie-restricted diet is generally unnecessary and can even be harmful unless the patient understands that the kilocalorie restriction is for control of weight gain, not for weight loss.

The blood sugar goals during pregnancy are very strict. Self monitoring of blood glucose (SMBG—see later discussion) is essential, as is checking for urine ketones. Occasionally a woman with GDM will require insulin to maintain good control of blood sugar levels. The detection of ketones may be a sign of the need for more food, or for insulin, or both. See Chapter 16 for more information on diabetes and pregnancy.

IMPAIRED GLUCOSE TOLERANCE

A higher than normal blood sugar level that is below the accepted values to diagnose diabetes is referred to as impaired glucose tolerance, formerly known as borderline diabetes (Table 9–3; values between "normal" and "acceptable" are diagnostic of impaired glucose tolerance). The higher than normal blood sugar level is related to cardiovascular disease and therefore should be taken seriously. Treatment remains the same as that for NIDDM: weight loss if needed, avoidance of concentrated sweets and fats, and an increased level of exercise. An increased intake of soluble fiber is often beneficial, especially if **hypertriglyceridemia** (excess triglycerides in the blood) is present. Hypertriglyceridemia often coexists with hyperinsulinemia and insulin resistance.

REACTIVE HYPOGLYCEMIA

In **reactive hypoglycemia,** simple carbohydrates cause the body to produce too much insulin. However, since the overproduction of insulin is delayed, the blood glucose level first rises too high and then falls too quickly (Fig. 9–3). This form of glucose intolerance may be a precursor to the development of diabetes.

Reactive hypoglycemia is characterized by serum glucose levels that fall to less than 50 mg/dL, with symptoms of hypoglycemia (Table 9–4) that are relieved by eating. The symptoms progress as the blood glucose level falls or when it reaches a low level. Persons with uncontrolled diabetes may experience feelings of hypoglycemia as their body adjusts to a lower, more normal level of blood glucose.

The person with reactive hypoglycemia needs to limit the intake of simple sugars and concentrated sweets and emphasize complex carbohydrates and frequent eating (about every 2 to 3 hours). Including a protein source

▲ TABLE 9–3

INDICES OF DIABETES OR IMPAIRED GLUCOSE TOLERANCE*

BIOCHEMICAL INDEX	NORMAL	ACCEPTABLE	POOR
Fasting plasma glucose (mg/dL)	≤115 (6.4)†	140 (7.8)	>200 (>11.1)
Postprandial (2 hr after glucose challenge) plasma glucose (mg/dL)	≤140 (7.8)	200 (11.1)	>235 (>13.1)

* Impaired glucose tolerance is indicated by values between "normal" and "acceptable"; diabetes, by values above the "acceptable" range.
† Values in parentheses are in millimoles (mM).
From the Physician's Guide to Non-Insulin Dependent (Type II) Diabetes: Diagnosis and Treatment, 2nd ed. Alexandria, VA, American Diabetes Association, 1988.

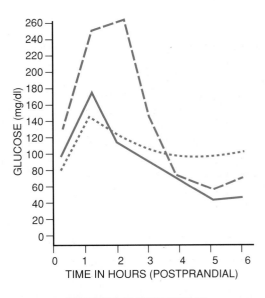

REACTIVE HYPOGLYCEMIA
(uncontrolled)
DIABETIC HYPOGLYCEMIC EPISODE
(uncontrolled)
NORMAL BLOOD GLUCOSE CURVE

▲ FIGURE   9 – 3

Comparison of blood glucose levels in reactive hypoglycemia and diabetes.

with meals and snacks helps to maintain appropriate blood glucose levels
because it slows carbohydrate digestion, causing only minimal stimulation
of insulin secretion (Table 9–5 lists high-protein snack ideas). Caffeine and
alcohol may exacerbate the symptoms of hypoglycemia owing to their effect
on liver glycogen and **glycogenolysis** (breakdown of glycogen into glucose).

▲   TABLE   9 – 4

COMMON SYMPTOMS THAT SIGNAL
HYPOGLYCEMIA

- Clammy skin
- Mental confusion
- Physical tremor
- Weakness
- Headache
- Rapid heart beat
- Double or blurred vision

▲ **TABLE 9-5**

HIGH-PROTEIN SNACK IDEAS FOR REACTIVE HYPOGLYCEMIA*

Graham cracker with peanut butter
Apple or banana slices with peanut butter
Celery with peanut butter
Cheese and crackers
Nuts and raisins (small amount of raisins)
Cottage cheese and fruit
Unsweetened fruit juice and cheese
Half sandwich (meat, peanut butter, or cheese)
Hard-cooked egg and small glass of milk
Hot cereal with melted peanut butter
Cold cereal with bite-sized chunks of peanut butter
Bagel and cream cheese
Parmesan muffin (English muffin with margarine and parmesan cheese)
Half a cantaloupe stuffed with cottage cheese

* Regular meals should be reduced in portion sizes to compensate for the added kilocalories consumed through snacks. Regular meals also need to be balanced, including a protein source and avoiding large quantities of concentrated sweets. Snacks should be consumed about 2 to 3 hours after regular meals.

What is Insulin?

Insulin is a hormone that is produced in the **beta cells** of the **islets of Langerhans** found in the **pancreas.** When these beta cells are damaged or when there is an increased need for insulin because of insulin resistance, the person's blood glucose level rises (see Fig. 9–1).

When hyperglycemia occurs from lack of internal production of insulin, insulin from an alternative source may become a requirement. Since insulin is composed of protein, oral intake is prohibited, as it would be digested before being used. Thus, injection is the primary route of administration, although insulin pumps are also used now to a limited extent. These pumps allow for continuous insulin supply rather than the large doses given intermittently through subcutaneous injections. Research continues on other forms of insulin delivery.

Different types of insulin may be given; the type and amount are determined by the physician based on blood glucose levels and individual glycemic (blood sugar level) responses to food intake. There are slow-acting, intermediate-acting, and rapid-acting types of insulin (see Table 9–1). Previously, these types of insulin were obtained only from beef or pork pancreas. Now human insulin is the main form used. This form of insulin is made either by genetic manipulation or by enzymatic manipulation of pork insulin so that it contains the same protein structure as human insulin. It does not come from humans.

It is now recommended that insulin injection be more frequent in an attempt to mimic Mother Nature. Normally each time we eat a meal the body produces insulin. The goal of intensive insulin therapy is normalization of blood sugar. Figure 9–4 shows different types of insulin and injection

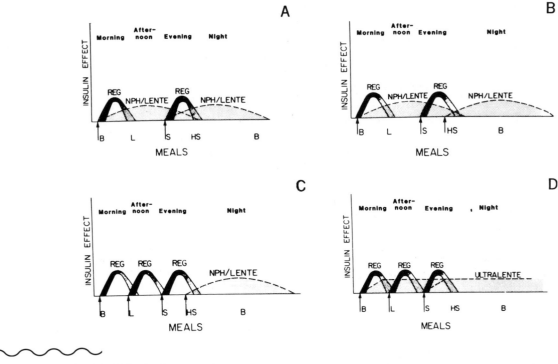

▲ FIGURE 9-4

Schema of ideal insulin effect provided by various subcutaneous insulin regimens with rapid-onset regular (REG) insulin, intermediate-acting (NPH or LENTE) insulins, or long-acting Ultralente insulin. A, Split-and-mixed insulin regimen consisting of two daily doses of regular and intermediate-acting insulin. B, Split-and-mixed insulin regimen in which evening intermediate-acting insulin was delayed until bedtime, resulting in peak action coinciding with pre-breakfast blood glucose measurement. C, Multiple-dose regimen providing three daily injections of regular insulin before meals and one injection of intermediate-acting insulin at bedtime. D, Multiple-dose regimen providing regular insulin before meals and long-acting relatively peakless Ultralente insulin for basal insulinemia. KEY: B = breakfast; L = lunch; S = supper; HS = bedtime snack; Arrow = time of insulin injection (30 min) before meals. From Schade DS, et al.: Intensive Insulin Therapy. Princeton, NJ, Excerpta Medica, 1983.

times. People with hectic lifestyles who cannot maintain regular meal timing may benefit from the use of Ultralente as the basal amount of circulating insulin, with regular insulin given at the time of meals, based on carbohydrate content. This approach mimics most closely what occurs in persons without diabetes. Its use in diabetes, however, requires a highly motivated individual who regularly monitors blood sugar levels and who can accurately estimate insulin needs based on meal composition and blood sugar levels. Special advanced patient training is necessary. All patients who use insulin should know when the likely peak time of action of their insulin occurs in order to plan a meal or snack and avoid exercise at these times (see Table 9-1).

Several **hormones** (chemicals produced by the body that regulate body functioning) act in concert to regulate blood glucose levels. Insulin, produced in the pancreas, is the only hormone that lowers blood glucose levels. There are many hormones that act to raise glucose levels, chief among them being glucagon, epinephrine (also called adrenaline), cortisol, and growth hormone. These are called **counter-regulatory hormones** because they work in an opposite manner to insulin. Any deviation in the balance of these hormones will cause fluctuations in blood glucose levels. Because of increased production of adrenalin, stress can lead to hyperglycemia by causing the liver to release glycogen (stored sugar).

FACT & FALLACY

FALLACY: A person can get AIDS from human insulin.
FACT: Since human insulin is made genetically, it is not possible to contract AIDS or any other disease from it. Insulin needles should not be shared, even by family members, as disease can spread through contaminated needles.

The warning signs of diabetes are unusual thirst; frequent urination; abnormal hunger; sudden weight loss (usually indicates IDDM only); skin disorders, infections, and delayed wound healing; blurred vision; and unexplained weakness and fatigue.

HYPERGLYCEMIA. Hyperglycemia is associated with the complications of diabetes. It also causes many of the symptoms of diabetes. Blurred vision can be caused when excess sugar in the eye changes the shape of the lens. Infections increase with hyperglycemia as the body's immune system does not work as efficiently. There are conditions under which the body normally raises the blood glucose levels, such as stress of infection, illness, or surgery. Sometimes a person with NIDDM will require insulin injections on a temporary basis until the stress has passed.

GLYCOSURIA. One way the body tries to lower blood sugar is to flush it out the kidneys. This is often described as "spilling over into the urine" and is known as **glycosuria.** Thus frequent urination and thirst are often associated with hyperglycemia. The level of blood sugar generally has to rise unacceptably high (>180 mg/dL) before glucose is detected in the urine. This is referred to as the **renal threshold.** Thus glycosuria tests are generally not recommended except as an easy screening test and for those persons who refuse, or are unable, to test blood sugars.

KETONURIA. Without insulin, carbohydrates are unavailable for energy utilization. Instead, the body calls upon fat as an energy source. Un-

A good assessment question to ask a patient is whether he or she has to get up in the middle of the night to use the bathroom and how often. Persons with undiagnosed diabetes are often relieved to hear they can again expect an uninterrupted night's sleep with improved blood glucose control. This can help with motivation to adhere to dietary and exercise prescriptions.

der normal conditions, the liver breaks down small amounts of fatty acids to form ketones. These ketones are further metabolized for energy. In uncontrolled diabetes, ketone production exceeds utilization. The excess is excreted in the urine. This is known as **ketonuria.** If the excess ketones are not removed adequately, the condition known as ketoacidosis develops. In ketoacidosis, the blood pH changes to a more acidic level, which can cause death. Treatment should be prompt and hospitalization will be needed if blood becomes too acidic. This condition generally occurs in IDDM but can also occur in persons with NIDDM who are under stress such as infection or surgery.

DEHYDRATION. The excess fluid loss associated with high levels of blood glucose causes water to be taken from body tissues. This can result in dehydration if water is not replaced and blood sugar controlled.

Dehydration with concentrated amounts of glucose in the blood can cause a condition known as **hyperglycemic hyperosmolar nonketotic coma (HHNK).** This condition is commonly found in elderly patients, in whom diabetes is much more prevalent and in whom there is a diminished sensation of thirst owing to the aging process. Because dehydration of the brain can occur, many elderly patients with HHNK have a history of lethargy, sleepiness, and confused state lasting several days to weeks (Kirk, 1993). Dehydration and HHNK are easily treated if caught in the early stages. All older patients, but especially those with diabetes, should be taught the importance of adequate water intake even if there is not a sense of thirst.

POLYDIPSIA AND POLYURIA. Increased thirst, known as **polydipsia,** is experienced as the body senses the need to replace excess fluids lost from frequent urination **(polyuria).** This is an attempt by the body to remove excess ketones and glucose.

POLYPHAGIA. Increased appetite, known as **polyphagia,** is the body's response to the need for energy. However, this need is not being satisfied, since carbohydrates are not available for energy without insulin. This can be another sign that a person has undiagnosed diabetes. A health care professional should inquire about a person's appetite and whether it has changed. Polyphagia may cause weight gain.

WEIGHT LOSS. Because the sugar is staying in the blood and is not used for energy, a feeling of weakness, hunger, and weight loss can be associated with hyperglycemia. Glucose that does not enter the body cells is excreted in the urine along with excess ketones. Both represent wasted energy sources. Weight loss results because energy demand exceeds available sources. This is more likely to happen with IDDM or in severe cases of NIDDM in which there is insufficient or no insulin production.

FACT & FALLACY

FALLACY: Diabetes is not life-threatening.

FACT: Although persons with diabetes can now expect increased longevity, morbidity from uncontrolled diabetes is still a major health problem. There is growing evidence that long-term complications such as blindness, kidney disease, amputation of feet and legs, and other complications are preventable through careful control of blood glucose levels. The Diabetes Control and Complications Trial (DCCT) sponsored by the National Institutes of Health and completed in 1993 showed that persons with IDDM could decrease the likelihood of eye, kidney, and nerve disease by about 60 per cent by maintaining an average blood sugar level less than 155 mg/dL and hemoglobin A_{1c} level of about 7.2 per cent (Dawson, 1993). A person with diabetes, however, needs to consult with a professional before determining personal ideal blood glucose levels because factors such as age and illness need to be considered.

NUTRITIONAL MANAGEMENT

Meal Planning

Balanced meals are essential for the management of diabetes. Pure carbohydrate meals will raise the blood sugar level faster since carbohydrates take no more than 1 hour for digestion. Food has to get through the stomach before it can significantly affect blood sugar levels. Including at least a small amount of protein with a meal or snack will slow down the process of digestion, thereby limiting its impact on blood sugar.

Kilocalories

The amount of kilocalories needed by a person with diabetes should be the same as the recommended dietary allowances (RDA) for a person without diabetes. Adjustments in kilocalories may be necessary to maintain or attain normal body weight and can be made as necessary. Generally, 20 to 30 kilocalories per kilogram body weight is adequate to maintain weight. A 500 kilocalorie reduction from this level should result in a weekly weight loss of 1 pound (see Chapter 20). The person with NIDDM is more likely to need weight loss, while the person with IDDM is more likely to need weight gain, especially at the time of diagnosis.

Protein

The percentage of kilocalories derived from protein should be up to 20 per cent. This allows the individual with diabetes from 1 to 1.5 g of protein per kilogram of body weight and should approximate the RDA. A level of protein intake at 0.8 g protein per kilogram body weight or less may be desirable to prevent or control kidney disease.

Carbohydrates

Carbohydrates are no longer restricted as much as they once were. The recommended allowance is 50 to 60 per cent of total kilocalories from carbohydrate. Complex carbohydrates are emphasized, as are high-fiber foods. Sugar may be tolerated in small quantities and should be counted as part of total grams of carbohydrate in a meal. Four grams of sucrose is the same as 1 teaspoon of sugar. Fructose and lactose (fruit sugar and milk sugar, respectively) are also simple sugars.

Fiber promotes normal blood glucose levels **postprandially** (after meals). It also can lower triglyceride levels. This is primarily the case with the soluble fiber found in oats, legumes, brown rice, barley, and many vegetables and fruit. The theory behind this finding is related to the increased time for digestion of food; however, it is also believed that fiber reduces insulin resistance at the cell level. Therefore, the use of available insulin is made more efficient and may allow for reduced need for medication. In terms of a real diet, a fresh orange would be more beneficial than the equivalent amount of orange juice. Whole oat bread would be better than refined wheat bread. Vegetarians, who typically have a high-fiber diet, are known to have lower rates than nonvegetarians of NIDDM (American Dietetic Association, 1988). Vegetarians are also generally of desirable body weight, which may be a contributing factor. The recommendation of the Dietary Guidelines for Americans for increased fiber is beneficial not only for the general public but also for the person with diabetes in particular. A goal of 20 to 30 grams of fiber should be promoted. Including whole grains, vegetables, and fruits according to the number of food servings recommended by the Food Guide Pyramid will provide this amount of fiber. Emphasis on legumes in the diet will be further beneficial.

Simple sugars (monosaccharides and disaccharides; Table 9-6) are generally not advocated for individuals with diabetes, nor for the general public. It is now recognized, however, that occasional small amounts may be safe and will allow feelings of greater normalcy for the individual with diabetes. The natural sugar content of fruit needs to be considered as well. One serving of fruit contains 4 teaspoons of sugar in the form of fructose. Many diabetes experts recommend that diabetic persons reduce fruit intake to one serving per meal and that women with GDM avoid fruit at breakfast. Regarding simple carbohydrates in particular, advice should be provided on an individual basis and in consultation with the patient's physician and a registered dietitian.

Sugar substitutes (see Table 9-6) are not always preferable. Sugar alcohols, such as sorbitol and xylitol, are often found in dietetic foods; they contain 4 kilocalories per gram, can cause the blood glucose levels to rise, and thus should not be considered "free foods." In addition, excess intake may

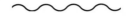

▲ TABLE 9-6

NUTRITIVE AND NON-NUTRITIVE SWEETENERS*

NAME	COMPOSITION	SOURCES
Nutritive Sweeteners		
Glucose	Monosaccharide	Found in blood as the end product of starch digestion
		Occurs naturally in fruit
Fructose	Monosaccharide	Found in fruit and honey
Sucrose	Disaccharide composed of glucose and fructose	Commonly known as table sugar and widely used in commercial foods
Lactose	Disaccharide composed of glucose and galactose	Found in milk and unfermented milk products†
Maltose	Disaccharide composed of two glucose molecules	Produced during brewing and breadmaking; also made commercially
Honey	Mainly fructose and glucose	Made from plants by honeybees
Maple syrup	Primarily sucrose	Made by boiling off the liquid found in sap of mature sugar maple trees
Corn syrup	Composed of glucose molecules of different chain lengths	Produced from cornstarch
High-fructose corn syrup	Contains 40–100% fructose	Produced enzymatically from cornstarch
Molasses	Contains 50–75% sucrose	Produced during the processing of table sugar
Sorbitol, mannitol, xylitol	Sugar alcohols	Found naturally in fruit and used as a sugar substitute
Aspartame	Methyl ester of two amino acids: phenylalanine and aspartic acid (aspartate)	Commonly known as NutraSweet and widely used in low-sugar food products; kilocalories are insignificant, since small amounts are used because it is intensely sweet (180–220 times as sweet as sucrose)
Non-nutritive Sweeteners		
Saccharin	Organic compound	Originally banned in 1977 after being implicated as causing bladder tumors in rats fed high doses; currently available as a sugar substitute
Cyclamate	Available as cyclamic acid, calcium cyclamate, and sodium cyclamate	Banned since 1969 after evidence showed it as a possible cancer-causing agent in rats; FDA may reconsider its use given more studies on its safety

* Nutritive sweeteners are those that provide kilocalories; non-nutritive sweeteners are entirely free of kilocalories because they are not metabolized.

† Lactose as found in milk is not harmful to diabetic individuals.

Modified from The Institute of Food Technologists' Expert Panel on Food Safety and Nutrition: Sweeteners: Nutritive and Non-nutritive. Contemp Nutr. 12(9): 1987.

lead to diarrhea. Saccharin, aspartame (NutraSweet), and acesulfame-K (a new sugar substitute) have no appreciable kilocalorie content in amounts commonly consumed but may be used in foods that contain other sources of kilocalories, such as fat. These foods may give a person with diabetes the false perception that if the food is sugar-free it is also kilocalorie-free. Commercial fructose offers only minimal advantage over sucrose for the person with diabetes, although both sweeteners may be tolerated in small amounts.

FACT & FALLACY

FALLACY: Although persons with diabetes need to avoid sugar, they can eat honey without problem.

FACT: Honey is composed of sucrose and fructose, two simple sugars, and as such cannot safely be used freely. Occasional moderate use, especially in a person who practices self monitoring of blood glucose (SMBG), may be appropriate.

Fat

Approximately 20 to 30 per cent of the total kilocalories for the patient with diabetes is derived from fat. Low-fat foods, lean meats, and unsaturated fats are emphasized to prevent cardiovascular disease (a common complication of diabetes). A low-fat diet helps the overweight person with NIDDM to lose weight and helps to keep blood vessels and arteries healthy in persons with either IDDM or NIDDM. Cholesterol restrictions are imposed if ordered by the physician. Choosing low-processed grain products such as bread, cereal, rice, and pasta along with moderate amounts of lean meat and low-fat milk, as recommended in the Food Guide Pyramid, can result in a healthy low-fat way of eating.

Calculating the Diet

Once the diet order is received from the physician, the diet can be calculated from protein, carbohydrate, and fat content. For example, if the diet order calls for 2000 kilocalories, it can be calculated as follows:

PROTEIN:

$$2000 \times 0.15 = 300 \text{ kcal} \div 4 \text{ kcal/g} = 75 \text{ g protein}$$

CARBOHYDRATE:

$$2000 \times 0.60 = 1200 \text{ kcal} \div 4 \text{ kcal/g} = 300 \text{ g carbohydrate}$$

FAT:

$$2000 \times 0.25 = 500 \text{ kcal} \div 9 \text{ kcal/g} = 55 \text{ g fat}$$

The calculations for protein, carbohydrate, and fat must now be translated into a meal pattern that will fit the person's lifestyle and insulin type. Meals are planned using **food exchange lists.** The foods in each list are grouped in terms of similarity of composition, and they supply approximately the same amount of protein, carbohydrate, and fat. One serving of any food may be exchanged for another serving in the same list. A concise, easily memorized form of the food exchange list is given in Table 9–7. The full exchange list is shown in Appendix 9. Adjustments can be made until the ideal diet plan is developed—one that is appropriate for diabetes management and good nutritional intake and is suited to fit individual lifestyles. Dietitians are best qualified to develop meal pattern guides based on patient food preferences and lifestyles, although other health professionals or persons with diabetes can be trained to calculate food patterns using the exchange list system.

It is important that the diet be individually planned to facilitate patient compliance. Thus, dissemination of preplanned diet guides is not in the best interest of persons with diabetes.

There are other forms of meal planning that may be appropriate. One is referred to as **carbohydrate counting.** Carbohydrate counting can be useful for someone who finds the exchange system too cumbersome. The person with diabetes learns how much carbohydrate is in foods and aims for a regular amount, such as 50 grams with each meal and 15 to 30 grams with each snack. It also helps the person with diabetes to understand how specific food choices affect blood glucose values. SMBG is imperative.

FACT & FALLACY

FALLACY: Diabetic individuals must give up the foods they love.
FACT: The rule of moderation applies to both the general public and the diabetic individual in achieving the goal of good nutritional intake. Moderate amounts of all foods are acceptable. All food consists of carbohydrate, protein, fat, or a combination, and therefore can be worked into the exchange list system. The potential problem with this approach is individual definitions of moderation. Assessment of weight control and SMBG are two methods that can indicate whether moderation is truly moderate. A referral to a registered dietitian is strongly advised in order to educate persons with diabetes about how to make appropriate changes in their diets and to help facilitate compliance in control of their diabetes. Some diabetes centers teach patients how to adjust insulin dose based on food and exercise choices in order to more fully meet the goal of good glycemic control.

Carbohydrate
Distribution

Carbohydrate should be distributed among the meals and snacks according to the type of insulin prescribed. For the person receiving oral hypoglycemic agents, meals and snacks should be guided by SMBG. Generally, an afternoon and an evening snack are desirable to prevent hypoglycemia for a person on diabetes medication. Distributing carbohydrate throughout the day will help prevent both hypoglycemic and hyperglycemic reactions.

Can a Person with
Diabetes Drink
Alcoholic Beverages?

Alcohol contributes about 7 kilocalories per gram (carbohydrate and protein yield 4 kilocalories per gram and fat yields 9 kilocalories per gram) and thus needs to be calculated into a diabetic diet. Mixed drinks, liqueurs, and sweet wines should be avoided entirely because of the high content of simple sugars. Beer, hard liquor mixed with water or diet soda, and dry wine may be tolerated in limited quantities but should be consumed only after consultation with the patient's physician and dietitian.

It is important that the patient eat appropriate foods such as whole-wheat crackers when having a drink, since alcohol can induce hypoglycemia. The person with diabetes should tell a companion that he or she has diabetes in case hypoglycemia develops while drinking alcohol. Hypoglycemia has been mistaken for intoxication. A drink of orange juice would be recommended if a person with diabetes appears inebriated.

How Can a Person
with Diabetes Eat at
Restaurants?

Restaurant eating poses no problem if there is adequate selection. Simple foods without gravy or other sauces may be desirable, and sweets and sweet alcoholic beverages should be avoided. Occasional high-fat choices are preferable to overconsumption of simple carbohydrate foods. Dessert might be shared with a friend and portions controlled by asking for a "doggy bag." Portions might also be controlled by ordering several appetizers rather than the entree, which generally is inappropriately large for persons trying to control their weight and blood sugar.

Eating "on the road" can be a particular challenge. Low-sugar snack foods should be packed for travel by car or when regular mealtimes may be difficult or impossible to achieve. Persons with IDDM need to receive instruction on how to make alternative choices of food based on carbohydrate, protein, and fat content. The use of the exchange system (Table 9–7) can facilitate this; in addition, fast food restaurants now make available the nutritional content of their food selections (see Appendix 4).

WHAT IS THE GLYCEMIC INDEX OF FOOD?

The body reacts differently to the various forms of complex carbohydrate foods and to combinations of foods found in meals. In other words, not all carbohydrate foods cause blood glucose levels to rise equally. This is referred to as the **glycemic index** of food. Research is still evolving as to the predictable glycemic responses with various foods and combinations of foods. Until more knowledge is acquired, specific indexes cannot be used appropriately for dietary guidance. However, it is generally known that legumes have a lower glycemic index than do root vegetables and grains. High-fiber foods have a lower glycemic index than do low-fiber foods.

ABBREVIATED FOOD EXCHANGE LIST*

Meat and Substitutes
  protein = 7 g
  fat = 5 g
    lean meat = 1–2 g
    fatty meat = 8–10 g

Each of these equals one meat choice (75 kilocalories)
  1 oz cooked poultry, fish, or meat
  ¼ c cottage cheese
  ¼ c salmon or tuna, water packed
  1 tbsp peanut butter
  1 egg (limit to 3/week)
  1 oz low-fat cheese, such as mozzarella, ricotta
Each of these equals two meat choices (150 kilocalories)
  1 small chicken leg or thigh
  ½ c cottage cheese or tuna
Each of these equals three meat choices (225 kilocalories)
  1 small pork chop
  1 small hamburger
  Cooked meat, about the size of a deck of cards
  ½ of a whole chicken breast
  1 medium fish fillet

Starch-Bread
  carbohydrate = 15 g
  protein = 3 g

Each of these equals one starch-bread choice (80 kilocalories)
  ½ c pasta or barley
  ⅓ c rice or cooked dried beans and peas
  1 small potato (or ½ cup mashed)
  ½ c starchy vegetables (corn, peas, winter squash)
  1 slice bread or 1 roll
  ½ English muffin, bagel, or hamburger or hot dog bun
  ½ c cooked cereal
  ¾ c dry cereal, unsweetened
  4–6 crackers
  3 c popcorn, unbuttered, not cooked in oil

Vegetables
  carbohydrate = 5 g
  protein = 2 g

Each of these equals one vegetable choice (25 kilocalories)
  ½ c cooked vegetables
  1 c raw vegetables
  ½ c tomato-vegetable juice

Milk
  carbohydrate = 12 g
  protein = 8 g
  fat = 0 g (skim); 5 g (2%)

Each of these equals one milk choice
The calories vary for each choice
  1 c skim milk (90 kilocalories)
  1 c low-fat milk (120 kilocalories)
  8 oz carton plain low-fat yogurt (120 kilocalories)

Fruit
  carbohydrate = 15 g

Each of these equals one fruit choice (60 kilocalories)
  1 medium fresh fruit
  1 c berries or melon
  ½ c canned in juice or without sugar
  ½ c fruit juice
  ¼ c dried fruit

Fat
  fat = 5 g

Each of these equals one fat choice (45 kilocalories)
  1 tsp margarine, oil, mayonnaise
  2 tsp diet margarine or diet mayonnaise
  1 tbsp salad dressing
  2 tbsp reduced-calorie salad dressing

* For a healthy diet, a person should have at least four choices from the starch-bread group, five meat or meat substitutes, two vegetable choices, two fruit choices, two skim milk choices, and not more than three fat choices totaling about 1200 calories/day.

Protein foods that are low in carbohydrate have a lower glycemic index. Fats have the lowest glycemic index. Thus cheese would not be expected to significantly raise the blood sugar but would be discouraged owing to the high saturated fat content and its contribution to heart disease. Low-fat cheeses are appropriate if the sodium is taken into account.

WHAT IS THE ROLE OF EXERCISE IN DIABETES MANAGEMENT?

Exercise is an integral component of treatment in NIDDM (Horton, 1991). It is a factor in weight control and has been found to lower blood glucose levels to the point of reducing or eliminating the need for oral hypoglycemic agents or insulin.

Exercise can be beneficial in IDDM, but greater caution is needed. For the ketotic or hyperglycemic patient (blood glucose level greater than 240 to 300 mg/dL), exercise will actually increase glucose levels further, primarily because insulin is a prerequisite for glucose usage in exercising muscles. Hyperglycemia is generally indicative of insufficient insulin availability. Exercise should be avoided unless blood glucose levels are under control. Even for the patient with well-controlled IDDM, however, a balance needs to be achieved between the extra energy demands of exercise and diet and insulin. The general rule of thumb is to eat slightly more food or decrease the amount of insulin, or both, and to avoid exercising at the times that insulin is acting at peak levels (see Table 9–1). These guidelines help prevent the development of insulin shock, which is caused by excess insulin in relation to the amount of blood glucose available. For anyone with diabetes, a complete physical examination by a physician is imperative before embarking upon an exercise program, but it is crucial for the insulin-dependent individual. SMBG is a valuable tool for determining the best way to adjust diet and insulin before, during, and after exercise. More food may need to be consumed for up to 24 hours after exercise as exercise-induced hypoglycemia can last this long.

MEASURES OF GOOD DIABETES MANAGEMENT

Self Monitoring of Blood Glucose

Self monitoring of blood glucose (SMBG) is a form of treatment in the sense that the patient can take responsibility for diabetes management. Because control of the blood glucose level is the chief goal of diabetes management, knowledge of its level is a valuable guide. Self monitoring consists of taking a drop of blood, which is then placed on a reagent strip. The reagent strip, after changing color, is matched against a predetermined color-coded guide or is inserted in a glucometer (digital reader) indicating the blood glucose level. There are many glucometers available, each with advantages and disadvantages to their use. Patients should be given information on available meters to select the one that best suits their needs. To achieve the maximum benefits from SMBG, the test should be done several times a day until control of glycemia is achieved. Recommended times to administer the test include before meals and 1 to 2 hours postprandially, at a minimum, in order to identify responses to foods. Typically, a meal can be expected to raise the blood sugar by 40 to 50 points. With a fasting blood sugar level of 100 mg/dL, an ideal meal should keep the blood sugar level to less than 150 mg/dL. If the blood sugar level goes higher than this, it is due to either excess carbohydrate in the meal or a need for medication. Keeping a journal of blood sugar levels is recommended in order to compare diet (specific quantity of foods and time consumed) with activity levels and, if applicable, administration of insulin or oral hypoglycemic agents. This information is used to decide the best course of action for the individual person with diabetes.

The advantage of SMBG is the flexibility it affords in diabetes management. Less guesswork becomes involved and SMBG allows the diabetic patient greater objectivity in decision-making.

> Questions such as "How do I adjust my diet and insulin for exercise?" or "Can I eat a piece of birthday cake safely?" can be addressed through self monitoring of blood glucose. Mr. Bernardo might find that a half piece of birthday cake with his evening meal may raise his blood sugar to an acceptable level. If his blood sugar goes above 200 mg/dL two hours after eating the cake, he might consider not eating more.

Drawbacks to SMBG are that the diabetic individual must deal with the restrictions of the disease several times a day and has to claim responsibility for the management of abnormal glucose levels. The benefits, however, far outweigh the drawbacks.

Ketone Checks

All persons with diabetes should know about ketones. For persons with GDM, ketones should be checked daily. Individuals with IDDM should check for ketonuria whenever their blood sugar is over 240 mg/dL on two or more occasions or when they are ill or under stress such as with surgery. Ketones are particularly important to assess during illness, when the likelihood of elevated blood glucose and dehydration occurs. Symptoms of nausea, vomiting, and deep labored breathing may be signs of impending ketoacidosis.

What is Hemoglobin A_{1c} and What is its Role in Diabetes Management?

Hemoglobin is a component of the red blood cells that is used to carry oxygen throughout the body. The amount of **hemoglobin A_{1c} (HbA_{1c}),** a portion of hemoglobin, is related to the average amount of blood glucose (versus daily or hourly amounts, which can fluctuate erratically), and thus gives an indication of overall control. Testing for HbA_{1c} is done only a few times a year, and if it is found to be high, the current individual plan of action for diabetes control should be altered. The goal is to maintain a normal level of HbA_{1c} (6 to 8 per cent maximum), thereby reducing long-term diabetic complications.

Lipid Screening

Lipid (blood fat) abnormalities go hand in hand with poor control of diabetes. An increased level of blood glucose is felt to contribute to these abnormalities. A high level of triglycerides (>200 mg/dL) with an associated low level of high-density lipoprotein cholesterol (<40 mg/dL) is generally found in persons with uncontrolled NIDDM. The cholesterol and low-density lipoprotein cholesterol may or may not be elevated (Hannah and Harper, 1993). There is usually improvement in the blood lipids upon improvement of diet, weight, and blood glucose levels. Medication is sometimes needed as well.

Albumin Screening

All patients with diabetes mellitus should have their urine tested for albumin. The test should be done annually in persons who have had IDDM for more than 5 years and in all persons with NIDDM (Hawthorne, 1989). Albuminuria (albumin in the urine) is associated with advancing kidney disease and should be treated aggressively. A moderate protein intake of 0.8 gram protein per kilogram body weight is the first dietary step, along with reduction in sodium intake (2 g sodium is generally adequate) if there is concomitant hypertension.

WHAT ARE COMPLICATIONS OF DIABETES?

Insulin Shock and Diabetic Coma

Insulin shock (insulin reaction) occurs when more insulin is injected than is needed (Table 9–8 describes dietary treatment of a conscious person). Insulin shock can result from omitting foods from the diet, increased activity and exercise (which burns more kilocalories than normal), or an error in insulin injection in relation to exercise (Table 9–9). The result is hypoglycemia, a lowering of the blood glucose level. The onset is usually sudden. If the hypoglycemia is not treated promptly, the diabetic patient becomes mentally confused and disoriented. If this situation is prolonged, seizures,

▲ TABLE 9–8

PORTIONS FOR DIETARY TREATMENT OF HYPOGLYCEMIC EPISODES IN CONSCIOUS PERSONS

15 g CARBOHYDRATE	30 g CARBOHYDRATE
3 oz apple juice	6 oz apple juice
4 oz orange juice	8 oz orange juice
5 oz regular soda pop	10 oz regular soda pop
4 tsp honey	8 tsp honey
4 tsp sugar	8 tsp sugar
¼ c sherbet	½ c sherbet

The 15:15 rule: check blood sugar; if low (less than 70 mg/dL) treat with 15 grams of carbohydrate. Recheck blood sugar in 15 minutes; if still low repeat with another 15 grams of carbohydrate. If the blood sugar is severely low (less than 50 mg/dL) treat with 30 grams of carbohydrate and recheck in 15 minutes.

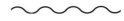

▲ TABLE 9-9

DIET DILEMMAS FOR INSULIN USERS

CONDITION	REMEDY	ADJUST MEAL PATTERN FOR ADDITIONAL CARBOHYDRATES
Insulin Reaction	15 g carbohydrate If lasts more than 15 minutes, take more carbohydrate	No
Exercise		
Light: (½-mile walk)	Do not increase food intake	No
Moderate: (golf, bowling)	10–15 g carbohydrate/hour of exercise	No
Vigorous: (skating, running)	20–30 g carbohydrate/hour of exercise	No
Delayed Meal	15–30 g carbohydrate will prevent reaction for 1–2 hours	Deduct from meal pattern
Illness	50–75 g carbohydrate every 6–8 hours	Replaces meal pattern

Data from El-Beheri-Burgess B. Diet dilemmas for insulin users. Diabetes Forecast. 1982; 35(5):10, © American Diabetes Association.

unconsciousness, and death can result. All family members should have on hand and know how to inject glucagon in order to raise blood sugar for an unconscious person. (**Glucagon,** as discussed earlier, is a counter-regulatory hormone that acts to release stored glycogen from the liver, thereby providing a blood sugar source; it is available with a physician's prescription.) Medical services should be sought in the case of insulin shock to help prevent another occurrence.

Diabetic coma is a potential result of ketoacidosis, discussed earlier in this chapter. In this condition, the blood glucose level becomes elevated, and glycosuria and ketonuria occur. The person experiences drowsiness, lethargy, and sometimes nausea with vomiting. The skin becomes hot and dry. There is a fruity odor to the breath (acetone). Breathing is deep and labored. Death can result if the patient is not treated promptly with insulin and fluids. Hospitalization is required.

What Are the Causes, Symptoms, and Treatment of Hypoglycemia?

Either insulin or **oral hypoglycemic agents** (diabetes pills; see Table 9–2) can cause the blood sugar to drop below a point at which the body can function. Feelings of hypoglycemia when no diabetes medication is being taken is not life-threatening and generally resolves on its own.

The individual with hypoglycemia may begin to perspire; experience hunger and nervousness; have skin that becomes pale, cold, and clammy; and experience mental confusion, physical tremor, weakness, headache, rapid heart beat, and double or blurred vision (see Table 9–4). When these symptoms are noted, the blood sugar level should be checked to verify hypoglycemia. However, not all diabetic individuals experience these symptoms, especially children, elderly persons, or persons who have had diabetes for many years. The health professional or close family member should suspect hypoglycemia, and treat accordingly, when a diabetic child becomes unusually quiet or fretful or when an elderly or other diabetic patient becomes weak or faint. A physician should be consulted if the cause is not readily apparent or if hypoglycemia happens frequently.

The treatment for a person who can swallow is to give 15 grams of a rapid-acting carbohydrate source such as 4 ounces of orange juice or 4 teaspoons of sugar mixed in water (see Table 9–8). The blood sugar should be rechecked in 15 minutes and the procedure repeated until the blood sugar returns to normal. This is referred to as the **15:15 rule.** For severe hypoglycemia, the amount of carbohydrate is increased to 30 grams of carbohydrate as long as the person can swallow. Squeezing cake icing or honey inside the cheek is appropriate only if the person can swallow.

A number of conditions and situations arise in which the individual with diabetes can anticipate the need for more carbohydrate to prevent a hypoglycemic episode (see Table 9–9). If the person becomes unconscious, glucagon can be injected or an intravenous solution of glucose may be administered in the hospital setting. Long-term treatment includes diet, activity, or insulin modification (see Fig. 9–4 for insulin action, and the chart on page 238 showing factors that raise or lower blood glucose levels) or education to help prevent future episodes.

Heart Disease

Seventy five per cent of deaths among persons with diabetes are related to cardiovascular disease (Bierman, 1992). The American Diabetes Association recommends that physicians measure blood lipids and treat associated problems as a primary intervention to reduce the risk of cardiovascular disease among persons with NIDDM (American Diabetes Association, 1989). See Chapter 8 for management of lipid disorders.

Kidney Disease

Persons with IDDM are at particular risk for kidney disease owing to small blood vessel damage. Kidney disease also occurs in NIDDM. The Diabetes Control and Complications Trial (DCCT) study found that maintaining good blood sugar control will greatly lessen the risk of kidney disease. Eating protein in more moderate portions is also believed to maintain kidney functioning by putting less stress on the kidneys. Controlling blood pressure is critical to preserving kidney functioning. Regular blood pressure screening is necessary, and antihypertensive therapy should begin when blood pressure reaches 140/90 mm Hg (Hawthorne, 1989). Borderline hypertension needs to be treated aggressively in persons with diabetes in order to preserve kidney function.

Eye Disease

Diabetic retinopathy (a disease of the back of the eye where visual images are conveyed to the brain) occurs in about half of all persons who have had diabetes for more than 10 years and in about 80 per cent of all persons who have had diabetes for more than 25 years. Controlling blood sugar levels significantly lowers the risk of retinopathy, according to the DCCT study. Hypertension should also be controlled. Regular eye exams, at least annually, with special tests to monitor for retinopathy are necessary to save vision. Treatment is available today that can preserve the sight of most persons with diabetes.

Nerve Disease

Nerve disease can occur at any location of the body but typically affects peripheral nerves (those at the periphery of the body such as the feet and legs) and the autonomic nervous system (comprising the nerves that send unconscious messages to the body, such as in the stomach, heart, or intestines). Problems with peripheral nerves **(peripheral neuropathy)** in the feet can cause burning, pain, and if severe, no feeling at all. It is paramount for persons with peripheral nerve problems of the feet to follow meticulous foot care. This can help prevent foot infections, which could lead to amputation. Any sign of a problem should immediately be taken care of by a physician or **podiatrist** (foot doctor).

Problems with the autonomic nervous system are referred to as **autonomic neuropathy. Gastroparesis** is partial paralysis of the stomach, resulting in diminished digestion and movement of food through the stomach. This can be a cause of unexplained hypoglycemia, since blood sugar levels can be raised only when food leaves the stomach. When this condition is suspected, a dye test is administered to determine the amount of time it takes for the food to leave the stomach. There is medication for this condition. Exercise may be discouraged for a person with autonomic neuropathy, as the heart may not be able to speed up to increase the oxygen intake. Another form of autonomic neuropathy affects the ability of the body to produce glucagon and epinephrine in response to low blood glucose. This is referred to as **hypoglycemic unawareness** because symptoms of hypoglycemia—shakiness, rapid heartbeat, and so on—will not be felt.

Are There Special Dietary Concerns During Illness?

The need for insulin increases when a person is acutely ill, even if there is a diminished intake of food. To prevent excess production of ketones, the person with IDDM must maintain adequate insulin injections and carbohydrate intake and contact a physician immediately when illness occurs.

The quality of the diet is less important than the quantity of carbohydrate consumed during severe illness; thus the intake of simple sugars such as those found in regular ginger ale may be recommended. Sipping juice or soft drinks throughout the day may be helpful when the intake of food is greatly diminished, as during an illness. To prevent loss of needed electrolytes, orange juice should be consumed for potassium and soup for sodium. Adequate fluid intake is imperative because dehydration compounds the undesirable effect of hyperglycemia and ketonuria. Table 9–10 shows a sample sick-day menu.

▲   T A B L E   9 – 1 0

EXAMPLE OF A CONCENTRATED DIET FOR A DAY OF MINOR ILLNESS

	HOUSEHOLD MEASURE	WEIGHT (g)	CARBOHYDRATE (g)	PROTEIN (g)	FAT (g)	KILOCALORIES
Breakfast						
Orange	Small	100	10	0	0	40
Egg	1	50	0	6	6	78
Bread	1 large slice	30	15	3	0	72
Margarine	1 tsp	5	0	0	4	36
Milk*	6 oz	180	9	6	6	114
Forenoon						
Orange	Medium	150	15	0	0	60
Lunch						
Oatmeal (cooked)	½ cup	120	10	3	1	61
Milk*	8 oz	240	12	8	8	152
Bread	1 large slice	30	15	3	0	72
Margarine	1 tsp	5	0	0	4	36
Orange	Medium	150	15	0	0	60
Afternoon						
Crackers, 2 × 2½ inches	2	10	7	1	1	41
Margarine	1 tsp	5	0	0	4	36
Milk*	6 oz	180	9	6	6	114
Supper						
Egg	1	50	0	6	6	78
Bread	1 large slice	30	15	3	0	72
Margarine	1 tsp	5	0	0	4	36
Milk*	6 oz	180	9	6	6	114
Orange	Medium	150	15	0	0	60
Bedtime						
Crackers, 2 × 2½ inches	2	10	7	1	1	41
Margarine	1 tsp	5	0	0	4	36
Milk*	6 oz	180	9	6	6	114
TOTAL			172	58	67	1523

* The caloric content of milk and thereby the percentage of calories derived from fat may be decreased by using 1% or 2% fat or skim milk rather than whole milk.

From Krall LP, Beaser RS: Joslin's Diabetes Mellitus, 12th ed. Philadelphia, Lea & Febiger, 1989.

Substitutions may be made according to principles previously outlined. Bread may be given as toast in amounts stated above. Fruit or fruit juice other than orange may be substituted in appropriate amounts (see Table 9–7).

COUNSELING STRATEGIES FOR THE NURSE AND OTHER HEALTH PROFESSIONALS IN DIABETES MANAGEMENT

The nurse or other health professional needs to determine what previous attempts have been made by the diabetic patient and what future barriers to change will have to be dealt with in order to assist most effectively in promoting good diabetes management. Positive verbal reinforcement for any attempt at control is always useful. Beyond that, the nurse can help patients to identify their perceived needs in relation to diabetes management, can make referrals as appropriate—for example, to the physician, dietitian, or diabetes support group—and can advocate gradual changes (small steps) in the control of diabetes. Simply being empathetic about the frustrations and challenges that are likely to be encountered by the individual with diabetes is an important role of the health care professional.

An important area to assess is the patient's knowledge of the physiology of diabetes mellitus, which is a prerequisite for effective decision-making in diabetes management. Does the individual have a basic understanding of what makes the blood sugar increase or decrease (see chart following)? Does the individual have the skills to determine what course of action is most appropriate for the various situations likely to be encountered, and does he or she have the ability to follow through in making adjustments in diet, insulin administration, or activity? Is the person able to accept the reality of having diabetes mellitus and to take responsibility for its control? How does the person's environment (social, economic, and so on) reinforce or inhibit diabetes management? By identifying areas of strength for positive reinforcement and areas of need for referral or personal assistance, the nurse or other health care professional can have an integral and valuable role in facilitating the potential for full and productive lives in individuals with diabetes mellitus.

FACTORS LOWERING BLOOD SUGAR LEVELS	FACTORS RAISING BLOOD SUGAR LEVELS
Weight loss or reduced intake of food	Weight gain or increased intake of food
Exercise	Excess carbohydrate intake, especially simple forms
Diabetes medication	Excess saturated fat intake
	Stress
	Infections and illness

* If there is insufficient insulin in the body, exercise will raise blood sugar levels. If blood glucose levels are consistently elevated above 240 mg/dL or in cases of ketonuria, exercise should be postponed until diabetes is better controlled.

STUDY QUESTIONS AND ACTIVITIES

1. How would you advise Mr. Bernardo, from the opening case study, regarding eating foods such as pizza, lasagna, or dried fruit?
2. Bring some convenience food labels into class. How can they be calculated into a diabetic person's diet?
3. Self monitor your blood glucose levels using Chemstrips for at least 1 day, prior to meals and 2 hours postprandially. Maintain a record of your eating habits, including amounts eaten and times, and time and duration of activities. Based on this experience, discuss in class how you feel about advocating SMBG for all individuals with diabetes.
4. Determine what changes, if any, you would have to make if you were personally diagnosed as having insulin-dependent diabetes

mellitus (IDDM). Could you consistently follow a low-fat, low-sugar meal plan? How would you feel if you had to give up eating sweets and greasy foods?

5. What are some reasons that Mr. Bernardo might develop hyperglycemia even though he currently has his blood glucose under control?

6. Describe why a person with hyperglycemia is at increased risk of heart disease and kidney disease.

7. Become a member of the American Diabetes Association (for about $24.00 per year) and receive their monthly publication, "Diabetes Forecast." Each publication contains a feature story about a person with diabetes along with other informative articles.

8. If a person with IDDM takes NPH insulin at 7:00 AM, what time will the insulin peak? If this person begins to feel shaky at 3:00 PM, what should he or she do?

9. Knowing that milk contains 12 grams of carbohydrate per cup and that the form of carbohydrate in milk is lactose, calculate how many teaspoons of sugar equivalent it contains. Why would milk be less likely to raise blood sugar than fruit juice? HINT: It has to do with protein and fat content.

10. Role play in class about the advice a nurse might provide for at least one of the following situations:

A person with IDDM who is hyperglycemic and who is determined to be a marathon athlete;

A person with non–insulin-dependent diabetes mellitus (NIDDM) who refuses to take responsibility for diabetes management;

A person with gestational diabetes who is losing weight because of attempts to follow a physician-prescribed 1800-kilocalorie American Diabetic Association (diabetic) diet.

REFERENCES

American Diabetes Association: Consensus statement: Role of cardiovascular risk factors in prevention and treatment of macrovascular disease in diabetes. Diabetes Care. 1989; 12:573–579.

American Dietetic Association: Vegetarian diets—technical support paper. J Am Diet Assoc. 1988; 88(3):353.

Bierman EL: Atherogenesis in diabetes. Arteriosclerosis. 1992; 12:647–656.

Dawson LY: DCCT and primary care: Prescription for change. Clinical Diabetes. July/August, 1993; 11(4):91–95.

Hannah J, Harper P: Nonpharmacologic treatment of diabetic dyslipidemia, introduction. Diabetes Spectrum. 1993; 6(5):290.

Hawthorne VM: Preventing the kidney disease of diabetes mellitus: public health perspectives. Am J Kidney Dis. 1989; 13(1).

Horton ES: Exercise. In Leibovitz HE, ed.: Therapy for Diabetes Mellitus and Related Disorders. Alexandria, VA, American Diabetes Association, Inc, 1991; p. 103.

Kirk JK: The risk of hyperglycemic, hyperosmolar nonketotic coma (HHNK) in elderly patients with diabetes. Diabetes Spectrum. 1993; 6(5):324.

Muntoni S, Songini M: High incidence rate of IDDM in Sardinia. Diabetes Care. 1992; 15(10):1317–1322.

CHAPTER 10

RENAL DISEASE

OBJECTIVES

After completing this chapter, you should be able to:
- Describe the basic functions of the kidneys
- Identify the clinical symptoms and serum parameters of renal disease
- Describe the principles of nutritional management, including the control of disease and promotion of good nutritional status
- Describe the role of the nurse and other health care professionals in the management of renal disease

TERMS TO IDENTIFY

Albumin
Albuminuria
Anuria
Azotemia
Blood urea nitrogen (BUN)
Carnitine
Continuous ambulatory peritoneal dialysis (CAPD)
Creatinine
Edema

End-stage renal disease (ESRD)
Erythropoietin
Glomerular filtration rate (GFR)
Hematuria
Hemodialysis
Hypercalciuria
Hypoalbuminemia
Hypotension

Nephron
Nitrogenous wastes
Oliguria
Osteomalacia
Osteoporosis
Positive nitrogen balance
Proteinuria
Renal insufficiency
Renal osteodystrophy
Uremia

Rita Bernardo was at her neighbor Fiona's house. They were discussing stomach pains. Fiona was being treated for kidney stones. She had had excruciating bouts of pain. The doctor was now hopeful the stone had passed. But Fiona continued to drink lots of water for now. Almost one gallon a day, just to be sure. And while Fiona thought she should be avoiding milk, the doctor thought her type of kidney stone did not require this restriction.

Rita thought to herself, no, my pain is different and seems to be getting worse. She thought perhaps it was time to see a doctor herself. She said no to her neighbor's offer of a bite to eat. Fiona had suggested to come in the house and try Sharwood's mango chutney with some digestive biscuits and cream cheese. These were a couple of food items from Fiona's native England. Rita wasn't quite sure she would like chutney made from mangos. She wasn't feeling well enough to try new foods today.

INTRODUCTION

Managing renal (kidney) disease is like a juggling act. Not just one but several nutritional components need to be controlled: protein, kilocalories, phosphorus, sodium, and potassium. Generally, all are restricted except kilocalories, which need to be maintained at a high enough level to prevent muscle protein from being broken down for energy needs. This breakdown causes additional stress on the kidneys because increased **nitrogenous waste** (excreted protein material) is filtered into the urine. However, once a renal patient begins dialysis, the restrictions are often reversed in order to compensate for the excess losses incurred. Managing renal disease is complex and difficult for the patient and the entire health care team. However, renal failure and the need for dialysis may be postponed or even prevented if the patient is willing and able to control the interrelated but diverse dietary factors, particularly that of achieving a low-protein, low-phosphorus diet (Ahmed, 1991).

The management of renal disease has come a long way. In the not-too-distant past, renal disease commonly led to uremia and death. Although the strategies of modern management of renal disease are complex and difficult, they do offer hope for an extension of life. The current dietary recommendations are likely to be modified in the future as technology develops and research advances.

WHAT ARE THE FUNCTIONS OF KIDNEYS?

Kidneys have three basic functions: (1) excretion of waste material, (2) reabsorption of important body constituents, and (3) a metabolic and hormonal role. Their most widely known function is as a filterer of body wastes, including drugs and toxins. This filtering process occurs in the **nephrons,** of which there are over 1 million (Fig. 10–1). For renal disease patients, medications need to be adjusted to reflect diminished clearance.

Selectively reabsorbing nutrients as necessary is another basic function of the kidneys. This function serves an important role in maintaining the

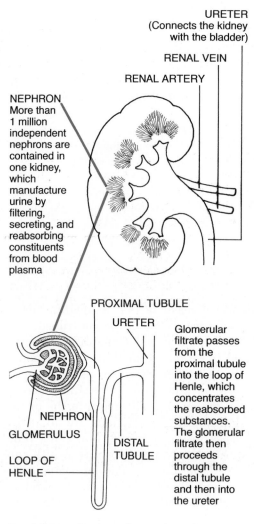

URETER
(Connects the kidney
with the bladder)

RENAL VEIN

RENAL ARTERY

NEPHRON
More than
1 million
independent
nephrons are
contained in
one kidney,
which
manufacture
urine by
filtering,
secreting, and
reabsorbing
constituents
from blood
plasma

PROXIMAL TUBULE

URETER

Glomerular
filtrate passes
from the
proximal tubule
into the loop of
Henle, which
concentrates
the reabsorbed
substances.
The glomerular
filtrate then
proceeds
through the
distal tubule
and then into
the ureter

NEPHRON

GLOMERULUS

DISTAL
TUBULE

LOOP OF
HENLE

Renal disease develops when nephrons lose
their capacity to filter, reabsorb, and secrete

▲ F I G U R E   1 0 - 1

Anatomy of a kidney. (Used with permission of
Ross Products Division, Abbott Laboratories,
Columbus, OH 43216. Redrawn from Renal Dis-
ease Dietary Modifications in Disease. © 1978
Ross Products Division, Abbott Laboratories.)

acid-base balance (pH level) and the balance of various body constituents.
Thus, kidneys help maintain appropriate levels of water, electrolytes, nitrogen, fixed acids, bicarbonates, and other body constituents through the two
functions of excretion of wastes and reabsorption of important nutrients.

The third and least well known function of kidneys is the metabolic and hormonal one. Kidneys convert the inactive form of vitamin D from foods and sun exposure into the active form. Kidneys also produce the enzyme renin, which affects systemic blood pressure, and the hormone **erythropoietin,** which stimulates red blood cell production by the bone marrow. Figure 10–1 portrays the composition of the kidneys.

HOW IS RENAL DISEASE DIAGNOSED?

The general criteria for diagnosing renal disease center around the functions of the normal kidney. Given that kidneys excrete excess nitrogen, protein, electrolytes, water, and other substances, tests for abnormal levels of these constituents provide an indication of whether renal disease is present and, if so, how severe it is. Renal disease progresses along a continuum (Table 10–1). Lack of urinary excretion **(anuria)** or decreased urinary output (oliguria) suggests renal obstruction, which may lead to irreversible renal damage. Other clinical manifestations of renal disease include **hematuria** (blood in the urine), **albuminuria (albumin,** a form of protein, found in the urine), **azotemia** (nitrogen in the blood), hypertension, edema, **hypoalbuminemia** (low levels of albumin in the blood), hyperlipidemia, and **proteinuria** (protein in the urine).

Specific serum indicators routinely used for assessing the degree of renal failure and response to dietary control are the **blood urea nitrogen (BUN)** level and **creatinine** (a nitrogenous compound formed in muscle), albumin, potassium, phosphorus, sodium, and calcium determinations. The **glomerular filtration rate (GFR)** also gives an indication of how fast the kidneys are functioning in excreting wastes. A normal GFR is 125 mL per minute; less than 25 to 30 mL per minute is equated with **renal insufficiency;** and less than 15 mL per minute is associated with uremia. Uremia is associated with high creatinine levels of over 5 mg/dL; normal creatinine is less than 1.5, and levels over 10 generally require dialysis.

▲ TABLE 10-1

STAGES OF CHRONIC RENAL DISEASE

STAGE	THERAPEUTIC DIETARY MEASURES
Glomerulonephritis	Protein restricted until kidney function improves; sodium restricted if hypertension or edema present; may be self-limiting or proceed to more severe renal disease
Nephrotic syndrome	May need to compensate for protein losses due to albuminuria; mild sodium restricted if edema present (3 g/day)
Diminished reserve	May need to control for hypertension with sodium restriction
Renal insufficiency	Restriction of protein, fluid, and electrolytes with adequate kilocalories required; level of dietary control based on renal functioning
Renal failure	Dialysis begun; diet needs to compensate for losses from dialysis; phosphorus restriction still needed
Uremia	Kidney transplant required unless uremia can be controlled through more frequent dialysis or stricter dietary control

SOME TYPES OF RENAL
DISORDERS AND THEIR
NUTRITIONAL
TREATMENT

Nephrolithiasis
(Kidney Stones)

There are several forms of kidney stones, each with its own medical and/or nutritional intervention. The best prevention of kidney stones is adequate intake of fluids ($1\frac{1}{2}$ to 2 quarts or liters per day). Adequate fluid intake helps keep the urine dilute, which helps prevent crystals that lead to stone formation. Once a stone has formed, treatment is best decided after a chemical analysis of the stone. The most common form of stone is calcium-based.

HOW ARE CALCIUM OXALATE STONES TREATED?

Calcium oxalate stones come in many forms. Medical input is necessary to determine nutritional intervention. Some calcium stones require medical or surgical intervention. Another form benefits with a low-oxalate diet. A dietitian should be consulted for such a diet, as foods high in oxalate are very nutritious (legumes and nuts, dark green leafy vegetables, berries, and citrus fruits). The diet to control stone formation from oxalates needs to be evaluated for adequacy. If **hypercalciuria** (high levels of calcium in the urine) is noted to be the cause of stone formation, treatment with a low-calcium diet may not be appropriate. Only one type of hypercalciuria will improve on a low-calcium diet. The calcium restriction is now more moderate—in the range of 800 to 1200 mg calcium per day. Patients with this form of hypercalciuria also need to follow a low-oxalate diet, such as avoiding legumes and dark green leafy vegetables. A magnesium supplement is also advised. This is the type of stone that Rita Bernardo's neighbor Fiona had. A mild sodium restriction (4 to 5 g/day) can decrease urinary calcium levels in another form of hypercalciuria. Adequate fluid intake and diuretic use (thiazide diuretics) is crucial (Mahan and Arlin, 1992).

URIC ACID STONES

Limiting protein to the level of the RDA (45 to 55 g/day) is useful for treating uric acid stones. Emphasis on milk instead of meat, eggs, and legumes for protein will help prevent acidic urine. Increased intakes of fruit (except cranberries, plums, and prunes) and decreased intake of bread products may also help prevent acidic urine.

CYSTINE STONES

Cystine stones require a high fluid intake (greater than 4 quarts or liters per day). Following the diet to avoid acidic urine may also help prevent future formation of cystine stones.

STRUVITE STONES

Struvite stones are not managed nutritionally. They are usually seen in women and require long-term antibiotic therapy with surgical or ultrasonic stone removal.

FACT & FALLACY

FALLACY: A person with kidney stones should follow a low-calcium diet.

FACT: Only recently it has been found that calcium restriction may be counterproductive for a person with kidney stones. Kidney stone formation now appears to be more related to oxalate intake with calcium binding to it. Oxalate is found in beets, chocolate, nuts, rhubarb, spinach, strawberries, tea, and wheat bran. Megadoses of vitamin C also contribute oxalate. The best course appears to be to avoid excess oxalate and protein while including the recommended amount of milk and increasing intake of potassium foods and water (Environmental Nutrition, 1993).

Nephrotic Syndrome

This disease involves loss of the glomerular barrier to protein in the nephron (see Fig. 10–1). Protein is thus lost in the urine. This in turn causes a decreased serum albumin level. A decreased serum albumin level leads to **edema** (fluid retention). Nutritional care is aimed at improving protein status. A **positive nitrogen balance** (the amount of protein needed in the diet to allow for tissue growth or intake of protein that exceeds output) will promote an increased serum albumin level and correction of the edema.

HOW MUCH PROTEIN IS NEEDED TO ACHIEVE A POSITIVE NITROGEN BALANCE?

The amount of protein recommended to achieve positive nitrogen balance is based on individual needs. In the past, patients were routinely given double the recommended protein intake (1.5 g/kg body weight as compared with the normal recommendation of 0.8 g/kg). Now it appears that the quality of protein is more important than the total amount. An intake of about 80 per cent of the protein from high biological sources (meat, eggs, and milk products) is recommended along with a high-kilocalorie diet (35 to 50 kcal/kg/day and up to 100 to 150 kcal/kg/day for children) (Mahan and Arlin, 1992).

HOW IS EDEMA TREATED IN THE NEPHROTIC SYNDROME?

Since the cause of edema in the nephrotic syndrome is secondary to hypoalbuminemia, typical treatment of edema (low-sodium diet and diuretic medications) does not apply. The underlying hypoalbuminemia and subsequent edema will be corrected by achieving a positive nitrogen balance through increased protein utilization. Sodium should be restricted only mildly to the 3 g/day range because further reductions can cause **hypotension** (abnormally low blood pressure). Hypoalbuminemia causes a low blood volume, which would be exacerbated with very low sodium intakes (less than 2 g/day).

Nephritic Syndrome

This syndrome includes a group of inflammatory diseases of the kidney, specifically of the glomerulus (see Fig. 10–1). A term used to describe this condition is glomerulonephritis, or nephritis. Hematuria, hypertension, and mild loss of renal function are common.

WHAT DIETARY CHANGES ARE MADE WITH THE NEPHRITIC SYNDROME?

No routine dietary changes are made for nephritic syndrome except to maintain health during the inflammation stage. This may require an increased intake of protein but should be based on serum lab values to ensure adequate functioning of the kidneys. Mild restrictions of protein and potassium may be indicated if there are signs of reduced renal function such as elevated serum levels of creatinine and elevated potassium levels. Sodium restriction of 2 to 3 grams per day would be appropriate to control hypertension.

Acute Renal Failure

Acute renal failure (ARF) occurs when there is a sudden decrease in glomerular filtration rate (GFR). **Oliguria** (reduced production of urine to less than 500 mL in 24 hours) may occur. Depending on the cause, ARF may be short-lived with no nutritional intervention necessary. If the patient goes on to develop **uremia** (a toxic buildup of protein byproducts in the blood causing such problems as nausea and vomiting) and other problems such as fluid and electrolyte imbalances, nutritional care becomes a primary treatment. *Chronic renal failure* is a term used to describe this condition.

HOW IS THE DIET MODIFIED IN ARF?

Protein intake is based on individual lab values. Recommendations can vary from as little as 0.3 g/kg to 1.5 g/kg (Mahan and Arlin, 1992). (See the sample menu for a 20-gram protein diet.) Energy needs are high (50 kcal/kg) to help prevent breakdown of body protein (for obese patients, weight needs to be adjusted as follows: [Actual body weight – Ideal body weight × 0.25] + Ideal body weight). Of the total protein, 60 to 70 per cent should come from high biological value protein unless essential amino acids are used (Wilkens and Brouns Schiro, 1992). Table 10–2 presents general dietary guidelines for renal disease.

The real challenge in treating ARF is to provide the body with the necessary protein and kilocalories while limiting fluid, sodium, and potassium. Monitoring of serum lab values is critical in order to determine changes in nutritional needs.

Usually a 1500 mg level of potassium is appropriate. A normal diet may contain as much as 3000 to 8000 mg because potassium is widely distrib-

SAMPLE MENU for a 20-gram PROTEIN DIET

▲

BREAKFAST
½ c. cranberry juice
½ c. cream of wheat cereal
2 slices bread, low-protein
2 tsp butter
2 tsp honey
¼ c. whole milk
2 tsp sugar
¾ c. coffee

▲

LUNCH
1 egg, scrambled
½ c. rice
½ c. cooked carrots
6 slices cucumber on 1 leaf lettuce
2 slices bread, low-protein
2 tsp butter
½ c. sweetened canned pears
1 tsp sugar
1 cup Kool-Aid

▲

SUPPER
Pineapple slice and peach half on lettuce
2 slices bread, low-protein
½ c. green beans
2 tsp butter
1 low-protein cookie
1 high-sugar, low-protein popsicle
1 tsp sugar
½ c. whole milk

From Howe P: Basic Nutrition in Health and Disease, 7th ed. Philadelphia, WB Saunders Co., 1981; p. 533.

uted in foods (meats, fruits, whole-grain breads and cereals, and dark green leafy vegetables). Cooking water and the juices from canned fruits and vegetables must be discarded because potassium is water-soluble. Table 10–3 gives a list of foods low in sodium, potassium, and phosphorus.

▲ TABLE 10-2

DIETARY GUIDELINES AND MODIFICATION FOR RENAL MANAGEMENT

DIETARY GUIDELINES	RENAL-MODIFIED GUIDELINES
Eat a variety of foods	Same, although dietary restrictions decrease allowed choices
Maintain desirable weight	Same
Avoid too much fat, saturated fat, and cholesterol	An increase in total fat may be necessary for weight control, but saturated fat and cholesterol should still be avoided
Eat foods with adequate starch and fiber	Same; low-protein bread may be used
Avoid too much sugar	An increase in sugar may be necessary for weight control (to help prevent weight loss)
Avoid too much sodium	Same
If you drink alcoholic beverages, do so in moderation	Alcohol may be allowed as a source of kilocalories to help prevent weight loss on an individual basis and under medical supervision

Restricting phosphorus to 600 to 1200 mg (the RDA for adults is 800 mg) should maintain desirable serum phosphorus levels. Phosphate binders can be used as well but should generally be avoided because of possible aluminum toxicity. The use of calcium carbonate can decrease serum phosphorus while increasing serum calcium (Wilkens and Brouns Schiro, 1992).

▲ TABLE 10-3

FOODS FOR MANAGEMENT OF RENAL DISEASE*

≤50 mg SODIUM, POTASSIUM, AND PHOSPHORUS	≤100 mg SODIUM, POTASSIUM, AND PHOSPHORUS
Fruits Cranberry juice cocktail, ≤2 c. Lemonade, ≤1 c.	**Fruits and Vegetables** Blueberries, ≤½ c. Grapes, ≤½ c. Lettuce, ≤½ c. Watermelon, ≤½ c.
Sugars Granulated, ≤8 c. Hard candy, ≤1½ lb Jelly beans, ≤5 c. Marshmallows, ≤3½ oz Jam, ≤2 tbsp Jelly, ≤3 tbsp	**Sugars** Honey, ≤½ c.
Fats Cooking oil (vegetable), unlimited Lard, unlimited Salt-free margarine, ≤1 c. Salt-free butter, ≤1 c.	**Alcohol** Beer, ≤12 oz Table wine, ≤4 oz

* Refer to food composition table (Appendix 5). Specific dietary advice should be given in conjunction with a registered dietitian and a physician. Foods contributing ≥2 g protein in common portions are not included.

Fluids are restricted for patients with kidney failure; a balance between intake and output must be achieved. The general guideline is 500 to 1000 mL (about 2 to 4 cups) plus the amount lost in daily urine production and other body fluids such as with vomiting. For example, if the patient has a daily urine and fluid output of 1000 mL, the recommended fluid intake would range from 1500 to 2000 mL per day; if there is anuria (no urine output), the fluid restriction would be 500 to 1000 mL per day. Thus the amount of fluid lost through urinary output needs to be estimated individually before recommended daily amounts can be determined.

During periods of stress, such as with infection, protein needs can be so high as to require parenteral nutritional support (see Chapter 14). Enteral liquid supplements have been developed to assist in providing amino acids (protein) and kilocalories while contributing low levels of the electrolytes sodium and potassium (see Appendix 8). If kidney function continues to deteriorate to end-stage renal disease (ESRD), dialysis or kidney transplantation may be required (see following section).

HOW DO THE DIETARY GUIDELINES RELATE TO MANAGEMENT OF RENAL DISEASE?

Although avoidance of sugar and fat is typically advised for healthy persons, their consumption may become mandatory for the renal patient to maintain adequate kilocalorie intake without contributing protein and electrolytes. The recommendation to increase sugar and fat may be met with resistance because of long-standing attempts to control health. A reduced sodium and moderate protein intake is recommended especially for the person with renal disease. Alcohol may contribute a major source of kilocalories but ideally should be avoided. Maintenance of ideal body weight applies to the renal patient as well as to the general population.

WHAT ARE SOME NUTRITIONAL COMPLICATIONS ASSOCIATED WITH RENAL DISEASE OR ITS TREATMENT?

Nutrient Deficiencies

Careful planning must be undertaken to help ensure that the renal patient's nutritional status is not jeopardized while trying to prevent further kidney damage through the use of the low-protein diet. Finding foods that are low in potassium is generally the most limiting restriction in terms of food choices for the person with renal disease, since potassium is found in meats, fruits, whole-grain breads and cereals, and dark green leafy vegetables. There are other foods low in only sodium and phosphorus. Other special low-protein products may also have low electrolyte content. These food restrictions can be compounded by food dislikes or intolerances and can predispose the person with renal disease to ingest inadequate nutrients. However, even with caution, the risk of vitamin and mineral deficiency is inherent in the restrictive diet. Until further research proves otherwise, it is prudent for some renal patients to have a water-soluble vitamin supplement that meets the RDA. Vitamin D supplement is generally required in ESRD since the kidney cannot activate dietary vitamin D. Supplementation with other vitamins and minerals should be based on lab values or other indices of deficiency (Wilkens and Brouns Schiro, 1992). However, the recommendation for vitamin and mineral supplementation should take place in conjunction with a physician consultation.

Carnitine deficiency becomes an issue for long-term hemodialysis patients because of the combined effect of two complications: decreased availability of lysine and methionine (amino acids) and of vitamin C, niacin, vitamin B$_6$, and iron (micronutrients) to synthesize carnitine; and decreased metabolic activity of the kidney combined with removal of carnitine by the dialysis procedure. Carnitine is a substance produced in the kidneys that has the role of fatty acid oxidation, primarily of the heart and skeletal muscle. Oral and intravenous supplementations of L-carnitine have been noted to decrease some of the complications of dialysis, resulting in improved muscle function, decreased hypotensive episodes, and improved protein catabolism (Ahmad et al., 1990). However, supplementation with L-carnitine is still considered experimental therapy (Wilkens and Brouns Schiro, 1992).

Concurrent Diabetes

About 30 to 40 per cent of people with insulin-dependent diabetes mellitus (IDDM) develop renal failure in an average of 20 years (American Association of Diabetes Educators, 1992). Persons with non–insulin-dependent diabetes mellitus (NIDDM) also can develop renal disease. Thus, while a high kilocalorie intake may be needed, especially for the person with IDDM, the source of kilocalories should not be in the form of concentrated sweets. The primary source of kilocalories is complex carbohydrates, unsaturated fats, and low-protein products. (An example of a creative, appealing solution used by a diabetic renal patient with whom this author once worked was low-protein bread fried in margarine, spiced with garlic, and toasted for use as salad croutons.)

Lipid Abnormalities

Another situation calling for a low-sugar diet is type IV hyperlipidemia, in which the triglyceride (very-low-density lipoproteins) level is elevated, whereas cholesterol levels are normal. This is a common occurrence in chronic renal failure and is treated with a low-sugar, high-fiber diet with moderate amounts of fat.

Renal Osteodystrophy

Renal osteodystrophy consists of a group of bone diseases resulting from the effects of chronic renal failure, such as poor bone development in children, **osteomalacia** (soft bones), and **osteoporosis** (brittle bones). Specifically, renal osteodystrophy is caused by a combination of high serum phosphorus levels, low serum calcium levels, and altered parathyroid function. Close monitoring and adherence to a controlled diet can help prevent or delay these complications.

Anemia

Problems with erythropoietin production may lead to diminished production of red blood cells and anemia. This condition is not responsive to iron supplementation; however, causes of iron deficiency should be ruled out before deciding not to treat with increased iron intake.

WHAT ARE THE SPECIAL NUTRITIONAL CONSIDERATIONS IN TREATING CHILDREN WITH RENAL DISEASE?

Children with renal disease have been noted to have stunted growth (achieving less than the fifth percentile on growth charts), which appears to be related to protein-energy malnutrition (Shapera et al., 1986) as well as to a disturbance in the calcium-phosphorus balance, resulting in insufficient availability of calcium for bone growth. Once phosphorus levels are under control, the calcium and vitamin D intake can be increased to help promote bone growth.

Making mealtime fun is important for good nutritional intake in children. Liquid supplements that are designed for renal management can be given popular names such as "Barney Milkshake" for young children. Health care professionals interacting with the child should try to make foods sound appealing, provide small portions frequently, and arrange for favorite foods.

WHAT ARE THE DIFFERENT FORMS AND PROCEDURES OF DIALYSIS?

Dialysis is often begun when a patient's creatinine level exceeds 10 to 12 and the BUN is above 100. This is indicative of **end-stage renal disease (ESRD).** Currently 90 per cent of dialysis patients reaching this stage have diabetes, hypertension, or glomerulonephritis (Mahan and Arlin, 1992).

There are two forms of dialysis, both of which have the goal of maintenance and balance of protein, electrolytes (potassium and sodium), and fluid levels. The traditional form is **hemodialysis,** which generally requires a renal patient to travel to a dialysis unit several times a week. For several hours, the patient's blood is extracted and filtered through a dialysis solution. The dialyzed blood is then returned through the patient's venous system.

FACT & FALLACY

FALLACY: With dialysis, the patient with renal disease need not restrict food intake.

FACT: It is true that in order to compensate for incurred losses, some of the dietary restrictions are reversed during hemodialysis (e.g., protein, potassium, and sodium for the normotensive patient) but the general rule is that there are still restrictions. In fact, the frequency and duration of hemodialysis can be reduced when strict dietary controls are adhered to. For patients using CAPD, a more liberal dietary intake may be possible. However, this method also has drawbacks. Because of the high glucose content of the solution, it may not be appropriate for persons with diabetes or for others with a glucose intolerance.

Continuous ambulatory peritoneal dialysis (CAPD) is a newer form of dialysis that was developed to improve the quality of life of the dialysis patient, as it does not require attachment to a machine. It entails filling the abdominal cavity with dialysis fluid, which has a high glucose content, which then absorbs toxins from the blood. After several hours, the dialysis fluid is drained, and fresh dialysis fluid is reinserted. This form of dialysis can also be performed intermittently, usually during sleep. This form of dialysis may not be appropriate for a person with diabetes because of the high sugar content of the dialysis fluid.

Dialysis has become commonplace since the U.S. Congress passed legislation allowing federal funds to be used for the procedure. Kidney transplants were also covered in this legislation, which was passed in 1972.

WHAT ARE SOME NUTRITIONAL RENAL TRANSPLANT ISSUES?

Steroid-induced weight gain can occur in conjunction with kidney transplants. Steroids are required to prevent rejection by the body of the new kidneys. Dietitians at renal transplant centers in the United States recommend 1.2 to 1.5 grams protein per kilogram body weight, 40 to 50 per cent of total kilocalories as carbohydrate, a fat intake less than 30 per cent of total kilocalories, and a kilocalorie intake aimed at achieving or maintaining ideal body weight. Restrictions of sodium to 2 to 4 grams is recommended, with potassium and phosphorus restrictions based on patient serum values. Reduced intake of simple sugars, cholesterol, and saturated fat minimize problems in post-transplant diabetic patients and associated hyperlipidemia (Edwards and Doster, 1990).

WHAT IS THE ROLE OF THE NURSE AND OTHER HEALTH CARE PROFESSIONALS IN THE MANAGEMENT OF RENAL DISEASE?

The nurse should be aware that nutritional treatment of kidney stones should not be undertaken lightly. Dietary changes may not be necessary, and restrictions can cause nutritional inadequacy and hardship for the patient. Nutritional advice should be made only in consultation with the patient's physician. Recommendations need to be based on the chemical composition of the stone and the underlying cause of its formation.

The patient with chronic renal disease has difficult decisions to make. Life expectancy with ARF or ESRD can be extended, but only at the expense of an impaired quality of life. As a consequence, it should be expected that a patient with newly diagnosed chronic renal failure will experience typical grief reactions: denial and anger first, with the need for information and acceptance of responsibility for management of the disease appearing only later.

Through a sensitive approach and strong communication and listening skills, the health care professional can begin to determine what stage the patient with renal disease is in and thereby develop an appropriate plan of action, with referrals being a cornerstone of therapy. A referral to a social worker might be indicated when the patient is exhibiting anger or denial. A referral to a dietitian is imperative when the patient is ready to accept responsibility for dietary control. A referral to a nurse at a dialysis center is beneficial in regard to dialysis issues, such as the control of dry mouth. The nurse can further help the renal patient identify the available options and the advantages and disadvantages of each. Finally, the health care professional can help motivate the patient to recognize that life is inherently valuable irrespective of the diminished quality.

For the patient who has begun to take responsibility for the control of chronic renal disease, the health care professional can help serve as a reality tester. The person with renal disease cannot make drastic long-term dietary changes easily and thus should be verbally rewarded for the attempts made and reassured that mistakes and overindulgences will happen but encouraged not to give up the fight.

STUDY QUESTIONS AND ACTIVITIES

1. What foods can the patient with renal disease generally consume freely, in moderate amounts, and in restrictive amounts?
2. Why does the patient with chronic renal failure need to restrict protein, electrolytes, and fluid?
3. What causes uremic symptoms to develop?
4. Record a 24-hour diet recall on yourself. Calculate the amount of protein, phosphorus, sodium, and potassium in your diet.
5. As a class, visit a dialysis unit. Arrange to have a nurse, a dietitian, and, if possible, a patient with renal disease consult with the class on the dietary control of renal disease as it pertains to dialysis.
6. Can you determine if Fiona's snack (in the opening case study) is appropriate for prevention of further kidney stones? What assessment questions might you ask?
7. Case Study:
    P. W. Herman, aged 35 years, is diagnosed as having albuminuria, hypertension, and edema. His glomerular filtration rate is 25 mL/minute. After his physician explains the diagnosis and the dietitian discusses dietary control, you observe him in the hospital cafeteria eating potato chips and drinking a large milkshake.
    What are some possible explanations for Mr. Herman's behavior? How should you, as his health care professional, respond?

REFERENCES

Ahmad S, Robertson HT, Golper TA: Multicenter trial of L-carnitine in maintenance hemodialysis patients. II Clinical and biochemical effects. Kidney Int. 1990; 38:912.
Ahmed FE: Effect of diet on progression of chronic renal disease. J Am Diet Assoc, 1991; 91(10):1266.
American Association of Diabetes Educators. Diabetes Education: A Core Curriculum for Health Professionals. Chicago, American Association of Diabetes Educators, 1992; p. 240.

Edwards MS, Doster S: Renal transplant diet recommendations: Results of a survey of renal dietitians in the United States. J Am Diet Assoc 1990; 90(6):843.

Environmental Nutrition. September 1993; 16(9):7.

Mahan LK, Arlin M: Krause's Food, Nutrition and Diet Therapy, 8th ed. Philadelphia, WB Saunders, 1992.

Shapera MR, Moel DI, Kamath SK, et al.: Taste perception of children with chronic renal failure. J Am Diet Assoc 1986; 86(10):1359.

Wilkens KG, Brouns Schiro K, eds: Suggested Guidelines for Nutrition Care of Renal Patients, 2nd ed., Chicago, The American Dietetic Association, 1992.

CHAPTER 11

GASTROINTESTINAL DISEASES AND DISORDERS

CHAPTER TOPICS

CHAPTER INTRODUCTION
PROBLEMS OF THE ORAL CAVITY
DISEASES OF THE ESOPHAGUS
DISEASES OF THE STOMACH
DISEASES OF THE INTESTINES
DISEASES OF THE LIVER
DISEASES OF THE GALLBLADDER
DISEASES OF THE PANCREAS
GENETIC DISEASES OF THE BLOOD
ROLE OF THE HEALTH CARE PROFESSIONAL IN CONTROLLING GASTROINTESTINAL DISEASES

OBJECTIVES

After completing this chapter, you should be able to:

■ Explain the role of diet in the treatment of diseases of the gastrointestinal tract
■ Explain how the normal diet is modified for these diseases
■ Describe the role of the nurse or other health care professional in managing conditions or diseases of the gastrointestinal tract

TERMS TO IDENTIFY

Achalasia	Dyspepsia	Jaundice
Ascites	Dysphagia	*Lactobacillus* culture
Celiac sprue	Esophageal reflux	Lactose intolerance
Cholelithiasis	Esophageal varices	Medium-chain triglycerides (MCTs)
Cholecystitis	Gastritis	Nontropical sprue
Cirrhosis	Gliadin	Peristalsis
Cleft palate	Gluten	Pernicious anemia
Constipation	Hiatal hernia	Residue
Crohn's disease	Hepatic coma	Sickle cell disease
Cystic fibrosis	Hepatitis	Steatorrhea
Diarrhea	Hyperchlorhydria	Thalassemia
Diverticulitis	Hypochlorhydria	Ulcerative colitis
Diverticulosis	Irritable bowel syndrome	Videofluoroscopy

Rita Bernardo sat in the doctor's chair. The nurse, Donna, had just come and gone with her temperature reading and blood pressure check. She wondered if she knew Donna's family since Donna was also Italian. She wouldn't be surprised.

Oh, another stomach pain. She'd had them before, but not like this. And she was feverish. Dr. Shaw came in. Diverticulitis. A prescription for antibiotics and a diet sheet for what she could and couldn't eat. What did this young doctor know? But she listened and figured she would give it a try. Anything to take this pain away. And he did say that when the fever was gone she would be able to eat all foods again. Low fiber for now but lots of fiber after the pain and fever subsided. She thought she had heard you weren't ever to eat fiber with this condition. Hadn't her son Antonio been talking about some fiber cereal? She would ask her son what his dietitian had told him.

INTRODUCTION

Think of the gastrointestinal (GI) tract as one long tube with a couple of attachments (liver, gallbladder, and pancreas). The GI tract is far more than a tube that allows food to pass through, however. It is one of the major endocrine glands, producing a wide variety of hormones and digestive enzymes that control how food is digested, absorbed, and metabolized. An individual's nutritional status is at risk of being affected whenever the gastrointestinal tract is functionally impaired. An adequate dietary intake is important but is sometimes difficult to maintain when the normal digestion and absorption process is interrupted. (See Chapter 4 for a full description of the digestive process.)

Physical disorders can begin where digestion begins—in the mouth, or oral cavity. Problems with the oral cavity such as **cleft palate** (an opening or hole in the roof of the mouth sometimes extending to the lip; see later discussion) or lack of teeth can prevent adequate ingestion of food. The esophagus transfers food from the oral cavity to the stomach. This process is complicated and can go awry with neurological or neuromuscular disorders. Swallowing problems, referred to as **dysphagia,** are often related to stroke, head injury, cerebral palsy, and other conditions (see Chapter 4, Fig. 4–6 regarding the swallowing process).

Organic disorders of the stomach result from a change in structural tissue. Examples include pathological lesions, peptic ulcer, hiatal hernia, carcinoma, and **gastritis** (inflammation of the gastric mucosa).

Functional disorders of the stomach (reflex disorders) involve a change in body functions without detectable changes in structural tissue. Examples include **dyspepsia** (indigestion), **hyperchlorhydria** (an excess of hydrochloric acid in the gastric juice), and **hypochlorhydria** (too little hydrochloric acid).

The small intestine, large intestine, liver, gallbladder, and pancreas all contribute to the digestive process and are susceptible to numerous diseases and disorders.

WHAT ARE PROBLEMS OF THE ORAL CAVITY?

Cleft Palate

Babies born with an opening in the roof of their mouth have difficulty creating a suction seal around their mother's nipple or a bottle nipple, which leads to inadequate ingestion of breast milk or formula. Severe cases may require surgical correction. Babies with less severe forms of cleft palate may benefit from special bottle nipples that do not require suction or from cutting a slightly larger hole in the bottle nipple. Mothers who are motivated to continue nursing until the problem is resolved should be encouraged to do so with supplemental bottle feedings as needed (see Chapter 16).

Dental Problems

Missing teeth or severe dental caries can adversely affect food choices made. Persons with dental problems may have a low fiber intake owing to difficulty in chewing. Without adequate nutritional knowledge, omitting food groups may not seem important to a person with dental problems. Alternatives should be discussed, such as eating applesauce in place of fresh apples, or eating cooked or soft vegetables in place of raw or hard-to-chew vegetables. Prevention of dental caries is addressed in Chapter 19.

Dysphagia

Dysphagia is an uncomfortable and potentially life-threatening condition that affects approximately 15 million people in the United States. Dysphagia is generally a neuromuscular problem. Patients who have had a cardiovascular accident (also called stroke; see Chapter 8) may not be able to swallow correctly, which may result in aspiration of food into the lungs. This can also occur in conjunction with other neurological damage.

Diagnosis of dysphagia can begin with asking patients about the following (from Dysphagia: A Review for Health Professionals, 1991):

- coughing or choking during or after eating
- food coming through the nose
- excessive drooling, especially immediately after eating
- frequent respiratory infection
- foods that are poorly tolerated

Dysphagia requires a review of the swallowing process in order to determine the best means of feeding. A speech therapist is trained to help assess swallowing problems. An x-ray examination called **videofluoroscopy** is used to objectively diagnose dysphagia. Liquids are usually the most difficult to swallow for persons with dysphagia. Table 11-1 shows categories of foods rated according to swallowing difficulty. A patient with dysphagia may benefit from having liquids thickened with a commercial product such as THICK-IT or with baby rice cereal or other thickener. Feeding positions can also help (see Chapter 18). Table 11-2 lists food consistency considerations.

▲ T A B L E   1 1 - 1

MAIN FEATURES OF DYSPHAGIA DIET CATEGORIES

Solid Foods*

Stage 1	All pureed foods, smooth hot cereals, strained soups thickened to pureed consistency, creamed cottage cheese, smooth yogurt, and puddings
Stage 2	All foods in previous stages plus soft moist whole foods such as pancakes; finely chopped tender meats, fish, and eggs bound with thick dressing; soft cheeses (e.g., American); noodles and pasta; tender cooked leafy greens; sliced ripe banana; soft breads; soft moist cakes
Stage 3	All foods in previous stages plus eggs any style, tender ground meats bound with thick sauce, soft fish, whole soft vegetables, drained canned fruits
Stage 4	All foods in previous stages plus foods with solids and liquids together (e.g., vegetable soup), all whole foods except hard and particulate foods such as dry breads, tough meat, corn, rice, apples
Stage 5	Regular diet

Liquids*

Thin†	Water, all juices thinner than pineapple, Italian ice, other clear liquids except gelatin desserts
Thick†	All other liquids including milk, any juice not classified as a thin liquid, sherbet, ice cream
Thickened	Liquids thickened with starch to pureed consistency for those who cannot tolerate any other liquids

* Progressing in swallowing difficulty from easiest to most difficult.
† Categories are unrelated in swallowing difficulty.
From Pardoe EM: Development of a multistage diet for dysphagia. © The American Dietetic Association. Reprinted by permission from J Am Diet Assoc. 1993, 93(5): 568–571.

WHAT ARE DISEASES OF THE ESOPHAGUS?

Achalasia

In **achalasia,** the lower part of the esophagus fails to relax, and swallowing difficulty occurs. Emotional stress tends to aggravate the disease. The individual senses fullness in the sternal region and may vomit; then there is danger that the contents of the esophagus may be aspirated into the respiratory passages. Weight loss may become a problem that requires nutritional intervention.

DIETARY MODIFICATIONS. A soft diet with low bulk is advised for mild cases of achalasia. Small meals should be eaten slowly along with frequent sips of fluids to facilitate swallowing. Smooth-textured foods (for example, pudding and pureed foods) are easier to swallow. When normal swallowing resumes, a regular diet following the guidelines given in Chapter 6 should be followed.

In more severe cases of achalasia, the esophagus may be dilated with inflatable bags, or surgery may be necessary. A high-protein, high-calorie liquid diet such as the one following may be prescribed.

According to the University of Iowa Hospitals and Clinics, "Kilocalories [can] be increased by approximately 800 kilocalories and protein by approximately 30 grams when additional [commercial] liquid supplements are consumed with the three meals and snacks. For additional kilocalories, butter

▲ TABLE 11-2

FOOD CONSISTENCY CONSIDERATIONS

TYPE OF DIET	EXAMPLE	POTENTIAL IMPACT ON ORAL FUNCTION
Thin foods and liquids	Soup broth, juice	More difficult to control within mouth, especially with limited tongue control, i.e., quickly runs to all areas of mouth. Often promotes excessive food loss
Thick foods	Pudding, yogurt, applesauce	Improved control within oral cavity due to reduced flow and increased sensory input (i.e., weight and texture)
Paste-like or sticky foods	Peanut butter, thick cheese sauce	May be more difficult to move in oral cavity with limited tongue movement May stick to the roof of the mouth, especially with a high, narrow palate
Slippery foods	Pasta, Jell-o	Often difficult to control and either triggers reflexive swallow too quickly or runs out of oral cavity before the swallow
Smooth textures	Pudding, pureed foods	Relatively easy to swallow; promotes minimal tongue and jaw movement, especially over periods of time
Coarse textures	Creamed corn, ground foods, Sloppy Joe filling	Increases sensory input to stimulate more jaw and tongue movements Coarseness of food should be carefully graded
Varied textures	Soups with noodles or chunks of vegetables	Difficult to manage in oral cavity, especially with limited tongue movement or decreased oral sensitivity (i.e., liquid is swallowed and solid pieces remain in the mouth)
Scattering textures	Grated carrots, rice, coleslaw, corn bread	Very difficult to manage with limited tongue movement and decreased oral sensitivity
Crisp solids	Carrot sticks, celery sticks	Requires sophisticated biting and chewing in order to grind pieces into consistency that is safe to swallow
Milk-based substances	Milk, ice cream	Appear to coat mucous membranes in oral-pharyngeal cavities to interfere with swallowing; appears to increase congestion
Broth	Meat broth, chicken broth	Appears to cut mucus in oral-pharyngeal cavity and facilitate swallowing
Dry foods	Bread, cake, cookie	May be difficult to chew or swallow with insufficient saliva
Whole soft foods	Slice of bread	Requires the ability to bite off appropriately sized pieces

Courtesy of the Occupational Therapy Department of the J.N. Adams Developmental Center, Perrysburg, NY.

or margarine may be added. . . ; powdered glucose polymers may be dissolved in fruit juices; and stick candy may be [appropriate]. For additional protein, dry milk powder or powdered protein supplements may be added to foods. Protein, vitamins, minerals, and kilocalories may be increased by supplemental formulas or milk-based nourishments. Adequate water must

SAMPLE MENU for HIGH-PROTEIN, HIGH-CALORIE LIQUID DIET*

▲

BREAKFAST
1 cup orange juice
1 cup farina
¼ cup half-and-half
1 cup eggnog
1 cup milk
2 tsp sugar
Coffee or tea
1 oz half-and-half

▲

MIDMORNING SNACK
½ cup pureed banana

▲

LUNCH
½ cup tomato juice
¾ cup cream of potato soup
½ cup pureed peaches
½ cup chocolate custard
⅓ cup vanilla ice cream
1 cup milk
1 tsp sugar
Coffee or tea
1 oz half-and-half

▲

MIDAFTERNOON SNACK
1 cup vanilla-flavored yogurt

▲

SUPPER
1 cup pineapple juice
¾ cup strained cream of chicken
soup
(½ cup soup with ¼ cup pureed
chicken)
½ cup sherbet
¾ cup chocolate milkshake
½ cup flavored gelatin
½ cup pureed pears
1 cup milk
1 tsp sugar
Coffee or tea
1 oz half-and-half

▲

EVENING SNACK
1 cup chocolate milk

* Approximate composition: Kilocalories = 3251; Protein, g =102; Fat, g = 105; Carbohydrate, g = 483.

Reprinted by permission from Recent Advances in Therapeutic Diets, Fourth Edition by the University of Iowa Hospitals and Clinics. © 1989 by Iowa State University Press, Ames, Iowa 50010.

be provided for excretion of the daily urinary solute load and to avoid dehydration" (the University of Iowa Hospitals and Clinics, 1989).

Esophageal Reflux

The condition of **esophageal reflux** is the opposite of achalasia: The lower esophageal sphincter is incompetent and allows stomach matter to regurgitate into the esophagus. "Chronic reflux may lead to esophagitis and subsequent ulceration, hemorrhage, or stricture. Normally the esophageal sphincter prevents reflux, but in relation to hormonal, drug, mechanical, or dietary factors, the sphincter pressure may become low, with resulting regurgitation. Reflux may also occur late in pregnancy, when an increase in progesterone results in muscle relaxation. Intra-abdominal pressure associated with obesity and constipation or even constricting garments can also result in regurgitation. Nicotine exposure is reported to be a factor" (the University of Iowa Hospitals and Clinics, 1989).

DIETARY MODIFICATIONS. Treatment may include weight loss to decrease abdominal pressure on the stomach, small frequent meals to avoid stomach distention, and avoidance of chocolate and fats, which reduce sphincter competence. Avoidance of caffeine and alcohol may be helpful to reduce stomach acidity. Drinking liquids between meals and remaining upright after eating also help.

A patient with esophageal reflux is likely to follow dietary advice if the rationale is given. This is due to the negative reinforcement of physical discomfort. Thus, you should explain that the goal of dietary treatment is to lessen physical discomfort. This is achieved through small frequent meals to help prevent an overly full stomach. Many individuals eat without thinking how full they are getting. The patient with esophageal reflux may need to be taught to chew thoroughly and slowly in order to better recognize feelings of fullness. It should be reinforced that gravity helps keep the food in the stomach. Thus, sitting up after meals is important.

Hiatal Hernia

A **hiatal hernia** is a protrusion of a part of the stomach through the esophageal hiatus (opening) of the diaphragm (Fig. 11–1). Persons with this disorder sometimes complain of heartburn because of the reflux of gastric contents into the esophagus. Medical treatment includes ingestion of antacids to neutralize or inhibit gastric secretions, and possibly surgery.

DIETARY MODIFICATIONS. Small, frequent meals that follow a normal balanced diet are recommended to reduce symptoms, although dietary modifications cannot eliminate the cause. Foods that are poorly tolerated are avoided, especially those that may irritate the mucous membranes (e.g., orange juice and tomato juice). Extremes in food temperature should be avoided. No food is allowed for approximately 3 hours before bedtime, and the person should remain in the upright position after eating. For the obese person, weight loss is indicated to help relieve pressure on the diaphragm. Any source of pressure on the abdomen such as bandages or clothes that fit too tightly should be eliminated. Table 11–3 shows recommendations for a diet for esophageal reflux or hiatal hernia.

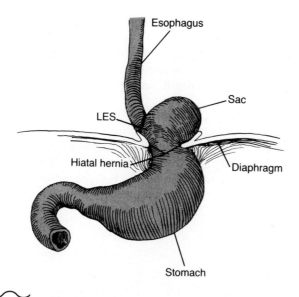

▲ FIGURE 11-1

Sketch of hiatal hernia. KEY: LES = lower esophageal sphincter. (From Hagarty G: A classification of esophageal hiatus hernia with special reference to sliding hernia. Am J Roentgenol. 1960; 84:1056. Adapted by Mahan LK, Arlin M for Krause's Food, Nutrition & Diet Therapy, 8th ed. Philadelphia, WB Saunders, 1992; p. 443.)

▲ TABLE 11-3

FOODS TO AVOID IN A DIET FOR ESOPHAGEAL REFLUX OR HIATAL HERNIA

Beverages	Coffee, decaffeinated coffee, carbonated beverages, and chocolate
Fats	Excessive amounts
Fruits, fruit juices	Citrus fruits and juices
Vegetables, vegetable juices	Tomato, tomato juice
Miscellaneous	Dill, peppermint, spearmint, and foods prepared with excess spices

Reprinted by permission from Recent Advances in Therapeutic Diets, 4th Edition by the University of Iowa Hospitals and Clinics. © 1989 by Iowa State University Press, Ames, Iowa 50010.

WHAT ARE DISEASES OF THE STOMACH?

Gastritis

Gastritis (acute or chronic) is an inflammation of the lining of the stomach that results in abdominal pain, nausea, and vomiting. It may be caused by food poisoning, overeating, excessive intake of alcohol, or bacterial and viral infections. A chronic condition may be related to other disease states. It often precedes the development of ulcers or cancer.

DIETARY MODIFICATIONS. Acute gastritis, which usually heals within a few days, is often treated first with antibiotics and neutralization of the stomach contents. The stomach is allowed to rest for a while, and then clear fluids are offered for the first day or two. The patient may then progress to small amounts of soft, low-fiber foods. It may be necessary to avoid highly seasoned foods, alcohol, caffeine, decaffeinated coffee, red (cayenne) pepper, and cola beverages.

SAMPLE MENU for a PEPTIC ULCER DIET

▲

BREAKFAST
Poached egg
Whole wheat toast
Orange juice
Milk

▲

MIDMORNING SNACK
Fresh apple slices

▲

LUNCH
Celery and carrot sticks
Macaroni and cheese casserole
Green beans
Fresh peach
Milk

▲

MIDAFTERNOON SNACK
Graham crackers
Milk

▲

SUPPER
Tossed salad with blue cheese dressing
Baked chicken
Sliced carrots
Bread and butter
Milk

▲

EVENING SNACK
Cheese and wheat crackers

Peptic Ulcer

A peptic ulcer is an eroded lesion in the lining (mucosa) of the stomach (gastric ulcer) or duodenum (duodenal ulcer). There are many theories as to the cause of peptic ulcers, including poor dietary habits (such as irregular and hurried eating), excessive smoking, excessive ingestion of aspirin, emotional stress, heredity, and excessive alcohol consumption. The consensus is that ulcers are actually caused by hypersecretion of gastric juices, hyperactivity of the stomach contents, reflux of the bile acid into the stomach from the duodenum, or (the latest theory) breakdown of the mucosal lining of the stomach with bacterial infection.

Symptoms include burning or gnawing pain in the pit of the stomach. Peptic ulcers are diagnosed by gastric analysis, x-ray or fluoroscopic studies, or gastroscopy.

DIETARY MODIFICATIONS. While an ulcer is bleeding, no food is allowed; instead, intravenous feedings of dextrose and amino acids may be given. As the condition improves, the patient usually progresses from a full liquid diet to a regular diet with the omission of irritants based on individual tolerances (see Sample Menu; individualization of this diet is suggested). Cigarette smoke is a non-dietary irritant of the gastric mucosa. Referral to a smoking-cessation program should be made as needed.

A liberal approach to dietary intervention is now being used by most clinicians, since it is now well known that a bland diet has little effect on the healing of ulcers. Nutritional advice should be individualized. If a patient feels that certain foods cause gastric pain they should be omitted until the person feels comfortable eating them again. Coffee, whether caffeinated or not, may cause gastric distress. Food omissions should be made carefully to prevent nutritional inadequacy. Table 11–4 lists some guidelines for dietary treatment of peptic ulcers.

Three types of drugs are used in the treatment of peptic ulcer disease: antacids to neutralize acid, antispasmodic agents to reduce gastric motility, and anticholinergic agents to reduce gastric acid secretion. New evidence shows that patients treated with antibiotics experience improved healing of ulcers and fewer recurrent ulcers. By decreasing the acid content of the

▲ TABLE 11-4

DIETARY TREATMENT OF PEPTIC ULCERS

GUIDELINE	RATIONALE
Eat three regular meals or six small meals	Inhibits stomach distention
Avoid caffeine-containing beverages, decaffeinated coffee	Decreases gastric secretions
Avoid alcohol	Reduces damage to stomach lining
Avoid black pepper, chili powder, cloves, nutmeg, curry powder, mustard seed	Reduces irritation of stomach lining
Avoid aspirin	Reduces irritation of stomach lining
Avoid cigarette smoking	Promotes healing of ulcer
Eat in a relaxed atmosphere	Reduces stress

stomach through medications, ulcer healing may be improved. This has been the mainstay of treatment. Antibiotic therapy shows promise, as it is now felt that infection may be the causal agent of the ulcer.

FACT & FALLACY

FALLACY: People with stomach ulcers need to avoid citrus juice.

FACT: Actually, the stomach produces hydrochloric acid, which is more acidic than any food. Therefore, orange juice cannot be considered harmful to the gastric mucosa, since it cannot increase the acidity of the stomach contents. However, caution should be used. The patient should be advised to try a small amount of orange juice (2 ounces) with a meal to ensure it is tolerated. Increased amounts can be consumed based on individual tolerance.

WHAT ARE DISEASES OF THE INTESTINES?

Lactose Intolerance

Congenital, or primary, **lactose intolerance** refers to the inability to digest milk sugar (lactose). It is caused by a deficiency of the enzyme lactase, which is necessary for converting lactose into glucose and galactose in the gastrointestinal tract. Symptoms include bloating, flatulence, cramping, and diarrhea.

Acquired lactase deficiency, also referred to as secondary lactose intolerance, is associated with chronic gastrointestinal disease and disorders such as gluten-sensitive enteropathy, Crohn's disease, and other conditions leading to atrophy of the villi of the intestines (see Chapter 4, Fig. 4–2) (Sinden and Sutphen, 1991). Different populations show variations in degrees of lactase deficiency, usually occurring after 5 years of age. Lactase deficiency is more common among persons of African, Asian, Mediterranean, Hispanic, and Native American heritage than among persons of Northern European heritage. See Chapter 3 for further discussion of lactose.

DIETARY MODIFICATIONS. Many persons with lactose intolerance do not have to eliminate lactose-containing foods entirely from their diets because they can produce small amounts of lactase (Table 11–5). Varying amounts of lactose are found in milk products; hard cheeses and yogurt have the least amount of lactose. When foods containing lactose are omitted, it is important to include other sources of calcium in the diet (see Table 1–3). If an individual whose genetic background predisposes to lactase deficiency reports these symptoms when milk is ingested, he or she should not be forced to drink it.

Lact-Aid is available commercially as an enzyme that can be added to milk, and it reduces the lactose content of milk by 70 to 90 per cent. The cost ranges from about 15 cents per day for drops to about 1 dollar for tablets for a day's supply. Lact-Aid will make the milk taste sweeter be-

GUIDELINES FOR A LACTOSE-RESTRICTED DIET*

FOOD GROUP	LACTOSE-FREE FOODS (ALLOWED IN ALL DIETS)	FOODS CONTAINING LACTOSE IN LIMITED AMOUNTS (ALLOWED IN SOME DIETS)	HIGH LACTOSE–CONTAINING FOODS (NOT ALLOWED)
Beverages	Coffee, tea, carbonated beverages, nondairy creamers, soy milk substitutes and beverages	½ cup regular milk; milk treated to reduce lactose,† powdered or tableted soft drinks	Milk and milk drinks
Breads	Crackers, rusk, homemade bread without milk, French or Vienna bread	Commercial bread and bread products containing milk or lactose (muffins, biscuits, pancakes)	
Cereals	All cereals except those containing milk or lactose	Instant Cream of Wheat, dry cereals containing milk or lactose	
Sugars and sweets	All except those listed as not allowed (see Desserts	Cream or chocolate candies, tableted candies, any commercial or homemade candies containing milk, lactose, or molasses	
Vegetables, vegetable juices	All except those listed as not allowed		Any prepared with milk or cheese
Desserts	Cookies, fruit ices, fruit pies and crisps, angel food or sponge cake, gelatin desserts, homemade baked products without milk	Commercial cake mixes, sherbet, yogurt	Ice cream, custard, pudding, cream pies, cheese cake
Eggs	All except preparations containing milk	Eggs prepared with small amounts of milk	Creamed eggs
Fats	Butter, milk-free margarine, vegetable oils, lard, shortening, mayonnaise, peanut butter, bacon, milk-free salad dressings, nondairy whipped topping	Margarine, whipped cream	Salad dressing made with milk, sour cream spreads and dips, cream cheese
Fruits, fruit juices	All except those listed as not allowed		Fruit drinks containing lactose
Meat, fish, poultry, cheese	Plain baked, broiled, roasted or stewed beef, fish, lamb, poultry, pork, or veal	Breaded foods	Creamed food, cheese and cheese products,‡ cold cuts, wieners
Potatoes or substitutes	White or sweet potato, hominy, macaroni, noodles, rice, spaghetti	Some commercial potato products	Any prepared with milk or cheese
Soups	Broth-based soups made with allowed foods		Cream soups, soups made with milk
Miscellaneous	Popcorn, vinegar, catsup, mustard, pure flavorings, salt, pepper, herbs, and spices		Cocoa mixes with dry milk solids, cream sauce, nonfat dry milk

* This diet does not meet the Recommended Dietary Allowances for calcium, riboflavin, and vitamin D. A supplementary source of calcium, riboflavin, and vitamin D (for children) should be prescribed.

† Examples are the sweet acidophilus milk and milk treated with Lact-Aid powder. Lact-Aid–treated milk has a greater reduction in lactose.

‡ Certain persons are able to tolerate a limited quantity of cheese (1 oz.).

Reprinted by permission from Recent Advances in Therapeutic Diets, 4th Edition by the University of Iowa Hospitals and Clinics. © 1989 by Iowa State University Press, Ames, Iowa 50010.

cause it breaks down the double sugar, lactose, into simple sugars. Lactose-reduced milk is also available in most grocery stores. Ensure and Sustacal are lactose-free nutritional supplements.

It is important to read all labels carefully to avoid foods containing lactose, whey milk, dry milk solids, and nonfat dry milk. According to the University of Iowa Hospitals and Clinics, "Small amounts of lactose may be tolerated, especially if consumed at body temperature with other food and spaced throughout the day. The amounts of lactose in chewing gum and most commercial bakery products are not of sufficient quantity to produce symptoms. Milk in fermented form such as yogurt or cheese in which the lactose has been converted to lactic acid is sometimes tolerated" (the University of Iowa Hospitals and Clinics, 1989). There will be no long-term

SAMPLE MENU for LACTOSE-FREE DIET*

▲ BREAKFAST
½ cup orange juice
½ cup farina
1 egg, soft cooked
1 slice Vienna bread toasted
2 tsp milk-free margarine
1 tbsp grape jelly
2 tsp sugar
Coffee or tea

▲ LUNCH
2 oz sliced chicken
½ cup rice
½ cup green beans
½ sliced tomato on lettuce
2 tsp mayonnaise
1 slice Vienna bread
2 tsp milk-free margarine
½ cup canned peaches
1 slice angel food cake
1 tsp sugar
Coffee or tea

▲ MIDAFTERNOON SNACK
1 cup 7-Up

▲ SUPPER
3 oz roast beef
½ cup cubed white potatoes
¼ cup beef broth gravy
½ cup cooked carrots
¾ cup tossed lettuce salad
1 tbsp French dressing
1 slice Vienna bread
2 tsp milk-free margarine
Small banana
1 tsp sugar
Coffee or tea

▲ EVENING SNACK
1 cup apricot nectar

* Approximate composition: Kilocalories = 1992; Protein, g = 70; Fat, g = 54; Carbohydrate, g = 309.
Reprinted by permission from Recent Advances in Therapeutic Diets, 4th ed. by the University of Iowa Hospitals and Clinics. © 1989 by Iowa State University Press, Ames, Iowa 50010.

health problem if lactose is accidentally ingested, however, because the condition is an intolerance, not an allergy. Lactalbumin, lactate, and certain calcium compounds do not contain lactose.

> The patient with lactose intolerance should be encouraged to try small amounts of milk products such as low-fat cheese or yogurt. These are often tolerated in mild forms of lactose intolerance. Lactose-reduced milk products should be promoted as needed. The rationale for inclusion of milk in the diet can be stressed. Milk provides not only calcium, but also protein, vitamin B_2 (riboflavin), potassium, and magnesium. Health benefits attributed to milk include prevention of osteoporosis and possibly control of hypertension. There is also some evidence that lactase enzyme activity can increase with regular intake of small amounts of milk products.

Diarrhea

Diarrhea is the passage of frequent stools of liquid consistency. It may be either acute, lasting 24 to 48 hours, or chronic, lasting 2 weeks or longer. When the condition is acute, the nutritional losses are easily replaced as food and fluid intake returns to normal. Chronic diarrhea results in more serious nutritional losses. The absorption of fluids, electrolytes, and nutrients may be impaired because of their rapid transit through the gastrointestinal tract.

DIETARY MODIFICATIONS. If diarrhea is severe, no food is given for up to 48 hours. This will give the intestinal tract a chance to rest. It may be useful to feed through most episodes of mild diarrhea, however (Sinden and Sutphen, 1991). Low-residue diets prescribed for acute diarrhea often restrict milk intake. Milk does not contain fiber and is a medium-residue food (leaves a moderate amount of **residue,** or undigested food matter, in the GI tract) and should not be restricted on a low-residue diet as long as the person can tolerate milk and is not lactase deficient (McDonald, Christian, et al., 1991). Intravenous solutions of dextrose, amino acids, electrolytes, and vitamins will help replace fluids and electrolytes and provide some nutrients. Clear liquid or an elemental diet may be given after this time. Once diarrhea has diminished, progression can be made to a diet that is restricted in residue and high in protein, calories, nutrients, and fluids. Table 11–6 shows how residue can be restricted using the food groups of the Food Guide Pyramid. These restrictions are gradually replaced by a regular normal diet as soon as the patient is able to tolerate it.

Antibiotic treatment can cause diarrhea because it kills helpful as well as the harmful bacteria. The intestinal tract normally contains certain types of bacteria that help to digest food matter. A person in this situation will benefit from consuming yogurt with live bacterial culture (***lactobacillus*** cul-

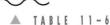

▲ TABLE 11-6

LOW-RESIDUE DIET AS MODIFIED WITH FOOD GROUPS FROM THE FOOD GUIDE PYRAMID

Grains	Emphasize refined grain products such as white bread, white rice, pasta, and cereals that are not whole grain
Vegetables/Fruits	Emphasize those without skins or seeds such as canned fruits and fruit juice
Milk	Two cups or more as tolerated per day
Meat	Emphasize tender meats; avoid fried meats or those with gristle
	Avoid legumes and nuts

ture). Carbohydrate foods low in roughage such as plain white rice, white bread, pasta, or peeled potatoes are generally well tolerated.

Constipation

Constipation is a condition in which the waste matter in the bowels is difficult to pass or the emptying time of the feces is so delayed that discomfort or uncomfortable symptoms result. Prolonged constipation is called *obstipation*. Symptoms include nausea, heartburn, headache, general malaise, or distress in the rectum or intestine as a result of the nerves reacting when the rectum is distended by the contained matter.

Atonic Constipation

Atonic constipation is characterized by the loss of rectal sensibility and weak peristaltic waves. It commonly occurs in elderly or obese persons, pregnant women, persons who abuse or overuse laxatives, and postoperative patients. Factors contributing to its occurrence include a low-fiber diet, irregular meals, inadequate fluid intake, lack of exercise, lack of time allowed for evacuation of stool, and prolonged use of chemical laxatives.

Spastic Constipation

This condition (also known as **irritable bowel syndrome,** spastic colitis, and mucous colitis) is characterized by irregular contractions of the bowel resulting in either diarrhea or constipation. Factors contributing to its occurrence include excessive use of laxatives or cathartics, irregular eating habits, antibiotic therapy, and nervous tension. Its treatment requires prolonged intervention.

DIETARY MODIFICATIONS. A high-fiber diet (see sample menu; Table 11–7) is used in the treatment of constipation, since it allows the feces to be easily and more quickly expelled. Figure 11–2 shows how this is accomplished. Fiber provides bulk by absorbing water and therefore aids in elimination of wastes from the body.

Dietary fiber is defined as a mixture of complex carbohydrates that are largely resistant to human digestion such as cellulose, hemicellulose, pectin substances, and a noncarbohydrate, lignin. These are found only in plant foods. The techniques for determining dietary fiber content are still being developed, and published data are limited (see Appendix 7). The recommended level of dietary fiber is 25 to 50 g per day (the University of Iowa Hospitals and Clinics, 1989).

▲ TABLE 11-7

GUIDELINES FOR A HIGH-FIBER DIET

FOOD GROUP	FOODS ALLOWED	FOODS TO AVOID
Beverages	All	None
Breads	Breads, crackers, and quick breads made from 100% whole-wheat or whole-rye flour; graham, wheat, and rye crackers	Refined white or rye bread or crackers
Cereals	Bran or whole grain cereals, two ½-cup servings daily	Highly refined cereals such as farina or cornflakes
Desserts	All, especially those containing fruits or nuts	None
Eggs	All	None
Fats	All	None
Fruits, fruit juices	All, especially fresh or dried, 3 or more servings daily	None
Meat, fish, poultry, cheese	All	None
Potatoes or substitutes	Baked potato with skin, fibrous sweet potato or yam, brown and wild rice	Hominy, macaroni, noodles, potato chips, spaghetti, white rice
Soups	All	None
Vegetables, vegetable juices	All, especially raw, 3 or more servings daily	None

Reprinted by permission from Recent Advances in Therapeutic Diets, 4th ed., by the University of Iowa Hospitals and Clinics. © 1989 by Iowa State University Press, Ames, Iowa 50010.

A variety of high-fiber foods from a variety of sources is recommended. Wheat bran, an insoluble fiber, increases bulk and facilitates the movement of feces along the intestinal tract. Large particles of coarsely ground bran are more effective than are finely ground fibers. Soluble fiber helps prevent constipation by absorbing water, thereby preventing dry stools that may be difficult to pass. There are many sources of soluble fiber such as oats, barley, brown rice, legumes, and psyllium. Psyllium is a grain grown in India. A commercial laxative product that contains psyllium fiber is Metamucil. When diarrhea occurs during spastic constipation, a minimal-residue diet may be beneficial (see Table 11-7).

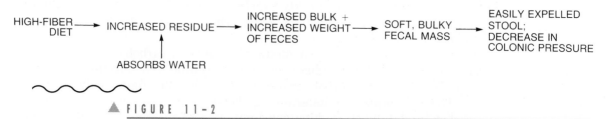

▲ FIGURE 11-2

How a high-fiber diet helps correct and prevent constipation.

FACT & FALLACY

FALLACY: Cheese causes constipation.
FACT: There is no evidence that supports the belief that cheese causes or aggravates constipation. A lack of dietary fiber and fluids is more likely to be the problem. Occasionally, a person may be allergic to dairy products and may experience constipation as a result. Cheese, however, may take longer to digest if it has a high fat content. Whole-grain breads and cereals, fresh fruits and vegetables, and at least 64 ounces of fluids daily should counteract any tendency toward constipation in most healthy individuals. Cheese and other dairy products are the best sources of calcium and riboflavin (vitamin B_2) and should be included in the daily diet. Cheese is a versatile food that can be eaten uncooked or used in recipes from many cultures. Cheese is provided by the WIC program (see Chapter 22).

Steatorrhea

Steatorrhea is diarrhea characterized by excess fat in stools and results from a malabsorption syndrome caused by disease of the intestinal mucosa or pancreatic enzyme deficiency. Steatorrhea usually indicates a more serious underlying organic disease. It may be seen in pancreatitis or following gastric or intestinal resection. It often is associated with diseases of the liver or gallbladder or with malabsorptive diseases such a nontropical sprue or regional enteritis. It sometimes occurs after gastrointestinal radiation. All of these disorders may involve problems with fat digestion or absorption. It is generally diagnosed from a fecal fat test, which may require 3 to 4 days of fecal material collection.

DIETARY MODIFICATIONS. The treatment of steatorrhea involves the use of **medium-chain triglycerides (MCTs),** which are fats that contain 8 to 10 carbon atoms (as opposed to the 12 to 18 carbon atoms found in long-chain triglycerides [LCTs]). MCTs are used in the treatment of steatorrhea because they are more easily digested, absorbed, and transported than are LCTs. They also help reduce fecal losses of water, electrolytes, and nutrients.

In diet planning, the emphasis is on low-fat foods to decrease the amount of LCTs in the diet. More than half of the allowed fat calories are in the form of MCTs. This can be accomplished with the use of commercially available products. The two principal forms of MCT are Portagen, which is a powdered formula that can be mixed and served as a supplement to meals, and MCT oil, which can replace vegetable oil in recipes.

SAMPLE MENU for HIGH-FIBER DIET*

▲

BREAKFAST
Fresh orange
½ cup bran cereal
1 slice toast, 100% whole wheat
1 tsp butter or margarine
1 tbsp jam
1 cup 2% milk
1 tsp sugar
Coffee or tea

▲

LUNCH
¾ cup creamed chicken
on 1 slice toast, 100% whole wheat
½ cup green beans
1 sliced tomato
¾ cup lettuce salad
½ cup canned peaches
Oatmeal-raisin cookie

▲

MIDAFTERNOON SNACK
Fresh apple

▲

SUPPER
½ cup lentil soup
2 oz roast beef
1 baked potato w/skin
½ cup cooked carrots
¾ cup tossed salad
1 tbsp French dressing
1 slice bread, 100% whole wheat
1 tsp butter or margarine
Date bar
1 cup 2% milk
Coffee or tea

▲

EVENING SNACK
½ cup bran cereal
½ cup 2% milk
1 tsp sugar

* Approximate content: Kilocalories = 2126; Protein, g = 103; Fat, g = 63; Carbohydrate, g = 303.
Reprinted by permission from Recent Advances in Therapeutic Diets, 4th ed., by the University of Iowa Hospitals and Clinics. © 1989 by Iowa State University Press, Ames, Iowa 50010.

Celiac Sprue

This malabsorptive disorder is also known as gluten-induced enteropathy. It is characterized by an allergy to a protein known as **gliadin** found in foods containing gluten. **Gluten** is the protein portion of wheat, oats, rye, and barley. The exact cause of this disease is unknown but it occurs more frequently among persons of British heritage than among other groups. There is some evidence that stressful events precede the onset of celiac disease. Symptoms include diarrhea, steatorrhea, and weight loss. Diagnosis must be confirmed with intestinal biopsy to determine the amount of damage to the villi of the intestine, which causes malabsorption and diarrhea. If celiac sprue is untreated, vitamin and mineral deficiencies become apparent. Depletion of vitamins B, D, and K and electrolytes can occur (O'Toole, 1992).

DIETARY MODIFICATIONS. A gluten-free diet is given, in which all products containing gluten or gliadin are eliminated (see Sample Menu; Table 11–8). Lactose intolerance often accompanies celiac sprue. Because some patients are extremely sensitive to trace amounts of gluten, all potential sources (including "gluten-free wheat starch" and white vinegar) should be avoided. The patient's condition improves dramatically on a gluten-free diet. Dietary counseling must include a discussion of foods allowed, reading labels for even small amounts of gluten in various foods, and using alternative flours (e.g., rice, corn, and potato) in recipes. Other substitutes include tapioca and soybean and arrowroot flours. "A possible substitute is amaranth, a pseudo-cereal (not in the grass family), which has been advertised as containing little or no gluten. Because gluten does not appear in other members of the Amaranthaceae family, the chance that amaranth contains gluten is remote. (The scientific studies and clinical trials to determine its presence had not been performed as of 1990.)" (The University of Iowa Hospitals and Clinics, 1989.) The gluten-free diet is a very tedious diet, and referral to celiac organizations is highly recommended (see Appendix 20).

Hydrolyzed vegetable protein, hydrolyzed plant protein, vegetable protein, starch, modified food starch, cereal, and millet are other ingredients that may contain gluten and are listed on food labels. The manufacturer of the product should be contacted to verify the presence of gluten. Celiac organizations are the best resources for current listings of acceptable foods.

▲ TABLE 11-8

GUIDELINES FOR A GLUTEN-RESTRICTED DIET

FOOD GROUP	FOODS ALLOWED	FOODS TO AVOID
Beverages	Milk, carbonated beverages, coffee, tea, decaffeinated coffee, fruit-flavored beverages, rum, brandy, tequila, dry table wines, dessert wines	Cereal beverages; malted milk; ale; beer; beverages containing wheat, rye, oats, barley, or malt, including whiskeys (scotch, bourbon, gin) and vodka unless made from potatoes or grapes
Breads	Breads made from cornmeal; corn, potato, rice, soybean, tapioca, and arrowroot flours	All bread and crackers containing wheat, rye, oats, or barley; "gluten-free" wheat starch,* triticale; millet and buckwheat†
Cereals	Cornmeal, rice, precooked rice cereal, dry cereals containing only rice or corn	All cooked and prepared cereals containing wheat, rye, oats, barley, malt, bran, or wheat germ
Desserts	Custard; gelatin desserts; fruit ice; pudding made with corn-cream; sherbet; cakes, cookies, and other dessert made with allowed flour or starches	Cakes, cookies, pastries, or commercial pudding mixes containing restricted flours; ice cream cones; fruit sauces thickened with wheat flour; commercial ice cream or sherbet containing a wheat stabilizer

Table continued on following page

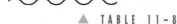

▲ **TABLE 11-8**

GUIDELINES FOR A GLUTEN-RESTRICTED DIET *Continued*

FOOD GROUP	FOODS ALLOWED	FOODS TO AVOID
Eggs	Baked, poached, soft or hard cooked, scrambled, fried	Creamed eggs, souffle, or fondue unless made with allowed flours
Fats	Butter, margarine, cream, vegetable oils and shortenings, lard, bacon, salad dressings thickened with allowed flours or starches	Salad dressings or gravies containing wheat, rye, oats, or barley
Fruits, fruit juices	All fresh, frozen, canned, and dried	None
Meat, fish, poultry, cheese	Baked, broiled, roasted, or steamed beef, lamb, liver, pork, veal; poultry; fish; cottage cheese, cream cheese, nonprocessed cheeses	Meat, fish, poultry, or cheese products containing restricted cereals (the following foods frequently contain these cereals: meatloaf, meat patties; breaded meat, fish, or poultry; canned meat products; cold cuts unless guaranteed all meat; cheese spreads)
Potatoes or substitutes	White and sweet potatoes, rice, hominy, potato chips	Creamed or scalloped potatoes unless made with allowed flours; macaroni, noodles, spaghetti
Soups	Broth-based and cream soups made from allowed foods	Soups containing wheat, rye, oats, barley, or products made from these grains; soups thickened with wheat flour
Sugar, sweets	Table sugar, syrup, honey, jelly, molasses, hard candy, chocolate, chewing gum	Commercial candies containing wheat, rye, oats, barley, or malt
Vegetables, vegetable juices	All fresh, frozen, and canned	None
Miscellaneous	Salt, flavorings, spices, cider vinegar, peanut butter, coconut, popcorn, olives, pickles, catsup, mustard, chocolate, cocoa powder, gravy or cream sauce if thickened with allowed flours or starches	Pretzels, distilled white vinegar,‡ gravy thickened with flours or starches other than allowed

* The current recommendation is to avoid wheat starch, since even "gluten-free" wheat starch may contain trace amounts of gluten.

† Although botanically different from other gliadin-containing grains, additional information is needed before these can be approved.

‡ Because grain is used as a starting material for white vinegar, it is possible that trace amounts of gluten may appear in the distillate.

Reprinted by permission from Recent Advances in Therapeutic Diets, 4th Edition by the University of Iowa Hospitals and Clinics. © 1989 by Iowa State University Press, Ames, Iowa 50010.

DIVERTICULOSIS

Diverticulosis is the formation of outpockets of small sacs (diverticula) protruding through the wall of the intestines. They are found mainly in the sigmoid colon. Low-fiber diets favor the development of diverticulosis because intraluminal pressure is exerted against the colon wall instead of longitudinally, resulting in pouches (Fig. 11–3). These outpockets do not disappear. Thus a person with diverticulosis will always have diverticulosis but can experience diverticulitis (the inflammation stage; see next section) in cycles. Diverticulosis is common among older persons.

DIETARY MODIFICATIONS.   The high-fiber diet (see Table 11–7) is used for diverticulosis. Insoluble fiber such as wheat bran tends to increase fecal bulk and soften the stool. The weight of insoluble fiber residue in the colon helps gravity propel fecal matter through the intestinal tract. Soluble fiber sources such as legumes and oatmeal provide moisture in the stool. The effect of fiber and liquids is expected to reduce the incidence and symptoms of diverticular disease by reducing pressure inside the intestinal tract. Until recently, the diet restricted intake of seeds, skins, and nuts.

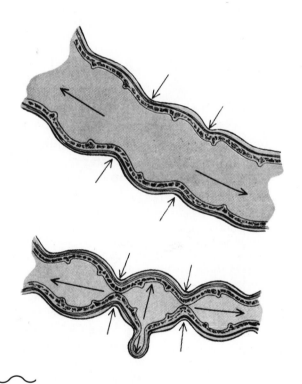

▲ FIGURE 11-3

Mechanism by which low-fiber, low-bulk diets might generate diverticula. Where colon contents are bulky (top), muscular contractions exert pressure longitudinally. If lumen is smaller (bottom), contractions can produce occlusion and exert pressure against colon wall, which may produce a diverticular "blow-out." (From Mahan LK, Arlin M: Krause's Food, Nutrition & Diet Therapy, 8th ed. Philadelphia, WB Saunders, 1992; p. 471.)

SAMPLE MENU for GLUTEN-RESTRICTED DIET

▲
BREAKFAST
½ cup orange juice
½ cup Cream of Rice cereal
1 egg, soft cooked
Cornmeal muffin
1 tsp butter or margarine
1 tbsp grape jelly
1 cup 2% milk
2 tsp sugar
Coffee or tea

▲
LUNCH
2 oz sliced chicken
½ cup rice
½ cup green beans
½ sliced tomato on lettuce
Rice muffin
1 tsp butter or margarine
½ cup canned peaches
Puffed rice bar
1 cup 2% milk
Coffee or tea

▲
SUPPER
3 oz roast beef
½ cup cubed white potato
½ cup cooked carrots
¾ cup tossed lettuce salad
1 tbsp French dressing
Rice muffin
2 tsp butter or margarine
1 cup 2% milk
Coffee or tea

Reprinted by permission from Recent Advances in Therapeutic Diets, 4th ed., by the University of Iowa Hospitals and Clinics. © 1989 by Iowa University Press, Ames, Iowa 50010.

Diverticulitis

Diverticulitis is an inflammation of diverticula, which may result from trapping of food particles or materials in the outpockets (described in the previous section) and attracting bacteria. Symptoms include abdominal pain, usually in the lower left quadrant, and occasionally fever. Other diseases with similar symptoms need to be ruled out, including colon cancer. There may be many tests before the diagnosis is made with assurance. Diverticulitis is a temporary condition of inflammation. This condition is what Mrs. Rita Bernardo has, as discussed in the opening chapter case study.

DIETARY MODIFICATIONS. During the acute phase, a clear liquid diet is given and progression is made to a restricted-residue diet (see Table 11–6). Once the symptoms have disappeared, gradual progression is made to a high-fiber diet (see Table 11–7).

FACT & FALLACY

FALLACY: A person with diverticulosis should avoid seeds, nuts, and skins.

FACT: These foods have a high fiber content and help keep the pressure down inside the intestinal tract, thus preventing further outpockets. The increased weight of fecal material in the colon from high-fiber foods helps prevent constipation, which further diminishes intestinal pressure. A high-fiber diet is recommended for individuals with diverticulosis. Thorough chewing is advocated to help the digestive process. Only during diverticulitis would these foods be restricted.

Crohn's Disease

Crohn's disease (regional enteritis) is another inflammatory bowel disease, the cause of which is unknown. However, it is becoming more common, especially in young adults, and is felt to be a autoimmune disease in which the body attacks itself. Crohn's disease can affect any part of the intestinal tract, but inflammation usually occurs in the terminal ileum. Diarrhea, abdominal cramps, fever, and weakness are common symptoms. Malnutrition is likely caused by inadequate dietary intake, decreased absorption of nutrients, and excessive losses from the gastrointestinal tract.

DIETARY MODIFICATIONS. The goal of dietary treatment is to maintain good nutritional status, promote healing, and reduce inflammation. A well balanced high-calorie, high-protein diet is indicated. However, an elemental diet may be used in the treatment of Crohn's disease. The theory behind elemental diets is that inflammation of Crohn's disease may arise from an immunologic response to dietary protein antigens. The use of an elemental diet, which provides nitrogen in the form of amino acids instead of whole protein, may lessen or avoid this response (Sullivan, 1993). A vitamin and mineral supplement that meets the RDA is beneficial because of the malabsorption that occurs with Crohn's disease. The prescribed diet is low in residue, especially during the acute stages. When a regular diet is resumed, foods that are not tolerated should be avoided. The patient should be taught the importance of documenting foods eaten in relation to symptoms. Particular attention should be paid to medications that may adversely affect the absorption of nutrients or increase nutrient needs. See Chapter 7 regarding food and drug interactions.

Ulcerative Colitis

Ulcerative colitis is a chronic disease characterized by inflammation and ulceration of the mucosa of the large intestine. The cause of this disease is unknown. In the 1970s, however, researchers found that patients with ulcerative colitis had high levels of prostaglandins (naturally occurring chemicals that regulate acid secretion in the stomach) in the stomach mucosa. Recent studies suggest that marine fish-oil supplements, which are high in omega-3 fatty acids, may reduce the inflammation associated with ulcerative colitis (Ross, 1993). Use of fish-oil supplements should be done only under a physician's guidance, as there may be undesirable side effects such as reduced clotting time of blood. Symptoms of ulcerative colitis include rectal bleeding, diarrhea, fever, anorexia, dehydration, and weight loss.

DIETARY MODIFICATIONS. When symptoms are evident, a tube feeding of an elemental diet (a liquid supplement that does not require digestion because the food material is already broken down), peripheral parenteral nutrition (PPN), or total parenteral nutrition (TPN) may be necessary (see Chapter 14). These forms of nutritional support will provide necessary nutrients without aggravating the condition. Once solid foods are tolerated, the patient progresses to a restricted-residue diet (see Table 11–6) that is high in calories, protein, vitamins, and minerals to replace nutritional losses and provide for tissue repair. Individualizing the diet to a patient's specific food tolerances is necessary to give optimal nutritional care. Vitamin and mineral supplements may be indicated to provide additional nutritional support.

WHAT ARE DISEASES OF THE LIVER?

Enzymes produced by the liver aid in the metabolism of protein, carbohydrate, and fat (see Chapter 4). The liver stores vitamins A and D and glycogen, detoxifies harmful substances, and synthesizes many needed substances. Liver diseases have major nutritional implications.

Hepatitis

Hepatitis is inflammation and injury to liver cells caused by infections, drugs, or toxins. Symptoms include anorexia, fatigue, nausea, vomiting, fever, diarrhea, and weight loss.

DIETARY MODIFICATIONS. The symptoms during the early stage of hepatitis make it difficult for the patient to consume adequate nutrients. PPN or tube feedings (see Chapter 14) may be indicated until oral intake of food is tolerated. Once oral intake is resumed, a diet high in calories, protein, vitamins, and minerals with moderate fat is planned for the patient. Several small meals are usually better tolerated than are three large ones.

Cirrhosis

Cirrhosis is a chronic liver disease in which normal liver tissue is replaced by inactive fibrous tissue. Because liver tissue is not able to function normally, there may be **jaundice** (a buildup of bile in the body causing yellowing of the skin and eyes), a prolonged bleeding time, fatty infiltration of liver tissue, lower serum albumin levels, and other complications, depending on the severity of tissue function impairment. Symptoms sometimes include nausea, vomiting, anorexia, **ascites** (accumulation of fluid in the abdomen), and **esophageal varices** (enlargement of the veins in the esophagus because of poor portal vein blood circulation).

An individual with cirrhosis may have a low energy level, which is related to inadequate metabolism of carbohydrate. Electrolyte imbalance is also common because of poor storage of minerals. A common cause of cirrhosis is chronic alcoholism. A nutritious diet does not prevent the development of cirrhosis but is still beneficial to promote health.

DIETARY MODIFICATIONS. Since carbohydrate metabolism is often affected in this condition, the diet for cirrhosis should be adequate in energy and nutrients to prevent further deterioration of the liver. As much as 300 to 400 grams of carbohydrate may be necessary, as well as 45 to 50 kilocalories per kilogram of body weight to spare protein. The fat intake may need to be modified because of malabsorption of fats. Protein is restricted to approximately 35 to 50 grams per day (see Sample Menu)—just the right amount to prevent a negative nitrogen balance as well as **hepatic coma** (a toxic effect on the brain due to diminished clearance of blood toxins; see following section). Vitamin and mineral supplementation is often necessary. Sodium and fluids are restricted if edema and ascites develop. It is not unusual for the sodium to be limited to 500 to 1500 mg per day. Fluids are restricted to 100 to 1500 mL per day, depending on the severity of the condition. Foods high in roughage (whole grains and vegetables and fruits with skin and seeds) may need to be restricted with esophageal varices to prevent rupture of these tiny blood vessels.

Hepatic Coma

When liver function becomes severely impaired, ammonia levels become abnormally high and toxic to brain tissue. The unconsciousness that may result is known as hepatic coma. Contributing factors include gastrointestinal bleeding, excessive dietary protein, severe infection, and surgical procedures. Symptoms include confusion, irritability, delirium, and flapping tremors of the hands and feet.

DIETARY MODIFICATIONS. The aim of this diet is to decrease the amount of ammonia that enters the general circulation. Antibiotics are administered to decrease the ammonia production from intestinal bacteria. Protein in the diet is restricted to 0 to 20 grams, depending on the severity of the condition (see Chapter 10, Sample Menu). The amount of protein is

SAMPLE MENU for a
35-gram PROTEIN MEAL*

▲

BREAKFAST
½ cup fruit or juice
½ cup cereal with ½ cup milk, sugar
1 slice toast with margarine and jelly
Coffee or tea

▲

LUNCH
1 small potato with margarine
½ cup vegetable
Tossed salad with Italian dressing
1 slice bread with margarine
½ cup fruit
½ cup milk

▲

SUPPER
1 oz meat or 1 egg
1 small potato
½ cup vegetable
Fruit salad
1 slice bread with margarine
½ cup fruit
½ cup milk
Coffee or tea

* On a 20-g protein meal pattern, 1 oz of meat and 1 cup of milk would be omitted. Extra margarine, concentrated sweets, low-protein bread and pasta, and possibly carbohydrate supplements help to provide adequate kilocalories in the diet.

gradually increased in increments of 10 to 15 grams as liver function improves. Supplements of branched-chain amino acids may be used (Hepatic-Aid). Kilocalorie intake must be kept high to prevent tissue breakdown. Kilocalories from carbohydrate and fat are emphasized. Sodium is restricted if ascites or edema is present. Additional vitamin and mineral supplements should be given.

WHAT ARE DISEASES OF THE GALLBLADDER?

Gallbladder diseases are related to stones and inflammation. The release of bile for fat digestion can cause severe pain.

Cholecystitis

Cholecystitis is an inflammation of the gallbladder. It can be caused by a bacterial infection or stones in the gallbladder. Symptoms include acute pain in the upper right quadrant, nausea, belching, vomiting, fever, and jaundice if the bile duct is blocked.

Cholelithiasis

Cholelithiasis is the formation of gallstones. Sometimes the gallstones block the bile duct and interfere with the flow of bile. Symptoms include pain in the right upper quadrant as the gallbladder contracts and jaundice if the bile duct is obstructed.

Obesity, diabetes, familial hypercholesterolemia, cardiovascular disease, multiple pregnancies, use of oral contraceptives, fasting (such as with very-low-kilocalorie diets) and TPN (see Chapter 14) are all associated with the increased incidence of gallstones. A high-fiber diet has been linked to decreased incidence of gallstones (Davis and Sherer, 1994).

DIETARY MODIFICATIONS. During an acute attack of cholecystitis or cholelithiasis, food may be withheld for up to 24 hours. Food is introduced gradually, starting with a clear liquid diet. As food tolerance improves, there is a progression to a minimum-fat diet (Tables 11–9 and 11–10) that contains approximately 30 to 50 grams of fat. As the patient's condition improves, progression is made to a low-fat diet (Table 11–9) containing approximately 50 grams of fat. Excess fat intake will cause the gallbladder to contract, which can be very painful if gallstones are present. Foods high in fat, therefore, may not be tolerated, including foods such as sausages, bacon, and peanut butter. Other food intolerances, such as with onions, may exist in certain individuals. If stone removal by surgery or ul-

▲ **TABLE 11-9**

DAILY FOOD ALLOWANCES FOR 50-GRAM FAT DIET

FOOD	AMOUNT	APPROXIMATE FAT CONTENT (gm)
Skim milk	2 cups or more	0
Lean meat, fish, poultry	6 oz or 6 equivalents	18
Whole egg or egg yolks	3 per week	3
Vegetables	3 servings or more, at least 1 or more dark leafy green or orange	0
Fruits	3 or more servings, at least 1 citrus	0
Breads, cereals	As desired	0
Fat exchanges*	5–6 exchanges daily	25–30
Desserts and sweets	As desired from permitted list (see Table 11–10)	0
	TOTAL FAT	46–51

From the American Dietetic Association: Handbook of Clinical Dietetics. New Haven, © Yale University Press, 1981, pp. E-4, E-5, and E-6.
* Each fat exchange equals 5 g fat. See Table 9–7.

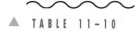

▲ TABLE 11-10

FAT-RESTRICTED DIET

FOOD GROUP	FOODS ALLOWED	FOODS EXCLUDED
Beverages	Skim milk or buttermilk made with skim milk, coffee, tea, Postum, fruit juice, soft drinks, cocoa made with cocoa powder and skim milk	Whole milk, buttermilk made with whole milk, chocolate milk, cream in excess of amounts allowed under fats
Bread and cereal products	Plain, nonfat cereals; spaghetti, noodles, rice, macaroni; plain whole grain or enriched bread	Biscuits, breads, egg or cheese bread, sweet rolls made with fat, pancakes, doughnuts, waffles, fritters, popcorn prepared with fat, muffins, natural cereals and breads to which extra fat is added
Cheese	Cottage, ¼ cup to be used as substitute for an ounce of cheese, or specially processed American cheese containing less than 5% butterfat	Whole milk cheeses
Desserts	Sherbet made with skim milk; fruit ice; gelatin; rice, bread, cornstarch, tapioca, or Junket pudding made with skim milk; fruit whips with gelatin, sugar, and egg white; fruit; angel food cake; meringues	Cake, pie, pastry, ice cream, or any dessert containing shortening, chocolate, or fats of any kind, unless specially prepared using part of fat allowance
Eggs	3 per week prepared only with fat from fat allowance; egg whites as desired; low-fat egg substitutes	More than 1 per day unless substituted for part of the meat allowed
Fats	Choose up to the limit allowed on diet among the following (1 serving in the amount listed equals 1 fat choice): 1 tsp butter or fortified margarine 1 tsp shortening or oil 1 tsp mayonnaise 1 tbsp Italian or French dressing 1 strip crisp bacon ⅛ avocado (4″ diameter) 2 tbsp light cream 1 tbsp heavy cream 6 small nuts 5 small olives	Any in excess of amount prescribed on diet; all others
Fruits	As desired	Avocado in excess of amount allowed on fat list
Lean meat, fish, poultry	Choose up to the limit allowed on diet among the following: poultry without skin, fish, veal (all cuts), liver, lean beef, pork, and lamb with all visible fat removed—1 oz cooked weight equals 1 equivalent, ¼ cup water-packed tuna or salmon equals 1 equivalent	Fried or fatty meats, sausage, scrapple, frankfurters, poultry skins, stewing hens, spareribs, salt pork, beef unless lean, duck, goose, ham hocks, pig's feet, luncheon meats, gravies unless fat-free, tuna and salmon packed in oil, peanut butter
Milk	Skim, buttermilk or yogurt made from skim milk	Whole, chocolate, buttermilk made with whole milk
Seasonings	As desired	None
Soups	Bouillon, clear broth, fat-free vegetable soup, cream soup made with skim milk, packaged dehydrated soups	All others
Sweets	Jelly, jam, marmalade, honey, syrup, molasses, sugar, hard sugar candies, fondant, gumdrops, jelly beans, marshmallows	Any candy made with chocolate, nuts, butter, cream, or fat of any kind
Vegetables	All plainly prepared vegetables	Potato chips; buttered, au gratin, creamed, or fried vegetables unless made with allowed fat; commercially frozen vegetables; casseroles or frozen vegetables in butter sauce

From American Dietetic Association: Handbook of Clinical Dietetics. New Haven, © Yale University Press, 1981; p. E-4.

trasonic or chemical dissolution is necessary, the patient should follow a low-fat diet until the procedure is performed.

After stone removal, a low-fat diet should be followed for several weeks until fat digestion is normalized. Thereafter, a normal diet is usually well tolerated and should be encouraged, although a 50-gram fat diet is appropriate for long-term use.

WHAT ARE DISEASES OF THE PANCREAS?

The pancreas produces digestive enzymes for metabolism of protein, carbohydrate, and fat; bicarbonate ions to neutralize chyme; and hormones such as insulin (see Chapters 4 and 9).

Cystic Fibrosis

Cystic fibrosis (also called cystic fibrosis of the pancreas) consists of an insufficiency or abnormality of some essential hormone or enzyme. Excessive thick mucus is produced by the exocrine glands and interferes with breathing and digestion. Fats are poorly digested and absorbed, and a common symptom is frequent fatty, bulky, and odorous feces. Recurrent respiratory infections and excessive loss of sodium and chloride from the sweat glands are common. Pancreatic insufficiency may develop. MCTs are more easily absorbed and therefore are the best source of fat in the diet for cystic fibrosis. Pancreatic enzyme tablets given at mealtimes, fat-soluble vitamins (A, D, E, and K), and a high-protein, high-kilocalorie diet are the cornerstone of diet therapy for this condition.

Children who have cystic fibrosis often have a good appetite, which allows for adequate intake of kilocalories and protein. If the appetite is low, recommendations for low-fat milkshakes can be made. For example, sherbet can be mixed with fruit juice for a high-calorie but low-fat drink. The addition of Carnation Instant Breakfast to skim or low-fat milk can provide a high-protein supplement that is low in fat.

Pancreatitis

Pancreatitis is inflammation of the pancreas. It is caused by digestion of pancreatic tissue by its own pancreatic digestive enzymes. The reason for this is not fully understood. Chronic alcoholism and triglyceride levels over 1000 mg/dL are often associated with pancreatitis. Symptoms include fever, malaise, nausea, and vomiting. Treatment is aimed at resting the pancreas. A low-fat diet is often implemented during acute pancreatitis. Pancreatic insufficiency may develop and is treated by administration of pancreatic enzyme at each meal.

Diabetes Mellitus

This disease is related to inadequate amounts of insulin produced by the islands of Langerhans (see Chapter 9). Since this is a complex disease, Chapter 9 has been devoted to a full discussion of its management.

WHAT ARE DISEASES OF THE BLOOD?

Sickle Cell Disease

Sickle cell disease is a serious hereditary, chronic condition that is found mainly in African-Americans but sometimes in persons of Mediterranean, Middle Eastern, and Asian Indian ancestry. The red blood cells (erythrocytes) in this disease are rigid and crescent- or sickle-shaped and have difficulty passing through the small arterioles and capillaries. The cells clump together and obstruct blood vessels, causing pain. The major symptoms are anemia, periodic joint and extremity pain (sometimes with edema), ankle ulcers, and severe bouts of abdominal pain with vomiting and distention. The patient is prone to infection.

Although there is no cure for sickle cell disease, preventive measures should be taken to avoid infections. Nutritional deficiencies must first be corrected (such as folate supplementation) and then good nutritional status maintained with a well-balanced diet (O'Toole, 1992).

Thalassemia

Thalassemia is a condition in which red blood cells are small and contain less hemoglobin than is normal. It is a hereditary disease. The relationship of vitamin E to β-thalassemia is being studied, especially since this vitamin has an antioxidant effect on cells and may improve red blood cell survival.

WHAT IS THE ROLE OF THE NURSE OR OTHER HEALTH CARE PROFESSIONAL IN MANAGING DISEASES OF THE GASTROINTESTINAL TRACT?

An important responsibility of all health care professionals is to be alert to problems of the GI tract. Problems of the GI tract should be identified through noting missing teeth, absence of or failure to use dentures, weight loss indicating either inadequate nutritional intake or problems with digestion or absorption of nutrients, and constipation or diarrhea. The health care professional should carefully assess and evaluate the person's need for nutritional intervention, which may include nutritional support measures (see Chapter 14). High-risk persons should be referred to their family physician and a registered dietitian for further assessment and intervention. The planning and implementation of nutritional care must always be individualized. The health care professional must be aware of the specific portion of the gastrointestinal tract involved and understand the digestive process in relation to the need for a modified diet. Remember that many of the modified diets recommended in this chapter are for short-term use only and that the return to a normal diet should be encouraged as soon as the individual's condition allows it. The various guides for good nutrition presented in Chapter 6 should be applied whenever possible.

For long-term dietary adherence, the Health Belief Model should be used. If the patient understands the rationale for the dietary change and recognizes that the result of those changes is feeling better and experiencing less discomfort, the likelihood of dietary compliance increases.

STUDY QUESTIONS AND ACTIVITIES

1. Why would a low-fiber and then a high-fiber diet be helpful for Rita Bernardo in the opening case study?

2. Refer to Maria Bernardo's grocery list from Chapter 3. What foods on that list should Rita Bernardo avoid during diverticulitis? What foods would be good for her once the inflammation has subsided? Why? Review Tables 11–7 and 11–8 for dietary recommendations.

3. Why is a 35- to 50-gram protein diet used to treat cirrhosis and a 0- to 20-gram protein diet used to treat hepatic coma?

4. Why is a low-fat diet used to treat gallbladder disease?

5. Plan a gluten-restricted menu for 1 day that meets the minimum recommended servings of foods in the Food Guide Pyramid.

6. Go to the grocery store and identify five nutrition labels that indicate the products contain gluten. Report your findings to the class.

7. How can a person with lactose intolerance consume adequate amounts of calcium?

REFERENCES

Davis JR, Sherer K: Applied Nutrition and Diet Therapy for Nurses, 2nd ed. Philadelphia, WB Saunders, 1994; pp 870–871.

Dysphagia: A Review for Health Professionals. Melrose Park, IL, Milani Foods, A Division of Alberto-Culver USA Inc., 1991.

McDonald Christian G, Alford B, Shanklin CW, DiMarco N: Milk and milk products in low-residue diets: Current hospital practices do not match dietitians' beliefs. J Am Diet Assoc. 1991; 91(3):341.

O'Toole M, ed.: Miller-Keane Encyclopedia & Dictionary of Medicine, Nursing, & Allied Health. Philadelphia, WB Saunders, 1992.

Ross E: The role of marine fish oils in the treatment of ulcerative colitis. Nutr Rev. 1993; 51(2):47.

Sinden AA, Sutphen AL: Dietary treatment of lactose intolerance in infants and children. J Am Diet Assoc. 1991; 91(12):1567–1569.

Spotlight: Mary Sullivan. RD. 1993; 14(3):2–3, 16.

The University of Iowa Hospitals and Clinics: Recent Advance in Therapeutic Diets, 4th ed. Ames, IA, Iowa State University Press, 1989.

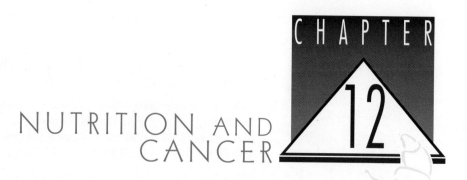

CHAPTER 12

NUTRITION AND CANCER

OBJECTIVES

After completing this chapter, you should be able to:
- Describe cancer prevention strategies
- Explain how cancer and cancer treatments affect nutritional status
- Describe the eating problems associated with cancer and possible solutions
- Explain why nutritional needs must be met during cancer treatment
- Describe the role of the nurse in counseling the patient for the prevention or management of cancer

TERMS TO IDENTIFY

Anorexia	Dysgeusia	Oncology
Cancer	Esophagitis	Radiation therapy
Cancer cachexia	Gluconeogenesis	Systemic
Chemotherapy		

Anna Bernardo hung up the phone. Her friend Oksana was home from the hospital. Her battle with cancer seemed to be over. Finally. How awful it had been. She had come to Anna's school last year after moving from the Ukraine. They suspected Chernobyl had been at least partly to blame for the cancer. After losing her beautiful long brown hair to chemo and losing lots of weight—she certainly was very thin—the latest news was that she's in remission. Finally, some good news in life.

INTRODUCTION

An estimated 30 per cent of Americans will eventually develop cancer (National Cancer Institute, 1989). The role of diet in the development of cancer is continuously being studied by the scientific community. Although there are still many questions to be answered, the best advice one can give the public regarding preventive nutritional practices is to follow the dietary guidelines that emphasize moderation, balance, and variety. Particular attention should be given to a reduced fat and alcohol intake and increased intake of fiber, foods high in vitamin C, and foods high in β-carotene.

This chapter will (1) discuss current knowledge regarding prevention of cancer; (2) discuss goals for the cancer patient; (3) explain how cancer treatment affects nutritional needs; and (4) review ways to cope with the nutritional problems that develop during cancer. Two changes that commonly occur in the course of the disease are in the way the body uses nutrients and in eating habits. These changes may be caused by the tumor itself, by the cancer treatment, or by the psychological impact of having cancer.

WHAT IS CANCER?

Cancer is characterized by the uncontrolled growth and spread of abnormal cells, which continue to reproduce until they form a mass of tissue known as a tumor. A malignant tumor interrupts body functions and takes away the food and blood supply from normal cells. Cancers develop in various sites and require different methods of management. **Oncology** is the study and the sum of knowledge of tumors.

What are the Causes and Prevention of Cancer?

There is strong evidence that reduction of fat intake to less than 30 per cent of total kilocalories will help lower the incidence of cancer. A further reduction to 20 per cent is entirely safe for most individuals and may further reduce the risk of cancer. The type of fat also seems to play a role. Saturated fat and a sedentary lifestyle have been linked to the development of colorectal (colon and rectal area) cancer (Whittemore et al., 1990).

Fiber is believed to lower cancer risk because insoluble fiber, otherwise called roughage, moves food faster through the gastrointestinal tract. This decreased time of transit of food decreases the amount of time carcinogens are in contact with the gastrointestinal mucosa. A recent study showed that 30 grams (1 oz or 2 tbsp) of barley bran flour decreased transit time by 8 hours (Lupton et al., 1993). Wheat bran can significantly lower serum estrogen concentration, which may help prevent breast cancer (Rose et al., 1991). Increased fiber intake to 20 to 30 grams daily may help prevent both colon and breast cancer (US Dept. of Health and Human Services, 1990).

Antioxidants such as β-carotene (found in dark green leafy vegetables and deep orange vegetables and fruits), vitamin E (found in seeds, nuts, and wheat germ), and vitamin C (found in citrus fruits and dark green leafy vegetables) appear to protect against cancer. Monounsaturated oils are preferred over polyunsaturated oils because they are less susceptible to oxidation. Thus olive oil or peanut oil (monounsaturated oils) would be expected to have a more protective effect against cancer development than corn or safflower oil (polyunsaturated oils).

Environmental factors such as alcohol intake and cigarette smoking are also linked to the development of cancer, especially that of the gastrointestinal tract and lungs. Individuals with a family history of cancer should be particularly careful to follow guidelines for cancer prevention. Exposure to radiation, such as following the Chernobyl explosion, may also induce cancer.

HOW DO CANCER AND CANCER TREATMENT AFFECT THE NUTRITIONAL STATUS OF THE HOST?

As the disease progresses in the cancer patient, the appetite and food intake are likely to decrease, which results in a form of malnutrition and emaciation commonly referred to as **cancer cachexia.** Figure 12–1 shows the pathways that contribute to cancer cachexia. The characteristics of cachexia include weakness, loss of appetite **(anorexia),** metabolic and hormonal abnormalities, a reduction in lean body mass, and a progressive loss of vital functions.

There are several reasons cachexia may develop. An altered sense of taste **(dysgeusia),** a lack of energy, a feeling of fullness, nausea and vomiting, food aversions, altered metabolism, and malabsorption of nutrients are commonly noted in cancer patients even before therapy begins. Side effects of treatment often add to the patient's discomfort. Chewing and swallowing problems, a sore mouth, **esophagitis** (inflammation of the esophagus), and decreased saliva production may occur, but most of these conditions will cease when treatment is finished. Metabolites, which are chemical substances produced by the tumor, may have an anorexic effect on the hypothalamus, that portion of the brain believed to regulate hunger and satiety.

Among the most common taste changes are a lowered threshold for bitter flavors and an elevated threshold for sweetness. This may account for the common aversion to meat and the difficulty in tasting sweet foods. Extra sugar on fruits and cereals is a frequent request of cancer patients. Thresholds for tasting sour and salty foods tend to increase. According to a study of 169 cancer patients, the most frequently reported symptoms affecting eating were alterations in taste and smell. Anorexia or food aversions or both often accompany subjective taste changes in cancer patients. The taste

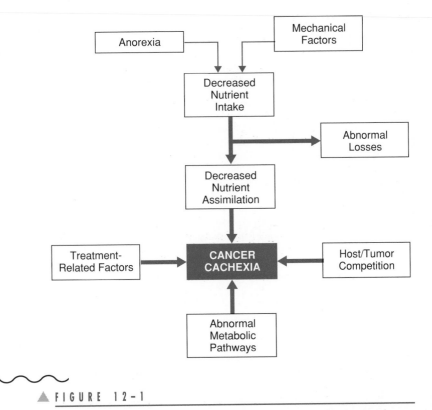

▲ FIGURE 12-1

The pathways contributing to cancer cachexia. (From Buzby GP, Steinberg JJ: Nutrition in cancer patients. Surg Clin North Am 1981; 61:694.)

for salt, sweet, sour, and bitter may be affected. Deficiency of vitamin B_{12}, thiamine, folacin, iron, and riboflavin have been associated with increased taste thresholds in cancer patients (Ames et al., 1993).

What are the Nutritional Problems Resulting from Cancer Treatment?

Cancer is usually treated by radiation, chemotherapy, and surgery, used alone or in combination. Each form of therapy imposes nutritional risks on the patient (Tables 12–1 and 12–2).

RADIATION

Radiation therapy (application of radioactive material) to the head, neck, thorax, esophagus, and abdomen can cause acute eating problems. For example, a dry mouth, sore throat, severe dental and gum destruction, and altered taste and smell sensations may develop after radiation to the head and neck. Swallowing difficulty (dysphagia) often results from radiation to the thorax, and when the abdomen is irradiated, malabsorption of many nutrients occurs if the damage to the gastrointestinal tract is severe. If damage is less severe, gastritis, nausea, vomiting, and diarrhea may result.

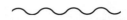

▲ T A B L E   1 2 - 1

CANCER SURGERY AND NUTRITION

AREA OF CANCER	SURGICAL PROCEDURES	POSSIBLE NUTRITIONAL PROBLEMS
Head, neck, tongue	Removal of all or part of the tongue (glossectomy)	Makes chewing and swallowing difficult
Jaw	Removal of lower jaw bone	Requires tube feeding
Esophagus	Removal (esophagectomy) with reconstruction using muscle from the intestine	Food can leak into the lungs or the new esophagus can narrow
Stomach	Removal (gastrectomy)	Food can travel to the intestines too quickly or hypoglycemia can develop
Small intestine	Opening created to outside the body (jejunostomy or iliostomy)	Poor absorption of nutrients, vitamin B_{12} deficiency, electrolyte imbalance, scars, intestinal blockage
Digestive organs	Removal of pancreas	Poor absorption of nutrients, diabetes
Large intestine	Removal (colectomy) with or without an opening created outside the body (colostomy)	Poor absorption of nutrients and water

From Foltz AT, Carty C, Nixon D, et al.: Nutrition of the Cancer Patient. Reprinted with permission from the American Institute for Cancer Research, 1987.

CHEMOTHERAPY

Chemotherapy is the use of drugs to cure or control cancer. It is **systemic,** meaning that it can affect the entire body rather than just a part of it. The drugs interfere with cells as they divide and reproduce themselves. Normal cells as well as cancer cells are affected, and when cells in the gastrointestinal tract are affected, diarrhea, constipation, or poor absorption of nutrients may occur. However, these side effects are only temporary, since the gastrointestinal tract cells replace themselves every 3 days.

Chemotherapy drugs cause nausea and vomiting. Steroids are sometimes used that cause water retention and bloating. After treatment, these conditions will disappear and the patient's nutritional status will improve. Steroids used in chemotherapy may require the use of dietary sodium and carbohydrate restrictions because of fluid retention and high serum glucose levels. The side effects experienced during chemotherapy treatments may make it difficult for the patient to consume the optimal amounts of nutrients. Chemotherapy-induced side effects are listed in Table 12–3. Anna Bernardo's friend Oksana probably lost weight because of the chemotherapy side effects.

SURGERY

Surgery is used in the treatment of cancer in an attempt to remove tumors or alleviate symptoms (e.g., obstruction). The nutritional problems that may develop are dependent on the type of procedure performed. Providing opti-

▲ T A B L E   1 2 - 2

RADIATION AND NUTRITION

AREA OF TREATMENT	SHORT-TERM EFFECTS	LONG-TERM EFFECTS
Head and neck	Irritation of mouth, tongue, esophagus	Dry mouth Tooth decay Stricture of esophagus Inability to taste
Abdomen	Irritation of stomach Diarrhea Milk intolerance Nausea and vomiting	Some of these symptoms may continue in some patients
Spine—upper areas	Irritation of stomach and esophagus	Some of these symptoms may continue in some patients
Spine—lower areas	Diarrhea	
Pelvis	Diarrhea Malabsorption	Some of these symptoms may continue in some patients

From Foltz AT, Carty C, Nixon D, et al.: Nutrition of the Cancer Patient. Reprinted with permission from the American Institute for Cancer Research, 1987.

mal nutrition may require dietary modifications based on the patient's ability or inability to consume, digest, and absorb nutrients. Table 12–4 lists common dietary modifications that are needed after certain surgical procedures.

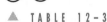
What are the Reasons for Preventing Weight Loss in the Cancer Patient?

In several tumor categories, patients who have not lost weight survive almost twice as long as those who have lost weight. Also, the response to chemotherapy in patients with breast cancer, lung cancer, colon cancer, and acute leukemia is more favorable if pretreatment weight loss has not oc-

▲ T A B L E   1 2 - 3

CHEMOTHERAPY-INDUCED SIDE EFFECTS

Irritation and inflammation of the mouth
Irritation and inflammation of the tongue
Irritation and inflammation of the throat
Diarrhea
Constipation
Nausea
Vomiting
Taste changes
Appetite changes (increased, decreased)
Weight changes (increased, decreased)
Milk intolerance
Food aversions

From Foltz AT, Carty C, Nixon D, et al.: Nutrition of the Cancer Patient. Reprinted with permission from the American Institute for Cancer Research, 1987.

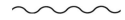

▲ T A B L E   1 2 - 4

SURGICAL PROCEDURES REQUIRING POSTOPERATIVE DIETARY MODIFICATIONS

PROCEDURE	NUTRITIONAL PROBLEMS	DIETARY MODIFICATIONS
Radical neck resection	Inability to chew or swallow	Nasogastric tube feeding
Gastrectomy	"Dumping syndrome"	Small frequent meals, liquids between meals, restrict concentrated carbohydrate
Small bowel resection	Diarrhea, malabsorption	Elemental diet
Ileostomy; colostomy	Fluid and electrolyte imbalances	Replacement of fluids and electrolytes

curred. Weight loss appears to negatively affect the response to therapy and likelihood of survival (Rombeau and Caldwell, 1993).

Why Does Weight Loss Occur in the Cancer Patient?

Decreased kilocalorie intake or increased kilocalorie expenditure (from energy demands of the tumor), or a combination, as well as decreased glucose tolerance and altered protein metabolism, all play a role in weight loss. Reduced gastrointestinal function with diminished movement of food from the stomach causes the individual to feel full too soon and further diminishes the appetite.

In conditions of stress (see Chapter 14), increased amounts of counter-regulatory hormones are produced that inhibit the action of insulin (see Chapter 9). This results in **gluconeogenesis** (production of blood glucose from protein). There is increased breakdown of proteins in the muscle of the cancer patient, which causes a loss of amino acids, resulting in muscle weakness and wasting. The ability to preserve muscle mass during periods of reduced food intake is diminished in a person with cancer. Thus, loss of muscle and protein stores is common during cancer. Significant hypoalbuminemia is frequently found (Rombeau and Caldwell, 1993).

WHAT ARE THE NUTRIENT NEEDS AND GOALS DURING CANCER TREATMENT?

The diet of the cancer patient must supply enough protein, fat, carbohydrate, vitamins, minerals, and fluids to meet the increased energy demands of a high metabolic rate to prevent weight loss, to rebuild body tissues, and to promote a sense of well-being during treatment. Little is known about specific requirements, but some researchers have suggested that energy and protein needs are increased by as much as 40 per cent (Consultant Dietitians in Health Care Facilities, 1990). Individual assessment of kilocalorie intake and weight stabilization will give insight into a particular patient's needs. Nutritionally complete liquid supplements in addition to meals are often needed to ensure adequate nutritional intake. As much as 3000 to 4000 kilocalories and 100 to 200 grams of protein may be necessary to prevent tissue breakdown and weight loss (see Chapter 14 for more information on nutritional support). It should be noted, however, that there is debate about which cancer patients will benefit with total parenteral nutrition

(TPN). It has been recommended that "routine use of TPN in patients undergoing chemotherapy should be strongly discouraged" (McGeer et al., 1990). General nutrition guidelines are as follows:

- No patient should be on clear-liquid diet/nothing by mouth (NPO) without nutritional support for more than 5 days
- All patients at moderate or high risk of malnutrition should be identified by screening and assessed within 72 hours of admission to a hospital
- Patients at moderate or high risk should be able to implement a nutrition care plan at discharge (Queen et al., 1993)

The intake of all vitamins and minerals should at least meet the recommended dietary allowance (RDA). Individual needs must be assessed carefully, since radiation, chemotherapy, and surgery impose nutritional risks.

Fluids are especially important to replace losses from fever, diarrhea, and vomiting and to aid the kidneys in the removal of waste products that result from cancer treatment.

The following are nutritional goals during cancer treatment:

1. Prevent weight loss (a short-term goal)
2. Achieve and maintain normal weight (a long-term goal)
3. Replace nutritional losses from side effects of treatment (i.e., fluid and electrolyte losses from vomiting, diarrhea, malabsorption)
4. Provide adequate kilocalories, protein, carbohydrates, fat, vitamins, and minerals

These goals cannot be achieved without an understanding of individual food tolerances and preferences.

FACT & FALLACY

FALLACY: The high-fiber, low-fat macrobiotic diet will cure cancer.
FACT: The macrobiotic diet is low in kilocalories and cannot support the high energy and nutrient needs of the cancer patient. Weight loss leading to cachexia would likely result; therefore, this diet is not recommended.

WHAT IS THE ROLE OF THE NURSE IN NUTRITIONAL COUNSELING FOR CANCER PREVENTION AND TREATMENT?

The nurse plays an important role in helping the cancer patient cope with eating difficulties that may arise. The nurse should establish a good relationship with the individual before explaining why it is important to eat well. Advice may then be given with sensitivity as to how to promote optimum nutrition at a time when the individual may be feeling poor physically, emotionally, and psychologically. Table 12–5 suggests possible solutions to problems such as lack of appetite, altered taste sensation, feeling full too soon, nausea, chewing and swallowing difficulties, and tiredness.

The cancer patient in the home needs encouragement to take advantage of the good days when favorite and well tolerated nutritious foods can be prepared in advance, frozen or refrigerated, and heated and served later at

▲ TABLE 12-5

SUGGESTED SOLUTIONS TO DIETARY PROBLEMS

Anorexia	Ice cream mixed with a carbonated beverage, milkshake, frozen yogurt, eggnog, blended sherbet and fruit juice
	Small frequent meals
	Snacks available during the day
	Bedtime snack
	Favorite foods; novel or ethnic foods
	Foods served attractively with garnishes, variety of color and texture
Dysgeusia	Substitute chicken, turkey, or fish for red meat if necessary; avoid strong-smelling fish
	Add bacon bits, sliced almonds, ham strips, or pieces of onion to vegetable for added flavor
	Tart foods may enhance flavors (lemonade, vinegar, or lemon juice)
	Wines, beer, or mayonnaise added to soups and sauces enhance flavor
	Marinate meat, chicken, or fish in sweet fruit juices, sweet wines, sweet and sour sauce, Italian dressing
	Many foods taste better if cold or at room temperature
Feeling full too soon	Small, frequent meals
	Chew foods slowly
	Limit greasy foods, butter, and rich sauces
	Liquids consumed should be nutrient-dense
	Limit the amount of liquids at meals
Nausea and vomiting	Antinausea medicine may be prescribed and taken ½ to 1 hour before eating
	Smaller portions of foods low in fat
	Salty foods recommended; very sweet foods avoided
	Clear, cool beverages recommended; liquids sipped slowly using a straw
	Liquids at mealtime not recommended—take ½ to 1 hour before meals instead
	Sit down rather than lie down after meals
	Fresh air and loose clothing may relieve nausea
Nausea and vomiting from the smell of food	Someone else may be requested to do the cooking
	Avoid greasy and fried foods
	Rather than cooking, warm already prepared foods from the freezer
Difficulty chewing and swallowing because of a sore or dry mouth	Physician may prescribe artificial saliva
	Eat soft foods—avoid rough, coarse, or dry foods
	Blend foods after cooking
	Add gravy to cut-up meats
	Use butter, gravies, or cream sauces on meats and vegetables
	Avoid very salty and acidic foods
	Add extra liquids to stews and casseroles
	Low-acid fruits and nectars may be easier to swallow
	Use a straw for liquids
	Rinse mouth as needed
	Avoid hot spices, hot food
	Use nutritional formulas to provide adequate calories if necessary
Too tired to eat	Cook easy to prepare foods (canned creamed soup, fruit and dairy foods, or a creamed sauce over fish or chicken)
	Small portions
	Make meals before tiredness is expected and freeze the food for future use
	Accept offers of food from friends
	Use Meals on Wheels

Modified from U.S. Department of Health and Human Services: Eating Hints. Public Health Service, National Institutes of Health, November, 1983.

mealtime. An effort should then be made to provide a pleasant dining atmosphere.

Visiting nurses, doctors, dietitians, and volunteers are often active in hospice care (a program for the terminally ill, including cancer patients) and assist in dealing with the last stages of life in the home setting, as discussed in Chapter 22. The nurse, however, has the primary responsibility in caring for the patient in the home setting and must learn what the nutritional needs really are and be able to know when to consult a dietitian or to personally counsel the patient wisely in order to promote comfort as long as possible.

Good nutritional status in the cancer patient is of utmost importance, as it greatly influences the effectiveness of therapy and overall comfort of the individual. The nurse must be aware of the various eating problems that may develop during cancer treatment; be able to give suggestions on how to deal with problems; and know when to consult with a dietitian, the nutrition expert.

STUDY QUESTIONS AND ACTIVITIES

1. Discuss some of the reasons that cancer patients experience anorexia.

2. Name some of the factors contributing to cancer cachexia.

3. What are some of the nutritional problems imposed by cancer therapies? What dietary modifications are necessary?

4. Why is it important to individualize the diet of the cancer patient?

5. Now that Oksana (from the opening case study) is in remission, what nutritional goals would be appropriate for her?

6. Case Study

    Mrs. Sweet is a 79 year old woman with diabetes who has recently been diagnosed as having stomach cancer. She has been undergoing chemotherapy and is complaining of a poor appetite and of feeling full too soon. She has an aversion to meat and has a strong desire for sweets. Even though Mrs. Sweet receives steroids, her blood glucose level has been maintained within the normal range by the administration of insulin in addition to her oral hypoglycemic agent for diabetes.

    What type of diet would you recommend, considering Mrs. Sweet's diagnosis and the conditions resulting from chemotherapy? What should the nutritional goals be for her?

REFERENCES

Ames HG, Gee MI, Hawrysh ZJ: Taste perception and breast cancer: Evidence of a role for diet. J Am Diet Assoc, 1993; 93(5):541.

Consultant Dietitians in Health Care Facilities, A Practice Group of The American Dietetic Association: Pocket Resource for Nutrition Assessment. The American Dietetic Association, 1990.

Lupton JR, Morin JL, Robinson MC: Barley bran flour accelerates gastrointestinal transit time. J Am Diet Assoc, 1993; 93(8):881.

McGeer AJ, Detsky AS, O'Rourke K: Parenteral nutrition in cancer patients undergoing chemotherapy: a meta-analysis. Nutrition, May-June, 1990; 6(3):233–240.

National Cancer Institute (NCI). What you need to know about cancer. Washington, DC USDHHS, National Institutes of Health, 1989.

Queen PM, Caldwell M, Balogun L: Clinical indicators for oncology, cardiovascular, and surgical patients: Report of the ADA Council on Practice Quality Assurance Committee. J Am Diet Assoc 1993; 93(3):338.

Rombeau JL, Caldwell MD: Clinical Nutrition, Parenteral Nutrition, 2nd ed., Philadelphia, WB Saunders, 1993; p. 513–514.

Rose DP, Goldman M, Connolly JM, Strong LE: High-fiber diet reduces serum estrogen concentration in premenopausal women. Am J Clin Nutr 1991; 54:520–525.

US Department of Health and Human Services, Public Health Service. Healthy People: Two Thousand National Health Promotion and Disease Prevention Objectives. DHHS Publication No. (PHS) 91-50212, 1990.

Whittemore AS, Wu-Williams AH, Lee M, Zheng S, et al.: Diet, physical activity, and colorectal cancer among Chinese in North America and China. J Natl Cancer Inst, 1990; 82(11):915–926.

CHAPTER 13

HIV AND AIDS

OBJECTIVES

After completing this chapter, you should be able to:
■ Define HIV, ARC, and AIDS
■ Describe nutritional concerns and interventions to delay the onset of AIDS
■ Describe nutritional interventions for persons with AIDS
■ Describe the nutritional needs of children with AIDS
■ Describe the role of the nurse or other health care professional in the nutritional delay
   and management of AIDS

TERMS TO IDENTIFY

Acquired immunodefi-
   ciency syndrome (AIDS)
AIDS enteropathy
AIDS related complex
   (ARC)

Dementia
Human immunodeficiency
   virus (HIV)
HIV positive

Kaposi's sarcoma
Person with AIDS (PWA)
Thrush

A FAMILY'S PERSPECTIVE ON NUTRITION

Tony Bernardo thought how fortunate it was he only had diabetes. At least it could be controlled. He could expect to live a long life. But his friend at work was another story. Poor Denise. She was such a nice person. Fun to work with. She had made his life a lot easier in the transition of jobs. But her boyfriend, who had a history of drug abuse, also had a history of HIV. Perhaps from drugs. But who knew how many sexual partners he had? So his good buddy Denise was HIV positive. He could deal with it. He was not concerned that he would get infected. It took close intimate contact for that to occur and he didn't think Maria would approve of that! No, Denise would remain a good friend only. He knew she was trying to eat wisely. Something about helping to maintain her immune system.

INTRODUCTION

As health care professionals we will all deal with **persons with AIDS (PWAs)** at some point in our career. You may already know someone who is **HIV positive** (infected with the human immunodeficiency virus) or who has **ARC (AIDS related complex)** or who has a full-blown case of AIDS. Perhaps you even have a family member who has already died from AIDS. There are at least 1.5 million people estimated to be HIV positive in the United States (Hecker and Kotler, 1990); however, the actual number of cases of AIDS is much smaller. To put AIDS into perspective, according to the National Center for Health Statistics, there were just over 25,000 deaths from AIDS in 1990, whereas there were half a million deaths from cancer and almost a million deaths from cardiovascular disease during that same year (Lynch, 1992).

AIDS is transmitted only through intimate personal contact in which body fluids are exchanged. HIV is spread through semen, vaginal fluids, and blood. You cannot catch HIV or AIDS from the drinking fountain or through casual contact such as handshaking. This is vital to remember when working with someone with AIDS, since a simple touch on the hand can have a very positive effect on the psyche of the person with AIDS.

AIDS, probably more than any other condition, presents with major biopsychosocial symptoms. Physiologically it is associated with severe weight loss resulting from elevated metabolism, reduced food intake, and increased gastrointestinal losses from diarrhea. Reduced social contact, because of social stigma, can have a profound negative psychological effect on a person with AIDS. AIDS can also cause a type of **dementia** (deranged mental functioning) such that the person with AIDS cannot make appropriate health care decisions. Care of the AIDS patient requires an understanding of the physiology as well as the psychological and social needs created by societal misconceptions and fears. All members of the health care team play a major role in the multifaceted needs of the AIDS patient.

WHAT IS AIDS?

Acquired immunodeficiency syndrome (AIDS) is a condition in which the body has lost its immune system. The **human immunodeficiency virus (HIV)** is felt to be the cause of the destruction of the immune system. A person with AIDS thus has no protective defense against infection.

A person who has been infected with HIV is said to be HIV positive. The time interval between HIV infection and AIDS is variable. AIDS related complex (ARC) precedes AIDS. Complications of AIDS include **Kaposi's sarcoma,** a malignancy that may be found on the skin, mucous membranes, lymph nodes, or gastrointestinal tract and can interfere with nutritional intake (Fig. 13–1). Good nutrition and weight maintenance are believed to delay the onset of full-blown AIDS by helping to preserve immune function. It may take 10 years or more before HIV infection develops into AIDS.

WHAT IS THE ROLE OF NUTRITION IN AIDS MANAGEMENT?

As soon as a person is diagnosed as being HIV positive, he or she should pay extra attention to nutritional needs. Ideally, a baseline nutrition and diet assessment by a registered dietitian should be undertaken. Since an adequate diet is a prerequisite to a healthy immune system, it is currently believed that good nutrition will at least delay and possibly prevent the onset of AIDS. This is why Denise, in the opening case study, is trying to eat well.

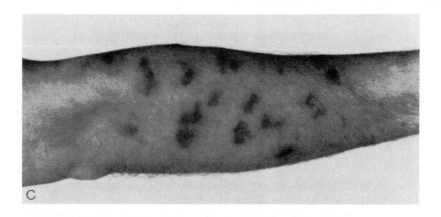

▲ F I G U R E   1 3 – 1

Nodular lesions of Kaposi's sarcoma. (From Kelley WN, et al.: Textbook of Rheumatology, 3rd ed. Philadelphia, WB Saunders Co, 1989; p. 1376.)

Adequate protein status is imperative for a fully functioning immune system. Assessment of protein status can be determined through:

- anthropometric measurements such as weight to height ratio, per cent weight loss from usual or last recorded weight, tricep skin-fold measures, and mid-arm circumference
- lab values such as serum albumin level
- a diet history to determine if adequate amounts of protein are consumed

Other nutritional concerns of newly diagnosed cases of HIV include adequate vitamins and minerals for a healthy immune system. Vitamins A and C are especially important. Other nutrients involved with a healthy immune system include vitamin B_{12}, copper, and zinc. Many other nutrients help maintain health and thereby reduce the stress on the immune system.

The same principles for an adequate diet for healthy persons applies to the person with AIDS or ARC. But the amount of kilocalories and protein will need to be increased when the metabolic rate increases from infections and other stressors. Generally, the person with HIV will not have additional requirements beyond the recommendations for all healthy persons until the advanced stage of ARC begins.

What Are Some Specific Nutrition Concerns Once HIV Has Progressed to ARC or AIDS?

Increased energy needs are a result of the stress and infections associated with ARC and AIDS. Other concerns have to do with either reduced food intake or malabsorption of nutrients with resulting diarrhea. Table 13–1 lists dietary considerations of nutrition-related complications. Loss of appetite can have biopsychosocial causes. Sores of the mouth and esophagus can make eating painful and difficult. **Thrush** (an infection of the mouth) causes an increased need for kilocalories owing to the accompanying fever as well as a diminished desire to eat. Medications for treatment of AIDS may also cause nausea. Abdominal discomfort and diarrhea associated with malabsorption of food nutrients compound the lack of desire to eat while increasing the need for additional nutrients. Physically there may also be difficulty breathing. Psychologically, dementia can cause such disorientation that the person with AIDS forgets to eat. Depression is often common and can reduce a desire to eat. Social isolation is a known aspect of decreased eating and desire to eat.

What Is the Role of Nutrition Support?

To maintain a very high intake of kilocalories, liquid supplements will often be required, often as high as 3500 kilocalories or more per day (see Fig. 20–3 for a sample menu with 3000 kilocalories; the addition of two cans of a commercial liquid supplement will supply the additional 500 kilocalories). It may be as simple as milkshakes or more expensive commercial supplements that are designed to provide high levels of kilocalories, protein, vitamins, and minerals. If oral intake is inadequate, even with liquid supplements, tube feeding may be required. The tube feeding may be in addition

▲ T A B L E   1 3 - 1

SUMMARY OF DIETARY CONSIDERATIONS* FOR NUTRITION-RELATED COMPLICATIONS†

Diarrhea	follow low-lactose, low-fat diet
	offer clear liquids with dilute juice (at most 12 to 24 hours)
	try Lactaid milk, milk products
	avoid gas-forming foods
	avoid hot foods, serve warm
	avoid caffeine-containing beverages
	try pectin and gum-type fiber (avoid bran-type)
	offer small, frequent meals
	offer liquids between meals; dilute juices
	replace K losses with high K foods, liquids
	consider flavored oral elemental diet
Nausea and Vomiting	emphasize low-fat foods
	try bland, soft foods
	offer small, frequent meals
	try dry, salty foods
	serve cold or room temperature foods
	offer foods when nausea is absent
	avoid concentration of very sweet foods
	offer high kilocalorie liquids between meals, use a straw
	offer meals before taking drugs that may cause nausea
	encourage eating slowly, relaxing
	avoid gas-producing or spicy foods
	encourage rest after meals, elevate head
Mouth Pain or Dry Mouth	offer soft or semi-solid foods or liquid or pureed food
	avoid acidic and spicy foods
	avoid hot foods, try cold or room temperature
	use straw to bypass painful area
	rinse mouth frequently
	try hard candies and gums
	provide artificial saliva (from dentist) for very dry mouth
	dip foods into beverage or soup to soften
	try popsicles before eating to numb mouth
Swallowing Difficulties	offer soft or semi-solid foods or liquid or pureed food
	offer moist foods
	offer adequate fluids, use straw
	add commercial thickening agents to foods before serving
	offer foods with even consistency versus uneven, combination foods
	avoid sticky foods
	offer acidic foods (may help thin saliva, aid chewing)
	tilt head back or move forward to aid swallowing
	see neurodiagnostics (speech pathology) for specific help with techniques and appropriate food consistency
Fever	offer high-calorie, high-protein diet
	increase fluids
	use nutritional supplements with infection or fever; when neutrophils less than 500/mm^3, neutropenic diet

Table continued on following page

▲ TABLE 13-1

SUMMARY OF DIETARY CONSIDERATIONS* FOR NUTRITION-RELATED COMPLICATIONS† *Continued*

Altered Taste	try new foods
	add herbs, spices, condiments
	marinate meats, poultry
	try alternative protein sources if meat does not appeal
	serve food cold or at room temperature
	adjust sweetness, saltiness and sourness to increase taste
Fatigue	prepare and freeze meals when feeling well
	keep easy-to-prepare items on hand (sandwiches, canned foods)
	use appliances, microwave, dishwasher
	eliminate cleanup with use of disposable plates, cups
	try take-out foods, home-delivered foods
	arrange for meals with family and friends
	check community resources for in-home help with meal preparation, meal delivery, food banks
	encourage adequate rest
	encourage small, frequent meals
	try calorie- and nutrient-dense foods and beverages
Anorexia	encourage small, frequent meals
	offer high-calorie, high protein snacks
	avoid low-calorie foods and beverages (e.g., coffee, tea)
	provide pleasant, relaxing atmosphere for meals
	drink liquids between rather than with snack or meal
	keep ready-to-eat snacks at side
	try schedule for meals, snacks: "eat by clock" regardless of appetite
	arrange for meals with family and friends
	try new foods to tempt appetite
	check with physician regarding small amount of wine before meals

* For oral intake only. Suggestions are not included for enteral and parenteral nutrition.

† When more than one complication is present, suggestions for one may be contraindicated by another (e.g., acidic juices may benefit those with an altered sense of taste but would likely cause pain when mouth sores are present).

From Schreiner J, Nutrition Handbook for AIDS, 2nd ed. Aurora CO, Carrot Top Nutrition Resources, 1990.

to oral feeding. When there are severe gastrointestinal problems such as digestive problems and malabsorption, oral feeding may be withheld and total parenteral nutrition (TPN) started (see Chapter 14). However, TPN should be used as a last resort because of the increased chance of sepsis at the site of infusion. Elemental formulas with tube feeding are generally well absorbed and should be tried before using TPN. The higher osmolarity of elemental formulas may require cautious increase in strength and rate of delivery (Schreiner, 1990).

How Are Kilocalorie Needs for PWAs Determined?

Studies of resting metabolic rates in persons with AIDS have had conflicting results (Hecker and Kotler, 1990), probably based on whether active infections such as pneumonia were present. Infection and fever will cause an elevated metabolic rate, resulting in an increased need for kilocalories. The general kilocalorie demands for most AIDS patients is about 40 to 50 kilocalories per kilogram of body weight. This kilocalorie need is about twice that of most healthy adults (20 to 30 kcals/kg). The kilocalorie needs for AIDS patients are further increased by about 13 per cent for each centigrade degree above normal body temperature (Schreiner, 1990). Estimated kilocalorie needs can be verified through weight monitoring. For example, if the patient shows an undesirable weekly weight loss of 1 pound, an increase of 500 kilocalories per day will be required to prevent further weight loss. This can be equated to the 3500 kilocalories required per pound of weight loss (see Chapter 20 for more information on weight management and kilocalorie goals).

What Are the Causes of and Nutritional Intervention for Diarrhea?

Diarrhea in the PWA can result from opportunistic infections of the gastrointestinal tract, medication side effects, inadequate digestion of food and malabsorption, and malnutrition with hypoalbuminemia (serum albumin level less than 2.5 g/dL) (Brinson, 1985). An unexplainable cause, which is generally referred to as **AIDS enteropathy,** might also be responsible.

Diarrhea may be controlled by reducing intake of lactose (lactose intolerance is common with gastrointestinal upsets, see Chapter 11), reduced fat or use of medium chain triglyceride oil (a commercial product available through pharmacies) if steatorrhea or fatty stool is present. Medium chain triglyceride oil does not require digestion and is well absorbed if fat maldigestion and malabsorption are present. A decrease in roughage or insoluble fiber along with an increase in soluble fiber may be of further benefit. Soluble fiber sources such as gums and pectin found in applesauce, pears, potatoes, oatmeal, and banana flakes can help diarrhea. Metamucil, which contains soluble fiber from psyllium seed, can also be helpful (Schreiner, 1990). Sometimes total bowel rest is indicated, and therefore the risks of TPN are outweighed by the positive nutritional benefits when the person's status is NPO (nothing by mouth). If diarrhea is persistent, dehydration can become an issue. The person with AIDS may need to be taught the symptoms of dehydration and constipation. Constipation can result with antidiarrheal medication and insufficient water intake.

Should the Person with AIDS Take Vitamins?

A multivitamin and mineral supplement is generally recommended in amounts supplying 100 to 200 per cent the RDA, especially if there are signs of maldigestion and malabsorption, such as diarrhea. This amount is felt to be adequate without causing harm. Megadoses of some vitamins and minerals (>1000% RDA) are felt to actually weaken the immune system (Schreiner, 1990).

HOW DO CHILDREN DEVELOP AIDS?

Women are increasingly developing AIDS through heterosexual contact and consequently passing the HIV infection to children prenatally. Twenty-five to 50 per cent of infants born to HIV infected mothers are infected through the placenta (Schreiner, 1990). Because of their immature immune systems, infants diagnosed with HIV have a life expectancy of less than 2 years (Schreiner, 1990). HIV can also be passed through breast milk (U.S. Dept. of Health and Human Services, 1991).

Infants with AIDS may require a high-calorie formula with 24 to 27 kilo-calories per ounce (Bentler and Stanish, 1987). Many of the same principles of nutrition care apply to infants and children. Kilocalorie and protein needs are more difficult to ascertain and should be based on individual needs using growth charts and nitrogen balance studies or by adding 50 to 100 per cent of the RDA for protein for the child's age (Bentler and Stanish, 1987).

In an attempt to increase kilocalories, any food that is tolerated and accepted by the child is appropriate. Thus general nutritional guidelines to avoid excess fat and sugar in the diet do not apply as strongly to the child with AIDS. As long as the child is consuming adequate amounts of protein, vitamins, and minerals (the child is eating at least the minimum recommended number of servings of the Food Guide Pyramid), added kilocalories can come from any source. Candy bars, soda pop, and potato chips provide significant amounts of kilocalories. Small amounts should be tried first to ensure tolerance to foods with a high fat content. More nutritious kilocalorie sources are preferable, such as milkshakes and puddings; these can be made to be low in fat if needed. Important to finding sources of additional kilocalories are the child's willingness to consume the food items and a physical tolerance of them.

WHAT IS THE ROLE OF THE NURSE OR OTHER HEALTH CARE PROFESSIONAL IN THE NUTRITIONAL MANAGEMENT OF HIV POSITIVE OR AIDS PATIENTS?

All health care professionals should encourage a person with HIV to eat well balanced meals to preserve immune function. The health care professional may need to assist in the patient's receiving meal trays in a timely fashion and may need to sit with the patient during the meal to provide emotional support. Prevention of weight loss is critical. It is much more difficult for a person with AIDS to regain lost weight than it is to maintain weight.

The nurse has a unique role in caring for AIDS patients because of the complex medical conditions. The nurse should be well versed in how to care for the AIDS patient and should be alert to problems that may compromise nutritional status. The nurse may need to become actively involved in feeding the person with AIDS when weakness prevents adequate self-care. All persons with AIDS should have a baseline nutritional assessment with referral to a registered dietitian for any high-risk conditions such as underweight or weight loss.

The health care professional can avoid acquiring HIV when dealing with HIV positive or AIDS patients by avoiding body secretions of the patients and using special care in handling needles used by the patient. Gloves should be worn and good hand washing is necessary after patient contact. Beyond avoiding bodily secretions, the health care professional does not need to worry about contracting AIDS. It is not spread through the air or through touch alone. In eliminating fears the nurse may have about AIDS transmission, sensitivity and compassion toward the patient are likely to increase.

STUDY QUESTIONS

1. What are the different nutrition management concerns for HIV and AIDS? What nutritional monitoring technique should Denise, in the opening case study, have done on a regular basis?
2. Why might a person with AIDS need to have a high kilocalorie intake?
3. How is diarrhea treated in AIDS?
4. CASE STUDY:

    Mr. Smith, diagnosed with AIDS enteropathy, is losing weight; his doctor determines a need for 3000 kilocalories per day. Mr. Smith, however, has no appetite and his mouth sores makes eating painful.

    What can you suggest to provide a high kilocalorie intake for Mr. Smith?
    How can you determine whether he is receiving adequate kilocalories?

REFERENCES

Bentler M, Stanish M: Nutrition support of the pediatric patient with AIDS. J Am Diet Assoc, 1987; 87:488.

Brinson RR: Hypoalbuminemia diarrhea and the acquired immunodeficiency syndrome (letter). Ann Intern Med, 1985; 102:413.

Hecker LM, Kotler DP: Malnutrition in patients with AIDS. Nutr Rev, 1990; 48(11):393–399.

Lynch D: The real risk of AIDS. American Journalism Review, January/February 1992.

Schreiner JE: Nutrition Handbook for AIDS, 2nd ed. Aurora, CO, Carrot Top Nutrition Resources, 1990.

US Department of Health and Human Services: Caring for Someone with AIDS. Centers for Disease Control and Prevention, NAIEP #498, May, 1991.

NUTRITIONAL SUPPORT IN PHYSIOLOGICAL STRESS

CHAPTER

14

CHAPTER TOPICS

CHAPTER INTRODUCTION
DEFINITION AND APPROPRIATE USE OF NUTRITIONAL SUPPORT
METHODS AND MONITORING OF NUTRITIONAL SUPPORT
THE NUTRITION RECOVERY SYNDROME
DISCONTINUATION OF NUTRITIONAL SUPPORT
THE ROLE OF THE NURSE OR OTHER HEALTH CARE PROFESSIONAL IN NUTRITIONAL SUPPORT

OBJECTIVES

After completing this chapter, you should be able to:
- Describe nutritional support
- Describe different types, methods, and uses of nutritional support
- Explain why the nutrition recovery syndrome might occur with nutritional support
- Describe the role of the nurse in nutritional support

TERMS TO IDENTIFY

Anabolic
Aspiration
Blood urea nitrogen (BUN)
Catabolic
D50W/D70W
Elemental
Enteral nutrition
Gastrostomy

Hyperalimentation
Jejunostomy
Nasogastric
Nasojejunal
Nutritional support
Parenteral nutrition
Peripheral parenteral
    nutrition (PPN)

Phlebitis
Physiological stress
Refeeding syndrome
Sepsis
Total parenteral nutrition
    (TPN)
Tube feeding

Kathryn Wade, certified nutrition support dietitian (CNSD), was in her office at Hamilton Memorial Hospital. She was calculating the nutrient and kilocalorie needs of Mrs. Maria Bernardo in anticipation of the need to start total parenteral nutrition. Mrs. Bernardo had been in the hospital too long to continue trying oral feeding. Considering this patient's hyperemesis and her major weight loss of over 10% of her body weight, feeding alternatives had to be planned. The hospital diet, even though it was low in fat and was given in six small meals to help empty the stomach sooner, just was not working. The patient was able to tolerate some sherbet, Jell-O, chicken broth, and crackers but could not eat enough to prevent further weight loss. Although her albumin level was acceptable at 4.5 g/dL, it was probably showing a high normal value (normal pregnancy value is 3.0 to 4.5 g/dL) owing to a state of dehydration. Once the patient was rehydrated, the albumin would probably decrease to an unacceptable level. Dehydration was also suspected based on an elevated blood urea nitrogen (BUN) level of 25 mg/dL and elevated sodium level of 150 mEq/L (normal values: BUN 5 to 15 mg/dL; sodium 135 to 145 mEq/L). The BUN level should come down with rehydration but she would be careful not to provide too much protein in the recommended feeding regimen until risk of renal impairment was ruled out. Mrs. Wade would also monitor Mrs. Bernardo's creatinine level to ensure kidney functioning was normal.

If tube feeding was begun, Mrs. Bernardo still ran a great risk of aspirating food into her lungs because of her severe vomiting. Her esophagus was also probably very irritated, which would only be made worse by inserting a nasojejunal tube. Given the seriousness of this situation, total parental nutrition would be the most appropriate feeding method. And this was what Mrs. Wade was going to recommend to Dr. Wong, Mrs. Bernardo's obstetrician. But first she had to calculate the recommended feeding regimen. The estimated total kilocalorie needs to promote a weekly weight gain of 1 pound were about 2500. Two liters of 5.5 per cent amino acids would provide adequate protein of 110 grams, as based on Mrs. Bernardo's current weight of 165 pounds. She would consult with the pharmacist, Linda Maus, regarding the best fat emulsion and whether D50W was available to meet Mrs. Bernardo's carbohydrate and fluid needs. She would also ask Linda her advice on the best vitamin, mineral, and trace element preparation. Home TPN would be considered if the local home health agency felt it was able to support this patient. She would call to see if this was appropriate. Otherwise, the patient would have to remain in the hospital until the hyperemesis was adequately resolved to allow for normal eating. Even then Mrs. Bernardo would need dietary instruction to promote good nutritional intake to achieve weight gain.

INTRODUCTION

Conditions of **physiological stress** (an insulin-resistant state in which increased amounts of stress-related hormones are present) are created through trauma, surgery, burns, fever, and infections (Table 14–1). Kilocalorie and protein needs can be dramatically increased under such conditions, causing weight loss and loss of muscle mass unless an adequate diet can be consumed. This is often not possible through meals alone. Thus, medical nutritional support is generally required during times of physiological stress. Oral intake or enteral nutrition through a tube into the gastrointestinal (GI) system is the preferred route. The rule of thumb states, "When the gut works, use it."

WHAT IS NUTRITIONAL SUPPORT?

Nutritional support can be as simple as providing between-meal snacks for institutionalized patients or as complex as total parenteral nutrition (TPN). **Nutritional support** is the provision of macronutrients (carbohydrate, protein, and fat) to promote healthy weight management and nutritional status. It is used during times of physiological stress, when the oral intake from standard meals cannot keep pace with the increased metabolic needs of the stress state. TPN is used when the GI tract is not functioning or is unavailable for feeding, such as following stomach surgery.

What Are Indications for Nutritional Support?

Nutritional support is essential for anyone who (1) has had an unplanned weight loss of 10 per cent or more within 3 months; (2) shows a significant loss of muscle mass; (3) has a serum albumin level of less than 3 g/dL or a serum transferrin level of less than 150 mg/dL, or both; or (4) is scheduled for major surgery, for example, a total gastrectomy or another procedure in which there is stress as well as a potential for starvation after surgery.

The nutrition assessment process may reveal a need for nutritional support. Recording a patient's food intake will give a fairly accurate estimate of kilocalories and nutrients consumed. From this information, an assessment can be made as to whether the patient's nutritional needs are being met orally, or if alternative methods of nutritional support should be considered. These techniques can be applied to certain stressful conditions resulting from surgery, burns, infections and fevers, radiotherapy, and chemotherapy. Hyperemesis, cancer, and AIDS often require nutritional support. Patients with pressure sores and chronic obstructive pulmonary disease also can benefit from nutritional support. Effective nutrition therapy that includes nutritional support is required for these conditions, which are listed in Table 14–1.

How Is Nutritional Support Delivered During Hyperemesis?

Hyperemesis (unrelenting vomiting) that occurs during pregnancy is a nutritional challenge. Oral feeding is the preferred method of meeting nutritional needs. Often low-fat, small, frequent meals are adequate to ensure nutritional intake. More intense contact with the patient will allow the dietitian to recognize what food the patient tolerates and to provide that food. The dietitian in the opening case study of Chapter 7 was in regular contact

▲ TABLE 14-1

PHYSIOLOGICAL RESPONSES TO STRESS

TYPE OF STRESS	POSSIBLE PHYSIOLOGICAL RESPONSE
Surgery	Blood loss, shock, hemorrhage
	Depletion of protein or increase in protein metabolism
	Negative nitrogen balance
	Dehydration
	Edema
	Nausea, vomiting, diarrhea
	Insulin shock in diabetes
	Electrolyte imbalance
Fractures of long bones and other trauma	Increase in protein metabolism
	Loss of phosphorus, potassium, sulfur
	Development of osteoporosis because of immobilization and loss of calcium
	Electrolyte imbalance
	Loss of fluids
	Renal failure and uremia
Burns	High loss of nitrogen
	Increased water loss
	Anorexia
	Fluid loss
	Weight loss
	Electrolyte imbalance
	Mineral losses
Infection	Increased metabolism
	Dehydration
	Fever
	Body tissue breakdown
	Nausea and vomiting
	Anorexia
	Poor synthesis of B-complex vitamins related to antibiotics given
	Loss of sodium and potassium if fever is present
Fevers, including those of short and long duration	Increased protein metabolism
	Depletion of body's energy stores
	Lowered sodium, chloride, and potassium levels
	Disturbance of appetite, digestion, and absorption
Radiotherapy and chemotherapy	Damage to gastrointestinal mucosa

with Mrs. Bernardo in attempts to increase her oral intake with between-meal nourishments. When oral intake is not sufficient, tube feeding or TPN should be considered. Because of Mrs. Bernardo's severe weight loss and hyperemesis, TPN was determined to be the appropriate course of action. Nasojejunal tube feeding (with the tube placed past the stomach into the duodenum) would be appropriate in cases of less severe hyperemesis.

How Can
Nutritional Support
Help Recovery from
Cancer?

The goal of nutritional support during cancer treatment is the maintenance of lean body tissue. Owing to the catabolic state induced by cancer, with rapid loss of muscle tissue with reduced intake of food, nutritional support may be critical to survival.

Enteral nutritional support is the preferred method if the GI tract is functioning. Tube feeding at rates of up to 150 mL/hour is usually tolerated (the flow rate should start at about 50 mL/hour and increase daily by about 25 mL/hour to ensure tolerance). Most liquid supplements provide 1 kcal/mL. Thus at 150 mL/hour for 24 hours, the intake will be 3600 kilocalories. This diet should meet the needs of the cancer patient. The dietitian, in consultation with the patient's physician, is the person who determines patient kilocalorie needs.

During the 1980s, TPN use in cancer treatment was common. Now there is an appreciation that TPN for some forms of cancer and types of treatment may be detrimental (see Chapter 12). If the antitumor therapy is expected to be successful, the patient should use TPN as indicated to prevent malnutrition. Children with cancer often are good candidates for TPN because of their high nutrient needs to support growth. TPN is not appropriate for terminal cancer patients.

A common problem among cancer patients is glucose intolerance, which should be considered in the provision of nutritional support. Glucerna is a commercial liquid supplement designed for persons with diabetes and may be an appropriate supplement to use for cancer patients if glucose intolerance is a problem (the patients' lab values for glucose should be monitored at least daily; glucose levels over 200 mg/dL can indicate a problem). TPN solutions can be modified to be lower in dextrose (sugar) and higher in fat content to provide adequate kilocalories. Insulin injection may be required, or insulin may be infused into the TPN solution.

Is Nutritional Support for AIDS Patients Appropriate?

The use of nutritional support is always appropriate. Provision of milk shakes, puddings, or commercial liquid supplements between meals can significantly increase kilocalorie and protein intake and help prevent weight loss. Tube feeding may also be desirable when oral intake is not adequate.

As with cancer, the question regarding the use of TPN has to do with the patient's prognosis. TPN should not be used for any terminally ill patients. If the person with AIDS has a reasonable life expectancy, and quality of life can be improved by correcting malnutrition but the person cannot achieve adequate nutrition with enteral support, TPN should be considered. Strict infection control guidelines should be adhered to with tube feeding and TPN.

How Does Preoperative Nutritional Support Help a Patient?

Even well nourished individuals under stressful conditions, such as surgery, experience a **catabolic** (cell breakdown) phase before the **anabolic** (cell growth) phase of healing occurs. For the patient to benefit from nutritional support, the anabolic phase must occur. This occurrence can be confirmed with the finding of a positive nitrogen balance (Jacobs and Scheltinga, 1993). When new tissue is formed to repair damage, a positive nitrogen and potassium balance is reached, and bodily functions such as digestion, urination, and hydration return to normal. This anabolic phase should be reached as quickly as possible by supply of sufficient nutrients and fluids to counteract the depletion caused by stressful situations.

To prepare a patient for such a stressful situation, preoperative dietary treatment may be required for a time, depending on the condition of the patient and whether the operation is major or minor. Patients at increased risk of mortality and morbidity postsurgically include those who have nutritional deficiency severe enough that there is a loss of reaction to skin antigens. One study found 36 per cent mortality and 52 per cent morbidity in patients with negative skin antigen test results, compared with only 2% to 7% in patients with positive skin antigen test results (Rombeau and Caldwell, 1993). Special attention is given to providing high-protein, high-carbohydrate meals, with mineral and possibly vitamin supplementation (particularly ascorbic acid) and fluids. Obese patients, anemic patients, and diabetic patients may need medical nutrition therapy.

WHAT IS THE USUAL PREOPERATIVE DIET PROCEDURE?

1. No food is allowed immediately before the operation; how long before is dependent on the type of operation and anesthesia.

2. For minor surgery, no food is allowed the day of the operation, unless surgery is scheduled for the afternoon.

3. For GI tract surgery, a fluid diet may be required for several days preceding the operation. Most surgeons will allow a more normal dietary intake followed by a "bowel cleansing" preparation the day before surgery. Special low-residue formulas may be used to maintain nutritional status. No fluid or food is allowed after midnight of the night prior to the operation.

What Are Nutritional Considerations After Surgery?

Adequate kilocalorie and protein intake should be the prime consideration in helping the patient reach the anabolic phase of healing after surgery. Otherwise, the patient will lose weight and become weak. Blood loss, dehydration, edema, nausea, vomiting, and diarrhea are all postoperative conditions requiring prompt nutritional intervention.

After major surgery, small amounts of clear fluid are offered first and the diet gradually progresses to normal as soon as the patient can tolerate it. Recommended nutritional guidelines after surgery are as follows:

- No patient is on a clear-liquid diet/nothing by mouth (NPO) without nutritional support for more than 7 days.
- No patient has weight loss greater than 10 per cent of admission weight at discharge; kilocalorie and protein and/or volume goals for patients on enteral or parenteral nutrition are documented in the medical record.
- Patients on enteral or parenteral nutrition receive at least 1000 kilocalories per day by the fourth day after an operation, although total kilocalorie needs will be greater than this (Queen et al., 1993).

How Can Nutritional Support Help Burn Patients?

Nutritional assessment and support are essential to promote wound healing and prevent weight loss in patients with burn injury. The increase in energy expenditure that accompanies burns exceeds that of any other injury.

These patients appear to become and remain hypermetabolic in response to a characteristic set of hormonal signals. The postburn elevated metabolic rate is proportional to the size of the thermal injury and lasts until the majority of the wound is closed. If the increased protein and kilocalorie requirements are not supplied externally through nutritional support, the patient's skeletal muscle is broken down for fuel. Inadequate nutritional support can result in weight loss, loss of lean body mass, negative nitrogen balance, delayed wound healing, skin graft failure, decreased immunological response, burn wound sepsis, and increased mortality.

Many methods exist for estimating the nutritional requirements of burn patients. All have some limitations. The Curreri formula is widely used to determine calorie requirements and is probably best at estimating peak energy expenditure.

Adult: (25 kcal × kg preburn weight) + (40 kcal × % of body burned)

Child
(≤12 years
of age): (60 kcal × kg preburn weight)+ (35 kcal × % of body burned)

Protein should be supplied in amounts to provide a nonprotein-kilocalorie-to-nitrogen ratio of 150 to 1. Additional protein may be required for patients with severe burns (more than 40 to 50% of body surface area). A goal of 1.5 to 2.0 grams of protein per kilogram of body weight can be used as a guideline. Patients should receive a high-kilocalorie, high-protein diet. Most also receive therapeutic vitamin and mineral supplementation. Adequacy of nutrient intake should be monitored by daily weight measurements and kilocalorie counts. Oral dietary supplements, tube feedings, or parenteral nutrition is included as needed.

No benefits to overfeeding have been demonstrated. In fact, overfeeding can be detrimental, as it has an adverse effect on the immune function (Lacy, 1993). Overfeeding a malnourished patient can also result in congestive heart failure. Maintaining the patient's weight within 10 per cent of preburn weight is suggested as a guideline to prevent the problems associated with over- or underfeeding (the University of Iowa Hospitals and Clinics, 1989).

How Can Nutritional Support Help Patients with Infections?

The goal of nutritional therapy for patients with infections is to combat the effects of increased metabolism, dehydration, and electrolyte imbalance. Fever often accompanies infections, and the patient's kilocalorie needs are increased by about 50 per cent over the basal metabolic needs. Protein needs are also increased when the body is trying to produce antibodies and lymphocytes to fight the infection. Extra fluids are necessary to match the increased kilocalorie needs associated with fever and increased metabolic rate (increase of 13 per cent with each degree centigrade above normal temperature). Fluids help the body eliminate toxins that enter the circulatory system and are carried out by the kidneys. Sodium chloride and potassium levels are lowered as a result of diarrhea and vomiting. Antibiotics used in treating the infections interfere with intestinal synthesis of B-complex vitamins. Nutritional support of patients with infection is summarized as follows:

1. An increase in kilocalorie intake (35 to 45 kcal/kg body weight)
2. An increase in protein intake (1.5 to 2 g/kg body weight)
3. An increase in B-complex vitamins as kilocalories are increased
4. Vitamin and mineral supplements
5. Frequent small feedings
6. Tube feeding as necessary

How Can Nutritional Support Help with Pressure Sores?

Patients with pressure sores need nutritional support to help with the healing process. Kilocalorie and protein needs may be doubled. Vitamin C and zinc are needed to help with wound healing. Liquid nutritional supplements or tube feeding can help meet this need.

How Can Nutritional Support Help Patients with Chronic Obstructive Pulmonary Disease?

This condition often results in weight loss, and nutritional support will be needed. A higher intake of fat and moderate amounts of carbohydrate may help ease the work required of the lungs because carbohydrate intake results in a greater production of carbon dioxide than does fat. It is especially important to avoid overfeeding the patient when attempting to wean him or her from a ventilator.

Special supplemental formulas, such as Pulmocare, are available that are low in carbohydrate and higher in fat content. If TPN is used, the percentage of dextrose should not exceed 50 percent of kilocalories, with fat up to 40 percent as tolerated.

WHAT ARE THE METHODS OF DELIVERING NUTRITIONAL SUPPORT TO THE PATIENT?

The techniques for providing the patient with optimal kilocalorie and nutrient requirements range from very simple to complex. Figure 14–1 shows how the type of nutritional support is determined. A patient receives nutritional support by oral feedings, tube feedings, peripheral parenteral nutrition, or total parenteral nutrition, all of which are discussed in the following sections.

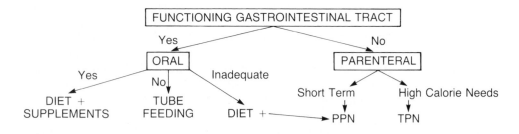

▲FIGURE 14-1

Determining the type of nutritional support for the patient.

Whenever possible, the patient should be encouraged to ingest a normal diet by an oral route. This is the preferred and most natural method of nutritional support. It has the psychological advantage of giving the patient control over at least one aspect of treatment. There is also the physical benefit of promoting continued GI functioning. High-kilocalorie/high-protein foods such as milk shakes, custards, and puddings are often used in conjunction with between-meal feedings. When more complete nutritional intake is needed, commercial liquid supplements should be used. These liquid supplements include the known vitamins, minerals, and other nutrients essential for health.

INDIVIDUALIZATION. Each person enters the hospital with eating habits that have developed since the introduction of solid foods as an infant. Cultural, social, religious, and economic influences play a major role in food selection.

Each patient should receive individual attention in planning meals according to the prescribed diet. Some hospital selections may be unfamiliar to the patient. Alternative food selections may be necessary in order to satisfy the patient's food preferences and tolerances. Every attempt should be made to provide the patient with adequate nutrients in familiar, well tolerated foods.

If the person will be consuming the supplement orally, taste is a major factor. Most supplements are very sweet, while a few are designed to be less sweet. If a person objects to sweet beverages but is having a difficult time consuming adequate kilocalories, the addition of extra fat to the diet may be appropriate. Using heavy cream instead of milk in cream soups or other milk-based foods might be the answer. High-fat sources, however, can suppress the appetite by delaying gastric emptying.

SUPPLEMENTS. Supplemental foods must also adhere to the diet order prescribed for the patient. When selecting these foods or liquid commercial supplements, it is important that the patient sample various supplements and choose those preferred for between meals. This has three advantages: (1) It gives the patient control over an aspect of treatment; (2) It increases the likelihood of the supplement's being consumed; and (3) It avoids intolerance of foods caused by changes in taste perception.

Commercial formulas as well as eggnog and milk shakes are among the most popular supplements. Commercial eggnogs should be used because they are pasteurized. Homemade eggnog with raw eggs has a higher risk of carrying salmonella (see Chapter 22). High-kilocalorie and high-protein puddings, gelatins, and soups have also been developed. The nutritional contents of some commercial products and specialized formulas are listed in Appendix 8.

Enteral nutritional support is also known as **tube feeding.** Tube feeding requires a functioning gastrointestinal tract. A tube feeding consists of blenderized foods or a commercial formula administered by a tube into the patient's stomach or small intestine. The enteral method of administering nutrients most closely resembles the body's own metabolic routes. The role of the liver in tube feeding is especially important because this organ extracts, processes, alters, and metabolizes the nutrients as they pass through it. Liver disease can inhibit the impact of nutritional support.

For temporary nutritional support, a small, flexible tube is inserted through the nose and placed either into the stomach (a nasogastric tube) or beyond the stomach into the duodenum. The latter approach is used when there are concerns about vomiting and **aspiration** (food or liquid entering the lungs). The duodenal or jejunal positioning of the tube is also appropriate at times when stomach emptying may be impaired, such as after surgery. The tube may be left in place for several days and changed on an occasional basis as needed. Or the tube may be removed daily and repositioned each night, for example in the case of home enteral nutritional support.

Long-term enteral nutrition may be required, such as with throat cancer or with neurological damage that causes swallowing difficulties. Long-term nutritional support is best done with the feeding tube implanted directly into the stomach (a gastrostomy) or the jejunum (a jejunostomy). Provision of the liquid supplement may be through gravity, by simply pouring the supplement at a slow rate directly into the tube (this is not recommended for jejunal feedings), or through the use of a pump set at the desired rate of flow. The supplement should not be excessively cold when administered.

INDICATIONS FOR USE. Enteral nutritional support is used when the patient cannot consume adequate nutrients and kilocalories orally but still has a functioning gastrointestinal tract. A tube feeding is commonly used for psychiatric patients who refuse to eat, anorexic cancer patients, patients who have had head or neck surgery, comatose patients, patients with obstructions of the esophagus or fractured jaws, or patients who are unable to chew or swallow for any reason.

Pediatric patients are increasingly being given tube feedings. Pediatric conditions that can benefit from tube feeding include bowel diseases such as Crohn's disease, cerebral palsy, cystic fibrosis, and congenital heart disease. A permanent G-tube (a tube placed surgically into the stomach—often called a "button") is more commonly used with chronic pediatric health problems. If the child's family has not come to terms with the child's diagnosis or need for home enteral nutrition support, there may be noncompliance with the goals of nutritional support (Zlotkin and Harrison, 1990).

WHAT ARE COMMON SITES FOR TUBE FEEDING?

The following are common routes for tube feedings (Fig. 14–2):

  1. **Nasogastric:** The tube is passed through the nose to the stomach.
  2. **Nasojejunal:** The tube is passed through the nose to the small intestine (also called nasoenteric).
  3. **Gastrostomy:** The tube is surgically inserted into the stomach.
  4. **Jejunostomy:** The tube is surgically inserted into the small intestine.

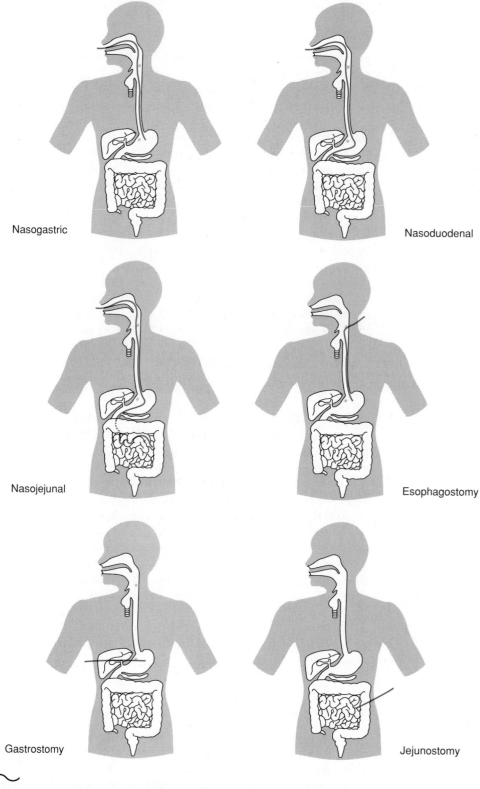

Nasogastric

Nasoduodenal

Nasojejunal

Esophagostomy

Gastrostomy

Jejunostomy

▲ FIGURE 14-2

Tube feeding routes. (Used with permission of Ross Products Division, Abbott Laboratories, Columbus, OH 43216. From Enteral Nutrition Handbook, © 1989 Ross Products Division, Abbott Laboratories.)

HOW IS THE TYPE OF LIQUID SUPPLEMENT DETERMINED?

Digestive and absorption processes and nutrient needs should be ascertained to determine the type of liquid supplement required. If the person has the ability to digest all nutrients and can absorb all nutrients, any liquid preparation that meets the RDA for the person's kilocalorie needs is appropriate. There are supplements designed for high-kilocalorie needs and other supplements designed for low-kilocalorie needs. Thus, the kilocalorie needs might dictate the appropriate type of supplement. Formulas that provide 2 kcal/mL are useful in the fluid-restricted patient.

Often in times of stress there is an inability to break down lactose, which will result in abdominal distention, bloating, and diarrhea. For this reason, many commercial supplements are lactose-free. Fat malabsorption is also common in many disease states. Medium-chain triglyceride (MCT) oil is another common ingredient in commercial supplements. MCT oil does not require bile salts so the fat is better absorbed.

A person's condition may require other diet restrictions such as low sodium, low sugar, low protein, or low potassium. There are specially developed formulas for these restrictions or related conditions, such as for kidney disease or diabetes. There are also formula modules that allow for following a "recipe" to meet the individual's needs.

HOW IS THE AMOUNT OR RATE OF FLOW DETERMINED?

The amount of liquid supplement is determined by assessing the person's need for kilocalories, protein, fluid, vitamins, and minerals. The rate of flow when a pump is used can be calculated by a mathematical equation to meet the needs. For example, if the person can easily have the pump run for 12 hours and the supplement desired contains 1 kilocalorie per milliliter, 125 mL per hour for 12 hours would be required to meet 1500 kilocalories (divide 1500 mL by 12 hours to equal 125 mL per hour). However, this is too high an amount to start. Thus, there would be a steady progression in flow rate starting at about 50 mL per hour and increasing by about 25 mL every 12 to 24 hours until the desired rate is achieved. Or the length of time of tube feeding could be increased to allow for a slower rate of delivery while meeting the kilocalorie needs sooner. Appendix 10 shows a sample tube feeding progression.

If a pump (Fig. 14–3) is not used, the flow rate is more difficult to manage; however, it can be done using a clamp and timing the flow rate. Manual delivery through a gastrostomy should take at least 15 minutes. To help with tolerance, the solution should not be excessively cold.

HOW ARE FLUID NEEDS DETERMINED?

A good rule of thumb is that 1 mL of water is needed for each kilocalorie provided. The actual water content of commercial liquid supplements can be obtained from the manufacturer (see Appendix 8 for phone numbers of

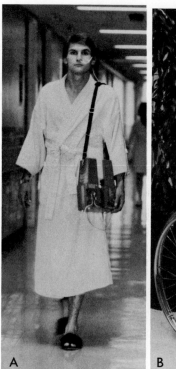
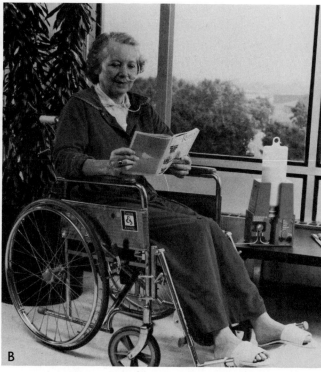

▲ FIGURE 14-3

Tube feeding systems have been developed so that patients are not confined to a hospital bed. Some may even be used in the home. (Used with permission of Ross Products Division, Abbott Laboratories, Columbus, OH 43216. From Enteral Nutrition Handbook, © 1989 Ross Products Division, Abbott Laboratories.)

the major suppliers) but usually is about 75 to 80 per cent of the total formula volume. Thus the volume of a 2000 kilocalorie solution is generally 2000 mL but only about 1600 mL of that is actual water content. Water flushes to keep the tube clean are recommended each time a bag of formula is used (a bag holds about 4 cans of formula). The amount of water for this purpose needs to be calculated into the patient's nutritional support regimen. All sources of fluid taken by the patient, including for medication delivery, need to be considered to avoid fluid overload.

WHAT TYPES OF FORMULAS ARE AVAILABLE?

A tube feeding may consist of blenderized foods or a commercially prepared formula. The current trend is toward the use of commercially prepared formulas, since they are more convenient, decrease the risk of bacterial contamination, offer a wide variety to meet the needs of different clinical situations, and allow the use of a smaller tube to administer the feeding. Commercial preparations can be expensive, however.

Commercial formulas vary in their composition of carbohydrates, proteins, fats, osmolality, and residues (see Appendix 8). The formula selected will depend on the clinical state of the patient. The dietitian is responsible for knowing when various formulas can and cannot be used. If the patient's gastrointestinal tract is fully functioning, a formula requiring digestion of all its components can be used (e.g., blenderized diet, Ensure, Sustacal, or other commercial liquid supplements). If the patient's gastrointestinal tract is not fully functioning, a formula containing digested nutrients can be administered. These formulas are referred to as **elemental** or defined formula diets (e.g., Vivonex, Vital). They are commonly used for short bowel syndrome, intestinal malabsorption, and pancreatitis, depending on the severity of the condition. These formulas are absorbed in the upper part of the small intestine. Elemental formulas generally are given via tube feeding, as most patients do not like their taste.

All formulas should be refrigerated once they are mixed or opened to prevent bacterial contamination. Any unused portion of the formula should be discarded after 24 hours.

HOW IS NUTRITIONAL SUPPORT MONITORED?

Serum glucose levels need to be monitored at least daily. In any physiological stress condition, glucose intolerance is common. Since many nutritional support preparations are high in sugar, a patient can easily reach unacceptably high levels of serum glucose. Modifications of supplement use, decreased rate of delivery, or implementation of insulin may be required to avoid hyperglycemia.

The serum albumin level should be monitored for all patients receiving tube feeding or TPN. If the level is low (less than 3.5 mg/dL), it may hinder the patient's ability to absorb the formula. Albumin may then be administered parenterally (intravenously), and the formula should be diluted to one-quarter strength until the desired albumin level is reached (if the formula is isotonic, dilution is not necessary). Blood urea nitrogen (BUN) is a lab value that can indicate how the body is accepting the increased protein intake. A very high level can indicate too much protein in the feeding regimen but can also be a sign of dehydration or excessive protein breakdown due to inadequate kilocalorie intake. A low BUN level may be indicative of excess fluid intake, severe malnutrition, or impaired liver function.

Patients receiving tube feedings should be weighed daily. This will indicate if the patient is receiving adequate kilocalories to promote weight gain. Adequate fluid intake is especially important with formulas containing high amounts of protein so that the kidneys can efficiently excrete nitrogenous waste products. Encouraging the patient to drink fluids as well as rinsing the tube with water between feedings will help increase fluid intake. Electrolytes and appropriate nutritional assessment tests should be monitored weekly.

FACT & FALLACY

FALLACY: If diarrhea develops with tube feeding, the feeding must stop immediately

FACT: The cause of diarrhea may be unrelated to formula use, especially if the formula is isotonic and lactose-free. Other problems should be ruled out such as the presence of hyperosmolar electrolyte solutions or sorbitol in some medications (Table 14–2).

What Is Peripheral Parenteral Nutrition and When Should It Be Used?

The simplest form of **peripheral parenteral nutrition (PPN)** is intravenous dextrose (a 5% sugar solution delivered into a vein of the arm). PPN is used in addition to oral intake and is often used in conjunction with delivery of a saline solution to treat dehydration. PPN can provide only minimal amounts of nutrition, as the route of access is a small vein. Therefore, although a patient may receive only PPN, it must be for a limited time period. For total parenteral nutrition, a large artery is used to deliver the nutrients.

INDICATIONS FOR USE. PPN should be used when a patient is unable to take an adequate oral or enteral feeding. It should continue for no more than 72 hours at each catheter site (Grant, 1992). Patients who cannot consume an adequate diet because of diagnostic tests or surgery should be considered for PPN. It is a short-term method of nutritional support.

COMPOSITION. Dextrose is the carbohydrate substrate used in PPN. Amino acid solutions provide protein. Fat is generally not provided in PPN, but if it is, it should be in solutions of soybean or safflower oil (10 to 20 per cent solutions). The solutions are mixed by the pharmacist (Fig. 14–4). The dextrose and amino acid solutions are mixed in one bottle and the fat solution in another bottle. Both bottles are connected at the site of infusion into the patient's peripheral vein (Fig. 14–5). Trace elements, vitamins, and minerals may be added.

MONITORING. **Phlebitis** (inflammation of a vein) is a potential complication of PPN, so the infusion site should be closely observed. Daily weights and weekly nutritional assessment tests, such as those for albumin and transferrin, are monitored. This is important to ensure that lean body mass is preserved. Triglyceride levels should be checked if there is lipid infusion to determine tolerance to fat intake.

What Is Total Parenteral Nutrition and When Is It Used?

The most aggressive form of nutritional support is **parenteral nutrition,** often referred to as **total parenteral nutrition (TPN)** or **hyperalimentation.** TPN is best used when the GI tract is not functioning or in cases of severe vomiting when potential aspiration is a concern, such as in hyperemesis of pregnancy as Maria Bernardo has in the opening case study (see Chapter 16 for more concerns of pregnancy). TPN solutions are delivered

▲ **T A B L E   1 4 – 2**

ENTERAL FEEDING COMPLICATIONS AND PROBLEM SOLVING

PROBLEM	CAUSE	PREVENTION/TREATMENT
Gastrointestinal		
Constipation	Inadequate fluid intake	Supplement fluid intake.
	Insufficient bulk	Select fiber-supplemented formula.
	Inactivity	Encourage ambulation, if possible.
Cramping, gas, abdominal distention	Nutrient malabsorption	Select formula that restricts offending nutrients.
	Rapid, intermittent administration of refrigerated formula	Administer formula by continuous method. Administer intermittent and bolus feedings at room temperature.
	Intermittent feeding using syringe force	Reduce rate of administration. Select alternate method of administration.
Diarrhea	Low-residue intolerance (lack of bulk)	Select fiber-supplemented formula.
	Rapid formula administration	Initiate feedings at low rate. Temporarily decrease rate.
	Hyperosmolar formula	Reduce rate of administration. Select isotonic formula or dilute formula concentration and gradually increase strength.
	Bolus feedings using syringe force	Reduce rate of administration. Select alternate method of administration.
	Hypoalbuminemia	Use elemental diet or parenteral nutrition until absorptive capacity of small intestine is restored.
	Lactose intolerance	Select lactose-free formula (most commercial formulas are lactose-free).
	Fat malabsorption	Select low-fat formula.
	Bacterial contamination	Follow approved institution procedures to ensure sanitary handling and administration of formula.
	Rapid gastrointestinal transit time	Select fiber-supplemented formula.
	Prolonged antibiotic treatment or other drug therapy	Review medication profile and eliminate causative agent if possible.
	Hyperosmolar electrolyte solutions; medications with sorbitol	Arrange alternative medication solutions.
Nausea and vomiting	Rapid formula administration Gastric retention	Initiate feedings at low rate and gradually advance to desired rate. Temporarily decrease rate. Select isotonic formula. Reduce rate of administration. Use half-strength formula. Select low-fat formula. Consider need for change in feeding route (e.g., feed into duodenum or jejunum).
Mechanical		
Aspiration pneumonia	Delayed gastric emptying, gastroparesis	Reduce infusion rate. Select isotonic or lower-fat formula. Regularly check gastric residuals.
	Gastroesophageal reflux; diminished gag reflex	Use small-bore feeding tubes to minimize compromise of lower esophageal sphincter.

Table continued on following page

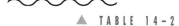

ENTERAL FEEDING COMPLICATIONS AND PROBLEM SOLVING *Continued*

PROBLEM	CAUSE	PREVENTION/TREATMENT
Irritation and leakage at ostomy site	Drainage of digestive juices from stoma site	Keep head of bed elevated 45° during and following feeding. Initially and regularly check tube placement. Feed into duodenum or jejunum, especially for high-risk patients. Attention to skin and stoma care. Use gastrostomy tubes with retention devices to maintain proper tube placement.
Nasolabial, esophageal, and mucosal irritation and erosion	Prolonged intubation with large-bore NG tubes; rubber or plastic tubes	Use small-caliber feeding tubes made of biocompatible materials. Tape feeding tube properly to avoid placing pressure on the nostril. Consider gastrostomy or jejunostomy sites for long-term feeding.
Pharyngeal irritation, otitis	Prolonged intubation with large-bore NG tubes	Use small-bore feeding tubes whenever possible.
Tube lumen obstruction	Thickened formula residue; formation of insoluble formula-medication complexes	Irrigate feeding tube frequently with clear water. Avoid instilling medications into feeding tubes. Irrigate tubes with clear water before and after delivering medications and formula.
Metabolic		
Dehydration	Inadequate fluid intake or excessive losses	Supplement fluid intake. Monitor fluid intake and output.
Hyperglycemia	Inadequate insulin production for the amount of formula being given; stress	Initiate feedings at low rate. Monitor serum and urine glucose. Use oral hypoglycemic agents or insulin if necessary.
Hypernatremia	Inadequate fluid intake or excessive losses	Supplement fluid intake. Monitor fluid intake and output.
Hyponatremia	Inadequate intake; fluid overload; inappropriate antidiuretic hormone secretion syndrome; excessive gastrointestinal fluid losses	Supplement sodium intake. Restrict fluids. Use diuretics if necessary. Replace with fluids of similar composition.
Overhydration	Rapid feeding; excessive fluid intake	Reduce rate of administration, especially in patients with severe malnutrition or major organ failure. Monitor fluid intake and output and patient condition.

directly into a large vein such as the subclavian vein below the collarbone (Fig. 14–6) since the formula does not need to be digested before entering the blood stream. TPN requires the use of a large vein because of the amount of nutrients provided and the high osmolarity of the solutions. TPN consists of a dextrose solution, such as **D50W** or **D70W.** D50W stands for 50% dextrose in water, which provides 1.7 kilocalories per mL water (see Appendix 11). A protein solution as well as vitamins, minerals, and trace el-

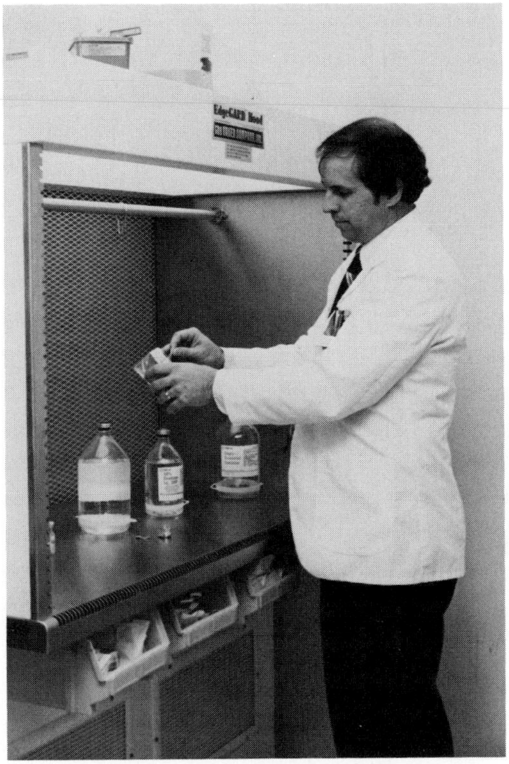

▲ FIGURE 14-4

The pharmacist mixes total parenteral nutrition and peripheral parenteral nutrition solutions under the laminar flow hood. (Courtesy of the Faxton Hospital, Utica, NY.)

ements in liquid form is also provided with the dextrose on a daily basis. The protein source is amino acids. Fat emulsions are generally given about twice a week or daily in order to provide essential fatty acids and supplement the kilocalories provided by carbohydrate (dextrose) and protein (amino acids). A person with TPN sometimes is still able to eat or may do so in the transition to an oral diet.

Two important goals of TPN are to maintain a positive nitrogen balance and to prevent electrolyte imbalance. Weight gain should be no more than ½ pound per day. In some stressed states, such as with cancer, achieving a positive nitrogen balance can be very difficult. One problem may be a too aggressive use of glucose administration (Rothkoph, 1990). A slow increase in glucose/dextrose delivery is important to allow for increased rates of insulin production without causing hyperglycemia.

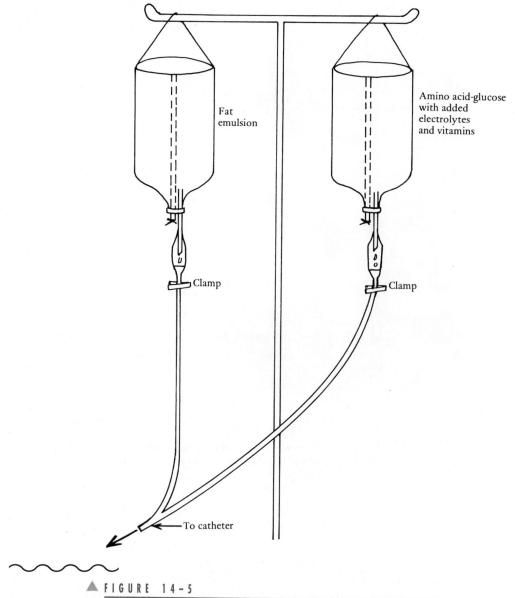

A Y-tube connects infusion sets from a bottle of amino acid–glucose solution and a bottle of fat emulsion with the central venous catheter or to a peripheral vein. (From Schneider HA, et al.: Nutritional Support of Medical Practice. Hagerstown, MD, Harper & Row Publishers, Inc., 1977.)

INDICATIONS FOR USE. TPN is used when a patient's GI tract is not functioning or when kilocalorie needs are extremely high. It is used in patients with inflammatory bowel disease, partial or total obstruction of the gastrointestinal tract, massive burns, severe malnutrition, and severe hyperemesis during pregnancy. When indicated, parenteral nutrition may be lifesaving for both mother and child (MacBurney and Wilmore, 1993).

The subclavian vein into which the total parenteral nutrition line is usually inserted. (From Mahan LK, Arlin M: Krause's Food, Nutrition & Diet Therapy, 8th ed., Philadelphia, WB Saunders, 1992; p. 519.)

COMPOSITIONS. The exact protein, fat, and carbohydrate composition of the solution depends on the nutrient needs of the individual. The major source of energy is glucose. Lipids supply essential fatty acids, and protein supplies essential amino acids. Both supply additional energy. Kilocalories vary depending on the strengths of the solutions; D70W provides about 2.4 kilocalories per mL and D5W provides less than 0.2 kilocalorie per mL (see Appendix 11). Lipid and amino acid solutions also vary in their nutritional composition (see Appendix 11). Vitamins, minerals, and trace elements are added, although their exact requirements in disease states are unknown at this time. Insulin is sometimes added to the TPN solution.

PROCEDURE. Usually the surgeon places the TPN line in the surgical unit, although some placements can be performed at the patient's bedside. The site of the TPN line is the subclavian vein (see Fig. 14–6). The nursing staff is called upon to pay strict attention to the care of the catheter to avoid **sepsis** (infection) at the site of the catheter, which is one of the more common problems associated with TPN. (This is different from catheter sepsis, which has systemic implications.) Prior to the placement of the TPN line, a plan of action should be determined. The dietitian often makes recommendations for the use of TPN and the rate of infusion based on a nutritional assessment. The attending physician must approve these orders and may be the person responsible for determining the amount of TPN solution to be supplied. The same basic nutrition needs apply when TPN is used, and the final solution is calculated based on the individual's kilocalorie and protein needs. The availability from the pharmacy of solutions for meeting these needs will determine the specific solutions supplied and how they are delivered. For example, a person with a fluid restriction would require a higher concentration of the TPN solution in order to meet the nutritional needs without causing overhydration. Appendix 11 provides kilocalorie and protein compositions of various TPN regimens.

MONITORING. Daily weights and the results of repeated nutritional assessment tests, performed as needed, will indicate if the patient is benefiting from the formula given. For more details, refer to the section *How is nutritional support monitored?* Experienced professionals must meticulously administer and monitor TPN.

A primary concern in connection with nutritional support for Mrs. Bernardo in the opening case study, is hyperglycemia. Pregnancy is a time of insulin resistance. Acceptable pregnancy serum glucose levels are also lower than those in the nonpregnant state. Recommended pregnancy fasting glucose levels are between 60 and 90 mg/dL and should never rise above 140 mg/dL. If Mrs. Bernardo's glucose levels exceed this standard, a decreased rate of TPN or adjustments in the amount of dextrose and fat used in the TPN solution may need to be made. If the carbohydrate intake is too low, however, ketone buildup can occur. Thus, frequent daily monitoring of blood glucose levels and daily monitoring of urine ketone levels and of body weight are essential to determine whether TPN adjustments are adequate or whether insulin administration should be instituted for Mrs. Bernardo.

WHAT IS THE NUTRITION RECOVERY SYNDROME?

Also referred to as the **refeeding syndrome,** the nutrition recovery syndrome can occur when nutritional support is provided too aggressively, particularly in the malnourished person. As the cells begin to be renourished, they take nutrients from the plasma first. Thus low serum phosphorus levels are common when nutritional support is undertaken, and death can result if they become too low. Monitoring of lab values is imperative to safe use of nutritional support.

Overestimation of kilocalorie needs can cause the refeeding syndrome. An increase in the heart rate, temperature, and respiration rate may occur. Critically ill patients may require less than the estimated 1.2 to 2.1 activity and stress factors used in the Harris-Benedict equation as noted in Appendix 12 (Hansen et al., 1992).

WHEN IS NUTRITIONAL SUPPORT DISCONTINUED?

Nutritional support should be gradually discontinued whenever the individual starts consuming enough food orally to maintain adequate nutritional intake. Small, frequent feedings are recommended. A low-residue diet may be necessary if diarrhea occurs, as is sometimes the case with patients who have been receiving TPN. If parenteral feedings are withdrawn too rapidly, hypoglycemia may result. Intravenous dextrose can help, or tube feedings may be needed to supplement the oral diet until the final adjustment to oral feeding is made. Kilocalorie intake studies and daily weight records will indicate whether nutritional support can be withdrawn.

WHAT IS THE ROLE OF THE NURSE OR OTHER HEALTH CARE PROFESSIONAL IN NUTRITIONAL SUPPORT?

Responsibility for identifying patients at risk for malnutrition is shared by all health care professionals. Routine weight assessments are critical. Unintentional weight loss should be a red flag, and a significant weight loss of 5 to 10 per cent of the usual body weight should be brought to the attention of the primary care physician and a registered dietitian.

Once nutritional support is implemented, the health care professional should be aware of any potential complications. The development of diarrhea, constipation, abnormal lab values, continued weight loss or excessive weight gain, or deviation from the prescribed regimen should be brought to the attention of all health care professionals working with the patient.

It is also of vital importance that all health care professionals provide positive patient support. Expressing negative comments related to taste of liquid supplements or squeamishness toward a catheter site is unprofessional and counterproductive to patient health.

STUDY QUESTIONS AND ACTIVITIES

1. Why is the diet for patients with fractures, burns, and infections high in protein?
2. What equation did Mrs. Wade, the dietitian referred to in the opening case study, use to calculate that Mrs. Bernardo required 110 grams of protein? (HINT: How many grams of protein based on kilograms of body weight?) Referring to Appendix 11, what TPN regimen might ultimately be used for Mrs. Bernardo based on a need of 110 grams protein and 2200 kilocalories from dextrose and amino acids?
3. Why did Mrs. Wade suggest TPN as opposed to tube feeding for Mrs. Bernardo?
4. Taste-test a variety of liquid nutrition supplements such as Carnation Instant Breakfast, Ensure, and Sustacal. Have a class recipe contest for developing the milk shake highest in kilocalories and protein that also tastes good.

REFERENCES

Grant JP: Handbook of Total Parenteral Nutrition, 2nd ed. Philadelphia, WB Saunders, 1992; p. 317.
Hansen MB, Krenitsky JS, et al.: Energy expenditure of critically-ill subjects: Use of predictive equations vs. indirect calorimetry. Poster Session, 1992 ADA Annual Meeting. J Am Diet Assoc (suppl). 1992; 92(9):A-31.
Jacobs DO, Scheltinga MRM: Metabolic assessment. In Rombeau JL, Caldwell MD, eds.: Clinical Nutrition: Parenteral Nutrition, 2nd ed. Philadelphia, WB Saunders, 1993; p. 245.
Lacy JA: Immune function and nutrition support. RD, Essential News for Dietitians From Sandoz Nutrition, 1993; 13(3):1.
Queen PM, Caldwell M, Balogun L: Clinical indicators for oncology, cardiovascular, and surgi-

cal patients: Report of the ADA Council on Practice Quality Assurance Committee. J Am Diet Assoc. 1993; 93(3):338.

Rombeau JL, Caldwell MD, eds.: Clinical Nutrition: Parenteral Nutrition, 2nd ed. Philadelphia, WB Saunders, 1993.

Rothkoph M: Fuel utilization in neoplastic disease: implications for the use of nutritional support in cancer patients. Nutrition. July-Aug, 1990; 6(4 suppl):14S–16S.

University of Iowa Hospitals and Clinics: Recent Advances in Therapeutic Diets, 4th ed. Ames, IA, Iowa State University Press, 1989.

Zlotkin SH, Harrison D: Home pediatric enteral nutrition. In Rombeau JL, Caldwell MD, eds.: Clinical Nutrition: Enteral and Tube Feeding, 2nd ed. Philadelphia, WB Saunders, 1990; pp 463–470.

PHYSIOLOGICAL AND PSYCHOLOGICAL FOOD ALLERGIES AND INTOLERANCES

CHAPTER 15

OBJECTIVES

After completing this chapter, you should be able to:
- Explain how food allergy and intolerance are diagnosed and treated
- Explain the difference between food allergy and food intolerance
- Identify common food allergens
- Describe assessment and intervention strategies for psychological eating disorders

TERMS TO IDENTIFY

Anaphylactic shock
Anorexia nervosa
Attention deficit hyperac-
    tivity disorder (ADHD)
Bipolar disorder
Bulimarexia

Bulimia
Elimination diets
"Fight or flight" response
Food allergens/antigens
Food allergy

Food intolerance
Immunoglobulin E (IgE)
    antibody
Purging
Schizophrenia

Rita Bernardo thought to herself, time to go talk to Fiona again. Different kind of stomach pains this time. The pain started after she ate pasta Alfredo the other night at the restaurant. Perhaps it was the cream sauce. She got real bloated in the abdomen and later had diarrhea. She would ask Tony to check with his dietitian, too. (Students may want to review the opening case study in Chapter 10.)

INTRODUCTION

Inadequate or inappropriate food intake can result from physiological or psychological problems, whether real or imagined. Food allergies are physiological problems involving the immune system. Food intolerances may be either physiological or psychological. For example, lactose intolerance is a physiological problem related to the inability to digest milk sugar. Anorexia nervosa is a psychological problem in which the person has a strong fear of eating. Persons with mental health problems may have altered thinking about food tolerances and intolerances.

The fields of medicine and psychology should be utilized in diagnosing and treating food allergies and intolerances. Problems need to be correctly diagnosed in order to plan the most effective intervention. Negative family functioning may be part of the cause of eating disorders or may be the result of dealing with food allergies and intolerances. Involvement of families in the assessment and planning stage promotes their support of the intervention plan. The school setting and peer pressure have an important impact on food choices. For example, how does the child with a wheat allergy deal with classroom birthday parties? This chapter explores physiological and psychological food intolerances and introduces some practical interventions.

WHAT IS A FOOD ALLERGY?

A **food allergy** is a condition that develops when a person is hypersensitive to certain proteins found in food. It is an immune response that can be mildly annoying or severe enough to induce death through **anaphylactic shock** (a life-threatening condition in which the breathing passages can be blocked). The immune system is designed to destroy harmful foreign substances in the body. With food allergies, the body reacts to certain food proteins as if they were harmful substances. In order to avoid this immune response, the offending foods need to be reduced in or entirely eliminated from the diet.

Food allergens/antigens are the proteins or other large molecules from food that induce an immune response. The immunoglobulin E (IgE) antibody is produced in response to these "foreign" substances in an attempt to rid the body of them. IgE causes the typical allergy symptoms. Symptoms involve the skin, nasal passages, and respiratory or gastrointestinal tract.

Hives, diarrhea, nausea, vomiting, cramps, headache, and asthma are common symptoms of food allergy. If the entire circulatory system is affected, shock occurs.

There are two major types of allergic reaction to foods: immediate and late. Immediate reactions are characterized by the rapid appearance of symptoms, often within minutes after the offending food is eaten or before the food is swallowed. The immediate allergic response is generally the more severe, and life-threatening, form of allergy. Late reactions are more subtle. Up to 48 hours may elapse between eating the allergenic food and the appearance of symptoms such as nasal congestion.

The foods that most often cause allergic reactions are milk, fish, shellfish, nuts, berries, eggs, chocolate, corn, wheat, pork, and legumes (green peas, lima beans, and peanuts) and some fresh fruits, such as those in the peach family.

HOW IS FOOD ALLERGY DIAGNOSED?

The diagnosis of food allergy is controversial. One of the concerns of the medical profession is the impact of the placebo effect. In other words, the mere thinking that a food is going to cause allergy can induce physical allergy symptoms. It is therefore imperative that proper medical testing be done before restrictive diets are implemented.

Medical Diagnostic Tests

Skin testing involves scratching or puncturing the skin with extracts of food. A skin reaction such as raised bumps around this area may be indicative of an immune response to the causative food extracts. The radioallergosorbent test (RAST) uses a blood sample. Both the skin test and the RAST can be incorrectly interpreted and thus are not considered infallible. The skin test should be done under medical supervision to avoid or safely treat anaphylactic shock that can ensue.

Nutritional Diagnostic Tests

A detailed allergic history is important in diagnosing and managing food allergy. Specific details of foods, beverages, and medications ingested are recorded along with any noted symptoms for a period of 2 to 4 weeks. This close observation may be able to pinpoint problematic substances in the diet.

Elimination diets are used to determine the causative food allergen. These diets contain a few carefully chosen foods, with common allergens omitted. The elimination diet should be followed for 1 to 2 weeks. Foods generally allowed on an elimination diet include rice, lamb, sweet potatoes, and carrots (Dobler, 1991). An improvement in physical symptoms may indicate that an allergenic food has been eliminated. Foods are slowly and cautiously put back into the diet, one food at a time for a few days. If no symptoms are noted, another food is added for another couple of days. This procedure is continued to ensure tolerance and identify those foods that are linked to the redevelopment of allergic symptoms.

Once food allergens are identified, a nutritionally adequate diet that eliminates the offending foods can be developed. Education is critical. A person
may know he or she has a milk allergy but not think of foods made with
milk such as cream soups, butter, cheese, and milk chocolate. Other terms
for milk protein on the food label such as lactalbumin, lactoglobulin, casein,
nonfat milk solids, or whey may not be familiar to the patient. The services
of a registered dietitian are helpful in patient education and may be required in the case of multiple food allergies in order to avoid nutritional inadequacies. Tables 11−8, 15−1, and 15−2 list common foods to be omitted

▲ T A B L E   1 5 − 1   EGG-FREE DIET*

FOOD GROUP	FOODS ALLOWED	FOODS EXCLUDED
Beverages	All plain milks, creams, and buttermilks	Egg nogs, malted beverages
		Beverages "cleared" with egg or shells
	Cocoa, tea, coffee	
	Carbonated beverages	
Soups	Creamed meat, fish, and vegetable soups prepared without egg (such as egg noodles)	Any soups "cleared" with egg or shells, egg powder, dried egg, and albumin
Protein sources	All plain meats, fish, and poultry (some severely allergic individuals cannot eat the meat of egg-laying chickens)	All breaded or batter-dipped foods if egg was used in the mix
	Cheese	Sausages, croquettes, or loaves using egg as a binding agent
Vegetables	Fresh, frozen, canned, raw, or cooked	None unless combined with egg
Fruit	All fresh, frozen, canned, or dried	None
	All juices	
Breads and cereals	Rye-Krisp, corn pone, beaten biscuits, and plain crackers	Gingerbreads, griddle cakes, muffins, waffles, fancy breads, pretzels, saltines
	Any homemade breads without egg	Commercial breads and rolls containing eggs or that have been brushed with egg
	Any breakfast cereal	
	Rice	
	Pasta made without egg	
Fats	All butters, creams, homemade salad dressings without eggs	All others unless label shows made without egg, albumin, or egg powder
Combination	Any made without egg or egg products	Any made with egg or egg products; avoid biscuit toppings, thickened sauces
Sweets and snacks	Plain fruit-flavored gelatins	Prepared mixes for pancakes, cakes, cookies (may contain egg powder), cream-filled pies, meringues, ice cream, sherbet
	Fruit pies	
	Ices	
	Cookies, frostings, cakes and puddings made without eggs	Some commercial candies that contain egg or albumin
	Popcorn, nuts, olives, pickles	
	Sugars, hard candy	

* Adequacy: Since a perfectly well balanced diet can be planned without eggs, if an individual eats the food provided, this diet can meet the Recommended Dietary Allowances (1989) for all nutrients.
Courtesy of Bureau of Nutrition Services, Office of Mental Retardation and Developmental Disabilities, Albany, NY.

▲ TABLE 15-2 MILK-FREE DIET

FOOD GROUP	FOODS ALLOWED	FOODS EXCLUDED
Beverages	Soft drinks Soya milk products Coffee, tea Decaffeinated coffee	All milk and milk-containing beverages
Soups	Any broth-based soup with no milk products	All creamed soups
Protein sources	All fresh meats Kosher luncheon meats, hot dogs, bologna, and salami labeled "Parve" (may be very spicy) All-beef hot dogs All poultry without stuffing All fish Eggs Dried beans, peas Peanut butter	Non-Kosher luncheon meats: bologna, salami, wieners, sausage, meat loaf, cold cuts Poultry with stuffing Meat balls, meat loaves Cheese Yogurt Breaded items that contain milk in batter or bread crumbs made with milk
Vegetables	Any fresh, canned, or frozen vegetables Pasta Rice	All creamed vegetables Any creamed sauces, including au gratin Mashed potatoes (unless made without milk)
Fruit	Any fresh, frozen, or canned fruit or juice	None
Breads and cereals	Rye-Krisp, homemade brands made without milk, rye breads Italian breads	Other baked goods
Fats	Poultry, meat, and pure vegetable fats and oils Dressings made without milk or milk products Margarine	Butter Any salad dressings containing milk or cheese Gravy made with milk or cream
Combination	Any made without milk or milk products	Any dishes containing milk or milk products
Sweets and snacks	Plain fruit-flavored gelatin Angel and sponge cakes Fruit ices Jellies and jams Sugars, hard candy	Prepared mixes: waffle, cake, muffin, pancake Puddings, creams, Ice cream, sherbet Milk chocolate candy

Courtesy of the Bureau of Nutrition Services, Office of Mental Retardation and Developmental Disabilities, Albany, NY.

on the wheat-, rye-, and oat-free diet, the egg-free diet, and the milk-free diet.

Individuals who are sensitive only to wheat products can follow a gluten-restricted diet (see Table 11–8), in which wheat, rye, oats, and barley are omitted. Food products with cornmeal or rice flour are acceptable for the diet. Cornstarch can be used as a thickening agent. A list of sources for allergy recipes may be found in Appendix 20. Many commercial products for allergy diets are available. Careful reading of the labels on such products is necessary to detect any specific allergen to be omitted in the diet.

Very often a person who is allergic to one food will be allergic to others in the same food family. For example, someone allergic to peanuts usually cannot eat peas or beans either, simply because they are members of the pea family.

HOW DO FOOD INTOLERANCES DIFFER FROM FOOD ALLERGIES?

Food intolerances do not involve the immune response; food allergies do. Since the immune response is not evoked, food intolerances are not life-threatening. Food allergies usually begin in childhood, while food intolerances can begin at any age. Food intolerances may have a biological basis, such as a lack of a digestive enzyme, or a psychological basis.

The general public often confuses intolerances and allergies. It is important to know the difference. For example, a person with milk allergy may become seriously ill with any trace of milk. But a person with lactose intolerance may be able to tolerate small quantities of milk or low-lactose forms of milk such as yogurt and cheese.

Psychosomatic illness, even though psychological in origin, can have physical consequences. This is due to the **"fight or flight" response** of the sympathetic system (the hormonal response to stress that induces increased heart rate and blood pressure). The overstimulation of the sympathetic nervous system can produce psychosomatic symptoms such as diarrhea, nervousness, and tremors (Brostoff and Gamlin, 1989). It is important to accurately diagnose physical intolerances as opposed to psychological ones so that effective intervention can be more appropriately planned.

WHAT ARE SOME COMMON FOOD INTOLERANCES?

There are well documented food intolerances and others that are not understood or recognized. A common food intolerance that is well known throughout the world is lactose intolerance. Rita Bernardo's symptoms may indicate lactose intolerance. If so, temporary avoidance of milk products may be helpful in controlling GI symptoms. Gluten intolerance is also common among people with British heritage. See Chapter 11 for further discussion.

Fat Intolerance

This condition is often related to pancreatitis and gallstones. Alcoholism is commonly associated with pancreatitis and problems digesting fat. Vegetarians or others who normally follow a low-fat diet often report nausea and indigestion as a result of increased meat or fat intake.

Intolerance to Vegetables and Fruits

This condition is highly individual. The problem may not be the food as much as the style of eating. Thorough chewing and eating slowly will lessen symptoms of intolerance. Many people avoid legumes (dried beans) because of excessive flatulence. Such people may benefit by slowly increasing amounts eaten. Chewing thoroughly and including adequate fluid in the diet is important. Some people find a commercial enzyme preparation such as Beano to be helpful. Older persons often find that lettuce causes indigestion or abdominal pain. Again, small amounts of lettuce that are thoroughly masticated may help. Jerusalem artichokes contain a type of carbohydrate that humans cannot digest. Undigested carbohydrate allows bacteria to multiply in the GI tract, which leads to flatulence. Apple skin may be a problem for some people. The cause of intolerance may be a sudden increase in the fiber content of these foods. Gradually increasing the amounts of fruits and vegetables eaten may be beneficial.

Intolerance to Hot, Spicy Foods

This condition is often associated with peptic ulcers, pancreatitis, and gallbladder disease. The intolerance may be physical or psychological in the case of persons who believe they cannot tolerate spicy foods. Intolerance to spicy foods is not diagnostic of peptic ulcers, although the amount of spicy food eaten may be related. Small amounts may be tolerated.

WHAT ARE SOME PSYCHOLOGICAL EATING DISORDERS?

Psychological eating disorders are increasingly recognized. Family relationships seem to contribute to the development of psychological and behavioral traits for risk of some eating disorders. Persons with eating disorders often are uncomfortable discussing problems with their guardians, don't feel that their problems are taken seriously, or perceive that their guardians are lecturing them (Larson, 1991).

It is estimated that anorexia nervosa affects about 1 per cent and bulimia 3 per cent to 19 per cent of young women (Larson, 1991). Adolescents with diabetes have an even higher prevalence of eating disorders, with estimates between 7 and 35 per cent. This increased percentage among diabetic adolescents is felt to reflect a compound problem of the usual causes, such as emotional state and parent-child interaction, coupled with the demanding meal requirements of diabetes management. In an adolescent, unexplained hypoglycemia and poor diabetes control should alert the health professional to a potential eating disorder (Connell and Thomas-Dobersen, 1991). Anorexia nervosa and bulimia not only are problems of weight control but also involve biological, psychological, and social factors. Obsessive dieting, refusal to eat, binging and gorging, purging, fasting, and laxative and diuretic abuse can lead to malnutrition, electrolyte imbalance, and cardiac arrhythmia, which can result in death.

Other psychiatric problems such as bipolar disorder and schizophrenia are associated with behavioral eating problems. It is felt that the systematic monitoring of weight and diet may be more important than generally thought in the management of psychiatric illness (Rao et al., 1991).

Anorexia Nervosa

Anorexia nervosa is characterized by a refusal to eat, stemming from emotional states such as anxiety, irritation, anger, and fear. Initially there is no real loss of appetite. However, once severe weight loss has occurred, hormonal changes take place that can alter hunger recognition and satiety cues. The syndrome occurs mainly in girls after puberty, but about 10 per cent of all cases of anorexia occur in boys and young men (Davis and Sherer, 1994). There is an increased risk of anorexia nervosa among high achievers and upper socioeconomic populations. The incidence of anorexia nervosa has increased fourfold since the 1950s (Czajka-Narins and Parham, 1990). The cause is generally felt to be of psychological origin, but treatment involves more than just psychotherapy. Some common correlates of anorexia are:

- an intense fear of becoming obese that does not lessen as weight loss progresses
- a disturbance of body image, such as claiming to feel fat even when emaciated
- weight loss of at least 25 per cent of original body weight
- refusal to maintain body weight over a minimal healthy weight for age and height
- no known physical illness that would account for the weight loss
- amenorrhea due to altered hormonal states
- bizarre eating habits such as cutting food into tiny pieces or limiting intake to only a few foods
- underlying low self-esteem
- compulsive exercise habits

DIETARY TREATMENT.　The goal of treatment should be to restore good nutritional status and resolve the underlying psychological problems. Outpatient treatment is the preferred method. The person with anorexia nervosa who is 30 per cent below normal weight, fails to gain weight, is in complete denial, or is suicidal should be hospitalized (Davis and Sherer, 1994). All members of the health care team must be aware of the need to individualize the care plan. The nurse's role includes closely supervising and encouraging the patient to eat all of the food provided. A trusting relationship between patient and health care professional is absolutely essential. It should be recognized that treatment will require a long-term, family-based approach with a considerable amount of time needed. Treatment is not always successful.

Bulimia

Bulimia is characterized by binge eating followed by purging through self-induced vomiting or abusive use of laxatives or both. The person is afraid of becoming overweight and is aware that the eating pattern is abnormal. However, the bulimic patient loses control over eating and often eats large amounts of food rapidly. High-kilocalorie, easily ingested foods are chosen during binge episodes. Fasting then follows, often resulting in a weight fluctuation of as much as 10 pounds. **Bulimarexia** is the term used to describe cycles of binge eating and **purging** (vomiting or laxative abuse) with undereating.

DIETARY TREATMENT. In the hospital, food intake should be normalized to appropriate mealtimes, with close supervision after eating to control vomiting. The patient must be counseled on the importance of the need to stop using laxatives and to accept a higher, but normal, body weight. Psychological assessment should take priority, and plans should be made for long-term, outpatient, family-based counseling with a health care professional trained in eating disorders. A total health care team effort is essential to ensure effective treatment. Outpatient dietary treatment of bulimia emphasizes regular mealtimes with appropriate food portions to satisfy hunger needs. Food is discouraged as a means of reward or comfort.

Attention Deficit Hyperactivity Disorder

Attention deficit hyperactivity disorder (ADHD) is the official term sanctioned by the American Psychiatric Association. The term attention deficit disorder (ADD) is an older but still used term. The central problem in this disorder relates to a child's inability to pay attention and to sustain effort. Professionals currently working with ADHD children are concerned more with the quality of the child's behavior than with the sheer quantity of movement. A high level of marital discord is observed in families with a child with ADHD, but this discord is probably a consequence of trying to manage a child who is unmanageable. Misdiagnosis is common. Children who have other problems, but similar symptoms, may be mistakenly labeled as having ADHD. Unnecessary medication of children and its resulting side effects is of concern.

Many dietary theories have evolved over the years. Discredited nutrition treatments include restrictions of sugar and food additives. Megavitamin therapy has also been advocated, but a carefully controlled study demonstrated that megavitamins were ineffective in reducing the symptoms of ADHD children while increasing blood levels of vitamins to toxic levels. Little evidence exists that dietary approaches normalize behavior for ADHD children (Gordon, 1991). It is still prudent for children with ADHD and their families to emphasize the dietary guidelines for less sugar and more complex carbohydrate along with well balanced meals.

Bipolar Disorder

Bipolar disorder is characterized by alternating periods of mania and depression. During the manic stage, such persons are hyperactive and may have grandiose ideas that they do not require food as most people do. In the depressive stage, appetite for nutritious foods may be diminished while appetite for sweets and other non-nutritious foods may be increased. Medication such as lithium may be helpful in the treatment of this condition.

Schizophrenia

Schizophrenia is a chronic mental disorder that causes bizarre perceptual disturbances such as visual hallucinations and delusions of hearing voices. A person with schizophrenia may feel that food has been poisoned. A health care team approach is strongly advised. Any attempts to encourage eating may cause the person to become even more suspicious that the food has been poisoned. A great deal of patience and a matter-of-fact approach are advisable when working with a person with schizophrenia.

WHAT IS THE ROLE OF THE HEALTH CARE PROFESSIONAL IN MANAGING FOOD ALLERGIES, INTOLERANCES, AND AVOIDANCES?

The nurse or other health care professional needs to be aware of the medical biases and unknowns when it comes to problems with food. The nurse should be supportive in listening to patients and their families describe food intolerances. Judgments should be avoided, such as the idea that psychosomatic illness is "all in the patient's head." The nurse should determine what valid testing has been undertaken to diagnose food allergies and intolerances. Assessment should include asking patients what foods they cannot tolerate. If major food groups, such as milk, are being omitted from the diet, the nurse or other health care professional should refer as needed to the patient's primary physician or a registered dietitian or both. The diagnosis should be confirmed when needed, and patient education should be provided to ensure good nutritional intake.

STUDY QUESTIONS AND ACTIVITIES

1. What are some symptoms of food allergy?
2. What is the difference between food allergy and food intolerance?
3. Why do Rita Bernardo's symptoms (in the opening case-study) more likely indicate lactose intolerance than milk allergy? If she had a true milk allergy, how might the symptoms be different?
4. What are the characteristics of anorexia nervosa and bulimia?
5. Plan a day's menu for someone who is allergic to wheat and milk.

REFERENCES

Brostoff J, Gamlin L: The Complete Guide to Food Allergy and Intolerance. New York: Crown Publishers, 1989.

Connell JE, Thomas-Dobersen D: Nutritional management of children and adolescents with insulin-dependent diabetes mellitus: A review by the Diabetes Care and Education dietetic practice group. J Am Diet Assoc. 1991; 91(12):1562.

Czajka-Narins DM, Parham ES: Fear of fat: Attitudes toward obesity, the thinning of America. Nutrition Today. January/February, 1990; p. 31.

Davis JR, Sherer K: Applied Nutrition and Diet Therapy for Nurses. Philadelphia, WB Saunders, 1994.

Dobler ML: Food Allergies. Chicago, The American Dietetic Association, 1991.

Gordon M: ADHD/Hyperactivity: A Consumer's Guide. DeWitt, NY, GSI Publications, 1991.

Larson BJ: Relationship of family communication patterns to Eating Disorder Inventory scores in adolescent girls. J Am Diet Assoc, 1991; 91(9):1065–1066.

Rao LO, Gruber LN, Baum MH, Hall WS: Dietary changes in psychiatric patients, poster session. J Am Diet Assoc (suppl) 1991; 91(9):A-125.

LIFESPAN AND WELLNESS CONCERNS IN PROMOTING HEALTH AND MANAGING ILLNESS

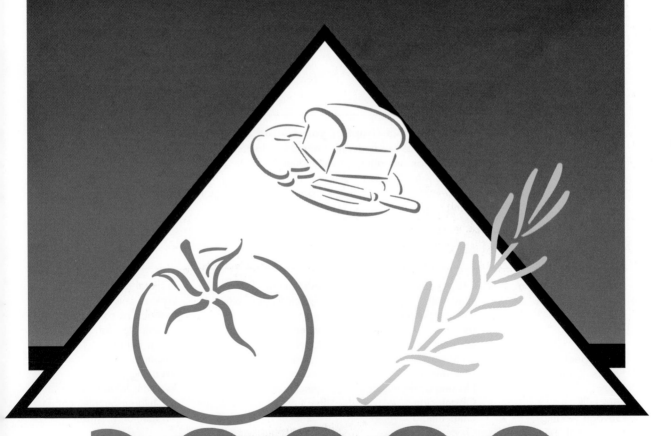

CHAPTER 16

MATERNAL AND INFANT NUTRITION

CHAPTER TOPICS

CHAPTER INTRODUCTION
IMPACT OF NUTRITION ON THE OUTCOME OF PREGNANCY
CLINICAL PROBLEMS OF PREGNANCY
IMPACT OF DIET ON THE NURSING MOTHER AND INFANT
LACTATION MANAGEMENT
BOTTLE-FEEDING ISSUES
FEEDING STRATEGIES FOR THE OLDER INFANT
INFANT GROWTH AND DEVELOPMENT
CLINICAL PROBLEMS OF INFANCY
OTHER NUTRITION ISSUES FOR WOMEN
ROLE OF THE NURSE OR OTHER HEALTH CARE PROFESSIONAL IN MATERNAL AND INFANT NUTRITION

OBJECTIVES

After completing this chapter, you should be able to:
- Describe nutritional needs during pregnancy, lactation, and infancy
- Describe lactation management techniques
- Describe infant feeding strategies
- Apply knowledge of nutritional needs during pregnancy, lactation, and infancy to meal planning

TERMS TO IDENTIFY

Antidiuretic hormone
Body mass index
Colostrum
Diuresis
Embryo
Esophageal sphincter
Failure to thrive
Fetus
Fore milk
Gavage feeding
Gestational

Growth spurts
Hind milk
Immunoglobulin A
Lactation
La Leche League
Let-down reflex
Milk anemia
Nursing-bottle mouth
Obstetrician
Otitis media
Oxytocin

Pediatrician
Physiological anemia
Pica
Pincer grasp
Placenta
Postpartum blues
Preconception
Preeclampsia
Pregnancy-induced hypertension
Premenstrual syndrome

Prenatal
Preterm milk
Products of conception
Unsaturated fat
Spina bifida
Toxemia
Weaning
Women, Infants, and Children Supplemental Nutrition Program

"Come on, baby Tony," Maria said. Antonio Augusto Bernardo III. They finally decided to give their new little baby boy the family name. Seven pounds, ten ounces and 19 inches long. He sure looked healthy.

But why did he not seem interested in nursing? Why was he so sleepy? The nurse came in and showed her how to tap his foot to wake him up. Maria had bottle-fed her first two babies but now she wanted to try breast-feeding. Although it sure wasn't as easy as a bottle. And she was starting to get engorged and sore. Maybe she should change to bottle-feeding, she thought to herself. She rang the bell to call the nurse again.

INTRODUCTION

The human species is fortunately very resilient, having survived over the centuries with wide differences in nutritional intake. For this reason, many adults are here today even though as infants they were fed under less than ideal circumstances. It has only been in this century that nutritional health, reproduction, and how to promote the healthiest babies have been fully understood. It is now widely accepted that nutrition plays a vital role in a healthy pregnancy and baby.

Growth of the **fetus** (the unborn baby; Table 16–1) may be affected by various maternal factors, for example, the ingestion, digestion, and absorption of food materials (nutrients) from the mother's intestinal tract. The fetus is dependent on these processes as well as on maternal metabolism of the absorbed nutrients and transfer of nutrients through the **placenta** (an organ that allows transfer of maternal nutrients to the fetus via the umbilical cord). An intact placenta of good size is critical for the ideal growth of the fetus.

The impact of maternal nutrition does not stop at birth. Breast-feeding, preparation for a future successful pregnancy, and even the infant's meal

▲   TABLE 16-1

FETAL DEVELOPMENT

FIRST TRIMESTER (EMBRYO; CRITICAL STAGE)	SECOND TRIMESTER (FETUS)	THIRD TRIMESTER TO BIRTH
Organs develop (4–12 weeks) Central nervous system develops (4–12 weeks) Skeletal structure hardens from cartilage to bone (4 weeks)	Growth and development continue (13–40 weeks) Teeth calcify (20 weeks) Fetus can survive outside womb (24 weeks)	Growth and development continue Storage of iron and other nutrients (36–40 weeks; premature babies often deficient in iron) Development of necessary fat tissue (36–40 weeks)

environment are all influenced by the mother's nutrition. A well nourished mother is better able to cope with the demands of infant care, and a well nourished infant can better display a pleasant disposition, facilitating the return of the mother's strength and vitality. Maternal and infant nutrition is very much a reciprocal relationship.

WHEN DOES NUTRITION MOST INFLUENCE THE OUTCOME OF PREGNANCY?

The development of the **embryo** (the fetus during the first trimester) is the critical period of pregnancy (see Table 16–1), although pregnancy is often not recognized until a significant amount of time has passed in the first trimester. It is for this reason that the **preconception** (prior to conception) nutritional status is now considered so important. This is especially true for a woman with diabetes (see later discussion). Maternal nutritional counseling should cover the preconceptual and postpartum periods as well as the more traditional **gestational** (time of pregnancy) period.

CAN BIRTH DEFECTS BE PREVENTED THROUGH NUTRITION?

Adequate nutritional intake without excess mineral or vitamin intake can help prevent some birth defects. For example, **spina bifida** (a birth defect in which the spine does not close) is associated with inadequate intake of folate. Adequate nutrient availability during the first trimester can help the embryo form well developed organs such as heart, lungs, liver, kidneys, and intestines. It is therefore important that the preconception nutritional status be good, since pregnancy is often not confirmed, or even suspected, until the end of the first trimester. Appropriate weight gain and avoidance of excess nutrients such as vitamin A during pregnancy are further associated with reduced morbidity and mortality.

Much more information needs to be learned about the prevention of birth defects. It is known that not all defects, for example, genetic disorders, are amenable to nutritional intervention.

WHAT WEIGHT GAIN IS ASSOCIATED WITH THE BEST OUTCOME OF PREGNANCY?

A major determinant of fetal outcome during pregnancy is maternal weight gain. Prior to 1960, weight gain was restricted to less than 15 pounds. Current research shows that more liberal weight gain improves fetal growth. A woman who is underweight prenatally needs to gain more weight than is typically recommended in order to best promote growth of the **products of conception** (Fig. 16–1). It is imperative that the placenta grow adequately in order to facilitate transfer of maternal nutrients to the fetus.

Ideal weight gain is now considered to be about 25 to 35 pounds for normal-weight women (**body mass index [BMI]** of 19.8 to 26.0—see Appendix 16; body mass index equals body weight divided by the square of the height), 28 to 40 pounds for an underweight woman (BMI < 19.8), and 15 to 25 pounds for an overweight woman (BMI > 26.0) with an average of about 1 pound gain per week in the second and third trimesters of pregnancy (The Subcommittee on Nutritional Status, 1990).

A **prenatal** (before birth) weight chart that takes into account the pre-

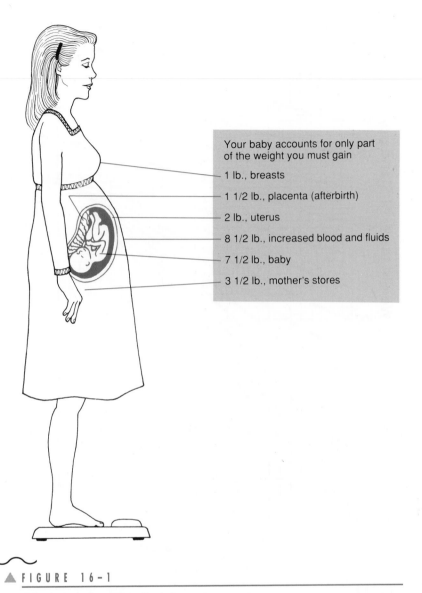

Your baby accounts for only part
of the weight you must gain

- 1 lb., breasts

- 1 1/2 lb., placenta (afterbirth)

- 2 lb., uterus

- 8 1/2 lb., increased blood and fluids

- 7 1/2 lb., baby

- 3 1/2 lb., mother's stores

▲ F I G U R E   1 6 – 1

Components of weight gain during pregnancy.

conceptual weight was proposed in 1985 by Rossa and is now used by the
Renal Dietitians Dietetic Practice Group for control of kidney disease during pregnancy (Wilkens and Schiro, 1992). To use this chart (Fig. 16–2),
one must first determine the percentage of standard weight of the mother
at 12 weeks of gestation from the nomogram for height and weight (Figs.
16–2 and 16–3). Women whose weight is equal to or less than 100 per cent
of the standard weight are advised to weigh 120 per cent of their standard
weight at term, whereas heavier women are advised to increase their
weight proportionally less than normal-weight or underweight women. Two
examples follow: A woman who is 5 feet 5 inches tall (162.5 cm) and weighs

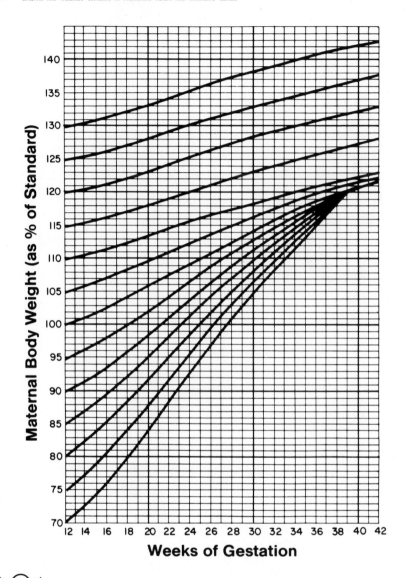

▲ FIGURE 16-2

Recommended weight gain percentile (for use in conjunction with Fig.16–3). After the mother's weight gain percentile at 12 weeks' gestation has been calculated, this chart indicates the appropriate amount and progression of weight gain over the total gestational period. The percentile figure at 40 weeks' gestation can be applied to Figure 16–3 to identify the recommended weight at the end of pregnancy. (From Rosso P: A new chart to monitor weight gain during pregnancy. Am J Clin Nutr, 1985; 41(2):649. © Am J Clin Nutr American Society for Clinical Nutrition.)

120 pounds (54.5 kg) at 12 weeks of gestation should gain about 34 pounds (93 per cent standard weight at 12 weeks to 120 per cent at term), whereas a woman who is 5 feet 3 inches tall and weighs 145 pounds should gain 23 pounds (120 per cent standard weight to 133 per cent at term). A more gen-

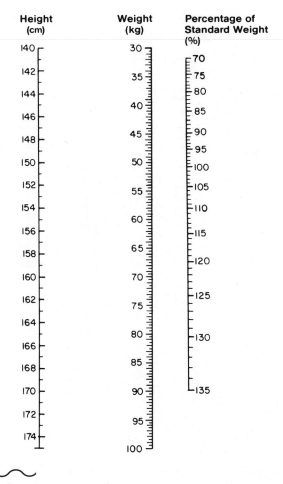

▲ F I G U R E   1 6 - 3

Nomogram to determine adequacy of weight for height and to calculate desirable total weight gain during pregnancy. To use the nomogram: Place a ruler on the correct height and weight at 12 weeks' gestation. Read over to the point where this line intersects with the percentage of standard weight. The percentage of standard weight at the beginning of pregnancy is then plotted on the chart shown in Figure 16–2 to determine the appropriate weight percentile at the end of pregnancy (40 to 42 weeks). This percentile can then be plotted on the nomogram to identify the recommended weight at the end of pregnancy. (From Rosso P: A new chart to monitor weight gain during pregnancy. Am J Clin Nutr, 1985; 41(2):648. © Am J Clin Nutr, American Society for Clinical Nutrition.)

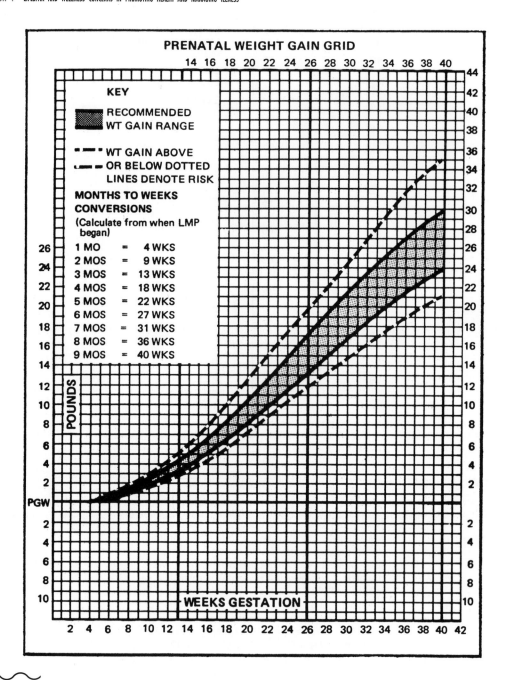

▲ FIGURE 16-4

Recommended prenatal weight gain. Chart to moniter weight gain throughout pregnancy. KEY: PGW = pregestational weight (weight prior to conception). (From the New York State Health Department, WIC Program.)

eral weight gain grid can also be used to plot weight gain throughout the pregnancy (Fig. 16–4).

FACT & FALLACY

FALLACY: Because a pregnant woman is "eating for two," she should eat twice as much.

FACT: It should be remembered that the second person is very small, being about 7 pounds at birth. Although some nutrient requirements increase dramatically during pregnancy, the overall kilocalorie needs increase only about 15 per cent, amounting to about 150 extra kilocalories a day during the first trimester and 350 additional daily kilocalories for the remainder of the pregnancy. Thus, it is important that a pregnant woman consume mainly nutrient-dense foods (foods that have a lot of nutrients for the amount of kilocalories).

WHAT NUTRITIONAL ADVICE IS APPROPRIATE FOR A SUCCESSFUL PREGNANCY?

To promote maternal and infant health, a pregnant woman should be encouraged to consume at least the minimum number of servings from the Food Guide Pyramid (Table 16–2), with a focus on the use of whole grains and unprocessed or lightly processed foods. Minerals such as zinc and magnesium are found in whole grains and legumes. Adequate consumption of dark green leafy vegetables and deep orange vegetables and fruits should be encouraged. These foods provide β-carotene (vitamin A). Vitamin C foods such as citrus fruits and dark green leafy vegetables should be increased during pregnancy and lactation. A well balanced diet will help the fetus grow well and allow for the mother to stay healthy for future pregnancies. Table 16–3 shows a sample menu.

In addition, adequate weight gain as determined by preconception weight should be promoted. A higher weight gain is necessary for those with low initial weight or for adolescents. Intake of nonessentials such as fats and sugars should be restricted unless a high level of kilocalories is needed to promote weight gain. Salt intake can be moderated but should not be rigidly restricted. Vitamin supplements should be used only as added insurance, not as a replacement for nutrients found in foods. Supplements should not exceed 100 per cent of the recommended daily allowance (RDA; Table 16–4). Iron is the only nutrient generally advised for routine supplementation in pregnancy. Good nutritional intake should be maintained after delivery for healthy lactation and in preparation for a future pregnancy.

Consultation with a registered dietitian or qualified nutritionist is recommended for women who have difficulty adhering to these guidelines or for other high-risk pregnant women.

▲ TABLE 16-2

CHANGES IN FOODS FROM THE FOOD GUIDE PYRAMID GROUPS DURING PREGNANCY AND LACTATION

FOOD GUIDE PYRAMID GROUPS*	NONPREGNANT WOMEN	PREGNANT WOMEN (SECOND HALF OF PREGNANCY)	LACTATING WOMEN
Milk			
Adult	2 cups or more	3 cups or more	4 cups or more
Adolescent	4 cups or more	5 cups or more	5 cups or more
Vegetable and fruit			
Citrus or substitute	1 serving	2 servings	2–3 servings
Dark green or deep orange vegetable	1 serving at least every other day	1 serving daily	1–2 servings daily
Other fruits or vegetables, including potatoes	3–4 servings	2 servings	2 servings
Meat or alternate	2 servings or more	3 servings or more (6 oz cooked or more) Include liver or heart every week	
Cereal and bread	6 servings or more	6 servings or more	6 servings or more
		If fortified milk is not used, obtain physician's instructions for vitamin D supplementation Use iodized salt Use water or other beverages—at least 6 to 8 cups daily	

* Additional servings of these or any other food may be added as needed to provide the necessary calories and palatability.

Modified from Howe, P.S.: Basic Nutrition in Health and Disease, 7th ed. Philadelphia, W.B. Saunders Co., 1981, p. 177.

FACT & FALLACY

FALLACY: A few cups of coffee per day poses no risk during pregnancy.

FACT: There is conflicting evidence about how much caffeine is too much during pregnancy. It is known that caffeine causes blood vessels to constrict, thus potentially limiting blood flow through the placenta to the growing fetus. Until more is known, the prudent approach is to cut back on caffeine intake gradually to no more than one cup daily.

Nausea

Nausea sometimes occurs in the first trimester and on occasion throughout the entire pregnancy. The cause of the nausea is not fully understood but is

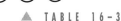

▲ T A B L E   1 6 - 3

SAMPLE MEAL PLANS FOR PREGNANCY

	PREGNANT WOMAN	PREGNANT ADOLESCENT*
Breakfast	Orange juice, 1 cup† Shredded wheat Scrambled egg Toast, 1 slice Milk, 1 cup Decaffeinated coffee	Orange juice, 1 cup† Shredded wheat Scrambled egg Toast, 2 slices Butter or margarine Marmalade† Milk, 1 cup
Lunch	Tuna sandwich Carrot and green pepper sticks Oatmeal cookies† Milk, 1 cup	Tuna sandwich on whole wheat bread Carrot and green pepper sticks Cheese cubes Oatmeal cookies† Fresh fruit Milk, 1 cup
Midafternoon	Milk, 1 cup	Chicken sandwich Milk, 1 cup
Dinner	Broiled steak Steamed broccoli Baked potato Tomato salad with French dressing Apple slices	Broiled steak Steamed broccoli with melted cheese Baked potato with sour cream Vegetable salad with French dressing Apple with peanut butter Milk, 1 cup
Bedtime	Hot milk or cocoa,† 1 cup	Milk or cocoa,† 1 cup

* Needs more kilocalories, protein, and calcium.

†For women with gestational diabetes, juice may be contraindicated for control of blood glucose; oranges or other vitamin C–containing fruit may be advised later in the day rather than at breakfast, and desserts should be restricted based on values obtained from the woman's self-monitoring of blood glucose levels (SMBG).

probably related to hormonal changes in pregnancy. One theory is related to low blood sugar levels, as nausea seems to increase when a woman has not eaten for a period of time. Eating high-carbohydrate foods, such as dry toast or crackers, before arising may alleviate the problem. Fried foods and other high-fat foods are a common cause of nausea and should be avoided unless tolerated and allowable within weight gain restrictions. A gradual increase of food intake during the late afternoon and evening can replace nutrients that were not consumed in the morning (a common time for nausea).

For severe nausea adversely affecting weight gain, all foods that are tolerated are considered acceptable. Nutrient density becomes a minor issue when kilocalories are paramount in promoting weight gain. Chocolate, potato chips, donuts, and other foods generally not considered the healthiest choices are appropriate if tolerated when increased total kilocalorie intake becomes necessary to prevent weight loss.

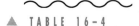

▲ TABLE 16-4

RDAs DURING PREGNANCY AND LACTATION

	NONPREGNANT WOMEN				LACTATION	
	15–18 Years	19–24 Years	25–50 Years	Pregnancy	First 6 Months	Second 6 Months
Kilocalories	2200	2200	2200	2500	2700	2700
Protein (g)	44	46	50	60	65	62
Vitamin A (RE)	800	800	800	800	1300	1200
Vitamin D (μg)	10	10	5	10	10	10
Vitamin E (mg TE)	8	8	8	10	12	11
Vitamin C (mg)	60	60	60	70	95	90
Folate (μg)	180	180	180	400	280	260
Niacin (mg)	15	15	15	17	20	20
Riboflavin (mg)	1.3	1.3	1.3	1.6	1.8	1.7
Thiamine (mg)	1.1	1.1	1.1	1.5	1.6	1.6
Vitamin B$_{12}$	2	2	2	2.2	2.6	2.6
Calcium (mg)	1200	1200	800	1200	1200	1200
Phosphorus (mg)	1200	1200	800	1200	1200	1200
Iodine (μg)	150	150	150	175	200	200
Iron (mg)	15	15	15	30	15	15
Magnesium (mg)	300	280	280	320	355	340
Zinc (mg)	12	12	12	15	19	16
Iodine (μg)	150	150	150	175	200	200
Selenium (μg)	50	55	55	65	75	75

From National Academy of Sciences National Research Council: Recommended Dietary Allowances, 10th ed. Washington, DC, National Academy of Sciences, 1989.

Hyperemesis

This condition is characterized by excessive and prolonged vomiting. It probably is more common than statistics show, since treatment may be in a physician's office rather than in a hospital setting. It can cause serious dehydration and weight loss—over 5 per cent weight loss is considered indicative of hyperemesis. Other effects of prolonged vomiting that have been reported include rib fracture, rupture of the esophagus, ruptured blood vessels in the eyes, electrolyte imbalances and depletion, and aspiration pneumonia (Erick et al., 1993). Charlotte Brontë, the famous writer, died of hyperemesis in 1855.

Hospitalization with administration of intravenous fluids may be necessary, as may more aggressive medical management. When total parenteral nutrition (TPN) such as Maria Bernardo received in the Chapter 14 case study is indicated, it can be lifesaving for both the mother and the fetus. Caution still needs to be exercised, as there are at least two published cases of maternal and fetal demise in connection with TPN.

Some women may respond to vitamin B$_6$ therapy for hyperemesis, but more studies are needed to support this approach. There are no clinical trials to date that implicate vitamin deficiency in hyperemesis. However, there is speculation that vitamin deficiency may exist (Erick et al., 1993).

FACT & FALLACY

FALLACY: Hyperemesis is psychological in origin.
FACT: There is little evidence that hyperemesis is caused by psychological problems. It is more likely that hyperemesis is the cause of psychological distress. Hyperemesis is known around the world. Reports of nausea and vomiting date back to the year 2000 BC. The evidence is much stronger that hormonal or other physical causes are the basis of the development of hyperemesis. Smells, odors, and motion often precipitate the nausea and vomiting (Erick et al., 1993).

Anemia

Anemia from iron deficiency may occur during pregnancy when iron intake and stores do not meet the demand. This is preventable and treatable by daily supplements of 30 to 60 mg of ferrous salts.

Anemia from folate deficiency may occur if the intake of food and nutrients is poor. A daily supplement of 400 μg of folacin and improvement in eating habits will correct the anemia.

Physiological anemia also results from the expanded volume of blood (plasma increases without a concomitant increase in red blood cells). There is controversy in the medical field over whether this form of anemia needs to be treated. However, until further research indicates otherwise, increased intake of iron is advised.

Constipation

Constipation can be related to iron supplementation as well as to decreased intestinal motility, which is believed to be a normal physiological process that assists in nutrient absorption during pregnancy. Adequate fiber, fluid, and appropriate exercise can help control constipation. Laxatives should only be used on the advice of an **obstetrician** (a physician specializing in pregnancy).

Heartburn

Heartburn in pregnancy is believed to be caused by the pressure of the growing fetus on the stomach, resulting in hydrochloric acid being forced into the esophageal area. For this reason, it may help to eat more frequent, smaller meals and to avoid a reclining position after meals. Excess fat intake can contribute to heartburn by allowing stomach contents to remain for longer periods in the stomach. Excess fat is also associated with relaxed muscle tone of the **esophageal sphincter** (the muscle connecting the stomach and esophagus), which further allows hydrochloric acid to be forced back up into the esophagus. The woman should not take over-the-counter medication for heartburn without consulting her obstetrician.

Pica

The practice of **pica** (eating nonfood items, especially clay or laundry starch) during pregnancy is a carryover from a tradition in Africa, where clay provided a source of calcium, iron, and other minerals. When clay is not available, laundry starch is sometimes substituted. Intake of these substances can interfere with consumption of adequate nutrients and their absorption.

Pica should be stopped to ensure optimal fetal development. However, the practice of pica is not often revealed, especially if the health care professional appears to have a judgmental attitude. Great sensitivity needs to be used by the health care professional in order to elicit an accurate assessment of the practice of pica. Since pica may be related to cultural heritage and beliefs, changing the practice may not be possible in a health care setting. Using objective measures such as the danger of anemia may help the woman understand the negative consequences of pica.

WHAT ARE SOME COMMON AND CLINICAL PROBLEMS DURING PREGNANCY?

Closely Spaced Pregnancies

Although many parents plan to space their children close together so that the children can be playmates, it is healthier for the mother and the fetus to wait at least 12 to 18 months between pregnancies. Longer spacing helps the mother to reestablish good nutritional stores.

Overweight

A weight reduction regimen should not be initiated at any time during pregnancy. Overweight women should observe the same principles of prenatal nutrition as do women of normal weight. The total weight gain, however, should be smaller, averaging about 15 to 25 pounds.

FACT & FALLACY

FALLACY: You can safely avoid gaining too much weight during pregnancy by taking calcium supplements instead of drinking milk.

FACT: Milk provides more nutrients than just calcium. A calcium supplement will not give you the extra 30 grams of protein found in the recommended four cups of milk. Riboflavin and other nutrients, such as potassium, magnesium, phosphorus, vitamins A and D, and other trace elements, are found in milk as well. Low-fat or skim milk can be used by weight-conscious women.

Pregnancy-Induced Hypertension

Pregnancy-induced hypertension (PIH), formerly known as **toxemia,** is a condition that may occur during the third trimester of pregnancy. Its cause is not known, but it is no longer felt to be a toxic condition; therefore, the term *toxemia* is no longer used. PIH is characterized by proteinuria, elevated blood pressure, and rapid weight gain caused by edema.

Preeclampsia is associated with symptoms of PIH. Eclampsia (the most severe form of preeclampsia) is associated with convulsions and coma. Some symptoms that can indicate its development include a sudden rise in blood pressure, severe headache, and blurred vision. Theories have been advanced that involve malnutrition, such as inadequate protein intake, as a factor in its cause. Women under 20 or over 30 years of age, those with multiple pregnancies (five or more), or with preexisting heart disease, diabetes mellitus, or hypertension are at increased risk of developing preeclampsia (O'Toole, 1992).

The former practices of restricting kilocalories and sodium to reduce the risk of PIH complications are now considered obsolete. To the contrary, there is a greater incidence of PIH among underweight women who fail to gain weight normally during pregnancy. The evidence indicates that the total amount of weight gain per se is not the significant factor. Sodium restriction is no longer recommended and may actually be harmful, since sodium needs are increased during pregnancy. However, avoidance of excessive intake of salt is recommended for pregnant women as well as for the general population.

Diabetes

Insulin-dependent diabetes mellitus (IDDM) was once considered an automatic cause for alarm if pregnancy developed. We now know that if the woman achieves near normal blood sugar control prior to conception and throughout the pregnancy, the likelihood of bearing a healthy, normal infant is as great as it is for a woman without IDDM. It is paramount, however, that tight control over blood sugar levels be obtained prior to conception to help prevent birth defects during the critical first trimester of organ development.

Gestational diabetes mellitus (GDM, a form of diabetes that occurs only during pregnancy) is not associated with birth defects, since the elevated blood sugar does not develop until after the critical first trimester is over. The consequences of uncontrolled GDM are more problematic at the time of birth. There is an increased likelihood of a large-sized baby who is very susceptible to hypoglycemia in the first few hours after birth. Strict control of blood sugar during pregnancy will increase the chances of normal labor and delivery of a healthy baby without complications. Routine screening for GDM now is done between the 24th and 28th weeks of pregnancy.

Control of either IDDM or GDM is best handled with a medical team approach so that the most appropriate plan and means of control are developed, including aspects such as insulin, diet, and home glucose monitoring. Maternal blood sugar levels should range between 60 mg/dL (fasting) and 120 mg/dL (2 hours after meals), with a maximum acceptable blood sugar level of 140 mg/dL 1 hour after meals. Higher blood sugar levels may be an indication for further carbohydrate restriction (breakfast often needs to be very limited in carbohydrate) or a need for insulin or both. Urine ketones also need to be monitored. Too little intake of carbohydrate, too little insulin production, or weight loss of any amount can cause the mother's body fat to be broken down excessively. The resulting ketone buildup is detrimental to the growing fetus and needs to be corrected with diet changes or insulin or both.

Alcohol Use

Fetal alcohol syndrome is caused by excessive alcohol intake by the mother during pregnancy. It is characterized by wide-set eyes, along with mental retardation and other physical characteristics. Since the safe limit of alcohol intake is not known, the best advice for the pregnant woman is to drink no alcohol. Professional counseling may be necessary.

Drug Addiction

The use of illegal drugs, as well as legal drugs such as tobacco and alcohol, impairs fetal growth. Women who are addicted before conception often deny the problem and present a challenge to the health care professional. Good nutrition is vital so that complications associated with drug use are not exacerbated.

Adolescent Pregnancy

Depending on the age of the teenager as well as other risk factors, an adolescent pregnancy may be perfectly normal or extremely high risk. Younger teenagers and those who become pregnant near the time of menarche are most at risk. There are an estimated 1 million teen pregnancies in the United States each year. And since pregnant teenagers tend to have eating patterns and food preferences similar to those of nonpregnant teenagers, nutrition concerns become evident. Dietary habits include frequent snacking on foods high in fat and sugar and low in essential nutrients, resulting in lower than recommended intake of nutrients that are especially important during pregnancy. A concern over body image may result in inadequate weight gain (Story and Alton, 1992).

Programs for pregnant teenagers are common in most communities and offer social support, encouragement to seek good medical care, and assistance in completion of school. The **Women, Infants, and Children Supplemental Nutrition Program (WIC)** (see Chapter 22) is generally available to all lower-income pregnant teenagers, and referral should be made by the health care professional.

Breast-feeding is possible for the motivated teenager; however, other life concerns may take precedence.

HOW DOES DIET INFLUENCE THE NURSING COUPLE?

The impact of maternal diet on infant growth does not end at delivery. This is true even for non-nursing mothers, who need to maintain their nutritional status in order to best cope with the demands of a new baby. During **lactation** (production of milk for breast-feeding; also referred to as "nursing"), adequate diet becomes more critical. Kilocalorie intake can affect the quantity of milk produced, and thus it is important for a breast-feeding woman to lose any excess weight slowly (an initial rapid loss will occur from fluid loss after delivery, which is unrelated to kilocalories). Other nutrients vary in their impact on the quality of breast milk. In general, problems are limited to the excessive intake of fat-soluble vitamins through the indiscriminate use of supplements in megadoses and insufficient intake of water-soluble vitamins. Minerals do not generally affect the quality of breast milk, since development of maternal deficiency and toxicity states is uncommon. Drinking milk is not a prerequisite for successful lactation, contrary to what is often believed. However, to help prevent maternal bone loss, other calcium-rich foods should be encouraged for the breast-feeding woman who cannot or will not drink milk, for example, cheese, yogurt, pudding, or soybean products such as tofu (see Table 16–2 for recommended intakes of food during lactation). Women who avoid drinking milk and who live in cloudy regions may have inadequate vitamin D, which is reflected in breast milk. A vitamin D supplement may be indicated in such situations.

Breast milk is an important source of vitamins for the infant. It provides all the necessary vitamins, as long as the mother's nutritional intake is adequate, with the possible exception of fluoride. Vegans who avoid all animal sources of food may have inadequate vitamin D and vitamin B_{12}. Supplements for their infants may be necessary. An additional health benefit to the infant from breast milk is increased immune responses. Breast-feeding is related to reduced incidence of **otitis media** (ear infections), owing either to an upright feeding position or to immunological factors (Sheard, 1993). In **colostrum** (the substance that precedes breast milk) and breast milk, a substance called **immunoglobulin A (IgA)** helps guard against the penetration of intestinal organisms and antigens, the latter of which are a cause of allergy development.

WHY IS LACTATION MANAGEMENT IMPORTANT?

Although many people believe that breast-feeding is both beneficial and natural, there are several important pieces of "how-to" information that are not widely known. Nurses who see lactating mothers during the first weeks following delivery can play a vital role in the success (or failure) of breast-feeding. Positive verbal encouragement and support are of crucial importance.

WHAT ARE SOME BREAST-FEEDING ISSUES?

Frequency of Feeding

A primary rule of thumb is that the more frequently a woman nurses, the more breast milk she will produce (Fig. 16–5). This is referred to as supply and demand. Since the quantity of breast milk production is difficult to ascertain, other guidelines are used to determine adequacy. These guidelines are: (1) adequate weight gain by the infant of 1 to 2 pounds per month, (2) eight to 12 nursings per 24-hour period, and (3) six or more wet diapers per 24-hour period (assuming that the infant is not given any bottles of water).

Infant Weight Gain

Some breast-fed infants gain more than the recommended 2 pounds per month, but generally this is not a cause for concern, since it is not possible to force-feed an infant who is fed only breast milk.

If the infant gains less than the recommended 1 to 2 pounds per month, great care must be taken not to discourage the lactating mother but to as-

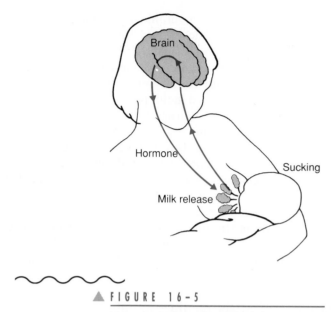

▲ FIGURE 16-5

Milk release during breast-feeding.

sess possible causes and provide appropriate counseling in a highly sensitive way. It is known that on average breast-fed infants gain weight more slowly than formula-fed infants after the first 2 to 3 months; however, this slower weight gain should not necessarily be viewed as a problem (Subcommittee on Lactation, 1991).

Inverted Nipples

A simple exercise can determine if a woman has inverted nipples (Fig. 16–6). Use of either the Hoffman technique or a milk cup (not a soft rubber shield) can be used to alleviate the problem (Fig. 16–7).

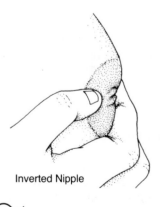

Inverted Nipple

INVERTED NIPPLE

An inverted nipple looks like a slit or a fold. A partly inverted nipple folds in on one side only.

A woman can tell if she has an inverted nipple by gently pinching the nipple at the base using the thumb and forefinger. If the nipple shrinks back, it is an "inverted" nipple.

Many women with inverted nipples have successfully breastfed, but special preparation is very helpful. Using the Hoffman Technique and wearing a hard plastic cup such as the Confi-Dry will encourage the nipple to stick out.

▲ FIGURE 16-6

Inverted nipple. (From Health Education Associates, Sandwich, MA.)

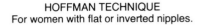

HOFFMAN TECHNIQUE
For women with flat or inverted nipples.

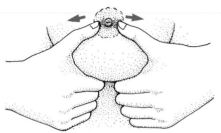

Place your thumbs opposite each other on either side of the nipple. Gently draw your thumbs away from the nipple. Then place your thumbs above and below the nipple and repeat.

Do this twice a day for a few minutes.

MILK CUP
For women with flat or inverted nipples

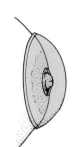

Begin by wearing the Cup under the bra for short periods of time and gradually work up to 8 to 10 hours a day.

You can allow your skin to breathe by removing the Cup for short periods, or by wearing only the base part.

Wearing the Cup is painless. It is not noticeable when worn in the bra unless the woman is wearing a tight-fitting jersey.

The Confi-Dry Milk Cup may be purchased from the Childbirth Education Association of Greater Philadelphia 5 E. Second Avenue, Conshohocken, PA 19428. (215) 828-0131.

▲ FIGURE 16-7

A, Hoffman technique. *B,* Milk cup. (From Health Education Associates, Sandwich, MA.)

WHAT ARE SOME FACTORS IN LOW WEIGHT GAIN AMONG BREAST-FED INFANTS?

Poor Let-down Reflex

Particularly for a first-time nursing mother, anxiety can be high and can inhibit the **let-down reflex. Oxytocin** (a hormone) promotes the let-down reflex. With let-down, the milk from the upper parts of the breast **(hind milk)** comes down to the areola (the darker skin around the nipple). A lactating woman can usually identify when the let-down reflex is occurring, as there is a momentary "pins-and-needles" feeling in the breast area.

The hind milk consists of a richer milk higher in fat content. Because of the high kilocalorie content of fat found in the hind milk, the let-down reflex is crucial for the infant's adequate weight gain. Relaxation techniques are thus important to successful lactation. Humor is useful in helping the nursing mother relax and should be encouraged by the nurse or other health care professional.

Insufficient Feedings

If the let-down reflex does not seem to be an issue (you can ask the mother if she feels a tingling sensation during nursing, which is a sign of let-down), the nurse should ask how often breast-feeding occurs. Very often, women try to maintain a feeding schedule and ignore the hunger cues of their baby, thinking "the baby can't be hungry yet," or the infant may be a "sleepy baby" who does not indicate his or her own hunger. Generally about every 2 hours is a good feeding schedule, but for infants who gain weight slowly, more frequent feedings may be in order until the milk supply and weight gain are increased.

During periods of **growth spurts** the baby may want to nurse more often than usual. Growth spurts often occur during the third week after delivery (just when the mother is likely to be going through **"postpartum blues"**—a feeling of depression) and at 6 weeks and 3 months. This is not a sign of needing to add formula; rather, it is Mother Nature's way of increasing milk production to meet additional needs. Good advice is to encourage bed rest with continuous nursing (although strong family support is a prerequisite for this approach). After a couple of days of very frequent nursing, the milk production will have increased and the baby will go for longer periods between feedings.

Another helpful point concerning frequency of feeding is that the total number of feedings is more important than their spacing. For example, an infant who sleeps through the night but feeds more frequently during the day and has the recommended 8 to 12 feedings will most likely gain weight as well as the infant who wakes up regularly all night and day but nurses the same number of times.

WHAT ARE SOME OTHER BARRIERS TO SUCCESSFUL BREAST-FEEDING?

Breast Engorgement

Breast engorgement is a common occurrence in the first few days after delivery. Temporary measures to release excess milk include taking a warm shower or leaning over a sink full of warm water with exposed breasts. By diminishing engorgement, the infant will be better able to grasp the nipple, thereby allowing emptying of the breasts. Short, frequent nursings can help keep engorgement under control. Eventually the amount of milk produced by the new lactating mother will even out to meet the infant's needs.

Sore or Cracked Nipples

Some comfort measures for sore or cracked nipples include:

1. relaxation techniques, such as deep-breathing, at the beginning of each feeding and warm washcloths with gentle breast (not nipple) massage to encourage milk flow prior to the infant's suckling;
2. nursing on the less sore side first;
3. changing feeding positions, using the football hold (baby's feet pointing outward from mother rather than inward toward mother), the regular position, or even lying down with the baby's feet pointing up toward the mother's head (awkward but effective in getting the baby's tongue off the sore spot on the woman's nipple);
4. giving short, frequent nursings (the major portion of breast milk is removed within about 5 to 10 minutes; frequent nursings will allow the baby to not be overly hungry, thereby lessening excessive suckling);
5. making sure the baby's mouth is well back on the areola, with the baby's tongue underneath the nipple;
6. making sure that the baby is removed properly from the breast, breaking suction with the mother's finger inserted into the corner of the baby's mouth;

7. air drying the nipples after each feeding; and
8. using cold compresses or washcloths between nursings.

FACT & FALLACY

FALLACY: A lactating woman who is experiencing sore nipples should be advised to wear a soft rubber nipple shield while breast-feeding.

FACT: Although this solution may provide relief in the short term, in the long term it can cause severe problems. Since tactile stimulation is necessary to continue producing milk, the physical barrier of the shield between the mother's nipple and the baby's jaw and tongue will inhibit milk production.

Twins

Many people believe that twins preclude the option of breast-feeding. However, since milk supply is most strongly influenced by frequency of feeding (supply and demand: the more one nurses, the more milk is produced), it is feasible to nurse twins.

Inappropriate Fluid Intake

Milk production necessitates increased fluid intake; however, the mother need drink only that amount of fluid necessary to satisfy her thirst. A sudden excess in fluid intake may actually decrease milk yield, as release of **antidiuretic hormone** (a hormone that regulates water loss through the kidneys) is inhibited when fluid intake is in excess of need, resulting in **diuresis**, excess water loss through the kidneys.

The Premature Infant

Premature infants or infants with cleft palate may be fed breast milk or commercial formula using bottles with special nipples. **Gavage feeding** (a form of force-feeding through a flexible tube or pump) may be required for those premature infants who do not have adequate suckling ability for survival. Premature infants have special nutritional needs, primarily because of immature gastrointestinal functioning. These infants now use either special formula or fortified breast milk. This breast milk ideally comes from the infant's own mother, and thus it is referred to as **preterm milk.** In addition, commercial fortifiers are added to the breast milk to increase the kilocalories and other nutrients.

The mother who is collecting milk for her premature infant probably will need extra support in order to maintain breast-feeding. She particularly needs extra support in order to relax in this high-tension situation. A picture of the baby that she can look at during the collection process can help elicit that good feeling of, "Oh, don't I have a beautiful baby!"—a feeling that is difficult to experience while the baby lies in the intensive care unit hooked up to tubes and other paraphernalia. A relaxed nursing staff is of particular importance; again, the use of humor is a positive approach to help encourage the let-down reflex. It is difficult to achieve the same high level of tactile stimulation to the nipple by artificial means, since no pumping machine fully mimics the action of the baby's tongue and jaw movements.

WHAT ARE SOME WEANING TIPS?

The **La Leche League** (a breast-feeding support group) generally advocates baby-led **weaning** (accustoming the baby to nourishment other than breast milk). If, however, the mother needs or wants to wean before the baby wants to, the following approaches are suggested:

1. Plan to wean gradually, one feeding at a time (for example, omit the midmorning feeding for a couple of days before proceeding further).

2. Substitute other nurturing activities for the omitted feeding, such as a story, a walk, or a drink of milk, juice, or water from a cup.

3. Avoid situations that the infant associates with nursing, such as a favorite chair used for nursing.

4. Consider continuing nursing at least once or twice a day, such as early morning or at bedtime; weaning does not have to be all-or-nothing (La Leche League, 1991).

NUTRITIONALLY SPEAKING, IS IT OKAY TO BOTTLE-FEED?

Although it is preferable to breast-feed because of the nutritional benefits, it is fortunate that commercial formulas have been developed that closely resemble breast milk for those women who cannot breast-feed because they are taking medications that contraindicate it, for women with medical problems, or for those who choose not to breast-feed. Although this may be the more practical method of feeding for the working mother, many mothers find that a combination of bottle- and breast-feeding works well, particularly if they work on a part-time basis. Expression of breast milk for use in a bottle can be an alternative, as shown in Figure 16–8.

It is helpful for a woman to hear that if she expresses only 1 or 2 ounces of milk initially, she is doing very well. Expressed milk cooled in the refrigerator can be added to previously frozen expressed milk in order to obtain full bottles (4-ounce bottles are the handiest for collecting and storing expressed milk). Visually, this is very interesting, with blue layers (**fore milk,** the milk from the front of the breast) and thick white layers (fat-rich hind milk) being formed. Being relaxed helps the let-down reflex, and expressing milk after a warm shower is helpful. After a woman is comfortable with the technique and her ability, she can easily express milk anytime, such as at work during her lunch break. The milk can then be stored in a portable ice chest if a refrigerator is not available. Expressed milk can be kept for 1 to 2 days in sterile bottles at refrigerator temperature, for 1 to 2 weeks in a freezer, or for up to 6 months if the freezer maintains a constant temperature of 0° F (about 17.8° C) or lower.

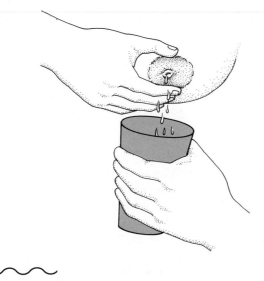

1. Do breast massage.

2. Place the thumb and index finger on the areola or darker skin around the nipple—about an inch back from the nipple. Press inward toward the chest wall and squeeze the thumb and finger together gently: *push back and squeeze.* Don't slide the thumb and finger. Don't pull the nipple out.

3. Keep the thumb and finger in that position and express until no more drops come out. Then move to another location around the nipple and repeat.

4. Lean over the sterile container and catch the milk. Switch to the other breast and again massage before beginning to express.

▲ FIGURE 16–8

Instructions for hand expression of milk. (From Health Education Associates, Sandwich, MA.)

ARE THERE PROBLEMS ASSOCIATED WITH BOTTLE-FEEDING?

Nursing-bottle Mouth

Nursing-bottle mouth (also known as baby-bottle tooth decay; see Fig. 19–2) is a condition in which the two front top teeth are severely decayed or completely eroded away in the older infant or child. It is caused by the infant's continuously suckling on a bottle that contains a source of carbohydrate. Sleeping with a bottle is particularly harmful because of decreased production of saliva that helps cleanse the teeth. As a general rule, juice should be given in a cup and only water bottles allowed at bedtime, if needed.

Milk Anemia

Milk anemia is caused when milk (not iron-fortified formula) is consumed to such a large degree that it replaces the intake of foods high in iron. A reduction in milk intake to that recommended in the Food Guide Pyramid may be in order, with substitute water bottles as necessary. By putting milk in a cup for the young child, the milk intake will often be decreased to the recommended amount. Juice intake, when excessive, can also contribute to anemia by replacing foods high in iron.

Microwave Heating

The excess steam that results when bottles are heated in a microwave oven can cause bottles to explode in the infant's face. Also, since "hot spots" in the liquid can develop, a seemingly safe temperature can actually cause the infant's mouth to be severely burned if there is contact with the hot spot. The safest way to heat a bottle is to allow very warm water from a faucet to flow over it until the chill is gone.

Use of Inappropriate Liquids

The only appropriate liquids for regular use in a bottle are expressed breast milk, formula, and water. Although occasional use of juice is acceptable (such as in a car when drinking from a cup is prohibited), the regular use of juice in a bottle can cause nursing-bottle mouth (see earlier discussion). Other sweet liquids such as Kool-Aid or soft drinks should be avoided entirely. Formula replacements, such as nondairy creamer or other milk products that are not specifically designed for infant use, should never be used. Formula should be mixed according to directions, not under- or overdiluted unless specifically recommended by a **pediatrician** (physician specializing in the care of infants, children, and adolescents) or a registered dietitian.

WHAT TYPES OF INFANT FORMULAS ARE USED?

Commercial Cow's Milk-Based Formulas

These formulas closely approximate human milk and are made from cow's milk. They are available in powder, liquid concentrated, and ready-to-feed types. Powdered forms are more economical but require mixing and careful measuring. Liquid concentrated formulas require proper dilution with water before using (a 1:1 ratio). Commercial formulas are fortified to meet all the vitamin and mineral requirements of the infant. Formulas containing iron are available and are recommended by the American Academy of Pediatrics. Examples of commercial formulas are Enfamil, Similac, and SMA.

Soybean-based Formulas

If the infant shows signs of allergy to cow's milk or when the parents are strict vegetarians (vegans), soybean-based formulas are used. Soybean-based formula is often the formula of choice as a supplement to breast-feeding owing to the reduced likelihood of allergies. Commercially prepared formulas are fortified with vitamins and minerals. Bottle-fed infants who have an intolerance to lactose can use soy formulas. Examples of soybean-based formulas are ProSobee, Neo-Mull-Soy, and Isomil.

Special Formulas

Special formulas may be necessary for infants with digestive disturbances, allergies, or inborn errors of metabolism. Examples are Portagen, Pregestimil, Lonalac, and Lofenalac.

WHAT ADDITIONAL FOODS ARE GIVEN DURING THE FIRST YEAR?

Neither breast milk nor a milk formula will furnish adequate amounts of all nutrients required by the infant in later months. One important reason for introducing some solid foods into the infant's diet is to replenish the depleting stores of iron between 4 and 6 months of age (Table 16–5 shows the RDAs for infants up to 1 year old). The general guidelines are as follows:

1. Introduce iron-fortified baby rice cereal at about 4 to 6 months of age.
2. Add pureed vegetables and fruits, one at a time, at about 6 to 8 months (starting with vegetables may help to increase acceptance by the infant not yet exposed to the sweet taste of fruits).
3. Add pureed meats at about 6 to 8 months.
4. Add juice when the infant is old enough to drink from a cup at about 9 months of age.
5. Add foods with more texture and finger foods at about 9 months of age (chopped meats, crackers, and so on).
6. Add allergenic foods, such as cooked eggs, whole milk, and orange juice, after 1 year of age (especially important for the infant with a family history of allergies or asthma).

▲ **TABLE 16-5**

RDAs FOR INFANTS: BIRTH TO 1 YEAR

	0-6 MONTHS	6-12 MONTHS
Energy	108 kcal/kg	98 kcal/kg
Protein	13 g	14 g
Vitamin C	30 mg	35 mg
Folate	25 μg	35 μg
Niacin	5 mg	6 mg
Riboflavin	0.4 mg	0.5 mg
Thiamine	0.3 mg	0.4 mg
Vitamin B_6	0.3 mg	0.6 mg
Vitamin B_{12}	0.3 μg	0.5 μg
Vitamin A	375 μg of RE	375 μg of RE
Vitamin D	7.5 μg	10 μg
Vitamin E	3 mg of TE	4 mg of TE
Calcium	400 mg	600 mg
Phosphorus	300 mg	500 mg
Iodine	40 μg	50 μg
Iron	6 mg	10 mg
Magnesium	40 mg	60 mg
Zinc	5 mg	5 mg
Selenium	10 μg	15 μg

KEY: RE = retinol equivalent; TE = tocopherol equivalent
Modified from National Academy of Sciences National Research Council: Recommended Dietary Allowances, 10th ed. Washington, DC, National Academy of Sciences, 1989.

WHAT IS THE HISTORICAL PERSPECTIVE OF THE INTRODUCTION TO SOLID FOODS?

Although many parents today feel that waiting until 4 months of age to start introducing cereal and other solid foods is too long, it was once a common practice. Prior to 1920, solid foods were seldom offered to infants before 1 year of age. As time progressed and with the increased reliance on bottle-feeding and the expanding knowledge of infant nutrition, the age at which solid foods were introduced declined to the point of weeks and months by the 1960s. This trend, however, was a rational response to the nutritionally inadequate formulas used at that time (often evaporated milk mixed with water and corn syrup). A vitamin C source, such as orange juice, and iron-fortified cereal were necessary then at an early age.

With the current return of breast-feeding and the development of highly nutritious commercial infant formulas, the risks associated with early introduction of solids (such as development of an allergy caused by the use of orange juice and cereal at an early age) outweigh any benefits.

There are also other reasons that the advice has changed and it is now recommended to wait until 4 to 6 months of age before starting solid foods. These are:

1. inability of the young infant to digest complex carbohydrates such as those found in cereal, vegetables, and fruits (thus infants can fill up without getting the nutrients they need to grow; breast milk is considered the ideal food and source of nutrients for young infants)

2. immature intestinal tract of the young infant that allows large, undigested food molecules to pass through the intestinal wall (which can activate an allergic reaction and may become a permanent condition)

3. inadequate physiological readiness of the infant to use tongue-thrust (it is felt that biologically the human species may have developed this characteristic to prevent inappropriate ingestion of food)

4. inability of the infant to indicate a desire for food by opening his or her mouth when a spoonful of food is presented or to indicate satiety by leaning back and turning away; it is felt that until an infant can respond in this manner (at about 5 months of age), feeding solid food may represent a type of force-feeding

---

FACT & FALLACY

FALLACY: Cereal helps babies sleep through the night.
FACT: There is no scientific evidence to support this belief. Many experienced parents admit that their babies wake up regardless of how much food they have eaten. Feeding cereal should be strongly discouraged until the infant is 4 to 6 months old, particularly for infants with a family history of allergies.

WHAT ARE SOME FOOD CONTRAINDICATIONS FOR INFANTS?

Aside from the special requirements for allergy-sensitive infants or for those who have metabolic disorders (a referral to a registered dietitian or a qualified nutritionist is in order in these cases), it should be stressed that parents should not give honey to babies because of the potential for botulism, since honey contains botulism spores (in a quantity too low to cause adverse effects in older children and adults).

The high sodium content of some processed foods (such as canned vegetables or cured meats) can be detrimental to the immature renal functioning of infants. For this reason, homemade baby food can be higher in sodium than commercial baby foods, which are now mostly low in sodium.

Foods that have a hard texture (such as a raw apple or carrot) or food in large pieces should also be avoided to prevent choking until the infant is old enough to chew adequately. Hot dogs should never be given to an infant and can also be problematic for older children.

WHAT ARE SOME FEEDING STRATEGIES FOR THE OLDER INFANT?

Solid foods should be introduced one at a time to ensure tolerance and acceptance. The meal environment is critical for long-term positive meal associations. Thus the introduction of new foods needs to take place when both parent and infant are in a good mood. Observing the infant for feeding cues is helpful to avoid overfeeding.

At about the time the growing infant develops the **pincer grasp,** the ability to put the thumb and index finger together (about 8 months of age), a sense of independence also begins to grow. This can be exasperating to a parent, particularly as the baby begins to spill food on the floor or decides to empty a full bowl of food on his or her head. Since it is felt that this is part of normal development, it is advised that the parent cope with this behavior through positive strategies. An old shower curtain can be placed under the high-chair to catch spills, a large bib can help prevent damage to the baby's clothes, and small quantities of food can be given at one time to lessen waste. Through the infant's being allowed additional servings, adequate intake can occur simultaneously with a lowered frustration level of the parents. Bribing and coaxing the infant to eat and not spill food can cause repetition of the negative behaviors as the infant learns he or she can control the parents' actions ("Let's see if I can get Mom and Dad to jump up and down if I drop this glass of juice"). Finger foods such as Cheerios are preferred by the older infant.

HOW DOES AN INFANT GROW AND DEVELOP?

A well nourished infant shows a steady gain in weight and height (with some fluctuations from week to week), is happy and vigorous, sleeps well, has firm muscles, has some tooth eruption at about 5 to 6 months with about six to twelve teeth having erupted by 12 months, and has good elimination characteristic of the type of feeding—breast or formula. The nutrients found in milk, especially the protein, are essential in the development of the new tissues that accompany this growth.

Each infant has an individual rate of growth, but all grow faster in weight than in height. A steady weight gain is more important than a large amount gained. In interpreting growth with the National Center for Health Statistics growth charts (see Appendix 13), percentiles are used. A child at the 50th percentile for age is considered average. There is no concern with growth if the length and weight for age is above the 10th percentile and is consistent (not dropping in percentile). Weight for height percentile should be between the 25th percentile and 90th percentile without showing a significant decrease or increase in percentiles.

WHAT ARE SOME CLINICAL PROBLEMS FOUND IN INFANCY?

Low Birth Weight and Premature Delivery

Babies born before they have had a chance to grow adequately are at nutritional risk. Babies less than 5½ pounds at birth generally stay in the hospital after delivery until they have reached at least this weight. Lung function may be compromised. The ability to suckle may be impaired because of immature muscle development. Special feeding devices, including tube-feeding, may be required until the infant is strong enough to suck. Guidance on the introduction of solid foods needs to take into account the amount of prematurity. For example, cereal is usually started at 4 months of age. If the infant was born 3 months prematurely, the introduction of cereal should be delayed until the infant is 7 months old. This is especially true if there is a strong family history of allergies.

Failure to Thrive

The **failure to thrive (FTT)** syndrome was first observed in infants raised in institutional settings in which they did not receive adequate amounts of attention (physical touch and emotional warmth). In recent years, this recognition has led to volunteers being used to cuddle premature infants in hospital settings in order to help their growth and survival.

Failure to thrive is associated with physical illness, poor nutrition, and maternal deprivation, which lead to severe retardation of physical growth and developmental delays. Failure to thrive is a medical diagnosis, but it includes a weight and height of less than the third percentile for age (see Appendix 13) and less than normal ability in the Denver Developmental Screening Test (O'Toole, 1992). A total health care team approach may be in order.

WHAT ARE SOME OTHER NUTRITION ISSUES FOR WOMEN?

Premenstrual Syndrome

Premenstrual syndrome (PMS) occurs the first few days of the monthly menstrual cycle and disappears after menstruation. The majority of American women experience some degree of PMS, with an estimated 10 to 15 per cent experiencing severe or disabling symptoms, including symptoms of hypoglycemia such as increased appetite, nervousness, irritability, and headaches. However, eating does not always relieve these symptoms as would be predicted in treating hypoglycemia. There are many theories about the cause, but at this time, "there is no evidence that PMS is caused by a poor diet or vitamin/mineral deficiency or that it can be prevented or cured by dietary therapy" (Casey and Dwyer, 1987). Eating balanced meals at regular times may, however, help to some degree.

Osteoporosis

This condition of brittle bones is more prevalent in women than in men. Women have less bone mass than men and often have inadequate calcium intake. Bone loss increases after menopause. Emphasizing milk or other calcium-rich foods in the diet helps to maintain bone integrity. The equivalent of 3 to 4 cups of milk is recommended to help prevent bone loss. Hormonal therapy with estrogen and weight-bearing exercise further help to maintain bone integrity (see Chapter 20 for the benefits of exercise). For more information on osteoporosis see Chapter 21.

WHAT IS THE ROLE OF THE NURSE OR OTHER HEALTH PROFESSIONAL IN MATERNAL AND INFANT NUTRITION?

During Pregnancy

A nurse or other health professional should be aware of potential barriers to adequate nourishment during pregnancy, such as poor attitude (denial of pregnancy or desire to maintain slimness), misinformation (belief that salt restriction and low weight gain are desirable), or physical barriers to adequate nourishment (insufficient food money, lack of adequate food preparation facilities, or hyperemesis). Once such a barrier is identified, referral to a registered dietitian or a qualified nutritionist, such as one associated with the WIC programs, may be in order, as well as immediate contact with the woman's obstetrician.

It is especially important for health care professionals to recognize the strong need of pregnant teenagers and all adolescents to rebel against authority figures. Rather than telling a pregnant teen what she must do, inform her of alternative actions and their likely outcomes. Work as the teen's advocate and ask her in a positive manner how you can best assist her. Ask her what her perceived needs are and how she feels about your concerns. Encourage her involvement in other supportive programs in your community. Be a good listener and a supportive advocate for her.

After Pregnancy

After delivering, women should be encouraged to maintain good nutritional status for themselves to help promote adequate energy for infant care as well as to help restore nutritional stores for subsequent pregnancies. Counseling can be provided as needed to encourage adequate spacing between pregnancies and nutritional intake to prepare a woman's body for a future healthy pregnancy.

> Two effective assessment questions concerning nutritional preparation for subsequent pregnancies could be, "Are you planning to have another pregnancy in the future?" and if so, "What have you heard is the ideal spacing between pregnancies?"

During Lactation

The obstetrical nurse plays an important role in promoting successful breast-feeding in the hospital setting. Of crucial importance is positive verbal encouragement and support. Flippant remarks can damage a woman's already sensitive emotions (related to hormonal changes associated with birth) and may impair her ability to breast-feed successfully.

The use of humor can help a tense new mother relax, which is important for a successful let-down reflex. All new breast-feeding women should be alerted to support and information services such as

- a local La Leche League
- the Women, Infants, and Children's Supplemental Nutrition Program (WIC), which supports breastfeeding education
- the Cooperative Extension's Expanded Food and Nutrition Education Program (EFNEP), which may have breast-feeding support available through trained Nutrition Teaching Assistants (see Chapter 22)
- the local hospital's obstetrics department, which will likely have nurses trained in lactation management—this can be especially helpful for problems that occur in the middle of the night

Breast-feeding "buddy systems" also exist in many communities. Volunteers experienced in breast-feeding are paired up with new breast-feeding mothers until breast-feeding is fully established. A nurse or other health professional can help set up such a system or make referrals to one already in existence.

For Bottle-fed Infants

In the case of a bottle-fed infant, it is important for the nurse or other health care professional to be aware of the parents' philosophy and knowledge about feeding. Do they adhere to rigid feeding schedules that impair the infant's intake of formula or do they go solely by the infant's crying with the potential for either over- or underfeeding? Are the parents receiving conflicting advice (which is likely) that undermines their confidence or that makes them follow inappropriate feeding practices? Do they believe that formula is made from "a bunch of chemicals" and that therefore whole milk is better? Do they realize that formula requires refrigeration after it has been prepared? Do they know how to properly prepare formula?

A good question to ask is, "Are you aware of what formula is made from?" followed by an explanation that it is cow's milk with the excess protein removed and vitamins and minerals added to make it more nutritious like breast milk. A further explanation can be provided by saying that there is so much protein in cow's milk to help the baby cow grow that it causes gastrointestinal irritation (stomach bleeding) in the human baby (a graphic depiction with the use of your hands of the size difference between a calf and a human baby can be very effective). This can support the continued use of formula versus changing to whole milk before the infant is physiologically ready to do so.

Is nursing-bottle mouth a potential problem? If so, recommend water bottles at bedtime (and for an older child, a choice: water bottle or no bottle).

Regarding the Introduction to Solid Food

Explaining why a grandmother or a mother-in-law may be giving one piece of advice while you are giving another can go a long way in building a new mother's trust in her own common sense. Since many new mothers are anxious and insecure in their first encounters with their infants, your efforts are best aimed at building confidence and strengthening decision-making skills.

In regard to the introduction of solid foods, a good question is, "Have you thought about when you are going to start solid foods such as cereal?" followed by "What have you heard from other people about when to start?"

STUDY QUESTIONS AND ACTIVITIES

1. What benefits may the mother-to-be expect if she is well nourished?

2. Based on birthweight and length given in the opening case study, could you reassure Maria Bernardo that her newborn son appears normal? Plot his height and weight using the growth chart in Appendix 13. Are they appropriate?

3. Why should the pregnant teenager be sure she receives adequate kilocalories as well as sufficient amounts of all important nutrients?

4. How and why do the foods needed in the daily diet during pregnancy and lactation differ from those needed by nonpregnant women? Does Maria Bernardo need to make changes in her diet during pregnancy in order to breast-feed successfully? Why or why not?

5. Name several different ways for the pregnant woman to incorporate milk in the diet if she does not find it possible to drink the recommended amount.

6. What should a nurse do for Maria Bernardo to support breast-feeding? What are immediate concerns versus long-term concerns and their possible solutions?

7. What guidelines would you give to Mrs. Bernardo to help her determine if breast-feeding is going well once she leaves the hospital?

8. Describe the likely impact of "growth spurts" on the nursing behavior of baby Tony.

9. What are the advantages of breast-feeding? Why is breast milk so suitable for the infant?

10. List some ways to encourage positive eating habits with baby Tony when solid foods are started.

11. What considerations for meal planning would be indicated for a pregnant or breast-feeding woman who has celiac sprue (see Chapter 11)?

REFERENCES

Casey V, Dwyer JT: Premenstrual syndrome: Theories and evidence. Nutrition Today, Nov/Dec, 1987; 22(6):4–12.

Erick M, Hintlian CC, Ecker JL: Morning Sickness: Myths, Miseries, and Management. Workshop. The American Dietetic Association Annual Meeting, Anaheim, CA, October 1993. (Information also found in Erick M: No More Morning Sickness: A Survival Guide for Pregnant Women. Penguin Books, 1993.)

La Leche League: The Womanly Art of Breastfeeding, 5th ed. New York, Penguin Books, 1991; pp. 254–256.

O'Toole M, ed.: Miller-Keane Encyclopedia & Dictionary of Medicine, Nursing, & Allied Health, 5th ed. Philadelphia, WB Saunders, 1992.

Sheard NF: Breast-feeding protects against otitis media. Nutrition Review, 1993; 51(9):276.

Story M, Alton I: Nutrition and the pregnant adolescent. Contemporary Nutrition, 1992; 17(5).

Subcommittee on Lactation from the National Academy of Sciences Committee on Nutritional

Status During Pregnancy and Lactation: Nutrition during lactation. Nutrition Today, May/June, 1991; p. 30.

The Subcommittee on Nutritional Status and Weight Gain During Pregnancy and The Subcommittee on Dietary Intake and Nutrient Supplements During Pregnancy: Nutrition during pregnancy, executive summary. Nutrition Today, July/August, 1990; p. 17.

Wilkens KG, Schiro KB: Suggested Guidelines for Nutrition Care of Renal Patients, 2nd ed. A Project of the Renal Dietitians Dietetic Practice Group of The American Dietetic Association. Chicago, The American Dietetic Association, 1992; p. 72.

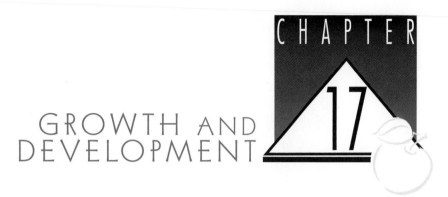

GROWTH AND
DEVELOPMENT

OBJECTIVES

After completing this chapter, you should be able to:
- Describe nutritional needs during childhood and adolescence
- Describe methods to promote good nutritional intake
- Apply knowledge of the nutrient needs to the meal environment

TERMS TO
IDENTIFY

Adipose tissue	Food distribution system	Hematocrit
Bone growth	Food jags	Hemoglobin
Development	Growth	Lean tissue

A FAMILY'S PERSPECTIVE ON NUTRITION

"No, Nanna Bernardo. Baby Tony does not have to stop nursing yet," Maria said, trying not to get upset as she answered the almost daily questioning from her mother-in-law. The pediatrician said breast-feeding past a year of age was perfectly normal. And both she and the baby were quite content to continue as a nursing couple. Baby Tony, who was 15 months old, ate many solid foods and used a cup but still seemed to want to nurse.

But Rita Bernardo was not convinced. Didn't the baby nurse all the time, every few hours and even at night? And she had given bottles to all her babies, including her son Antonio, by 6 months of age. How could Maria expect baby Tony to grow well with breast milk at this age? And he must be hungry if he wanted to nurse all the time. She would speak with her son. He would listen to her.

Maria was very grateful that her pediatrician had warned her that her mother-in-law might give her advice contrary to what was now considered the best feeding method for infants. In fact, he said that in many countries women often nurse for two or three years, but he clarified that the addition of solid foods by the first year of age was recommended. He had also warned her that babies have a strong need to suckle and that nursing helped meet this need. She hoped she could make it. Maybe she would call La Leche League again. They were so helpful when she first began to nurse. She hoped they could help her through this latest dilemma. After all, baby Tony was only nursing in the mornings, evenings, and occasionally in the night. She did not feel this was excessive.

She also hoped she would survive her adolescent children's eating habits. Joey seemed never to find time to eat except when Nanna made sure he did. His school activities always seemed to interfere with mealtimes. She wondered to herself if there was anything wrong, as he just didn't seem to have a normal appetite for a teenaged boy. She was sure wrestling had a negative impact on how much he would eat. Although his appetite did pick up after a wrestling match. And Anna seemed to be trying to starve herself in her attempt to lose weight.

INTRODUCTION

Although the rapid growth that occurs prenatally and during infancy slows in childhood and only later picks up in adolescence, developmental changes are rapid. From learning to walk to climbing trees, from uttering first words to chattering nonstop and monopolizing phone lines, from being totally dependent to growing into independence, the changes that take place from early childhood to adolescence are truly remarkable.

Nutrition plays a key role in this process. Sources of food that provide good nutrition change throughout the period of childhood. Breast-feeding may continue for the first few years. Some young children need to rely on bottle use beyond the first year, although this is generally discouraged ow-

▲ T A B L E   1 7 – 1

AGE-RELATED CHILDHOOD FOOD GUIDELINES

AGES (YEARS)	FOOD SUGGESTIONS
1 to 2	Provide plain, simple finger foods Place small amounts on the plate (about 1 tbsp of each food for each year of child's age) Provide cups with handles that do not tip easily, large-handled silverware, and plates with edges (for pushing food against) Trust child's hunger cues, as appetite can vary from day to day
2 to 3	Encourage the "one-taste" rule to expose children to new foods but do not force child to eat Make mealtimes pleasant and enjoyable Offer structured food choices to allow for a growing sense of independence Recognize that "food jags" (eating the same food day after day) is common at this age and beyond Continue to increase the variety of foods offered
3 to 5	Begin to include the child in food shopping (the young child can recognize numbers on food labels; give guidelines such as cereals with less than 6 grams sugar per serving) Include child in simple cooking techniques such as stirring and pouring Avoid using food as a bribe or as a reward Continue to increase the variety of foods offered
5 to 10	Continue to provide breakfast, which is especially important for better school performance Help child categorize foods into groups of the Food Guide Pyramid Be sensitive to the effects of food advertising; help the child understand that many foods advertised are high in fat and sugar
10 to 18	Recognize that increased body fat often precedes puberty Be sensitive to the influence of friends on food and beverage choices Provide information on healthy food choices at fast food restaurants and for snacks Help child find time to eat breakfast and to eat around sports and school events

ing to concerns of dental health. The texture of foods becomes increasingly more solid as the child develops the full ability to chew. Peer pressure becomes more of a deciding factor in food choices as childhood advances (Table 17–1).

The human body is a complex system that includes the control of satiety. If a parent or caregiver trusts this physiological hunger system and learns to distinguish feeding cues of young infants, appropriate food intake can continue through later years. By understanding the psychology of eating, the trials and tribulations of preschooler food jags and adolescent food avoidances can be overcome in a positive manner. Short-term solutions never outweigh long-term consequences. Forcing a child to eat a vegetable today can result in an adult who never again eats that same food. Eating is part of socialization. Eating nutritious foods helps the full potential of heredity to be realized.

WHAT IS MEANT BY GROWTH AND DEVELOPMENT?

Growth is the increase with age in weight and height, or *size* as it is popularly designated, that comes about as a result of the multiplication of cells and their differentiation for many different functions in the body. Growth is a continuous but not uniform process from conception to full maturity. During fetal life and infancy, the rate of growth is very rapid. This period is followed by one of slower growth during early and middle childhood. Another period of very rapid growth occurs during adolescence, followed by a tapering off until the growth period ends.

Development refers to the increasing ability of body parts to function. For example, being able to use a knife and fork successfully is a fine-motor skill that is age-dependent (see Table 17–1). Factors affecting the rate of growth and development include heredity, or inborn capacity to grow, and environment. An extremely important environmental factor is nutrition. Better diets, which accompany improved economic conditions, are credited for the taller stature of children and adults in the United States today. Adults were significantly smaller in past decades. In technologically advanced countries, the average height and weight of children of any given age have increased over the last 100 years, which is evidence that well nourished children reach the potential set by their heredity, not only in physical growth but also in mental development.

WHAT IS THE IMPORTANCE OF NUTRITION TO HEALTHY GROWTH AND DEVELOPMENT?

Without an adequate supply of nutrients, optimal growth and development to adulthood would not be possible. Nutrients supplied by food that the child consumes provide energy and the necessary building blocks for synthesis of new tissues. Foods for growth include those in the three lower levels of the Food Guide Pyramid.

Breast milk can continue to provide good nutrition for several years. Breast milk is a source of protein as well as calcium and other nutrients needed for good growth. With the ample food supply in the United States, the nutritional component of breast-feeding is secondary to the emotional needs provided by close contact with the mother in the older years. All children will eventually become weaned (stop nursing or using the bottle) without assistance (see Chapter 16 for weaning guidelines).

Brain growth stops in early childhood, but other important organs continue to grow. Although the weight of the child (specifically **adipose tissue**—body fat) is more affected by the total quantity of kilocalories consumed, **bone growth** (the growth that occurs in length and thickness of bones) and **lean tissue** (muscle) growth are affected by both the quantity and quality of the diet. Parents should strive for a high-quality diet as well as an adequate quantity of foods. Cookies and cupcakes alone do not make a strong child.

Every child is different in his or her nutrient requirements based on factors such as chronological age, individual growth rate, stage of maturation, level of physical activity, and the efficiency of absorption and utilization of nutrients. There are guidelines, such as recommended dietary allowances (RDAs) and the Food Guide Pyramid, that give general indications of needed nutrients for growth. Growth charts are another important tool (see Appendix 13). If the child's growth is appropriate, it can be generally assumed that nutritional intake is adequate. Health problems unrelated to growth can occur, for example, anemia (as discussed later). Health problems can lead to poor growth.

Since the human is a social being, appropriate interaction is important for growth and development. Food often serves as a social link, such as at mealtimes. Children should eat as part of a family unit, ideally at the table. Eating with others can stimulate appetite and reinforce that eating is a pleasurable experience.

FACT & FALLACY

FALLACY: All children should take a multivitamin and mineral supplement.

FACT: Although commercial vitamin and mineral supplements contain much of what is needed for good health, food contains even more. A balanced diet consisting of a variety of foods is more likely to supply all the necessary nutrients for growth and repair than a vitamin preparation will. In addition to being unnecessary most of the time (and therefore a waste of money), excess vitamin intake can be fatal. If a parent feels safer giving vitamins, he or she should make sure that the content does not exceed 100 per cent of the RDA.

WHICH CHILDREN ARE AT HIGH RISK OF UNDERNUTRITION?

Children at high risk of undernutrition or inadequate food intake are:

- from low-income families
- those with special health care needs
- those whose primary caregiver is mentally ill or drug- or alcohol-dependent (Splett and Story, 1991).

WHAT ARE THE EFFECTS OF MALNUTRITION ON GROWTH AND DEVELOPMENT, LEARNING, AND BEHAVIOR?

Children who do not get enough to eat and are malnourished tend to be smaller and are more likely to become ill than well fed children. They also may be less able to learn. The extent to which malnutrition occurs in the United States means that many children will not be able to achieve their full potential. For developing nations worldwide, in which children may constitute a large percentage of the population, malnutrition may constrain the country's future social and economic development.

A prolonged lack of one or more nutrients retards physical development or causes specific clinical conditions to appear. For example, anemia, goiter,

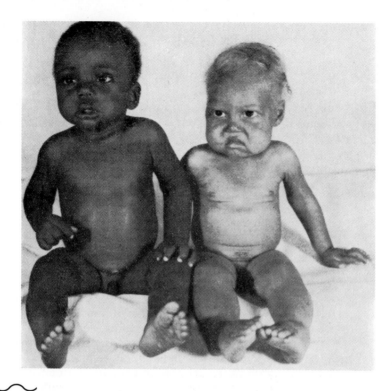

▲ FIGURE 17-1

Right, Infant with "sugar baby" kwashiorkor, attributed to a high-sugar, low-protein diet. The infant has stunted growth, edema of the feet and hands, fatty liver, moon face, and dyspigmentation of the skin and hair. *Left,* normal infant. (From Jelliffe DB: Hypochromotrichia and malnutrition in Jamaican infants. J Trop Pediatr 1955; 1:25; by permission of Oxford University Press.)

and rickets reflect a state of malnutrition. Severe malnutrition, which is characterized by clinical manifestations, is of two basic types: *kwashiorkor* (protein deficiency) (Fig. 17-1) and *marasmus* (overall deficit of food, especially kilocalories; also known as PEM—Protein Energy Malnutrition) (Fig. 17-2). Kwashiorkor generally occurs at or after weaning, when milk high in protein is replaced by a starchy staple food providing insufficient protein. A child with this type of malnutrition usually has stunted growth and edema, skin sores, and discoloration of dark hair to red or blond. Infantile marasmus is frequently the result of early cessation of breast-feeding, overdilution of formula, or gastrointestinal infection early in life, and it is accompanied by wasting of tissues and extreme growth retardation. See Chapter 3 for a more detailed discussion of kwashiorkor and marasmus.

Undernourished children are identified most often by biochemical and clinical signs, but the value of these signs is limited to identifying an extremely inadequate diet. Chronic long-term undernutrition generally results in stunting of growth (Fig. 17-3). The degree of malnutrition is often proportional to the degree to which the child is subnormal in height or weight.

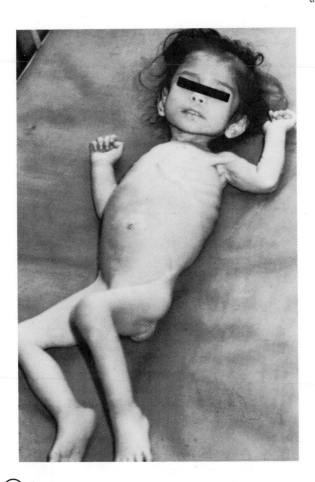

▲ FIGURE 17-2

Marasmus in a child 2 years and 4 months old. (From
Cotran RS, Kumar V, Robbins SL: Robbins Pathologic Basis
of Disease, 4th ed. Philadelphia, WB Saunders, 1989.)

Therefore, anthropometric measurements (height, weight, and amount of
fat; see Chapter 7 for more on anthropometrics) are the most commonly
used indices of undernutrition.

Types of moderate malnutrition include (1) that caused by chronic food
reduction (manifested by growth retardation) and (2) that resulting from vitamin or mineral deficiency and accompanied by clinical symptoms such as
rickets or pellagra. Malnutrition is most often associated with poverty resulting from a **food distribution system** (how food is allocated to the
world's population) that is based on purchasing power. Exact determination
of the effect on the individual is difficult, since other factors influence human growth and behavioral development, including individual innate potential, health status, and environment.

In the United States, three of the extensive surveys of nutritional status
conducted in recent years have reached similar conclusions: Marasmus and

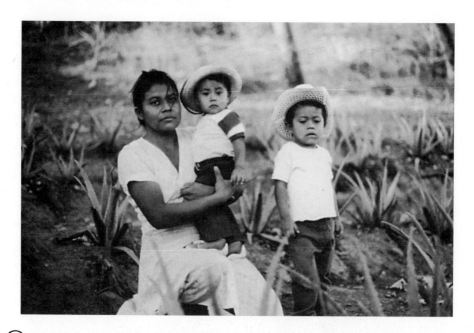

▲ FIGURE 17-3

Stunting (severe growth failure in height) is common in Guatemalan children. (From Nutrition Today, Jan/Feb., 1993; p. 11. Photo credit: Margarita de Martinez.)

kwashiorkor are quite rare, but chronic undernutrition and iron deficiency are surprisingly common. A child's growth record is a more accurate measure of whether a child is receiving sufficient nutrients than are RDAs because the gross estimates of nutritional needs are not designed to assess an individual's nutritional status.

Malnutrition impairs the body's defense against disease. Therefore infection, which is rampant in underdeveloped regions of the world because of poor sanitary conditions, occurs more frequently in malnourished children. Very severe malnutrition in infancy, if of long duration and followed by childhood undernutrition, produces irreversible effects in behavior, which in turn can impair a child's ability to learn.

WHY IS IRON-DEFICIENCY ANEMIA SO COMMON AMONG CHILDREN?

Young children are particularly susceptible to iron-deficiency anemia because of the rapid use of iron during growth and the difficulty in obtaining adequate iron from the diet. Other reasons include blood loss and parasites. Lead poisoning is associated with iron-deficiency anemia (see Chapter 5). Teenaged girls are at an increased risk of anemia because of the start of menstruation, the rapid growth of adolescence, and not enough iron in their diets.

In regard to diet, children often find eating meat difficult. This may be because it is too tough from being overcooked (meat cooked at low tempera-

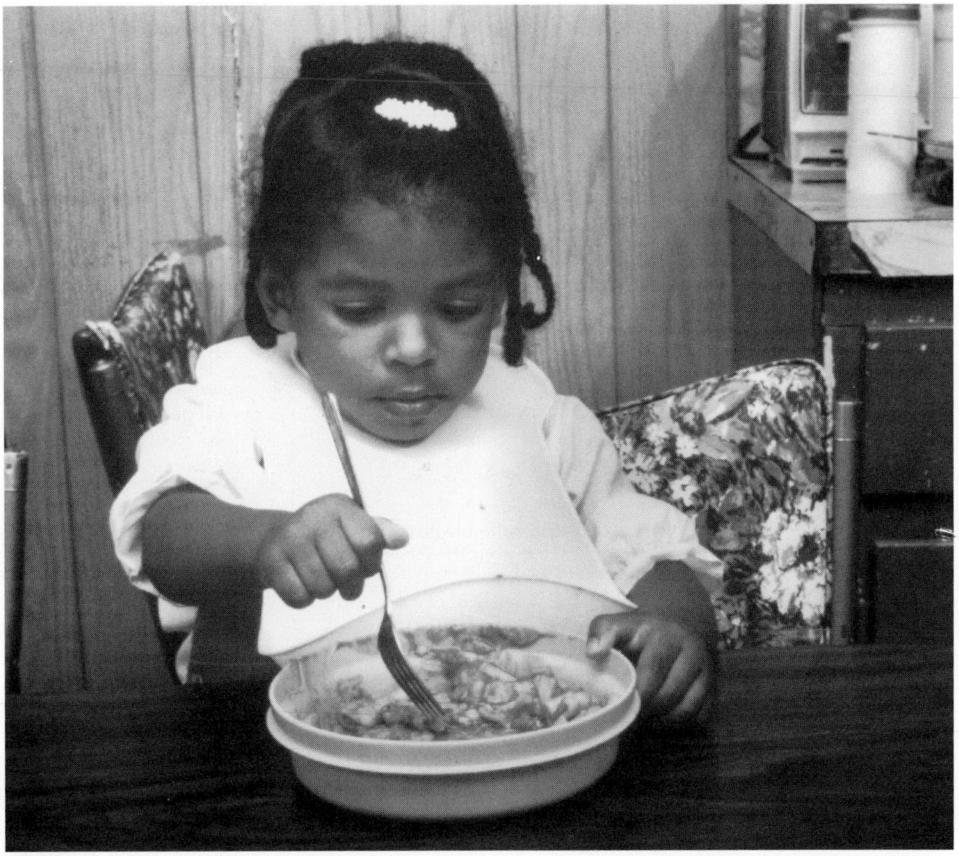

▲ FIGURE 17-4

Pasta is a favorite dish of young children. (Courtesy of Cornell University Photography, Ithaca, NY 1993.)

tures using moist methods, such as in stews, is more tender), because they have not acquired a taste for it (such as with liver), or because the family avoids it for economic, religious, moral, or other reasons. Pasta dishes are favorites of young children but are low in iron (Fig. 17-4).

Prevention of Iron-
Deficiency Anemia

Aside from increased meat intake, other foods that are high in iron should be consumed freely. As noted in Chapter 5, the iron found in meat, referred to as heme iron, is well absorbed, whereas other food sources of iron (called nonheme iron) need to be eaten with a vitamin C food in order to enhance absorption. For example, iron-fortified cereal sweetened with molasses (a source that is naturally high in iron) followed by a glass of orange juice or other food high in vitamin C will greatly enhance the absorption of iron (see Chapter 5 for other iron sources and Table 17-2 for other vitamin C sources).

▲ TABLE 17-2

HOME-PACKED SCHOOL LUNCH IDEAS

Choose one food or a combination of foods from each group to meet one third of the RDA

Vitamin A ½ cup or equivalent	Vitamin C ½ cup or equivalent
Apricot or apricot nectar	Cabbage (for coleslaw)
Broccoli (raw florets)*	Cauliflower (raw florets)
Cantaloupe*	Grapefruit or juice
Carrot sticks or juice	Orange or juice
Peaches	Strawberrries
Spinach (raw for a salad)*	Tangelo or juice
Sweet potato (as in a pudding)	Tangerine or juice
Tomato slices, juice, or soup*	
Watermelon (½ slice)*	

Protein 1 oz or ¼ cup or equivalent	Calcium 1 cup or equivalent
Any meat, chicken, or fish	Milk
Peanut butter	Yogurt
Egg (hard-cooked or egg salad)	Hard cheese (1 oz)
Cottage cheese	Cottage cheese
Hard cheese	Cream soup
(Meat and peanut butter are also high in iron and B vitamins)	(These foods are also high in protein and vitamins D and B_2)

Other foods are important, for example, whole-grain or enriched white flour products such as muffins, graham crackers, bread, noodles, rice, or pasta and other foods, for variety and to contribute other essential nutrients.

* Also contributes one third of the RDA for vitamin C.

Diagnosis and Treatment of Iron-Deficiency Anemia

Since iron-deficiency anemia continues to be a major health problem in the United States, there is widespread screening among children (particularly children from low-income families, who tend to have difficulty obtaining adequate amounts of iron in their diets). Programs such as the Well Child Clinic (operated out of Public Health Departments), the Women, Infants, and Children Supplemental Nutrition Program (WIC), and other programs commonly screen for iron-deficiency anemia using either the test for **hemoglobin** (the part of the blood that carries oxygen and is rich in iron) or the test for **hematocrit** (the amount of packed red blood cells) values.

Controversy exists regarding the blood levels that constitute iron-deficiency anemia. Generally, hemoglobin values greater than 12 g/dL and hematocrit values greater than 37 per cent are considered normal. Hemoglobin readings of less than 11 g/dL and hematocrit readings of less than 33 per cent should be evaluated further, and complete blood counts will often show low transferrin saturation levels (transferrin is an important constituent of red blood cell formation). Hemoglobin values of less than 10 g/dL (which is roughly equivalent to a hematocrit value of less than 30 per cent) are signs of iron-deficiency anemia and require immediate medical attention with iron supplementation. A test dose of iron may be used to help determine if anemia is due to iron deficiency. Increased focus on dietary intake of iron is also imperative to help resolve the anemia and prevent future episodes.

IS CHILDHOOD OBESITY RELATED TO ADULT OBESITY?

Obesity in children by itself is not predictive of adult obesity. However, it does tend to run in families and most children of obese parents tend to be overweight. While the increased rate of childhood obesity is an important public health issue, the lack of predictable variables in determining correlation with adult obesity and the lack of successful weight loss methods indicate that caution should be used in trying to treat childhood obesity (McNutt, 1991).

Great care needs to be taken to ensure that an overweight child's self-esteem is not damaged in attempting to control weight gain. A positive approach with emphasis on good nutritional choices can be helpful. However, care needs to be used to avoid labeling foods as good or bad. The reasons behind weight gain should be assessed, such as inactivity (excess television watching) or eating for emotional reasons. The reasons behind the obesity need to be assessed and addressed rather than simply giving a diet sheet for weight loss (see Chapter 20).

IS HYPERACTIVITY RELATED TO NUTRITION?

There is a widespread belief that sugar and food additives cause hyperactivity among children, although research has shown this to be generally false. Food additives may cause hyperactivity, but this is rare and is felt to be limited to children who are allergic to the additives. Sugar may actually slow a child down through its role in the production of serotonin in the brain. Often a very active child is falsely labeled as being hyperactive (see Chapter 15). Part of the public's confusion with the belief that sugar causes hyperactivity is that often sweets coincide with stimulating activities such as school recess, birthday parties, or holidays (at which time the activity or excitement, and not the sugar, causes excess activity).

WHAT ARE IMPORTANT CONSIDERATIONS IN FEEDING THE PRESCHOOL-AGED CHILD (1 TO 5 YEARS OLD)?

As children grow, their eating habits change. These changes are reflective of their stage in development. Among toddlers, finger foods are a favorite (see Table 17–1 and Fig. 17–5). When compared with the infant, the preschool-aged child experiences a slowing rate of growth and development. A decrease in the consumption of food parallels this decrease in metabolic rate. A parent should not become alarmed if the following changes in eating behavior occur; rather, these changes are considered normal for the preschool child:

- wanting foods plain with no sauces and not mixed together
- varying interest and lack of interest in food, with appetites up and down
- **food jags**—eating only a few foods day after day or week after week until the next food jag starts

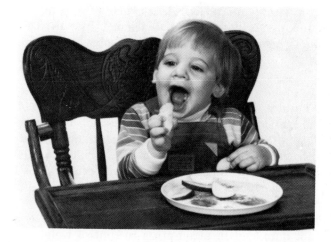

▲ F I G U R E   1 7 – 5

Finger foods are popular among preschool children.

WHAT ARE IMPORTANT CONSIDERATIONS IN FEEDING THE PRESCHOOL-AGED CHILD (1 TO 5 YEARS OLD)?

Keeping a record of food portions may help to allay parents' fears that their child is not eating enough. Being able to see the whole day or a whole week very often makes it apparent that the child is eating the recommended food servings of the Food Guide Pyramid. This knowledge, along with comparison of the child's growth with a growth chart, can be very helpful in calming parents' fears of nutritional inadequacy. A healthy appearance in children is further evidence of good nutritional status (Fig. 17–6).

If the child's diet does appear to be lacking in a food group that is affecting growth, offering previously omitted foods at the times when the child is most hungry can help. Food acceptance may take time and patience with children. A child may need to be exposed to the food on several occasions before deciding that the food is worth eating. Seeing the food in the grocery store or being prepared in the kitchen and a small portion served on the plate all help. The use of choice also helps.

For example, a parent might ask, "Would you like your carrots cooked or grated?" Or "Would you like your carrots on this side of the plate or this other side?" By being given a choice, children can gain a sense of control over their environment. Children should never be forced to eat.

Preschool-aged children seem to prefer foods that are simply prepared. Mixed foods are generally unpopular with this age group. Differences in

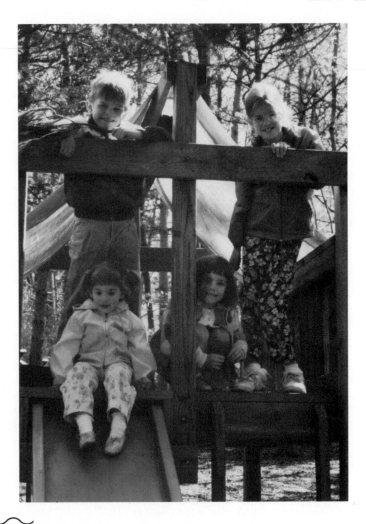

▲ FIGURE 17-6

Healthy children love to play.

food textures interest children. Each meal might include something soft (such as macaroni and cheese), something chewy/crunchy (such as pineapple chunks), and something dry (such as peas).

Mealtime needs to be a pleasant experience in order for the child to develop positive eating attitudes and behaviors. The atmosphere should be relaxed and conducive to pleasant conversation. The child should be equipped with eating utensils and dishes that are easy to handle. The child should be offered only small amounts of food at a time. Even giving one bite of each food served, with second or third helpings allowed, can stimulate a child's interest in eating, in part because of feelings of accomplishment and control. By eating with the family, children are likely to develop an interest in food that mirrors that of their parents. By the age of 4 or 5 years, the child may be able to dish food onto a plate in accordance with his or her appetite. Being forced to eat may encourage a habit of overeating or may even lead to undereating if the child perceives that he or she is eating only to please the parents instead of eating for his or her own pleasure and needs.

Snacks should be planned to enhance the nutritional value of the diet (Table 17–3). They should be served at least 1 hour before the meal to allow sufficient intake of food at mealtime. However, sometimes a compromise is needed if the child is very hungry. Consider a premeal snack to be an appetizer before dinner. Good choices might include a dish of applesauce or yogurt, both nutritious choices for the young child.

For a guide to the foods that should be included and amounts that should be provided for the preschool-aged child, see Table 17–4. Good food habits developed at this time will help ensure an adequate diet throughout life.

FACT & FALLACY

FALLACY: Once a picky eater, always a picky eater!

FACT: It takes time for food likes to develop. Many foods are not liked when first tried, but with repeated exposure in a positive environment, even the most finicky eaters can learn to appreciate a wide variety of foods. Children should be encouraged to have one taste of all foods served but beyond that, forcing or begging a child to eat has no place in the development of long-term food preferences. It may be helpful for the anxious parent to remember that the parent's responsibility is to offer nutritious foods in a positive meal setting, but that it is the child's responsibility to determine how much and what he or she eats (Satter, 1987). Children seem to eat better if they perceive they are eating because it makes them feel good and not simply to please their parents.

WHAT ARE SOME NUTRITION ISSUES IN THE PROCESS OF GROWTH AND DEVELOPMENT?

A Growing Sense of Independence Among Preschoolers

Promoting Sound Food Values

A growing sense of independence occurs naturally in preschoolers. Parents will be well advised to offer the preschooler structured choices to allow for a sense of independence. This applies to food as well as to other daily activities (for example, "Are you going to put on your shoes or am I?"). Recognition of this facet of the growing child can foster positive parent-child interaction and healthy food selection. A structured food choice at the dinner table might be, "Would you like an apple or a banana for dessert?" A structured food choice at the super market might be to allow the child a choice of cereals with less than 6 grams (1.5 teaspoons) of sugar.

The manner in which food is offered is fundamental to the development of interest in a variety of nutritious foods. If you reflect for a moment on the

▲ TABLE 17-3

SUGGESTED SNACKS AND FINGER FOODS

Fruits
- Apple wedges
- Banana slices
- Berries
- Dried apples
- Dried apricots
- Dried peaches
- Dried pears
- Fresh peach wedges
- Fresh pear wedges
- Fresh pineapple sticks
- Grapefruit sections (seeded)
- Grapes
- Melon cubes or balls
- Orange sections (seeded)
- Pitted plums
- Pitted prunes
- Raisins
- Tangerine sections

Vegetables
- Cabbage wedges
- Carrot sticks
- Cauliflower florets
- Celery sticks*
- Cherry tomatoes
- Cucumber slices
- Green pepper sticks
- Tomato wedges
- Turnip sticks
- Zucchini or summer squash strips

Meats and Meat Substitutes
- Cheese cube
- Cooked meat cubes
- Hard-cooked eggs
- Small sandwiches (quartered)
- Toast fingers
- Whole-grain crackers

* May be stuffed with cheese or peanut butter.
From U.S. Department of Agriculture: A Planning Guide for Food Service in Child Care Centers, FNS-64. Food and Nutrition Service, Washington, DC.

types of holiday foods promoted, such as chocolate on Valentine's Day and candy at Halloween, you will quickly realize the value our society places on food. However, it is possible to promote nutritious foods. Kiwi fruit might be offered in Easter baskets and dried fruit at Halloween.

One woman captured this idea well. When the wide variety of vegetables her children liked was commented on, her reply was, "Do you know how I did it? Whenever I offered a reward I would say, 'If you are good you can have a vegetable!'" Rewarding with food is not recommended, especially as it is often done with candy. Rewarding with vegetables in this scenario, however, allowed the children to develop a strong appreciation for a healthy food group.

Parents are the most effective nutrition educators of their children. They teach by example and by attitude (Worsham, 1991). Parents should be encouraged to promote positive food choices in an enjoyable manner.

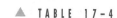

▲ T A B L E 1 7 – 4

PATTERN OF FEEDING

MEAL	CHILDREN 1 TO 3 YEARS	CHILDREN 3 TO 6 YEARS
Breakfast		
Milk, fluid*	½ cup	¾ cup
Juice or fruit	¼ cup	½ cup
Cereal or bread, enriched or whole-grain† cereal or bread	¼ cup‡	⅓ cup§
	½ slice	½ slice
Midmorning or Midafternoon Supplement		
Milk, fluid* or juice or fruit or vegetable	½ cup	½ cup
Bread or cereal, enriched or whole-grain† bread or	½ slice	½ slice
cereal	¼ cup‡	⅓ cup§
Lunch or Supper		
Milk, fluid*	½ cup	¾ cup
Meat or meat alternate¶		
Meat, poultry, or fish, cooked **	1 oz	1½ oz
Cheese	1 oz	1½ oz
Egg	1	1
Cooked dry beans and peas	⅛ cup	¼ cup
Peanut butter	1 tbsp	2 tbsp
Vegetables and fruits††	¼ cup	½ cup
Bread, enriched or whole-grain†	½ slice	½ slice

* Includes whole milk, low-fat milk, skim milk, cultured buttermilk, or flavored milk made from these types of fluid milk, which meet state and local standards.
† Or an equivalent serving of an acceptable bread product made of enriched or whole-grain meal or flour.
‡ ¼ cup (volume) or ⅓ ounce (weight), whichever is less.
§ ⅓ cup (volume) or ½ ounce (weight), whichever is less.
¶ Or an equivalent quantity of any combination of foods listed under Meat and Meat Alternates.
** Cooked lean meat without bone.
†† Must include at least two kinds.
From U.S. Department of Agriculture: A Planning Guide for Food Service Child Care Centers, FNS-64. Food and Nutrition Service, Washington, DC, p. 5.

FACT & FALLACY

FALLACY: Once a sweet tooth, always a sweet tooth.
FACT: Children whose diets are continually high in sugar can lose their ability to appreciate the natural taste of foods. As with salt and other substances, the taste for sweetness can be both learned and unlearned. Gradual reduction in quantities used is the easiest and surest way to overcome a "sweet tooth."

Coping with Food Advertisements

Since many television or written advertisements promote foods that are not very nutritious (when was the last time you saw an ad for broccoli?), children need to be empowered to resist the negative messages. One approach is to divide food into two categories: foods that help you grow and those that do not; or foods that make you grow tall versus those that make you grow wide. This approach can help the child appreciate that the adult is being helpful by providing nutritious foods that are not advertised on television.

Working Mothers

Two parents working or single mothers working can put added stress on mealtime. Finding time to prepare meals and to offer meals in a relaxed, positive manner can be difficult. However, there is some evidence that nutrient intake is not directly related to maternal employment status (Johnson et al., 1992).

WHAT ARE THE IMPORTANT CONSIDERATIONS IN FEEDING SCHOOL-AGED CHILDREN (5 TO 11 YEARS OLD)?

Meeting the nutritional requirements of the 5- to 11-year-old child takes larger amounts of the same foods needed by the preschool-aged child. Growth during prepuberty is slow and steady, with gradual increases in height and weight.

With the introduction of school into the child's daily routine, the child's meal pattern is likely to change. Breakfast may have to be eaten earlier to allow sufficient time to get to school. Children who skip breakfast are less well fed, since it is difficult to make up missed nutrients at other meals. If the family has good breakfast habits, the child will likely continue this practice. The child may be taught to prepare a simple but nutritious breakfast. Parents should eat breakfast with their children, even if it is only 5 minutes for eating a quick bowl of non–sugar-coated cereal.

At school, the child is introduced to group feeding. Peers and teachers may influence eating behavior, and the child may be more or less willing to try an unfamiliar food, depending on the eating behavior of others in the group. A child who has been exposed to a wide variety of foods at home is more likely to try new foods at school or at a friend's house.

Whether the child brings a lunch prepared at home or buys lunch from the National School Lunch Program, it should supply approximately one third of the RDA for all nutrients (see table inside front cover). Nutrition education may occur at school through such means as cooking and identifying foods. Ideally, this food exposure at school should positively promote sound food choices without labeling foods as good or bad.

HOW DO THE CHANGES OF ADOLESCENCE AFFECT EATING PATTERNS?

Although children may be best friends and equals in elementary school, the onset of adolescence creates vast differences. One girl may become voluptuous by junior high school, whereas another girl still has her "baby fat" and another is concerned she is too thin and underdeveloped (Fig. 17–7). Girls especially tend to increase their amount of body fat just prior to puberty and their "growth spurt" (the time of increased long-bone growth). Their male peers, who do not reach puberty as early and retain their boyish frames, may begin to question their masculinity. Eventually boys catch

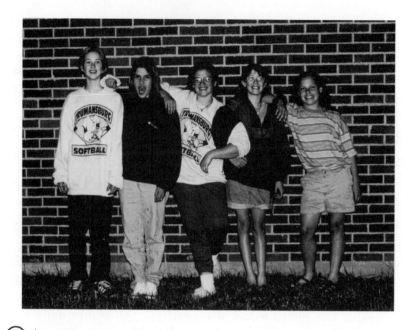

▲ FIGURE 17-7

A group of seventh grade friends shows their differences in growth and developmental stages.

up to the girls with increased muscle mass and long-bone growth. All this is happening as the adolescent's face begins to look like a war zone covered with acne—or so it is perceived even if there is only one pimple. All of these changes are hormonally related.

Intense concern with nutritional intake develops as a consequence of these changes, but too often in a negative way. Some teenagers try weight-control diets either to lose their baby fat or to regain a sense of control over their rapidly changing bodies. This can result in conditions such as anorexia and bulimia (see Chapter 15). Others ignore sound nutritional practices (such as eating potato chips in place of fruits or drinking soft drinks or even beer in place of milk) in order to feel accepted among their peers. The need for a sense of self-worth and of identity can take priority over good nutritional practices.

Other barriers adolescents encounter in good nutritional intake include the following:

1. *Society's emphasis on slimness.* Television advertisements now promote "the perfect size 6." Women still aspire to the 19-inch waists once common among 19th-century women, who achieved their hourglass figures by wearing tight-laced corsets. We tend to forget that we are 20th-century women who are taller and proportionally larger than our earlier counterparts. Good nutrition can suffer, particularly among female adolescents, in the attempt to achieve this unrealistic image.

2. *Access to jobs and spending money.* This allows the adolescent greater freedom in purchasing food as well as restricting the time to eat, since teenagers often dash to part-time work directly from school. Fast food outlets are a common lure for this population. Adolescents' sense of immortality can overshadow their knowledge of the importance of good nutrition, which can result in an increased intake of fat and sugar.

3. *More time spent away from home.* Adolescents are increasingly in a position to determine what or if they eat. This, coupled with adolescent rebellion, can result in their consuming the opposite of what they know they should.

4. *Alcohol as a rite of passage.* Alcohol increasingly becomes an issue for teenagers. Television advertising can lure them into thinking that alcohol, such as beer, brings with it fun and glamour. Alcohol used by teenagers can make them feel more adult and independent. Many teenagers regularly drink beer and wine. Alcoholism occurs in teenagers. Alcohol can seriously impair the final stages of growth and development by replacing foods or more nutritious beverages such as milk and juice. Chronic alcohol intake can impair the body's ability to absorb and use food nutrients.

What Are the Nutritional Requirements of the Adolescent (12 to 18 Years Old)?

During the rapid growth period of adolescence, calorie and nutrient needs are higher to provide for increases in bone density, muscle mass, and blood volume and for the developing endocrine system. There is an increased need for kilocalories, calcium, iron, and iodine (see table inside front cover). Nutrient needs can be met easily by increasing the serving size or number of servings, as recommended in the Food Guide Pyramid. (The maximum number of servings in this guide will meet most adolescents' nutritional needs without promoting inappropriate weight gain.)

WHAT IS THE ROLE OF THE NURSE OR OTHER HEALTH CARE PROFESSIONAL IN PROMOTING GOOD NUTRITION DURING CHILDHOOD?

For Children

The terminology used with children needs to be concrete and nonscientific. Abstract concepts cannot be understood, such as the role of nutrients in foods, even though a young child can pronounce the words. Therefore, it is more appropriate to focus on promoting positive attitudes toward eating nutritious foods. Children can appreciate the concept that eating is fun, and this concept should be applied to nutritious foods. One method that strongly appeals to children (and even to the parents who may be present) is the use of puppet shows. Stick puppets are made easily with food pictures, and with the addition of paper eyes and mouths they "come alive." Children's books such as "Green Eggs and Ham," or "Stone Soup" can also favorably influence a child's willingness to try new foods.

For Teenagers

A sensitive approach to teenagers' needs, recognizing their need for autonomy and acceptance by their peers, should be used in counseling or educational settings. The use of appropriate humor can help the teenager to recognize that the health care professional is a caring human being, not

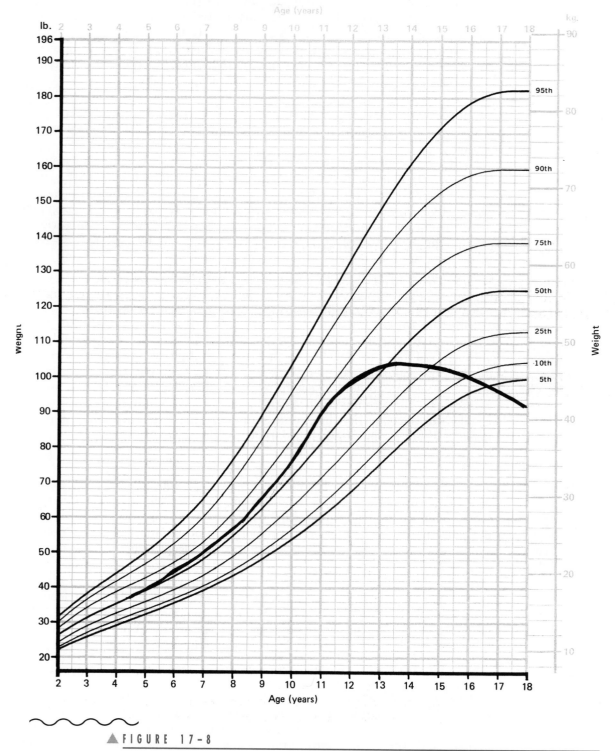

GIRLS FROM 2 TO 18 YEARS
WEIGHT FOR AGE

Age (years)

lb.

kg.

95th

90th

75th

50th

25th

10th

5th

Weight

Weight

Age (years)

▲ F I G U R E 1 7 – 8

Sample growth fall from normal curve as assessed using the weight-for-age chart for girls 2 to 18 years of age.

merely an authority figure. Comments should be positive ones that help promote positive self-worth and do not undermine a teenager's already fragile self-image. Teenagers should be told about realistic body perceptions and eating patterns such as those represented in growth charts and the Food Guide Pyramid.

Nutrition counseling is especially important for the teenager who has failed to develop good food habits up to this point and for the teenager who has strayed from previously good habits. Information should be presented in an interesting and motivating manner. Since teenagers are very interested in their physical appearance, it should be emphasized that adequate nutrients allow for optimal growth and development of their body. A teenaged girl who feels that she is overweight and starts to lose weight too rapidly can use a growth chart to gain a better sense of normalcy. This tool can be particularly helpful to a teenager with anorexia or bulimia when she can visualize her growth fall from the normal curve (Fig. 17–8). Although relatively rare, boys are also known to experience anorexia and bulimia (see Chapter 15).

It is important that the counselor respect the independence of the teenager. Presenting the adolescent with flexible eating styles instead of a rigid eating pattern will increase the effectiveness of counseling. Special problems of teenagers, such as obesity, alcoholism, anorexia nervosa, and pregnancy, should be an important focus of nutrition counseling, as should prevention of heart disease, cancer, diabetes, and other diseases that may occur later in life.

STUDY QUESTIONS AND ACTIVITIES

1. How would you explain the terms *growth* and *development?*
2. Should Maria Bernardo wean her toddler? Why or why not? What advice would be good for her? How does Nanna Bernardo's perception of the frequency of breast-feeding differ from Maria's? (You may want to refer back to the section on breast-feeding in Chapter 16.)
3. List all the reasons that a good breakfast is important from early childhood throughout life.
4. What suggestions could you give the Bernardos if they find it difficult to get their teenagers Anna and Joey to eat an adequate breakfast? To get one-year-old Tony to try new foods?
5. Plan three different adequate lunches the Bernardos could pack for their older children, based on the family shopping list described in the Chapter 3 case study.
6. What effects might be expected later in life from foods inadequate in quantity and quality during the growing period?

7. Why is it particularly important for an adolescent girl to have a nutritious diet? What are some barriers Anna Bernardo might face (refer to Chapter 6 case study)?

8. What issues would a young teenager face who has diabetes (refer back to Chapter 9)?

REFERENCES

Johnson RK, Smiciklas-Wright H, Crouter AC, Willits FK: Maternal employment and the quality of young children's diets: empirical evidence based on the 1987–1988 Nationwide Food Consumption Survey. Pediatrics, August 1992; 90 (Part 1):245–249.

McNutt K: Are we pickin' on the kids? Nutrition Today, May/June 1991; p. 43.

Satter EM: How to Get Your Kid to Eat . . . But Not Too Much. Palo Alto, Bull Publishing, 1987.

Splett PL, Story M: Child nutrition: Objectives for the decade. J Am Diet Assoc. 1991; 91(6):665.

Worsham L: Good nutrition can make the difference for your children. N C Med J. Sept 1991; 52(9):439–442.

NUTRITIONAL CARE OF THE DEVELOPMENTALLY DISABLED

CHAPTER
18

OBJECTIVES

After completing this chapter, you should be able to:
- Define developmental disability
- Describe specific nutritional problems and conditions of the developmentally disabled
- Discuss the role of each health care team member in feeding and weight control programs
- Discuss mealtime skills and feeding techniques in relation to eating problems

TERMS TO IDENTIFY

Autism
Cerebral palsy
Developmental disability
Down syndrome
Epilepsy

Hyperkinesis
Inborn errors of metabolism
Mental retardation
Neurological impairment

Prader-Willi syndrome
  (PWS)
Spasticity
Tongue thrust

A FAMILY'S PERSPECTIVE ON NUTRITION

Maria Bernado was thinking about her clients at work. Her job at the Developmental Disability Center was so rewarding. She loved working with Amy, the teenaged girl who had cerebral palsy. Even if she couldn't talk she knew how to do puzzles. Never ceased to amaze her, Maria thought to herself, that Amy could point out the puzzle piece before she herself could find one to fit. Maria also wondered about Frank and John, who always said good morning to her. Like adult children in some respects. She was sure they missed seeing her since she had been out on maternity leave. But she also knew they would be quick to forgive her for being gone so long. Exhausting but rewarding work. There was no doubt the Center's dietitian would be glad to see her back at work to help make sure Amy ate enough food.

INTRODUCTION

The developmentally disabled population is at nutritional risk because of feeding problems, food and drug interactions, altered growth patterns, and metabolic disorders. The maintenance and promotion of good nutritional status ultimately spare society an economic burden through facilitating independent living versus care through institutions. It also helps society realize a moral obligation to help ensure that all citizens are allowed the pursuit of a high-quality life.

Caregivers of persons with developmental disabilities have to deal with issues such as difficulty in understanding and implementing diet instructions, inappropriate feeding practices, lack of nutritional information, lack of knowledge regarding appropriate food selection and preparation, and difficulty in setting limits around food choices and amounts eaten (ADA Position Paper, 1992).

Appropriate nutrition programs and services can have a positive impact on the health of the developmentally disabled population by helping to prevent further disabilities, improving overall health and nutritional status, and maximizing educational, vocational, and social potential. "The spectrum of clinical nutrition services includes a) screening for nutrition-related problems; b) assessment of dietary practices, anthropometric data (using tools specific for the population), biochemical measures of nutrients, feeding skills, medications, and clinical examinations; c) planning and implementation of family-centered, community-based care plans; and d) monitoring the outcome of care plans and periodic reassessment of nutritional status" (ADA Position Paper, 1992). This chapter will address numerous disabilities and associated nutritional problems.

WHAT IS MEANT BY A DEVELOPMENTAL DISABILITY?

The term **developmental disability,** according to the Developmental Disabilities Assistance and Bill of Rights Act, refers to a severe, chronic disability that:

1. is attributable to a mental or physical impairment or a combination of mental and physical impairments;

2. is manifested before the person reaches the age of 22 years;

3. is likely to continue indefinitely;

4. results in substantial functional limitations in three or more of the following areas of major life activity: self-care, receptive and expressive language, learning, mobility, self-direction, capacity for independent living, and economic self-sufficiency;

5. reflects the person's need for a combination and sequence of special interdisciplinary or generic care, treatment, or other services that are lifelong or of extended duration and individually planned and coordinated.

The subcategories of developmental disabilities are **mental retardation** (a general term for a wide range of conditions resulting from many different causes, some of which are directly related to various diseases); **autism** (characterized by extreme withdrawal and an obsessive desire to maintain the present status; temper tantrums and language disturbances are evident); **cerebral palsy** (characterized by a persistent qualitative motor disorder caused by nonprogressive damage to the brain; may involve sensory

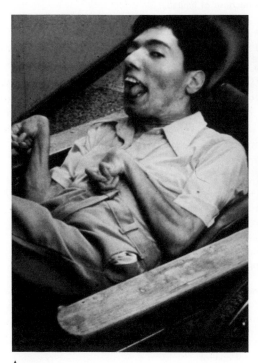
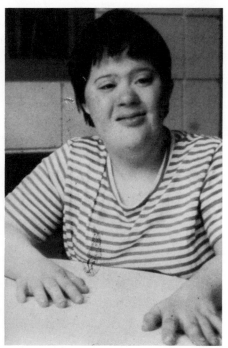

A   B

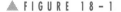

▲ FIGURE 18-1

A, Client with Down syndrome. *B,* Client with cerebral palsy. (Courtesy of Ross Laboratories, Columbus, OH.)

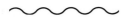

▲ T A B L E 1 8 - 1

DESCRIPTION AND NUTRITIONAL IMPLICATIONS OF SOME CONDITIONS

COMMON CHARACTERISTICS	NUTRITIONAL IMPLICATION
Down syndrome (caused by chromosomal abnormalities)	Chewing, swallowing, sucking and tongue control may be affected
Reduced muscle tone in varying degrees	Appetite and behovior at mealtime may be affected
Growth retardation:	Weight control
Small flattened skull	
Narrow nasal passage	
Delayed tooth development	Dental caries
Narrow palate	Eating problems
Cerebral Palsy	
Neuromuscular impairment:	Weight control
Motor disability	
Poor occlusion	Difficulties in chewing, swallowing, tongue control, and drooling
Types:	
Spastic: disharmony of muscle movements, overweight possible because of limited movement	
Athetoid: involuntary movements of extremities, underweight possible	
Ataxic: inability or awkwardness in maintaining balance	
Hypotonic: muscles to fail to respond to stimulation	
Hypersensitivity	Sensitivity to taste temperatures and consistency of food
Prader-Willi syndrome (endocrine, hypothalamic disorder)	
Hyperphagia	
Obesity	Weight control
Short stature	
Small hands and feet	
Hypogenitalism	
Mild mental retardation	
Bizarre eating behaviors (gorging, food stealing, eating inappropriate foods, e.g., pet food)	
Poor sucking ability and failure to thrive in infancy	Feeding difficulties in infancy
Rapid weight gain after 1 year of age	
Slow motor development	Dental caries
Obesity-related diabetes in later childhood	
Frequent lack of emotional control	

deficits and mental retardation; exhibits varying levels of **spasticity** [movements of the body]; Figure 18–1 shows individuals with cerebral palsy and Down syndrome); **epilepsy** (a group of symptoms or conditions that overstimulate nerve cells of the brain, resulting in seizures); and **neurological impairment** (involves sensory, mentation, and consciousness functions; Table 18–1).

<table>
<tr><td>

HOW IS THE NUTRITIONAL STATUS OF THE DEVELOPMENTALLY DISABLED INDIVIDUAL ASSESSED?

</td><td>

The same steps in the nutrition assessment process that were discussed in Chapters 2 and 7 are followed for the developmentally disabled population, but standard criteria are not yet available, thus making it more difficult to assess nutritional status. Growth charts, except in the case of **Down syndrome** (a genetic defect that consists of an extra gene and results in varying levels of retardation, short stature, and characteristic facial features; Fig. 18–1), have not been developed, and ways to determine dietary needs have not been clearly established. Height is used in determining energy needs of a child with developmental disabilities (Table 18–2).

</td></tr>
</table>

Weighing and measuring someone with bony deformities and severe contractures may be more difficult than it is for a normally developed person. Segmental measurements taken from joint to joint with a flexible metal tape are totaled, giving an approximate length, which is then plotted on a growth chart. Nonambulatory persons can be weighed in a sling-type balance such as a Hoyt lift (Fig. 18–2).

When assessing the nutritional status of the developmentally disabled individual, several areas are addressed by the dietitian, as shown in Figure 18–3. Figure 18–4 shows a flow chart for attaining nutritional goals. A detailed assessment is necessary if any of the following are present or suspected:

- unusual food habits
- inadequate or imbalanced dietary intake

▲ TABLE 18–2

ENERGY REQUIREMENT CHART FOR INDIVIDUALS WITH DISABILITIES

DIAGNOSIS	ENERGY REQUIREMENT
Cerebral Palsy (mild spasticity), 5–11 years old	13.9 kcal/cm
Cerebral Palsy (severe spasticity), 5–11 years old	11.1 kcal/cm
Down Syndrome, boys	16.1 kcal/cm
Down Syndrome, girls	14.3 kcal/cm

From Rhudy NT, Kristopher L., Miller A, Murphy P: Calculating Nutritional Requirements for Individuals with Disabilities. Morgantown, WV, Nutrition and Dietary Services, University Affiliated Center for Developmental Disabilities (UACDD).

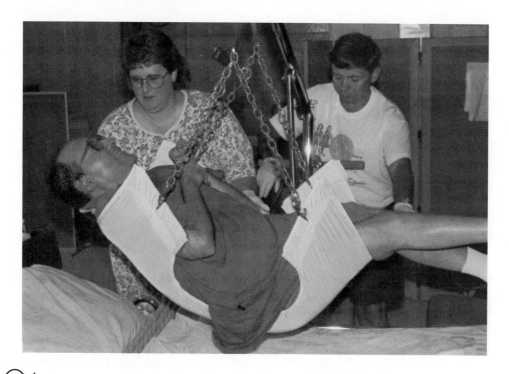

▲ FIGURE 18-2

Weighing a nonambulatory person in a Hoyt lift. (Courtesy of Tompkins Day Treatment Program, Broome Developmental Services, Ithaca, NY.)

- inadequate feeding skills
- problems with sucking, swallowing, or chewing
- marked overweight or underweight

WHAT ARE THE NUTRITION-RELATED PROBLEMS AND CONCERNS?

Eating Problems

Eating problems may result from neuromuscular dysfunction, obstructive lesions, psychological factors, or a combination of factors (ADA Position Paper, 1992). *Neuromuscular dysfunction* refers to abnormal sensory input and muscle tone and is manifested in sucking, swallowing, and chewing movements that are hampered when oral muscles do not function properly. When chewing reflexes are lacking, ways must be found to stimulate them. For example, sweet and cold foods are found to be effective. Also, the act of chewing stimulates saliva production and facilitates swallowing. Neuromuscular dysfunction is common in cerebral palsy, Down syndrome, and the Prader-Willi syndrome.

Anatomic defects and *malformations,* such as cleft palate, may cause food to pass into the nasal passages. Choking is a major concern in such a condition. Poor lip closure and tongue control, a strong bite reflex, tongue thrust, excessive drooling, choking, and delayed hand-to-mouth coordination are likely to cause inadequate nutrient intake. **Tongue thrust** is a term

SUBJECTIVE DATA

FOOD HABITS: _____

_____

FLUID INTAKE: _____
ACTIVITY/HABITS: _____

OBJECTIVE DATA

DIET RX:_____   DX: _____

_____   NUTRITION HX: _____

MEDICATIONS:_____

_____

_____

_____   AGE:_____ MALE/FEMALE HEIGHT:_____

BOWEL/BLADDER FUNCTION:_____   WEIGHT HX: _____

_____

LABORATORY VALUES: _____   WEIGHT:_____ DWR: _____

_____   PHYSICAL INDICATORS:_____

_____

_____

MEAL OBSERVATIONS:_____

_____

MEDICAL FACTORS AFFECTING NUTRITIONAL STATUS:_____

_____

_____

_____

_____

PHYSICAL LIMITATIONS:_____

_____

_____

_____

PROGRAM INFORMATION: _____

_____

SOCIAL/BEHAVIORAL:_____

_____

_____

SUMMARY OF CARE PLAN:_____

_____

_____

RECOMMENDATIONS:_____

_____

_____

_____

▲ FIGURE 18-3

Nutrition Assessment Form. (Courtesy of Broome Developmental Services, Ithaca, NY.)

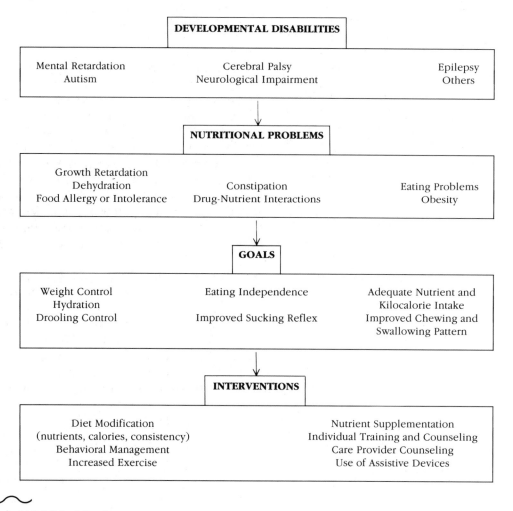

▲ FIGURE 18-4

Flow chart for attaining nutritional goals for the developmentally disabled population.

used to describe the condition in which the teeth are not brought together to initiate swallowing, the tongue pushes out saliva, and drooling occurs. It should be noted that special feeders are available for babies with anatomic defects and that surgery can largely correct cleft palate.

Just as a period of anxiety can cause gastric distress in the normally functioning population, *behavioral problems* such as tantrums, agitation, rocking, and flailing of arms (forms of self-stimulation) can result in esophagitis, aspiration of food, dehydration, and malnutrition in the developmentally disabled. Pica behavior (the ingestion of nonfood items) may cause malabsorption of certain nutrients or even intestinal blockage. Food stealing is another behavioral problem that often occurs in conditions such as the Prader-Willi syndrome.

Dental Problems

Poor oral hygiene or the inability to perform self-help skills, or both, as well as the excessive intake of sweets, result in dental caries. Certain medications can cause gum hyperplasia (especially anticonvulsants); therefore, good dental hygiene and regular checkups, as well as intake of foods that stimulate gums, should be encouraged. Sweet, sticky snacks should be discouraged and not used as rewards. Appropriate food reinforcers are sometimes needed, however, to help modify behavior (see later discussion).

Dental caries and periodontal disease are major problems. Suppressed immune function, drug therapy, oral motor dysfunction, and modified diets put the developmentally disabled person at high risk for oral infections. Three fourths of congenital anomalies affect the head and facial regions of the body. Cleft lip, cleft palate, misaligned jaws and teeth, and malocclusion can have a serious effect on speech, socialization, chewing ability, the enjoyment of eating, and nutritional status. The tissues of the oral cavity are all sensitive to nutrient imbalances. Caregivers are often so overwhelmed with medical, physical, psychological, and feeding concerns that regular home care is often neglected (Nutrition Focus, 1992).

To alleviate dental problems, sugar and sweets should be restricted and vegetable consumption encouraged. Soft foods and modified texture are necessary if gums are swollen and chewing is painful.

Individuals with Down syndrome have a normal size tongue, but because of their facial structure, the oral cavity is frequently too small to accommodate the tongue, which may have deep fissures that can retain food particles. Consequently, tongue brushing should be part of daily oral hygiene (Nutrition Focus, 1992).

Autistic children may pouch their food rather than swallow it and prefer soft foods that require little chewing. This puts them at greater risk for dental caries.

Growth Problems and Weight Disorders

Growth retardation, underweight, and obesity are common problems among developmentally disabled persons and require nutritional intervention. Nutritional factors influencing growth and weight abnormalities include

- inadequate dietary intake caused by feeding problems (such as oral abnormalities), reflux, or food scarcity;
- chronic conditions such as congenital heart disease that increase nutrient needs;
- lack of weight-bearing resulting from a disability that prevents mobility;
- metabolic disorders such as phenylketonuria and maple syrup urine disease;
- inability to absorb food, such as in celiac disease and galactosemia.

Excessive weight compounds the health problems already present. The goals of independent care and mobility are impaired with excess weight. Health care costs will be increased for those individuals requiring braces and wheelchairs if they have to be modified as weight increases. And, as in the general population, hypertension, diabetes, hyperlipidemia, and decreased pulmonary function may develop.

Persons with Down syndrome and the **Prader-Willi syndrome** (**PWS;** a genetic condition of unknown etiology) are frequently identified as being obese. Obesity is likely to occur whenever there is limited mobility, poor muscle tone, altered growth, lack of nutritional knowledge, hyperphagia, and feeding and eating problems, unless a preventive approach is taken by caregivers and parents. Unfortunately, some well-meaning people believe that food is the only source of enjoyment for those who are physically and mentally disabled. Such an attitude will only lead to more health problems.

People with PWS need fewer kilocalories than are normally required to maintain weight. The guidelines are 10 to 14 kilocalories per centimeter of height for weight maintenance and 7 to 8 kilocalories per centimeter of height for weight loss (Hoffman et al., 1992). Large, soft cage balls, Sitter-cize records, simple dance routines, and walks are all effective in promoting weight loss (Fig. 18–5). Kilocalorie needs are increased with **hyperkinesis** (excessive movement) and seizure activity. Persons with cerebral palsy, such as Amy in the opening case study, have very rigid muscles, which can increase kilocalorie needs.

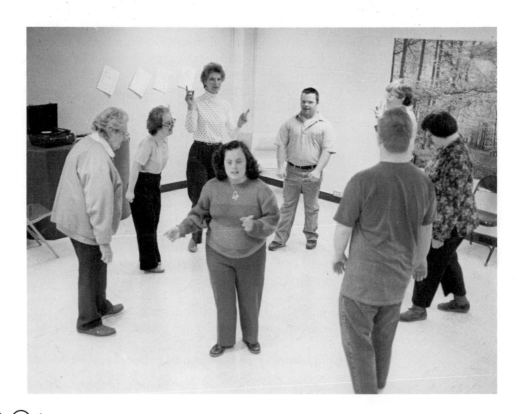

▲ F I G U R E   1 8 – 5

Clients exercising to promote weight loss in a simple dance routine. (Courtesy of Tompkins Day Treatment Program, Broome Developmental Services, Ithaca, NY.)

What Are Some
Common Drug-
Nutrient Interactions
in the Developmentally
Disabled?

Long-term drug therapy is frequently needed for controlling seizures, behavioral problems, recurrent infections, chronic constipation, and attention deficit disorders. The medications that are prescribed include anticonvulsants, central nervous system stimulants and depressants, and laxatives. These drugs may affect nutritional status in different ways (Pronsky, 1993).

Chronic use of anticonvulsants can result in abnormal nutrient and bone metabolism and gingival hyperplasia. These drugs may also result in folate deficiency and may increase serum iron levels and decrease serum ferritin. Therefore, consumption of dark green leafy vegetables, whole grains, and dried peas and beans should be encouraged.

Central nervous system stimulants can cause a loss of appetite (anorexia), insomnia, and stomach pains, which may result in weight loss. Antidepressants and tranquilizers are known to promote weight gain attributable to fluid retention and an increase in appetite.

Laxatives, bulk preparations, stimulants, and stool softeners for bowel management programs require additional fluids and fiber-rich foods in the diet. The excessive use of laxatives for constipation may affect nutrient absorption. Mineral oil may decrease the absorption of fat-soluble vitamins, calcium, and phosphate.

Inactivity (physical and peristaltic), inadequate fiber and fluid intake, and certain medications contribute to the problem of constipation in the developmentally disabled population. Chewing and swallowing difficulties caused by the disability may mean that fibrous fruits and vegetables are not tolerated. However, bran and prune juice (natural laxatives) can be incorporated into the daily diet.

The individual who experiences drooling or who is prone to urinary tract infections is especially in need of extra fluids. Some developmentally disabled individuals are unable to express their thirst or are unaware of the need for fluids and must be encouraged and assisted in obtaining beverages. It must be remembered, however, that plain water satisfies thirst best and that sweetened beverages and salty liquids may increase the body's need for fluids. At least 64 ounces (about 2000 mL, or 1 mL of fluid for each kilocalorie in diet) of fluids should be offered daily, and physical activity as tolerated should be encouraged to promote bowel regularity. Thickened liquids may be necessary to ensure adequate intake if there are swallowing problems. There are appropriate commercial thickeners and baby rice cereal, or yogurt may also be used to thicken liquids.

It is important, therefore, that nutrition counseling be provided. Vitamin and mineral supplements may be recommended to offset any nutritional problems that result from long-term drug therapy. Table 7–8 shows drug-nutrient interactions, including drugs that are commonly prescribed for conditions of the developmentally disabled individual.

What Are
Conditions of
Inborn Errors of
Metabolism?

The term **inborn errors of metabolism** refers to a group of diseases that affect a wide variety of metabolic processes. Certain enzymes are lacking because of a genetic defect, requiring the diet to be modified to prevent toxicity from the excessive accumulation of by-products. Failure to detect inborn errors of metabolism at an early age results in a variety of severe problems such as damage to the central nervous system and many body organs if an effective treatment is not started soon after birth. Many inborn errors of metabolism require specific diets for treatment. A specific diet order from the physician should be obtained, and the dietitian should provide a list of acceptable foods for various special occasions.

GALACTOSEMIA. Features that characterize galactosemia include a lack of transferase (a liver enzyme that converts galactose to glucose), toxic levels of galactose in the blood, diarrhea, drowsiness, edema, liver failure, hemorrhage, and mental retardation.

The lack of the enzyme transferase requires elimination of all milk products or other milk ingredients such as lactose, nonfat dry milk solids, casein, whey, and whey solids (see Table 15–2). Acceptable infant formulas are Isomil, Neo-Mull-Soy, ProSobee, Soylac, meat-based formulas, Nutramigen, and Pregestimil. Additional nutrients are provided according to the RDA.

It is very important that all ingredient labels for processed and packaged foods be read carefully. Any foods containing milk, lactose, nonfat dry milk solids, casein, whey, or whey solids cannot be tolerated. Lactate, lactic acid, and lactalbumin are acceptable. The complete list of ingredients may not be found on some foods, such as bread and imitation milk. Therefore, frequent monitoring of red blood cell levels of galactose and galactose-1-phosphate is recommended to assure adherence to the diet.

PHENYLKETONURIA. Phenylketonuria (PKU) is characterized by a lack of the enzyme necessary to metabolize phenylalanine, one of the essential amino acids. As phenylalanine is not metabolized, high levels accumulate and there is a characteristic excretion of phenylketones in the urine. Infants are usually blond, blue-eyed, and fair and often have eczema. All infants are now tested at birth for PKU. When untreated, the infants are hyperactive and irritable with an unpleasant personality and a musty or gamy odor. Severe retardation results if treatment is delayed. However, some studies have shown improvement in behavior in untreated individuals later in life even when the diet was not started at birth.

Special infant formulas are necessary to prevent buildup of toxic levels of phenylalanine. Lofenalac, Phenyl-Free, and PKU-Aid are acceptable. A 10 to 30 per cent increase of protein over the RDA is necessary to assure adequate absorption of amino acids. Kilocalories need to be adjusted for the age, appetite, and growth pattern of the child. Special tables showing the phenylalanine content of various foods are available. Only one fourth of the phenylalanine provided by the protein of the RDA should be consumed. Many products on the market contain aspartame, which is a source of phenylalanine and can be a problem for individuals with PKU.

HOMOCYSTINURIA. This disease is characterized by a lack of the enzyme necessary for sulfur amino acid metabolism. The purpose of the diet for homocystinuria is to lower blood methionine and homocystine levels. Adequate L-cystine must be supplied. It is used to prevent the buildup of methionine and homocystine in the plasma and homocystine in the urine. Typically, the untreated child is retarded, with a fair complexion and detached retinas. Death usually occurs from spontaneous thrombosis.

TYROSINOSIS. This disorder is a result of an error in tyrosine metabolism. The purpose of the diet for tyrosinosis is to reduce plasma tyrosine and phenylalanine levels and to prevent liver and kidney damage. It may prevent mental deterioration if started early in life.

MAPLE SYRUP URINE DISEASE. In maple syrup urine disease (MSUD) there is an inability to utilize branched-chain amino acids. The purpose of the diet for this disease is to reduce leucine, isoleucine, and valine plasma levels to normal. The diet is used to prevent neurological damage and rapid death by reducing these branched-chain amino acids in the diet.

HISTIDINEMIA. This condition is caused by a lack of the enzyme for histidine metabolism. The purpose of the diet is to lower the plasma histidine level and to treat the symptoms of histidinemia, which results in speech disorders and mental retardation. Special formulas are available for homocystinuria, tyrosinosis, MSUD, and histidinemia.

WHAT IS A SUCCESSFUL FEEDING PROGRAM?

The success of a feeding program is dependent on several factors:

1. Selection of an appropriate diet (see Chapter 7)
2. Proper positioning
3. Use of appropriate feeding techniques and devices
4. Relaxation of individual before feeding
5. Staff's abilities to interact and handle the disabled individual

Proper Positioning

An individual is properly positioned for eating if

- the head and upper trunk are as upright as possible
- the feet are adequately supported
- the hip and knees are flexed to approximate an 84-degree angle
- the head is tipped slightly forward
- the table height is appropriate
- the arms are centered close to the body and are resting comfortably on the lap
- the person is seated close to the table

Figure 18–6 shows a properly positioned person. If a patient must eat in bed, wedges and pillows can be used to achieve a nearly upright position. Figure 18–7 is a sample form that may be used in screening eating skills.

Feeding Techniques and Environmental Conditions

Feeding techniques and dietary considerations include the following (Table 18–3):

WRONG   RIGHT

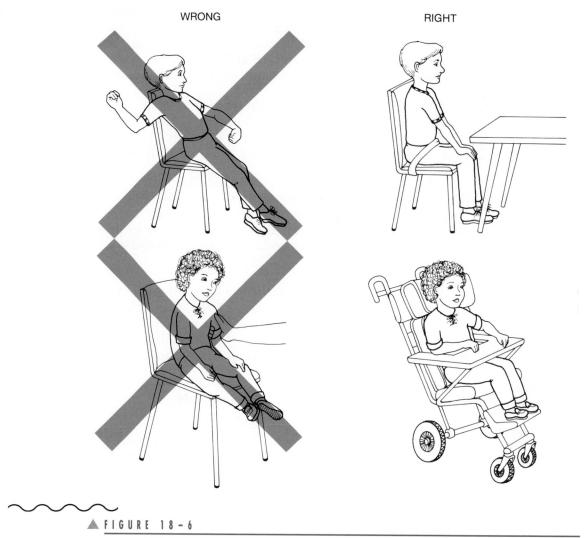

▲FIGURE 18-6

Proper positioning. (From Crump IM: Nutrition and Feeding of the Handicapped Child. Boston, College Hill Press, 1987.)

- food consistency modification (thickened liquids are easier to swallow and manage than thin liquids; Table 18–4)
- vitamin and mineral supplementation as either a milk-based beverage or tablets
- small, frequent meals
- provision of straws for beverages
- provision of plate guards, special spoons, forks, knives, and other adaptive devices (Fig. 18–8)
- encouragement and reminders to eat
- feeding techniques specialized for abnormal reflex responses and problems

EATING SKILLS SCREENING FORM (SAMPLE)

Client Name: _____   Date of Intake: _____

Date of Birth: _____   Age: _____   Sex: _____   Height (in.) _____   Weight (lb.) _____

General Status of Health: Excellent ❑   Good ❑   Fair ❑   Poor ❑

POSITION OF INDIVIDUAL FOR FEEDING:
_____ Upright Unsupported
_____ Upright Supported
_____ Held
_____ Bed/Lying Down

METHOD OF FEEDING:
_____ Independently spoon feeds
_____ Spoon feeds with asistance
_____ Finger feeds
_____ Fed by caregiver

PRESENT DIET:
_____ Blended
_____ Soft
_____ Chopped
_____ Regular
_____ Dietary Restrictions

SAMPLE DAILY INTAKE:
(Explain on reverse side, including
snacks and schedule.)

APPETITE:
_____ Good
_____ Fair
_____ Shows preference for certain foods
_____ Allergies

PRIOR FOOD EXPERIENCES:
(Explain on reverse side.)

ALERTNESS:
_____ Focuses attention on eating
_____ Responds to presence or absence of food
_____ Responds to environment
_____ Unresponsive or apathetic

SENSORY FUNCTIONS:

Intact	Impaired	
_____	_____	Visual
_____	_____	Auditory
_____	_____	Tactile

EATING SKILLS:

Good	Fair	Poor	
_____	_____	_____	Head/Trunk Control
_____	_____	_____	Jaw Control
_____	_____	_____	Lip Closure
_____	_____	_____	Tongue Movements
_____	_____	_____	Swallowing
_____	_____	_____	Chewing

ORAL REFLEXES:
_____ Rooting
_____ Suckling
_____ Bite Reflex
_____ Hyperactive Gag
_____ Hypoactive Gag
_____ Tongue Thrust
_____ Hypersensitivity around mouth

MOTOR DEFICITS AFFECTING SELF-FEEDING:
(Explain on reverse side.)

DENTAL CARE AND STATUS:
(Explain on reverse side.)

SUDDEN AND/OR LARGE WEIGHT CHANGE:
_____ Loss   _____ Gain

COMMENTS: _____
_____
_____
_____
_____

▲ FIGURE 18-7

Sample of an eating skills screening form. (Courtesy of Ross Laboratories, Columbus, Ohio.)

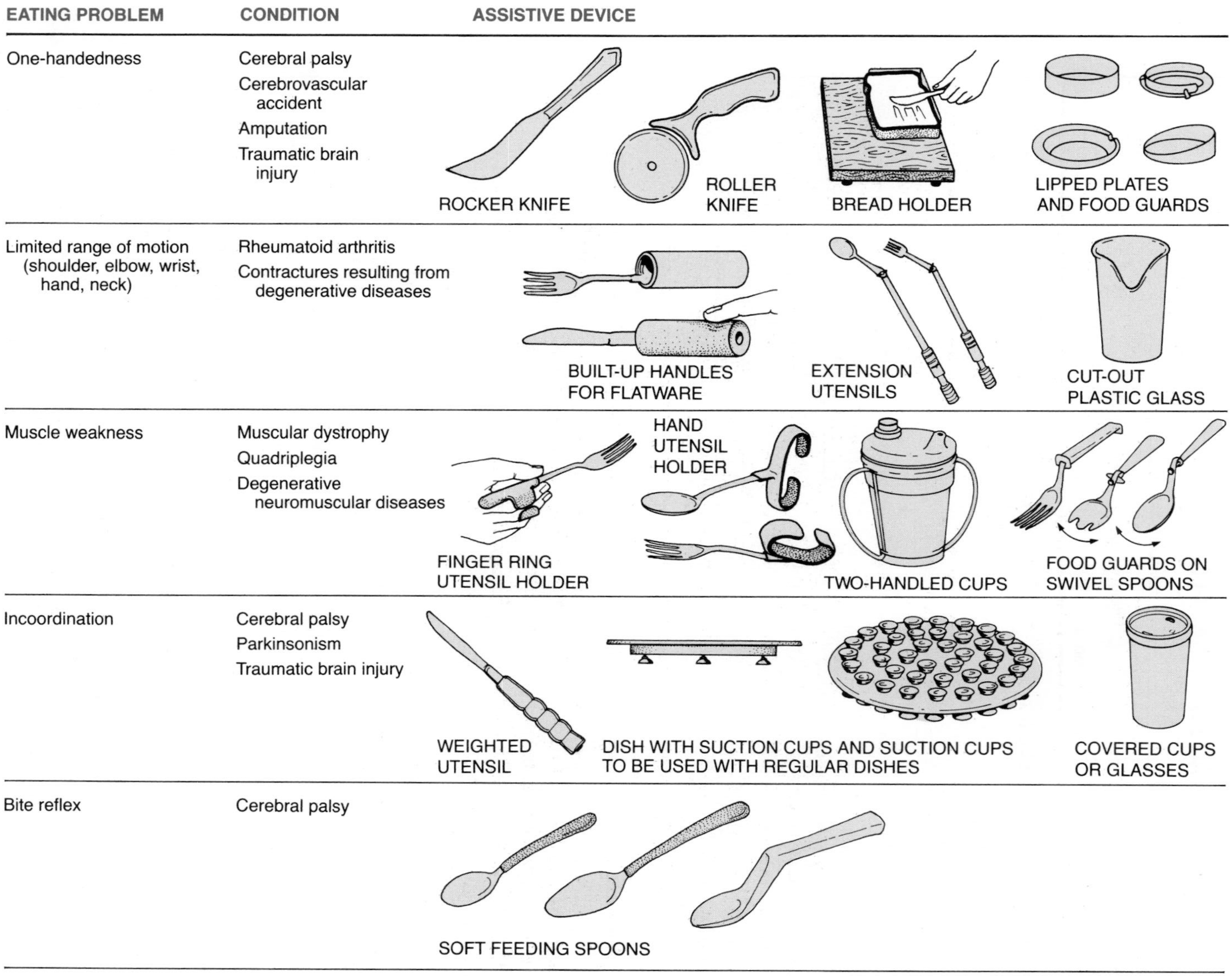

EATING PROBLEM	CONDITION	ASSISTIVE DEVICE
One-handedness	Cerebral palsy Cerebrovascular accident Amputation Traumatic brain injury	ROCKER KNIFE　ROLLER KNIFE　BREAD HOLDER　LIPPED PLATES AND FOOD GUARDS
Limited range of motion (shoulder, elbow, wrist, hand, neck)	Rheumatoid arthritis Contractures resulting from degenerative diseases	BUILT-UP HANDLES FOR FLATWARE　EXTENSION UTENSILS　CUT-OUT PLASTIC GLASS
Muscle weakness	Muscular dystrophy Quadriplegia Degenerative neuromuscular diseases	FINGER RING UTENSIL HOLDER　HAND UTENSIL HOLDER　TWO-HANDLED CUPS　FOOD GUARDS ON SWIVEL SPOONS
Incoordination	Cerebral palsy Parkinsonism Traumatic brain injury	WEIGHTED UTENSIL　DISH WITH SUCTION CUPS AND SUCTION CUPS TO BE USED WITH REGULAR DISHES　COVERED CUPS OR GLASSES
Bite reflex	Cerebral palsy	SOFT FEEDING SPOONS

FIGURE 18-8

Assistive devices for eating problems. (From Consultant Dietitians in Health Care Facilities: Feeding Is Everybody's Business: A Manual for Health Care Professionals Involved in Feeding Programs. Mead Johnson Nutritional Division.)

▲ **TABLE 18-3**

FEEDING TECHNIQUES FOR RESOLVING AND IMPROVING FEEDING PROBLEMS

POSSIBLE ABNORMAL REFLEX OR PROBLEM	FEEDING TECHNIQUE
Rooting Reflex Mouth opens and head turns in the direction of the stimulus when cheeks or lips are touched beyond 3 months of age.	Avoid stimulation to face between swallows or bites, such as wiping face with a cloth.
Suck-Swallow Rhythmical suck and simultaneous swallowing movement that continues as long as stimulus is present.	Occupational therapy program for oral normalization such as mouth and tongue stimulation, lip closure, stroking the throat, and so on. Follow OT program to progress from sucking to chewing. When using stimulation techniques, use firm, deep pressure rather than light pressure, which may tickle or irritate. Gradually increase texture and thickness of food.
Tonic Neck Reflex Develops at 4 weeks. Stimulated by receptors in the neck, it aids in eye-hand coordination. Position of the arms depends on position of the head.	
Asymmetrical Tonic Neck Reflex When the head is turned toward the right, the right arm extends outward. If to the left, the left arm extends. Prevents individual from keeping the head in position to be fed and interferes with jaw control. When self-feeding, it prevents proper hand-to-mouth coordination.	Position head and whole body in midline. (Refer to Positioning discussed previously.)
Gag Reflex Prevents passage of food into the windpipe. Present from birth on through life, although it weakens in later life.	Gagging is a "yellow light, not a red light." The feeder may think that gagging on a new food means that the individual is not ready for more complicated textures. This may not be so but just a warning to take things more slowly. To prevent behavioral problems, handle gagging in a very matter-of-fact way. Simply place hand over the child's mouth and close it until he swallows. Be careful to prevent food from entering the windpipe. Keep the head forward. Neck extension can cause aspiration.
In hypertonicity, a gag is elicited by tactile stimulation to the anterior half of the tongue. Caused by hypersensitive tongue, and difficulty in swallowing.	Tongue stimulation at other than mealtime to decrease hypersensitivity to touch. To control tongue activity, place food on the middle of the tongue with a slightly downward pressure of the spoon.

Table continued on following page

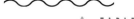

▲ T A B L E 1 8 – 3

FEEDING TECHNIQUES FOR RESOLVING AND IMPROVING FEEDING PROBLEMS *Continued*

POSSIBLE ABNORMAL REFLEX OR PROBLEM	FEEDING TECHNIQUE
In hypotonicity, no gag response occurs regardless of what part of the tongue is prodded.	Feeder must be extremely careful in feeding this individual to prevent choking. Feed slowly. Walk the tongue with a tongue depressor or fingers in small steps to the point of gag, then withdraw depressor, close client's mouth, and wait for a swallow.
Bite Reflex Rapid rhythmical opening and closing of the jaw as long as the stimulus is present. This reflex is integrated by 4 months.	Use small Xylon spoon when feeding to prevent injury to oral structures. Wait for relaxation before removing spoon (do not try to pull spoon out).
Chewing Rotatory movement in which food is positioned between the teeth for mastication and then repositioned for swallwing. Do not mistake tongue mashing (mashing food against the roof of the mouth) for chewing.	To encourage chewing, place dried fruit, beef jerky or cracker between the molars. Use jaw control to stimulate chewing while giving a slight tug on the food. Placement of food should be alternated from one side of the mouth to the other.
Tongue Thrust Food is pushed out of the mouth in an upward forward motion. Caused by inability to control tongue movements, improper positioning (head too far back), mouth breathing or being given too large a spoonful of food at one time.	Position client as described in positioning. Do not let client push his head back. Exercise jaw control. Use thickened pureed food. Place pressure on the tongue with the spoon. Hold the pressure briefly to stop tongue from protruding. Hold mouth closed until a swallow occurs. If mouth breather, allow time for breathing between bites.
Jaw Control Necessary to facilitate chewing. In hypertonia, jaw deviation is due to persisting asymmetrical tonic neck reflex. Will also have poor jaw control if head is tilted back too far.	Follow procedure for good positioning. When the client has poor head control, the feeder sits beside or behind the individual. The jaw is controlled with the nonfeeding hand (See Diagram *A*). For the client with good head control, the feeder sits in front of him (See Diagram *B*).

Table continued on following page

▲ T A B L E   1 8 – 3

FEEDING TECHNIQUES FOR RESOLVING AND IMPROVING FEEDING PROBLEMS *Continued*

POSSIBLE ABNORMAL REFLEX OR PROBLEM	FEEDING TECHNIQUE

DIAGRAM A

DIAGRAM B

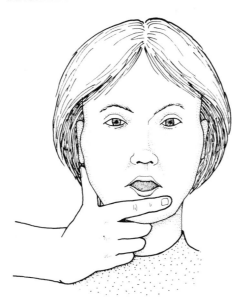

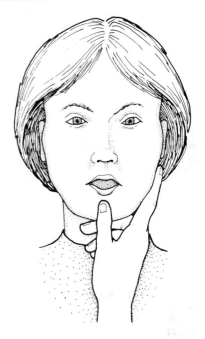

Jaw control (arm around client's head) with thumb on jaw joint, index finger between chin and lower lip.

Lip Closure
Necessary for removing food from the spoon and for preventing drooling.

Jaw control (applied from front) with thumb between chin and lower lip, index finger on jaw joint, middle finger applied firmly just behind the chin.

Prefeeding stimulation of lips and jaw control in which the index finger is above the upper lip, pulling downward slightly as the spoon is removed. Never scrape food off the spoon with the client's teeth. A spoon with a flat bowl will work better than a deep-bowled spoon.

Do not try to scrape any excess food from the lips with the spoon or wipe the client's mouth or chin after every bite. This may give the client the wrong signal to open his mouth, rather than keeping it closed to masticate and swallow. Allow for a little messiness while the client learns that the touch of the spoon means that he is to open his mouth and withdrawal of the spoon means he is to close his mouth.

Table continued on following page

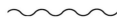

▲ T A B L E 1 8 - 3

FEEDING TECHNIQUES FOR RESOLVING AND IMPROVING FEEDING PROBLEMS *Continued*

POSSIBLE ABNORMAL REFLEX OR PROBLEM	FEEDING TECHNIQUE
Tongue Mobility Used in moving food to the back of the mouth for swallowing and relocating food from the sides of the mouth.	Encourage lip-licking with the tongue by placing something tasty on the lips such as peanut butter. Also place small pieces of cereal between the lips and gums.
Drooling Caused by ineffective swallowing of saliva. It is evident when there is poor jaw and tongue control and poor lip closure.	The therapist must solve the drooling problem indirectly by correcting the other feeding problems first.
Refusal to Eat Solid Food Hypersensitivity to touch. Dislikes change. May have very tight mouth.	Eliminate canned pureed food. Introduce wide variety of regular table food that has been pureed. Gradually introduce thickened consistency. Then food with general lumpiness such as rice pudding rather than discrete lumps. When introducing vegetables, initially avoid vegetables with an outer shell such as corn, peas, and lima beans.
Refusal to Drink from a Cup Poor coordination to suck-swallow. Previous experience from choking on liquids.	Begin cup drinking by using thickened liquids that flow more slowly and give the client more time to swallow. Alternate spoonfuls of thickened liquid with spoonfuls of client's other food at the meal. Gradually increase the number of spoonfuls of liquid given in succession but give client enough time to swallow between spoonfuls. Gradually thin down liquid. Ex.: Add apricot nectar to pureed apricots. Then reduce strained fruit gradually until the client is drinking juice alone. Use jaw control to close lips and jaw, and reinforce "normal" swallowing pattern.

Information approved by an occupational therapist of Broome Developmental Services, Ithaca, NY, 1990.

Food consistency should be appropriate to the individual's ability to chew and swallow. It can be classified as grainy, lumpy, smooth, heavy, light, or mass consistency (one texture of food or a mixed consistency). Table 18–4 lists the effects that various food textures have on oral function; for example, certain foods stimulate sucking and other foods such as solids and chopped foods stimulate the lips and tongue to promote chewing and prevent choking. Foods that hold some shape also stimulate the swallowing reflex.

The temperature of the food served should also be considered. Extremely hot or cold foods should be avoided when the mouth is hypersensitive in order to avoid burning or numbing the tongue.

▲   T A B L E   1 8 – 4

FOOD CONSISTENCY CONSIDERATIONS

TYPE OF DIET	EXAMPLE	POTENTIAL IMPACT ON ORAL FUNCTION
Thin foods and liquids	Soup broth, juice	More difficult to control within mouth, especially with limited tongue control, i.e., quickly run to all areas of mouth Often promote excessive food loss
Thick foods	Pudding, yogurt, applesauce	Improve control with oral cavity owing to reduced flow and increased sensory input (i.e., weight and texture)
Paste-like or sticky foods	Peanut butter, thick cheese sauce	May be more difficult to move in oral cavity with limited tongue movement May stick to the roof of the mouth, especially with a high, narrow palate
Slippery foods	Pasta, Jell-o	Often difficult to control and either trigger reflexive swallow too quickly or run out of oral cavity before the swallow
Smooth textures	Pudding, pureed foods	Relatively easy to swallow; promote minimal tongue and jaw movement, especially over periods of time
Coarse textures	Creamed corn, ground foods, Sloppy Joe filling	Increase sensory input to stimulate more jaw and tongue movements Coarseness of food should be carefully graded
Varied textures	Soups with noodles or chunks of vegetables	Difficult to manage in oral cavity, especially with limited tongue movement or decreased oral sensitivity (i.e., liquid is swallowed and solid pieces remain in the mouth)
Scattering textures	Grated carrots, rice, coleslaw, corn bread	Very difficult to manage with limited tongue movement and decreased oral sensitivity
Crisp solids	Carrot sticks, celery sticks	Require sophisticated biting and chewing in order to grind pieces into consistency that is safe to swallow
Milk-based substances	Milk, ice cream	Appear to coat mucus in oral-pharyngeal cavities to interfere with swallowing or appear to increase congestion*
Broth	Meat broth, chicken broth	Appears to cut mucus in oral-pharyngeal cavity and facilitate swallow
Dry foods	Bread, cake, cookie	May be difficult to chew or swallow with insufficient saliva
Whole soft foods	Slice of bread	Require the ability to bite off appropriate-sized pieces

* However, there is no scientific evidence to support this belief by some people.
Courtesy of the Occupational Therapy Department of the J.N. Adams Development Center, Perrysburg, NY 14129.

If acidic foods such as citrus juice increase salivation to the extent of excessive drooling, they should be offered at the end of the meal rather than at the beginning. Sweets are also known to increase saliva production.

Mealtimes should be relaxing in order to aid digestion and increase the enjoyment of food. Unless the mealtime environment is pleasant, even appealing food may be rejected. Avoidance of loud noises, bright lights, and sudden movements will help individuals with developmental disabilities to eat better.

Food and Nonfood
Rewards

Sometimes a specific reinforcer is needed to help someone modify his or her behavior. When the interdisciplinary team agrees that food items are the most effective means of reinforcing client behaviors, the following health issues should be addressed and considered:

▲ **TABLE 18-5**

THE TEAM APPROACH TO HEALTH CARE IN FEEDING

HEALTH CARE PROFESSIONAL	RESPONSIBILITY
Dietitian	Meal planning
	Supervision of food and modified diet preparation
	Delivery of meals
	Execution of diet orders
	Diet modification
	Nutrition counseling
	Nutrition assessment
Nurse	Mealtime supervision
	Proper positioning
	Charting of food and fluid intake
	Communication with dietitian and physician regarding acceptance of food served
	Implementation and integration of total care plan
Occupational therapist	Assessment of oral motor function
	Instruction of staff on appropriate alignment for feeding
	Assessment of need for assistive devices
	Working with client on chewing, swallowing, and other functional skill necessary to achieve feeding independence
Physical therapist	Evaluates mobility deficits
	Prescribes appropriate feeding activities
	May assist in evaluating oral motor problems
Speech pathologist	Provides assessment of oral motor functions and recommends appropriate treatment
	May provide help in solving problems and work with problems of bite reflex and tongue thrust
Psychologist	Evaluates specific behaviors that affect nutrition (such as food stealing, pica behavior, obsessive eating, and bizarre eating habits) and plans ways to manage them
Social worker	Collects social history and demographic data regarding patient and family
	Summarizes client's financial status and reaction to proposed therapy
	Provides financial information if needed by client in acquiring funds
Dentist	Provides assessment of patient's dental health (condition of gums, oral structure, and sensitivity related to teeth)
Physician	Identifies feeding problems
	Requires consultation in writing to appropriate health care professional
Recreational therapist	Provides premeal activities (music for dining, socialization)

Data from Consultant Dietitians in Health Care Facilities: Feeding Is Everbody's Business—A Manual for Health Care Professionals Involved in Feeding Programs. Mead Johnson Nutritional Division, Evansville, IN 47721.

- maintenance of dental health (see Chapter 19)
- avoidance of empty kilocalories, especially when overweight is a problem
- the negative consequence of food as a reward must be outweighed by the positive behavioral outcomes

Appropriate foods that may be used for reinforcers include popcorn or nuts for those persons without chewing or swallowing problems, fruit sections, low-fat cheese cubes, unsweetened cereal pieces such as Cheerios, pretzels, fruit juice popsicles, or diet soda. The dietitian needs to approve specific individual food reinforcers if they are deemed necessary.

Food rewards should gradually be replaced with other items such as stickers and stars, grooming supplies, and other small items. Verbal praise and outings are often excellent rewards that can be used instead of food. The staff's positive attitude about nonfood reinforcers increases the value of such rewards.

HOW DO HEALTH CARE PROFESSIONALS WORK AS A TEAM IN FEEDING AND WEIGHT REDUCTION PROGRAMS?

Table 18–5 shows the varied responsibilities of the health care team in working with the developmentally disabled population. Various health care professionals need to be involved with weight control interventions, for example, increased exercise, dietary modification, and behavioral management. However, it is a challenge to develop good eating habits and appropriate levels of exercise in the developmentally disabled person.

STUDY QUESTIONS AND ACTIVITIES

1. Define developmental disability and name some specific diseases.
2. How are nutritional problems of the developmentally disabled population grouped?
3. Name the growth retardation characteristics of Down syndrome.
4. With what type of cerebral palsy is obesity likely to develop? What type may involve underweight? Why may the cerebral palsy be the cause of Amy's need to eat enough food in the opening case study?
5. As a class activity, try to drink water in the following positions: head tipped to one side; head facing downward; trunk leaning backward with no support; correct position as described in this chapter.
6. Describe the techniques used when feeding a person with tongue thrust.
7. How does the environment play a role in the mastery of mealtime skills?
8. Describe how the assessment process is different in the developmentally disabled population.
9. How might hypertension be controlled in an adult with a developmental disability? What dietary advice might be appropriate?

REFERENCES

American Dietetic Association, Position Paper: Nutrition in comprehensive program planning for persons with developmental disabilities. J Am Diet Assoc 1992; 92(5):613–615.

Hoffman CJ, Aultman D, Pipes P: A nutrition survey of and recommendations for individuals with Prader-Willi Syndrome who live in group homes. J Am Diet Assoc 1992; 92(7):823–833.

Nutrition Focus for children with special health care needs: Dental nutrition concerns of children with special health care needs. July-Aug 1992; 7(4).

Pronsky ZM: Powers and Moore's Food Medication Interactions, 8th ed. Published and distributed by Food-Medication Interactions, Pottstown, PA, 1993.

ORAL AND DENTAL HEALTH

OBJECTIVES

After completing this chapter, you should be able to:
- Describe the causes of dental decay
- Identify the factors related to dental health
- Describe public health measures to control dental decay
- Identify good snack foods for dental health

TERMS TO IDENTIFY

Baby-bottle tooth decay	Dental enamel	Periodontal disease
Cariogenic	Dental erosion	Purging
Decalcification	Dental plaque	Salivary glands
Dental caries	Fluoride	Xerostomia

A FAMILY'S PERSPECTIVE ON NUTRITION

Ms. Wimberg had Joey in the dental hygienist's chair cleaning his teeth at his annual check-up. It was really odd, she thought. There certainly appeared to be extreme dental erosion. Not the normal amount of dental decay that might be detected at a yearly dental check-up. This was much more serious. And he was very thin. She would discuss this further with the dentist and have him check Joey's teeth before he left the office.

Finally, thought Joey, he had gotten out of the dentist's office. The dentist sure did seem concerned about him. What was the big deal? So he had a little dental decay. He hurried on home because he knew his Nanna had dinner waiting.

"Mangia, Joey, mangia" Nanna exclaimed. But how could he eat more, Joey thought to himself. He had to make weight for tomorrow's wrestling match. All that pasta meant added weight for sure. No, he couldn't risk it, he thought. "Joey, stai bene?" Nanna asked, concerned. Joey knew full well what was going through Nanna's mind, "He's not eating; he must be ill!" What was he to do? But he knew what he was going to do. He'd been doing it for quite some time now. It wasn't so bad really. And he got to please Nanna while enjoying the pasta he loved and still make weight for wrestling. He sure hoped no one caught on to his post-meal bathroom ritual. But his dentist already had.

INTRODUCTION

Dental caries develops from a complex process of demineralization of the tooth (**decalcification**—removal of calcium from the tooth structure) and acid destruction. Acid is formed from the combination of carbohydrate and oral bacteria. Saliva helps neutralize this normal acid production. But when acid is continually in contact with **dental enamel** (the outer hard surface of the teeth) the structure can be quickly decalcified. Another source of acid destruction is related to erosion of the dental enamel. **Dental erosion** does not involve bacterial action but happens in cases such as bulimia, in which constant purging of meals allows the acid contents of the stomach to cause severe erosion of the dental enamel. A new role for the dental profession in diagnosing bulimia has evolved as a consequence of this nation's obsession with weight.

Dental decay is difficult to control through food choices alone. Limiting the frequency of carbohydrate snacks can help. Snacks containing sucrose should be limited in particular. Including a protein source at snack time can also help. Good dental hygiene with regular dental check-ups and the use of topical fluoride are the most effective and appropriate preventive measures. The role of the dental professional should include the assessment of eating disorders (see Chapter 15) and between-meal snacking patterns.

HOW DOES DENTAL DECAY DEVELOP?

It has long been believed that sugar causes cavities. While this is true, we know today that there is a more complex cause of dental caries. Tooth decay is caused by loss of calcium from the tooth enamel. This process is exacerbated by acidic destruction of the dental surface, the enamel. Bacteria, normally present in the oral cavity, feed on all forms of carbohydrate including starch. The combination of bacteria and carbohydrate results in acid production that decalcifies tooth enamel. Thus, the acidic demineralization of dental enamel normally occurs after the consumption of carbohydrate foods and drinks. Erosion also occurs through other means of acid contact with teeth, including the repeated purging of acidic stomach contents associated with bulimia or excess intake of acidic beverages such as some soft drinks.

Bacteria, found in **dental plaque** (a buildup on dental surfaces that provides a medium for bacteria to grow) on and between the dental surfaces, use carbohydrate to grow. The chemical end product of this carbohydrate "meal" by the bacteria is acid. This process occurs whether the carbohydrate is sugar or starch. Thus, oral bacteria and carbohydrate act in concert to cause acid destruction of dental enamel.

Given an ideal situation of a plaque-free mouth, the carbohydrate in our foods would not cause dental decay, even if the diet consisted entirely of sugar. Since a bacteria-free oral cavity is not feasible, the elimination of carbohydrate from our diet would also prevent dental decay. However, as we need carbohydrate for good health, a series of compromises needs to occur in order to control and prevent dental decay.

WHAT STEPS CAN BE TAKEN TO PROMOTE GOOD DENTAL HEALTH?

The optimum approach to good dental health is thorough, frequent cleansing of the mouth, regular dental visits to remove plaque buildup, limiting the intake of carbohydrate foods and drinks to meals and snacks that include a protein source, and using fluoridated toothpaste or mouthwash or both after each meal. If toothbrushing cannot or does not occur immediately after eating, the mouth should be rinsed with water after eating. Chewing sugar-free gum after meals stimulates the flow of saliva. Other means to protect the enamel surface of the teeth include avoiding harsh abrasives on the teeth, not chewing ice (which can chip the teeth), not opening bottles with the teeth, and using pliable mouth guards in sports.

Proper diet, which includes adequate amounts of calcium, contributes to strong enamel formation. The formation of enamel begins in utero; thus a pregnant mother's diet should contain adequate amounts of calcium (the equivalent of 3 to 4 cups of milk daily: 1000 mg or more). A strong and thick enamel dental surface helps resist the destructive effect of acid production in the mouth.

Fluoride helps promote the formation of strong enamel in childhood and can be obtained through fluoridated drinking water or fluoride drops or tablets until about the age of 12 years. Once the adult teeth are fully formed, fluoride rinses continue to be an effective preventive treatment through promoting retention of the enamel surface. Fluoride is believed to actually promote remineralization of the dental surface.

To control loss of dental enamel, aside from the use of fluoride, promotion of good dental hygiene and control of carbohydrate foods are in order. All carbohydrate foods, especially sugar, contribute to acid production in the presence of oral bacteria. Foods containing sugar should be limited to mealtimes to decrease their time of exposure to the dental surfaces. Eating sweet foods with a meal containing protein or fat or both will further help to promote dental health. Eating carbohydrate foods with a thoroughly clean mouth will also be of great benefit. Acid production begins shortly after eating is begun, so toothbrushing and flossing before eating may be as helpful as brushing after a meal. Limiting the time of exposure to acidic beverages is also important.

The supporting structure of the teeth, the gums or gingiva, requires a good nutritional status to remain strong and healthy. Irritants, such as plaque, can increase the risk of gingivitis. Regular toothbrushing and daily flossing along with at least annual dental visits for plaque removal can help decrease the risk for **periodontal disease** (a painless gum disease that results in tooth loss in adulthood).

WHAT IS THE ROLE OF PURGING IN DENTAL DECAY?

Purging (intentional vomiting) after eating can ultimately cause irreversible enamel erosion by increasing the acid content of the mouth (Fig. 19–1). **Xerostomia** (diminished or absent production of saliva) and irritation of the lining of the mouth can also occur in connection with frequent purging. Dehydration and a resulting dry mouth are caused by other forms of purging such as laxative and diuretic abuse. Persons with bulimia (see Chapter 15) report being thirsty on a regular basis and can further con-

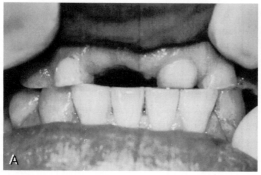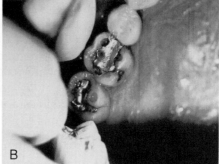

▲ FIGURE 19–1

Two examples of bulimia-induced dental erosion. *A*, loss of tooth structure, *B*, dished-out areas around the fillings due to acid destruction related to purging. (From Ruff J, Abrams R: Oral signs and symptoms in the diagnosis of bulimia. J Am Dent Assoc. 113(5):761–764, © 1986. Reprinted by permission of ADA Publishing Co., Inc.)

tribute to dental decay by frequently consuming acidic or sugared beverages (Howat and Wampold, 1990). Hyperemesis of pregnancy (see Chapter 16) can also contribute to severe dental decay through frequent vomiting and dehydration. Frequent mouth rinsing with water is important if a person cannot drink even water because of severe nausea and vomiting.

In the opening case study scenario, Joey Bernardo frequently purges to control his weight for wrestling. Sports-induced bulimia is a challenge to correct. The school has a vital role in assisting Joey, and others, to aim for realistic weight goals in sports. A health care team approach is important. This would include the school coach, school physician, and school psychologist along with Joey's family and dentist, at a minimum. School policy toward nutrition and weight for school sports needs to be examined to prevent future problems. A registered dietitian can help Joey learn how to eat the family foods in a more healthy way. (See Chapter 20 for healthy weight management strategies in sports.)

HOW DOES SALIVA PRODUCTION HELP PREVENT DENTAL DECAY?

Saliva surrounds the dental surfaces, acting as a lubricant. More importantly, saliva serves to neutralize the acidic pH level induced by the combination of oral bacteria and carbohydrate foods. Saliva also contains calcium, which helps prevent the loss of dental calcium in the enamel surface. Finally, saliva helps rinse the teeth of food debris.

Individuals at high risk of dental decay should be encouraged to use their natural saliva production to bathe each tooth with the tip of the tongue. The action of chewing or biting down can also release saliva from the salivary glands. High-risk individuals may need to chew sugar-free gum or eat other crunchy foods such as vegetable sticks or salads to promote saliva production.

What Is the Impact of Xerostomia on Dental Decay?

Xerostomia is a diminished or absent production of saliva. Severe and rapid dental decay has been observed in individuals with xerostomia, such as in patients with throat cancer whose radiation therapy damaged the **salivary glands** (glands near the mouth that produce saliva). This same effect can be induced through medications that cause dryness of the mouth such as antihistamine medications, diuretics, and others (Pronsky, 1993). Breathing through the mouth can also cause dryness of the mouth. Patient complaints of dry mouth should be taken seriously in regard to prevention of dental decay. In the geriatric population, there is a diminished sense of thirst, which increases risk of dental caries.

WHAT ARE SOME OTHER CONTRIBUTORS TO DENTAL DECAY?

Acidic drinks such as some soft drinks (e.g., cola drinks, citrus fruits or juices) can quickly erode tooth enamel. The length of exposure to the acid is important. Drinking a glass of orange juice or cola in 10 minutes is less detrimental than sipping the drink for an hour. Chewable vitamin C tablets, also known as ascorbic acid, have also been found to be destructive to dental enamel.

ARE SOME FOODS MORE CARIOGENIC THAN OTHERS?

All foods containing carbohydrate can be utilized by oral bacteria to allow acid production. Thus all carbohydrate foods are **cariogenic** (able to induce dental caries or cavities). Potato chips and other sources of cooked starches may be just as harmful to dental health as candy. Harm done is due in part to the public not knowing that starch can cause decay and so not as readily undertaking preventive toothbrushing when starches are eaten versus candy. Sugar and cooked starches are the most cariogenic foods. Sticky carbohydrate foods are also more cariogenic because of their prolonged contact with the dental surface.

Foods containing protein generally are low in carbohydrate (exceptions are milk and legumes) and provide some fat (exceptions are egg whites and skim milk). The fat content of protein foods can coat the teeth and provide some protection to the dental surfaces. Thus, not only are protein foods and fats the least cariogenic food sources, they may also help prevent dental caries through their protective action.

WHAT IS BABY-BOTTLE TOOTH DECAY AND ITS SIGNIFICANCE?

Baby-bottle tooth decay (also referred to as nursing-bottle mouth) occurs in babies and young children who use a bottle excessively, especially at bedtime (Fig. 19–2). Sweet liquids such as juice and other soft drinks are felt to be the primary culprits in baby-bottle tooth decay. But even formula and cow's milk contain sugar in the form of lactose. Bedtime bottles are the most harmful since there is a decreased production of saliva during sleep. Water bottles are acceptable for bedtime if there is no sugar added to the water. It is best, however, if the infant does not take a bottle to bed at all. The teeth that are most at risk are the upper front teeth (see Fig. 19–2).

The physical significance of baby-bottle tooth decay is that removal of the decayed teeth can cause jaw misalignment, preventing normal spacing for adult teeth as they erupt. The pain of dental decay is not pleasant for the infant or child and can cause crying and screaming. Further, a young child

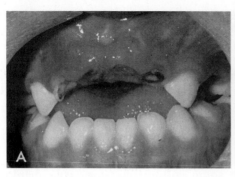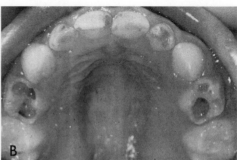

▲ FIGURE 19-2

Examples of baby-bottle tooth decay. (From Johnsen D, Nowjack-Raymer R: Baby Bottle Tooth Decay (BBTD): Issues, assessment, and an opportunity for the nutritionist. J Am Diet Assoc. 1989; 89(8):1113. © The American Dietetic Association. Reprinted by permission.)

with dental decay experiences a frightening and painful first dental visit. It is best to prevent dental caries in infants and young children for the sake of the child, the parent, and the dental professional. A visit to the dentist by the age of one or two for a dental check-up and cleaning is a good idea. Baby-bottle tooth decay is entirely preventable (Johnson and Nowjack-Raymer, 1989).

WHAT ADVICE SHOULD A NURSE OR OTHER HEALTH CARE PROFESSIONAL PROVIDE FOR DENTAL HEALTH?

Suggesting good oral hygiene with specific advice is appropriate for all health care professionals. The importance of good dental care spans all ages, from infants to the very old. Emphasizing good oral hygiene with regular dental check-ups for plaque removal is in order. Infants can have their teeth cleaned with a wet washcloth. Young children can be taught to brush their teeth or have their parents do it for them. Older adults or others at risk of inadequate saliva production or other dental concerns need special care in promoting dental health (see Chapter 18 regarding the dental needs of the developmentally disabled). The use of fluoride can be promoted for all ages if it is not in the local water supply. Children can use fluoride tablets, as prescribed by a dentist, and adults can use fluoride rinses.

Dietary advice is a bit trickier. Assessment of dietary practices is important, especially that of between-meal snacking habits. Sugar is a known cariogenic food. If sweetened foods are eaten at mealtimes, they are less

GOOD SNACK FOODS FOR DENTAL HEALTH

▲

Carrot and celery sticks
Zucchini "matchsticks"
Radishes
Green and red pepper rings
Cucumber slices
Peanuts and other nuts (for children over 3 years, to avoid choking)
Cheese, regular in moderation or low-fat varieties
Hard-cooked egg, with or without the yolk (for cholesterol control)
Grain products (crackers, toast, bagels) with peanut butter or cheese
Apple wedges with peanut butter
Milk or yogurt

cariogenic. Cheese as part of a snack can help prevent dental decay, possibly because of the calcium and phosphate content (Gedalia et al., 1991); however, in the attempt to prevent dental caries we do not want to promote heart disease. To avoid excess intake of fat, food models might be used to show what 1 ounce of cheese looks like. A referral to a registered dietitian would be in order for someone with a strong family history of cardiovascular disease to make sure he or she does not eat too much fat or the wrong type of fat in an attempt to control dental decay.

Health care professionals need to be aware of the existence of bulimia and its detrimental effect on dental health. A health care team approach is advised for bulimia but also for dental care in general. Local educational programs on dental health are usually offered by the health department or the WIC program (see Chapter 22). These programs generally focus on children's dental health. The health care professional should be aware of local programs in order to make referrals.

STUDY QUESTIONS AND ACTIVITIES

1. Why is it important to prevent baby-bottle tooth decay?
2. Why is Joey at high risk of dental erosion? What steps should be taken by his dental hygienist, dentist, and parents?
3. What are some strategies to make snacking less harmful to dental health?
4. Contact your local health department to determine if the water supply is fluoridated. If not, what means are available for children to receive fluoride supplementation in your area?

REFERENCES

Gedalia I, Ionat-Bendat D, Bem-Mosheh S, Shapira L: Tooth enamel softening with a cola type drink and rehardening with hard cheese or stimulated saliva in situ. J Oral Rehabil, 1991; 18:501–506.

Howatt PM, Varner LM, Wampold RL: The effectiveness of a dental/dietitian team in the assessment of bulimic dental health. J Am Diet Assoc, 1990; 90(8):1099–1102.

Johnson D, Nowjack-Raymer R: Baby bottle tooth decay (BBTD): Issues, assessment, and an opportunity for the nutritionist. J Am Diet Assoc, 1989; 89(8):1112–1115.

Pronsky ZM: Powers and Moore's Food Medication Interactions, 8th ed., Published and Distributed by Food-Medication Interactions, Pottstown, PA, 1993.

PHYSICAL FITNESS AND HEALTHY WEIGHT MANAGEMENT IN ACHIEVING WELLNESS

CHAPTER

20

OBJECTIVES

After completing this chapter, you should be able to:
- Relate the importance of physical fitness to healthy weight management
- Describe the nutritional needs of the physically active and the athlete
- Describe obesity and underweight and discuss treatments of each condition
- Calculate the energy value of foods

TERMS TO IDENTIFY

Aerobic exercise	Fad diet	Metabolism
Amenorrhea	Fat cell theory	Obesity
Anaerobic exercise	Hyperinsulinemia	Overweight
Behavior modification	Hyperplasty	Physical fitness
Body mass index (BMI)	Hypertrophy	Set point theory
Carbohydrate loading	Lipogenic	Sports anemia
Desirable weight	Lipolysis	Underweight
Energy balance		

A FAMILY'S PERSPECTIVE ON NUTRITION

Anna Bernardo read the notice. A weight support group for teenagers to be held in the school nurse's office. She did have a scale in her office. Would Anna have to have her weight checked in front of the other girls? If so, she wouldn't join. But it did sound good. Ongoing weekly meetings in the nurse's office after school and the use of the school gym equipment at off-hours for privacy. But she hoped it wouldn't be too "tell all." She wasn't sure she was ready for other girls to know that her weight bothered her. It was much easier making jokes about it. But she really wanted to look nice for her senior prom. She would certainly get a date if she was thin. She figured at her height of 5'2" that she should lose about 50 pounds since she now weighed about 150 pounds.

She picked up a brochure describing the program. Where was the type of diet she would follow? It sounded so vague. "Learn to eat in a sensible way." How could she lose weight if it wasn't a diet? She had been trying to starve herself and it didn't seem to be working. She decided to call the school nurse, Mrs. Jones, in the morning.

INTRODUCTION

Physical fitness and nutrition are closely related. An adequate diet in combination with physical exercise has long been recognized as essential for building and maintaining strong, healthy bodies and maintaining stamina. Being physically fit helps achieve good weight management.

One fourth of the adult population in the United States is estimated to be overweight. In a large population of adolescent females, 75 per cent perceived themselves as overweight and 55 per cent reported being terrified about being obese (Czajka-Narins, 1990). Millions of dollars are spent trying to control weight in the United States with little positive impact. In the United States and Canada, overnutrition is much more prevalent than is undernutrition. Many persons are easily allured by dieting gimmicks because they feel helpless to control their intake of food. They refuse to make food choices and so are able to rely on the rigidness of a **fad diet** (a diet that promises quick weight loss and an easy cure). When the desired weight loss is achieved, most overweight persons will regain the lost weight. This can be very costly psychologically. In addition, chronic dieting impairs health, especially when diets are nutritionally inadequate.

Unfortunately, in today's society, extremes of behaviors are sometimes encouraged. This is certainly true with athletic competition and weight control. Aiming for a very low body fat percentage and high lean muscle mass can be detrimental to health if not done in a sensible manner. The use of anabolic steroids by some athletes in an attempt to build muscle is a detrimental practice. And popular culture's emphasis on high-fat, high-sugar foods can create conflict in the fitness-minded person. Anorexia and bulimia have increasingly become problems of our athletic youth as is the case with Joey Bernardo (see Chapter 15 for more on these psychological eating disorders).

All persons, whether athletes or not, benefit from a diet that contains a wide variety of foods to ensure an adequate intake of nutrients. Energy needs depend on the percentage of lean body tissue present and the level and duration of activity performed. Optimum health and performance are promoted by a diet with 55 per cent or more of the kilocalories supplied by complex carbohydrate, approximately 15 per cent by protein, and no more than 30 per cent by fat, with ample water to prevent dehydration. Weight control and increased muscle stores can be achieved by carefully adjusting diet and exercise patterns.

FACT & FALLACY

FALLACY: "Diet pills" allow a person to eat as much as desired and still lose weight.

FACT: There are different types of so-called diet pills ranging from amphetamines to over-the-counter drugs promising quick results. Some cause loss of appetite but may also irritate the heart muscle and negatively affect the nervous system. The use of pills may also lead to dependency and abuse. No medication of any kind should be used as an aid to lose weight without strict medical supervision. Even with medical supervision, there is the matter of permanency. No changes should be made unless they can be maintained for life.

WHAT IS PHYSICAL FITNESS?

Physical fitness, according to the President's Council on Physical Fitness, is "the ability to carry out daily tasks with vigor and alertness, without undue fatigue, and with ample energy to enjoy leisure time pursuits and to meet unforeseen emergencies." Physical fitness increases cardiovascular endurance, muscle strength, stamina, and flexibility of muscles and joints in the full range of movement. A body that is physically fit utilizes more kilocalories (muscles require more energy to be maintained than adipose tissue does). A physically fit person feels better and can cope more easily with stress.

WHAT IS HEALTHY WEIGHT MANAGEMENT?

Healthy weight management means achieving a weight that is conducive to physical health as well as psychological health. **Desirable weight,** however, may be higher than ideal body weight according to predetermined weight-for-height charts. For this reason, the term "healthy weight" is increasingly gaining acceptance. Other factors such as age, general health status, and potential for obtaining and maintaining weight loss are also considered when determining desirable weight.

Aiming for an unrealistic weight that cannot be permanently maintained is not a healthy goal. Losing weight only to gain it back is far worse than never losing any weight at all. Generally, a 10 per cent weight loss for the overweight person is feasible and can have a significant impact on health. Slow weight loss of approximately 1 pound per week is more likely to be permanent and therefore falls within the boundaries of healthy weight management.

WHY IS EXERCISE SO IMPORTANT FOR WEIGHT MANAGEMENT?

The first and most obvious reason that exercise is important for weight management is that it "burns" kilocalories. The duration of the activity, the intensity of the activity, and the weight of the individual performing the activity are all factors that affect just how many kilocalories are expended.

Activity is also important because it causes more kilocalories to be expended even *after* the exercise is finished. Research shows that physical activity can increase the metabolic rate by as much as 10 per cent for as long as 24 hours after the activity ceases. This is especially true of aerobic exercise.

Regular exercise, either alone or in combination with dietary modification, can have an important role in weight management. Exercise is a necessary component of daily living but one that is forgotten all too often. Exercise will help:

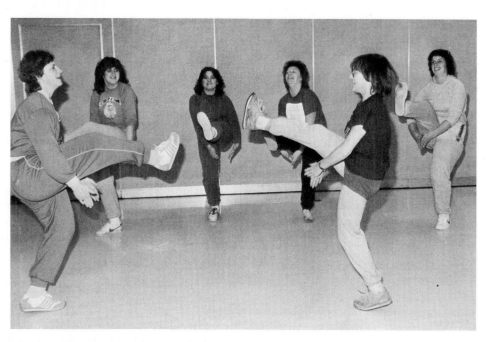

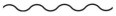

▲ FIGURE 20-1

Exercise is an important part of weight management. (Courtesy of St. Elizabeth Hospital, Utica, NY.)

- decrease body fat while helping to preserve and tone muscle tissue
- relieve stress
- increase energy levels
- provide a sense of control over health and lifestyle
- control appetite

The amount of exercise for persons with health problems will depend on the physician's advice. Figure 20–1 shows exercise as an important part of weight control. The approximate number of kilocalories per hour it takes to perform each of the five different types of activity is given in Table 20–1. These figures include the basal kilocalories needed.

▲ T A B L E   2 0 – 1

KILOCALORIES EXPENDED PER HOUR FOR VARIOUS TYPES OF ACTIVITIES

TYPE OF ACTIVITY	KCAL/HOUR*	TYPE OF ACTIVITY	KCAL/HOUR*
Sedentary Activities Reading, writing, eating, watching TV or movies, listening to radio; sewing; playing cards; typing, office work, and other activities done while sitting that require little or no arm movement.	80–100	**Moderate Activities** Making beds; mopping and scrubbing; sweeping; light polishing and waxing; laundering by machine; light gardening and carpentry work; walking moderately fast; other activities done while standing that require moderate arm movement; and activities done while sitting that require more vigorous arm movement.	170–240
Light Activities Preparing and cooking food; doing dishes; dusting; handwashing small articles of clothing; ironing; walking slowly; personal care; miscellaneous office work and other activities done while standing that require some arm movement; and rapid typing and other activities done while sitting that are more strenuous.	110–160	**Vigorous Activities** Heavy scrubbing and waxing; handwashing large articles of clothing; hanging out clothes; stripping beds; other heavy work; walking fast; bowling; golfing; gardening.	250–350
		Strenuous Activities Swimming; playing tennis; running; bicycling; dancing; skiing; playing football.	350 and more

* A range of caloric values is given for each type of activity to allow for differences in activities and in persons. Of the sedentary activities, for example, typing uses more kilocalories than watching TV. And some persons will use more kilocalories in carrying out either activity than others; some persons are more efficient in their body actions than others. Values closer to the upper limit of a range will give a better picture of kilocalorie expenditures for men and those near the lower limit a better picture for women.

From U.S. Department of Agriculture: Food and Your Weight. Home and Garden Bulletin No. 74. Washington, DC.

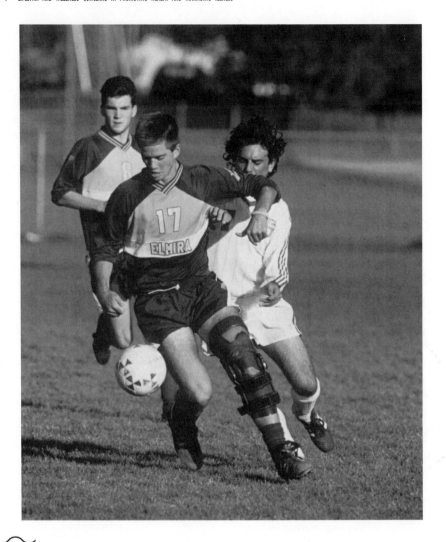

▲ FIGURE 20-2

Soccer is a form of aerobic exercise. (Courtesy of Cornell University Photography, Ithaca, NY.)

Aerobic Versus
Anaerobic Exercise for
Weight Management

Aerobic exercise is any exercise that requires more air (just like the term sounds: "air-o-bic"). It is this type of activity that tends to use the highest percentage of body fat for fuel, thus promoting the most beneficial weight loss. Aerobic exercise involves large muscle groups and builds cardiovascular endurance (Fig. 20–2). Aerobic exercise includes cycling, jogging, walking briskly, cross-country skiing, rowing, and dancing. When such activity is performed continuously for at least 20 minutes three to five times per week, there is considerable benefit for weight management and cardiovascular health. But there is increasing acceptance that even "5 minutes here or there" is better than no exercise and can encourage a person to slowly increase physical activity.

A good analogy to use in patient education is that of a fire in a fireplace that is going out. You can say, "When you blow on the fire it burns faster. And while it is true that we do not have a fire in our stomachs, we still use air (oxygen) to burn our food kilocalories. Aerobic exercise causes us to take in more air and thus we burn food kilocalories faster."

Walking and swimming are generally safe exercises that can promote weight loss without injury. High-risk individuals, such as those with a history of heart disease, hypertension, or diabetes should first contact their physician before embarking on any exercise regimen.

Anaerobic exercise means without air. Weight training is an example of anaerobic exercise. It will produce an increase in lean body mass. An increase in lean body mass will indirectly help in weight management since muscle requires more energy than adipose tissue. For the short term, muscle development can be associated with weight gain. This is a healthy gain and is often in conjunction with decreased inches related to loss of body fat. (A pound of muscle takes less space, as it is denser than an equivalent pound of body fat; thus weight loss may not occur even though inches decrease.)

Other Benefits
of Exercise

Exercise is associated with improved blood sugar control for the person with diabetes, reduced blood pressure, increased amounts of the good high-density lipoprotein cholesterol, and improved bone density. Weight-bearing exercise can slow down bone loss after menopause. Prior to or close to menopause, lifting weights actually increases bone density (Johns Hopkins Medical Letter, 1994).

WHAT STANDARDS ARE USED TO DETERMINE DESIRABLE WEIGHT?

The Metropolitan Life Height and Weight Tables (see Appendix 15) are commonly used tools for determining desirable weight; however, they should not be used without taking into account their shortcomings. Several considerations to bear in mind when using the Metropolitan Life tables follow:

1. Tables are not representative of the whole population, especially not of minority populations.
2. Tables are based on mortality data. Morbidity is not considered.
3. Frame size was not measured. Thus a small-framed person may appear underweight on this table while large-framed persons may appear overweight when they are not.
4. Weight tables do not provide information on the amount of weight contributed from muscle, fat, and bone. Thus a person whose weight is mostly from bone and muscle (such as a body builder) may appear overweight.

The **body mass index (BMI)** is considered one of the simpler tools that more accurately determines appropriate body weight. The formula used for the BMI was developed over 100 years ago by a mathematician named Quetelet. As only a mathematician can do, he realized that dividing a person's weight in kilograms by the square of the height in centimeters gives a better sense of body proportion. A healthy BMI is between 21 and 24 with an upper limit of 27—see Appendix 16 for a nomogram version of the BMI (American Dietetic Association, 1993). A BMI under 30 may be acceptable if there are no health problems.

Even more precise methods of determining body fat percentage include:

- skin-fold measurements taken at different body sites
- bioelectric impedance machine, which sends an imperceptible electrical current through the body
- underwater weighing (usually done only at research centers)

In some sports activities, such as wrestling, there is often great pressure for the athletes to attain a weight lower than their usual weight. In order to achieve peak performance and maintain health, the athlete must be well nourished and have a healthy minimal fat reserve. Athletes, especially teenaged ones, should never be encouraged to lose weight by excessive loss of body mass or body fluids. Methods such as starvation, the use of diuretics or cathartics, the restriction of fluids, and prolonged sauna sessions are dangerous. Such methods lead to nutritional deficiencies and dehydration, with increased risk of heat stress and renal problems. Rapid weight loss and restricting the diet prior to competition can actually lessen the wrestler's ability to compete. This is due to loss of muscle through rapid weight loss and depleted glycogen stores with precompetition fasting. Adequate glycogen is needed to fuel the muscles during the sports event (see Fig. 20–2).

In determining appropriate body weight, measuring levels of body fat is a more helpful method than using height and weight tables, which may indicate, for example, that a muscular football player is overweight. Average levels of fat for the general population are 15 to 18 per cent of body weight for men and 20 to 25 per cent of body weight for women. The usual range of per cent body fat is 5 to 12 per cent for male athletes and 10 to 20 per cent for female athletes. A body fat percentage less than 4 per cent for men and 10 per cent for women is a possible indicator of an eating disorder (American Dietetic Association, 1993). A health professional trained in anthropometry can calculate the percentage of body fat that should be lost before the season of competition starts and can plan how to accomplish this goal safely.

If body fat percentage is greater than acceptable, the school nurse (or health educator) can assist the coach by counseling the athlete to lose weight gradually through moderate reduction in the amount of food consumed while moderately increasing activity. If sudden or excessive weight loss occurs, serious organic illness or psychological problems should be ruled out.

If weight gain is recommended to improve performance, the weight should be in the form of increased muscle mass. It should be recognized that the desired weight gain may simply not be attainable because of the level of physical maturity. An additional intake of 800 to 1000 kilocalories per day may need to be consumed to support the energy needs.

WHAT ARE THE NUTRITIONAL NEEDS OF THE PHYSICALLY ACTIVE?

Energy Requirements

An individual who is physically active uses more energy. The increased energy needs for the physically fit person are related in part to increased muscle mass. Muscles require more energy to be maintained than does body fat. Exercise of the large muscles of the body (thighs and upper arm muscles) requires the most energy. Thus, walking and upper arm exercises can contribute to weight management.

Specific energy needs depend on one's age, sex, type of exercise, and degree of exertion. According to the Food and Nutrition Board of the National Academy of Sciences, the adult energy requirement for maintaining weight with moderate activity is about one and a half times the basal energy requirement. For very active persons, such as athletes, the allowance may be two times the basal energy requirement or more (National Academy of Sciences, National Research Council, 1989). As many as 6000 kilocalories may be needed to maintain weight. With a few exceptions, a male teenaged athlete should eat no fewer than 2000 kilocalories per day, and a female teenaged athlete should eat 1700 to 1800 kilocalories per day.

The distribution of energy-producing nutrients in the athlete's diet is similar to that in the nonathlete's diet. There should be at least 55 to 60 per cent carbohydrate, of which less than 10 to 15 per cent is simple carbohydrates (sugar), up to 15 per cent protein, and less than 30 per cent fat (University of California at Berkeley, 1993). This recommendation is similar to that for the general population.

Calculation of Kilocalorie Needs

A 24-hour diet recall is one way to estimate current kilocalorie intake. A weight loss of 1 to 2 pounds per week should result from a reduction of 500 to 1000 kilocalories per day from the current intake.

A simple formula can also be used to calculate approximate kilocalorie needs as follows:

20 kcals/kg body weight for low activity (10 kcals/lb body weight)
30 kcals/kg body weight for high activity (15 kcals/lb body weight)
38 kcals/kg body weight for adolescent females
45 kcals/kg body weight for adolescent males

Carbohydrate Needs

During exercise, most of the energy that is used comes from carbohydrate. Carbohydrate is the nutrient that is most readily digested, stored, and metabolized. Its storage form, glycogen, is found in both the liver and muscle and is readily available during exercise, assuming the glycogen stores are not depleted. For endurance events, carbohydrate intake at regular intervals should be emphasized. Although the body can use fat and protein for energy, carbohydrate is the most efficient fuel.

Carbohydrate Loading for the Sports Person

Fat cannot be metabolized effectively without carbohydrate. While we have almost unlimited amounts of body fat that can be used for energy, our storage of carbohydrate is limited to what our liver and muscles can hold. For these reasons, carbohydrate storage is the limiting factor in the length of time exercise can be sustained. **Carbohydrate loading** is a means of manipulating diet and exercise in an effort to maximize glycogen stores during an endurance competition. It is most often practiced by long-distance runners, cyclists, and swimmers.

The safest and simplest way of achieving high glycogen stores requires that the athlete consume about 800 grams carbohydrate (6 to 10 grams carbohydrate per kilogram of body weight) per day for at least 3 days prior to a sports event lasting more than 90 minutes. Complete rest is required the day before competition (American Dietetic Association, 1993). Exhaustion is delayed simply by increasing muscle glycogen stores.

Role of Protein for Physical Fitness

Protein's major role is to build and repair body tissues. Recent evidence suggests that the RDA of 0.8 grams protein per kilogram body weight is too low for an athlete. The suggested protein requirement is now set at 1 to 1.5 g/kg/day. This protein level is easily met by a diet containing 1800 to 2000 kilocalories per day. Thus protein supplements are not necessary and are potentially detrimental to health and athletic performance. Dehydration and renal complications may result, for example. Also, a high-protein diet is often high in fat and kilocalories and can increase the risk for cardiovascular disease and obesity (American Dietetic Association, 1993).

FACT & FALLACY

FALLACY: Athletes require large amounts of protein for building muscles.

FACT: Muscle mass can be increased only by appropriate exercise. The only athletes who require slightly more than 0.8 grams of protein per kilogram of body weight are those who swim, jog, or bicycle and do other aerobic activities. However, the additional 0.5 grams per kilogram of body weight that these people need is met by the typical American diet, which usually supplies more protein than required.

Role of Fat for Healthy Weight Management and Physical Fitness

Fat is a major source of fuel during endurance activity, including light exercise such as walking. A trained athlete is able to use a higher percentage of fat for fuel, thereby sparing glycogen stores and running longer before exhaustion. However, fat used during exercise can be taken from body fat stores; for this reason, most athletes do not need to increase dietary fat consumption to meet needs. Exceptions are extremely lean athletes or anorexic athletes who have very low body fat stores. These individuals may require greater amounts of fat to gain or maintain weight during training.

The Role of Vitamin and Mineral Supplementation in Sports Nutrition

For women with **amenorrhea** (no menstrual period), a calcium intake of 120 per cent of the RDA (about 1400 mg) is recommended (American Dietetic Association, 1993). Food is still the recommended source. No supplementation is necessary for women with normal menses who have a balanced diet, including the recommended calcium intake, and perform weight-bearing exercises that promote bone resorption of calcium.

Sports anemia is a condition observed in healthy athletes. The cause appears to be related to an increase in plasma volume (thereby diluting the amount of iron in the blood) that is associated with the initiation of training. Sports anemia is not a clinical iron-deficiency anemia. Adequate iron intake, according to the recommended dietary allowance (RDA), should be ensured. Iron status should be evaluated periodically in athletes before a supplement is prescribed (American Dietetic Association, 1993).

FACT & FALLACY

FALLACY: Competitive athletes benefit from megavitamin supplements.

FACT: Taking megadoses of vitamins can be dangerous, and there is no good scientific evidence that shows that supplements are helpful. An overdose of fat-soluble vitamins can be harmful, and an excess of water-soluble vitamins is excreted in the urine and may also be harmful (see Chapter 5).

What Is the Role of Water and Electrolytes in Sports Activities?

Water is probably one of the most critical nutrients for athletic performance, yet it is the nutrient that so many active individuals tend to forget about or ignore. (About 50 to 75 per cent of the human body is water; it is essential for circulation, urine production, and temperature control.)

As the athlete exercises, heat is produced by the muscles. This heat needs to escape in order for a safe internal body temperature to be maintained. Body heat cannot escape fast enough unless sweat is produced. When sweat evaporates, heat is released from the blood circulating near the skin, and the body is cooled. This "water-cooling mechanism" is extremely effective in maintaining the necessary body temperature. However, if adequate hydration is not maintained, sweating will diminish or cease entirely. As a result, body temperature quickly rises and heat exhaustion, heat stroke, and death may result. The warning signals that occur during dehydration are:

- pronounced thirst
- loss of coordination
- mental confusion with irritability
- dry skin
- decreased urine output

Electrolytes such as sodium, potassium, chloride, and magnesium are all lost in sweat. However, in most cases, electrolytes lost during exercise can be replaced easily by increasing the intake of potassium-rich foods such as citrus fruits, bananas, dark green leafy vegetables, lean meats, dried beans, potatoes, and milk. If exercise is prolonged or undertaken in extreme heat or humidity, a sports drink with added electrolytes may be desirable (American Dietetic Association, 1993).

FACT & FALLACY

FALLACY: Salt tablets should be taken by the athlete.
FACT: Salt supplementation is not recommended. Salt tablets can remain whole in the stomach and cause irritation to the stomach lining. Excess salt also draws fluid away from the body cells where it is needed. Thus salt tablets are not necessary and are potentially harmful. Eating foods will naturally replace the amount of sodium lost in sweat from exercise.

How Is Dehydration Prevented?

Thirst should never be relied on as an accurate gauge for fluid needs, since the feeling of thirst is not triggered until the athlete is already considerably dehydrated. Water should be consumed frequently and regularly by the athlete before, during, and after exercise. The following regimen is recommended before, during, and after an endurance event:

- 2 hours before competition, drink at least 2 cups fluid
- 15 minutes before competition, drink another 2 cups fluid
- during hot/humid weather, drink ½ to ¾ cup cool fluid every 15 minutes
- after the endurance event, drink 2 cups of fluid for every pound of body weight lost (American Dietetic Association, 1993).

Cool or cold water is the ideal fluid, since it empties from the stomach most quickly. Other fluids, such as juices and soda pop, have a high sugar concentration, resulting in a slower gastric emptying time. Athletes should experiment prior to competition to find out what works best for them. Diluted juice may be fine, but generally water is the preferred fluid. Commercial sports drinks may be desirable to help maintain blood glucose and electrolyte levels during exercise. It should be noted that beverages containing caffeine or alcohol cause increased urine production and water depletion and therefore should not be considered as fluid replacement (Clark, 1990).

The Precompetition
Meal for Athletes

A light meal that includes some well liked foods rich in complex carbohydrates with approximately 500 to 600 kilocalories is recommended by experts and should be eaten at least 3 hours before the competition to allow complete digestion to occur and to prevent any feelings of hunger throughout the event. Diluted juice can be consumed just prior to the sports event if there are concerns for low blood sugar. All food groups from the Food Guide Pyramid should be represented in the meal, including low-fat or skim milk.

Caffeine should be avoided because of its diuretic effect. Foods high in fat slow the rate of digestion and are not recommended for the presports meal. A drastic increase in the amount of fiber and complex carbohydrates for the meal may result in gastrointestinal distress, especially when the athlete may already be nervous about the competition. Carbonated beverages should be avoided, but 2 to 3 cups of other liquids are recommended, and fluids should be consumed up until the competition begins in order to guard against dehydration. Athletes who experience nausea before an event may prefer to take the precompetition meal in the form of a well balanced liquid that can be digested quickly.

A sample precompetition meal containing 500 to 600 kilocalories may be:

> 1 cup spaghetti with low-fat meat sauce
> 1 cup skim milk
> 1 slice Italian bread
> 1 cup sliced pears
> 1 cup water

or

> 1 light-meat turkey sandwich on whole-grain bread
> 1 large banana
> 1 cup skim milk

FACT & FALLACY

FALLACY: Milk causes "cotton mouth" (dryness and discomfort in the mouth).

FACT: Milk supplies valuable nutrients and is a good source of extra energy, vitamins, and minerals. It does not cause "cotton mouth" or discomfort.

FALLACY: Candy bars are a good source of quick energy before a sports event.

FACT: The fat in the candy bars slows the rate of digestion and the sugar that is quickly absorbed causes an increase in insulin production, leading to hypoglycemia, premature fatigue, and decreased performance.

The Postevent
Sports Meal

The athlete should consume carbohydrate foods or drinks as soon as possible after an endurance event. The first several hours after the exercise are most conducive to restoration of glycogen stores. Up to 600 grams of carbohydrate may be needed (American Dietetic Association, 1993). Fruit juice may be most easily consumed, although it would take about a gallon of juice to make up this amount of carbohydrate. This could be achieved by drinking 1 cup juice every 15 minutes for about 4 or 5 hours after the sports event. When the appetite returns to normal, sandwiches, fruit, and milk, which all contribute carbohydrate, may be appealing to the hungry athlete.

WHAT ARE THE CAUSES AND TREATMENTS OF OBESITY AND OVERWEIGHT?

Obesity versus
Overweight

Overweight refers to an excess of body weight and is usually determined by comparing a person's weight against a standard height and weight chart, such as the Metropolitan Life tables (see Appendix 15). If a person's weight is 10 per cent greater than the standard, he or she is considered to be overweight. It is important to note that an excess of body weight may be, but is not necessarily, an indication of too much body fat. Overweight may also be caused by fluid retention or extensive muscle development. A professional football player is a good example of an individual who may be overweight according to height and weight tables but who carries his extra weight in muscle mass, not fatty tissue.

Obesity is a term used to describe an excess of body *fat*. Although weight alone does not indicate the degree of body fat, an individual is still classified by many health professionals as obese if weight is 20 per cent or more than the standard weight for height. A more accurate means of determining obesity is by first estimating the percentage of body fat in relation to total weight. Individuals with a body fat content of more than 25 per cent of total body weight for men and 30 per cent for women are considered obese (American Dietetic Association, 1993). Obesity is associated with hypertension and hypercholesterolemia, both of which are major risk factors for cardiovascular disease. Obesity also tends to impair glucose and plasma insulin regulation, which is linked to diabetes.

Causes of Obesity

The causes of obesity are numerous and complex and are not thoroughly understood. Most simply, obesity occurs as a result of long-term positive **energy balance.** In other words, weight gain occurs when kilocalorie intake exceeds kilocalorie expenditure over an extended period of time. This can explain the increased occurrence over the past 2 or 3 decades of obesity in children and youth, many of whom also lead a sedentary lifestyle (Pate, 1993). There are many factors that can affect energy balance in any individual. Eating habits, cooking methods, family customs, emotional problems, peer pressure, food advertising, and food availability all have their influence on kilocalorie intake. Factors such as age, gender, heredity, body composition, job type, and exercise habits all affect energy expenditure.

Beyond energy balance, it is now believed that as much as 79 per cent of human obesity has a genetic component (Community Nutrition Institute,

1993). This explains the propensity toward obesity; however, environmental triggers are still needed, such as excess kilocalorie intake compared with energy needs.

As a general rule of thumb, a gain of 1 pound of body fat is the result of approximately 3500 kilocalories that have been ingested above energy needs. On the same note, a deficit of 3500 kilocalories must be achieved in order to lose 1 pound of body fat. Therefore, effective treatment of obesity is aimed at decreasing kilocalorie intake and increasing energy expenditure.

The two most common theories about obesity, although controversial, are the **fat cell theory** and the **set point theory.** These theories have been proposed by researchers who hope to explain why many people have difficulty controlling their weight even when they are highly motivated.

THE FAT CELL THEORY.   During childhood, excess kilocalorie intake can result in increased numbers of fat cells **(hyperplasty).** At any age, but especially after puberty, enlargement of fat cells **(hypertrophy)** can occur. Once a fat cell is created, it exists for life. Therefore, when an obese person loses weight, fat cells do not disappear, they only shrink. It is felt that a person with hyperplastic obesity has more trouble losing weight and an increased likelihood of regaining any lost weight (Davis and Sherer, 1994).

THE SET POINT THEORY.   This theory holds that each individual has a "natural" weight, which is predetermined by a number of biological factors. Attempts to change weight below the set point are thwarted by various mechanisms in the body. In other words, the body defends its set point, even though it may be a greater weight than what is considered ideal. The set point is also felt to contribute to normal weight and underweight as well; thus attempts to change one's predetermined biological weight may be thwarted by physiological mechanisms (Davis and Sherer, 1994).

OTHER THEORIES.   There are other controversial theories that also attempt to explain the development and maintenance of obesity. The malfunctioning hypothalamus theory views obesity as a result of overeating that is caused by a defective hypothalamus. The sluggish metabolism theory holds that owing to heredity, certain individuals have bodies that function on less energy than is normal. The brown fat theory is based on the premise that a special type of fat (brown fat) in the body gets rid of extra calories through heat generation, and obese people have less brown fat than do nonobese people.

A new theory is beginning to emerge among some health care professionals related to insulin production. It is increasingly being recognized that families with a history of diabetes (especially non–insulin-dependent diabetes) have an underlying genetically based insulin resistance. Excess insulin is produced by the body to compensate for the inherited insulin resistance. Insulin is known to be **lipogenic** (promoting body fat) and inhibits **lipolysis** (breakdown of body fat) (Grant, 1992). This **"hyperinsulinemia"** (excess insulin in the blood) is known to coexist with obesity. But it has not yet been thoroughly researched to determine which comes first, the obesity or the excess insulin production, as obesity is known to cause hyperinsulinemia. But there is evidence that normalizing insulin production will promote weight loss. "With reduction in caloric intake, insulin secretion decreases, allowing mobilization of body fat" (Grant, 1992). A study with rats concluded that "hyperinsulinemia is a pathological driving force in producing incipient obesity by overstimulating white adipose tissue" (Cusin et al., 1992). Hyperinsulinemia with or without insulin resistance is commonly found in hypertensive individuals and may be a common pathophysiological feature of obesity, hypertension, and glucose intolerance (Modan et al., 1985). Some overweight individuals thus may benefit from a decreased sugar intake in addition to reduced fat intake for effective weight loss or management and control of hypertension. Reduced sugar intake will promote decreased insulin production. Researchers in Japan have shown that the combination of fat and sugar in a meal, such as with cake, cookies, and ice cream, may cause more weight gain than expected by kilocalories alone (Lepke, 1993).

FACT & FALLACY

FALLACY: Obesity is caused by lack of willpower.
FACT: Many overweight persons do not consume a total amount of kilocalories in excess of what their thinner counterparts consume. There may be metabolic differences between the obese and the thin person and the obese person may be better able to conserve kilocalories consumed. More research is needed to fully establish the metabolic differences contributing to obesity.

Obesity Treatments

Obesity is a very difficult condition to treat successfully in the long term. "Up to 95 per cent of formerly obese patients have regained all or most of weight lost in 2 to 5 years" (Community Nutrition Institute, 1993).

The majority of all obese persons can be categorized as mildly obese, that is, a weight of 20 to 30 per cent greater than the ideal. For these mildly obese individuals, the comprehensive treatment plan includes some basic components, which will be discussed on the following pages: (1) a nutritionally adequate diet plan; (2) physical activity; (3) behavior modification; and (4) cognitive-behavioral therapy.

Extreme morbid obesity has been treated with various surgical techniques, such as gastric bypass, jaw wiring, gastric stapling, fat suctioning, and modified fasting. These treatments had limited success and are not currently routinely recommended.

Food intake for any individual attempting to lose weight should meet the body's needs for all nutrients but not kilocalories. It takes a deficit of about 500 kilocalories per day to lose 1 pound of fat in 1 week. For safe and permanent weight loss, an individual should lose no more than 1 to 2 pounds per week. This is a much slower weight loss than most people are willing to accept. However, this rate is most closely associated with permanent weight loss. Persons with a history of diet failures or weight cycling may be more accepting of this newer approach. Because of the way the body uses fuel from carbohydrate, fat, and protein, a faster weight loss than this will compel the body to use protein for energy instead of fat. This is highly undesirable because it decreases muscle mass, which will lower the person's needs for kilocalories. Weight cycling can change the body's composition so that muscle percentage decreases (muscle loss with each dieting attempt) and body fat percentage increases (regain of mostly body fat with each failed dieting attempt).

Experience has shown that in order to lose weight at the optimal 1 to 2 pounds per week, most women need to consume about 1200 kilocalories per day; men will lose this amount with an intake of about 1500 to 1800 kilocalories per day. These kilocalorie levels may vary, however. And too much emphasis on kilocalories can be counterproductive. Reducing fat and sugar intake and learning to eat based on internal hunger cues rather than for non-hunger reasons can go a long way toward normalizing intake and weight management. Vitamin and mineral supplementation should be ordered when energy intake is less than 1200 kilocalories per day. Before embarking on any weight loss program, an individual should be examined by a physician. The dieting plan should also be individualized and flexible (Table 20–2).

Some correlates with successful weight loss include losing at a slow rate (as little as ½ pound per week is considered significant, and a maximum of

▲   TABLE 20-2

DIETING TIPS

1. Eat regularly, choosing foods low in fat and sugar.
2. Chew thoroughly and slowly.
3. Stop eating when stomach is comfortably full.
4. Make diet changes that can be maintained for life; temporary quick-fixes are counterproductive for healthy weight management.
5. Wait 15 minutes before having second helpings.
6. Include exercise for healthy weight management.
7. To deal with the "clean your plate" practice, remember that excess food goes either to waste or to the waist.
8. When faced with an indulgence, ask yourself, "How will I feel tomorrow if I don't eat this food today?" Give yourself permission to eat if feelings of deprivation may arise.
9. When ready to give up on dieting efforts, remember Ann Landers' quote, "The difference between a successful person and an unsuccessful person is that the successful person never stops trying."
10. For individualized meal-planning tips, consult a registered dietitian, the expert in nutrition.

1 to 2 pounds per week recommended), regular exercise, and ongoing support through family, friends, or a therapist specializing in weight management. Improving the likelihood of long-term weight loss may result in a shift toward a chronic disease model of care with extended patient contact. This implies that a person attempting to lose weight should have ongoing professional support rather than enrolling in a short-term weight loss program (Wing, 1992). Once weight loss is significant, relapse prevention training is considered important (Baum et al., 1991). In other words, maintaining weight loss can be more difficult than losing weight in the first place.

FACT & FALLACY

FALLACY: Skipping meals is a good way to lose weight.
   FACT: Studies have shown that three to six meals a day is the best and most healthful way to eat. Skipping meals tends to suppress **metabolism** (the rate at which food kilocalories are burned) and to cause overeating later in the day.

Meal Planning

In addition to keeping the number of kilocalories low, it is also important to plan the foods from which the kilocalories are coming. Carbohydrate, fat, protein, and alcohol are the only sources of kilocalories. Carbohydrate and protein provide 4 kilocalories per gram, fat provides 9 kilocalories per gram, and alcohol provides 7 kilocalories per gram. There is growing acceptance, however, that fat may actually contribute the equivalent of 11 or 12 kilocalories per gram in relation to how the body uses it. In other words, ounce for ounce, dietary fat provides two to three times as many kilocalories as either protein or carbohydrate. Fat should be very limited in the diet for this reason, as well as for its association with heart disease and cancer. Fat should contribute no more than 30 per cent of total kilocalories, whereas protein should contribute 10 to 15 per cent and carbohydrates at least 55 to 60 per cent. These proportions are similar to the Dietary Guidelines for Americans discussed in Chapter 6. Alcohol in moderation (1 to 2 ounces or drinks) may be included in a weight loss plan as long as the minimum number of servings of the Food Guide Pyramid are included in the daily diet. A small glass of wine or one light beer provides about 100 kilocalories (roughly the equivalent of 2 teaspoons of added fat).

Any long-term eating plan for weight management must be easy to follow if it is to be successful. Variety, flexibility, and consideration of an individual's lifestyle and food preferences must be a part of the plan. Changes in eating habits must be viewed as a permanent change in lifestyle or "way of eating" rather than a diet, which implies a temporary and restrictive change. Most individuals who successfully lose weight and maintain their weight loss have made lifelong changes in eating patterns.

The food exchange system is the tool most often used in reducing kilocalorie intake. Originally developed by the American Diabetes Association and the American Dietetic Association, the exchange system aims to control carbohydrate intake and kilocalorie intake in the management of diabetes (see Appendix 9). This system is also used for weight management alone. The exchanges break all foods into six separate groups. Foods in the same group have similar proportions of carbohydrate, fat, and protein and about the same number of kilocalories. The exchange list for each food group provides the portion size of each food that is nutritionally equivalent to all other foods in the group. By allowing a given number of exchanges in each group, a daily diet pattern can be developed that offers the dieter a choice of a variety of foods within the given pattern. The famous Richard Simmons' "Deal A Meal" card system is based on the exchanges. Weight Watchers also uses the exchange system.

The Food Guide Pyramid shows a kilocalorie range of as little as 1000 to 1200 kilocalories if only lean meats and skim milk and no added fats or sugars are consumed (Table 20–3). The upper limit of recommended servings of the Food Guide Pyramid is about 2000 kilocalories. Additional amounts of food or added fats and sugars can make up the high kilocalorie needs of the athlete or sports-minded adolescent. Table 20–4 shows how a normal 3000-kilocalorie diet may be modified to give one family member a 1200-kilocalorie diet without preparing separate meals. Some items are omitted, some are served in smaller portions, and some are served in modified form, for example, skim milk instead of whole milk or black coffee instead of coffee with cream and sugar.

Any meal plan, but especially one that is low in kilocalories to begin with, must emphasize nutrient-dense foods. These are foods that "pack in" plenty of vitamins, minerals, or protein with a relatively small number of kilocalories. Conversely, weight loss regimens should avoid "empty-calorie" foods that contribute few nutrients but are high in sugar or fat kilocalories. Candy, soft drinks, most cookies, butter or margarine, and potato chips are examples of empty-calorie foods. Foods such as skim milk, spinach, cantaloupe, and fish are examples of nutrient-dense foods. Table 20–5 gives examples of specific kilocalorie content of foods in the Food Guide Pyramid food groups.

Behavior Modification

Behavior modification principles are used to assist the obese individual in identifying the personal eating behaviors that have been promoting weight gain and maintaining obesity. Once these factors are recognized, various techniques can be used to minimize their effects or remove them from the environment. For example, the sight of freshly baked cookies in a bakery window may be a strong enough stimulus to cause an individual to buy a dozen and eat them all on the way home. Behavior modification techniques could be employed that would suggest that this person take an al-

THE FOOD GUIDE PYRAMID AS A HEALTHY WEIGHT LOSS PLAN

FOOD GROUP	SERVING SIZE	COMMENTS
Bread, Cereal, Rice, and Pasta Group (6–11 servings)*	1 slice of bread 1 ounce of ready-to-eat cereal (check labels: 1 ounce = ¼ cup to 2 cups, depending on cereal) ½ cup of cooked cereal, rice, or pasta ½ hamburger roll, bagel, english muffin 3–4 plain crackers (small)	Count each serving of starch as 80 to 100 kilocalories Based on carbohydrate content and kilocalories, count dry vegetables (potatoes) and sweet vegetables (sweet corn, sweet peas, and sweet winter squash) as a starch
Vegetable Group (3–5 servings)*	1 cup of raw leafy vegetables ½ cup of other vegetables, cooked or chopped raw ¾ cup of vegetable juice	One serving of vegetables is about 25 kilocalories Vegetables that are low in carbohydrate and kilocalories are high in water content and are not sweet
Fruit Group (2–4 servings)*	1 medium apple, banana, orange, nectarine, peach ½ cup of chopped, cooked, or canned fruit ¾ cup of fruit juice	One serving of fruit is about 60 kilocalories Fruits that are dry (bananas) or are in portions greater than ½ cup contain more kilocalories (see Table 20–5 for examples)
Milk, Yogurt, and Cheese Group (2–3 servings)*	1 cup of milk or yogurt 1½ ounces of natural cheese 2 ounces of processed cheese	One cup of skim milk contains about 80 kilocalories One-per-cent milk has 100 kilocalories, 2-per-cent, 125 kilocalories, and whole milk, 170 kilocalories Two ounces of full fat cheese contains 200 kilocalories
Meat, Poultry, Fish, Dry Beans, Eggs, and Nuts Group (2–3 servings)*	2–3 ounces of cooked lean meat, poultry, or fish (1 ounce of meat = ½ cup of cooked dry beans, 1 egg, or 2 tablespoons of peanut butter)	One ounce of most meats contains 75 kilocalories Lean meat contains 50 kilocalories per ounce and high fat meat contains 100 kilocalories One tablespoon peanut butter contains 100 kilocalories and is counted as 1 ounce meat in the Exchange System One ounce equals ¼ cup; 3 ounces is the size of a deck of cards

* Recommended number of servings per day. Serving size information taken from a publication of the New York State Dietetic Association (NYSDA), Albany, NY.

▲ **T A B L E   2 0 – 4**

MODIFIED 3000-KILOCALORIE DIET

1200 KILOCALORIES		3000 KILOCALORIES	
Breakfast			
Orange juice	½ cup	Orange juice	½ cup
Soft-cooked egg	1 egg	Soft-cooked egg	1 egg
Whole wheat toast	1 slice	Bacon	2 medium strips
Butter or margarine	1 tsp	Whole wheat toast	2 slices
Skim milk	1 cup	Butter or margarine	2 tsp
Coffee (black), if desired	1 cup	Whole milk	1 cup
		Coffee	1 cup
		Cream	1 tbsp
		Sugar	1 tbsp
Lunch			
Sandwich		Tomato soup with milk	1 cup
Enriched bread	2 slices	Sandwich	
Boiled ham	1½ oz	Enriched bread	3 slices
Mayonnaise	2 tsp	Boiled ham	3 oz
Mustard	free	Mayonnaise	2½ tsp
Lettuce	1 large leaf	Mustard	free
Celery	1 small stalk	Lettuce	2 large leaves
Radishes	4 radishes	Celery	1 small stick
Dill pickle	½ large	Radishes	4 radishes
Skim milk	1 cup	Dill pickle	½ large
		Apple	1 medium
		Whole milk	1 cup
Dinner			
Roast meat	3 oz	Roast meat	4 oz
Rice, converted	½ cup	Rice, converted	⅔ cup
Spinach	¾ cup	Spinach, buttered	⅔ cup
Lemon	¼ medium	Lemon	¼ medium
Salad		Salad	
Peaches, canned	1 half peach	Peaches, canned	2 halves
Cottage cheese	2 tbsp	Cottage cheese	2 tbsp
Lettuce	1 large leaf	Lettuce	1 large leaf
		Rolls, enriched	2 small
		Butter or margarine	1 tsp
		Plain cake, iced	1 piece, 3 × 3 × 2 inches
Between-Meal Snack			
Apple	1 medium	Saltines	4
		Peanut butter	2 tbsp
		Whole milk	1 cup

From U.S. Department of Agriculture: Food and Your Weight. Home and Garden Bulletin No. 74. Washington, DC.

ternate route home from work, thereby removing the stimulus from his or her environment and preventing the eating response. By focusing on small, gradual behavioral changes, the individual learns to gain control of eating behaviors.

▲ **TABLE 20-5**

CALORIE CONTENT OF SPECIFIC FOODS OF THE FOOD GUIDE PYRAMID

Milk Group	Kilocalories	Meat Group	Kilocalories
Milk, whole, 1 cup	165	Meat, cooked, 4-oz serving	
Milk, skim, 1 cup	90	Beef, veal	250–425
Buttermilk, 1 cup	90	Lamb	300–475
Cheese, American, cheddar, 1 oz	115	Pork	375–450
Cheese, cottage, ½ cup	100	Note: variation depends on fat content	
Cereals and Bread		Poultry, cooked, 4-oz serving (without added fat)	
Bread, whole wheat or enriched,		Broiler-fryer	175
bakery, 1 slice	65	Roaster	225
homemade, 1 slice	100	Hens	350
Breakfast cereals, whole grain,		Liver—1 tsp fat	235
¾ cup cooked	100	Heart	150
Breakfast cereals, whole grain,		Tongue	300
dry, 1 oz	100	Fish	
Cornmeal, farina, spaghetti,		Lean—broiled, baked,	125
macaroni, noodles, rice, ¾ cup		haddock, cod	
cooked	100	Fat—broiled, baked,	225
Crackers, graham, 2 medium	55	halibut, salmon, tuna	
saltines, 3	50	Shrimp	150
Flour, whole wheat or enriched		Oysters, ½ cup	100
1 cup	400	Eggs, one	75
1 tbsp	25	Dry beans, peas, ½ cup cooked	100
		Nuts, 1 tbsp	50
		Peanut butter, 1 tbsp	100

Vegetables and Fruits (½ cup servings)

15 Kilocalories	25 Kilocalories	50 Kilocalories	75 Kilocalories
Asparagus, green	Broccoli	Grapefruit juice	Peas
Peppers, green	Carrots	Orange juice	Lima beans
Snap beans, green	Greens, cooked	Lemon juice	Sweet corn
Salad greens	Tomato, 1 medium	Strawberries	Apple, 1 medium
Cabbage, raw	Tomato, canned or fresh cooked	Peach, 1 medium	Apple juice
Peppers, raw	Tomato juice	Pears, canned with water	Sweet potato, ½ medium
Cantaloupe	Beets	Pineapple, raw	Banana, 1 medium
Celery	Brussels sprouts	Onions	Pear, 1 medium
Cucumbers	Cabbage, cooked	Parsnips	Apricots, dried
Eggplant	Cauliflower	Applesauce	Watermelon, 4-inch wedge
Lettuce, head	Rutabagas	Blackberries	Pineapple, canned or frozen
Radishes	Turnips	Blueberries	Pumpkin (¾ cup)
Squash, summer	Apricots, canned with water	Grapes	Winter squash
	Peaches, canned with water	Pineapple juice	
		Plums	
		Raspberries	

Cognitive-Behavioral Approach

This is a new approach that seeks to diminish weight cycling, which often occurs when only a behavioral approach is taken. This method includes helping the patient develop a support system of peers who are available to promote appropriate eating and exercise habits. Cognitive-behavioral treatment focuses on how thoughts, moods, dieting, and social pressure to be thin affect control of eating (Goodrick and Foreyt, 1991). This approach has been found to be effective in the short term in helping obese, nonpurging bulimic patients (Telch, 1990).

Fasting

Any severe restriction of food or limiting of food intake that results in weight loss can be referred to as fasting. This loss is mostly from lean body mass and poses great risks to health. Protein in the lean body tissue is used for energy when the body's stored glucose is depleted. This is not recommended, although some groups do practice periodic fasting for religious reasons. Owing to the health risks, fasting should not be used to lose weight.

WHY IS UNDERWEIGHT A HEALTH PROBLEM?

Underweight (10 per cent below recommended weight for height or a BMI of less than 19) associated with undernutrition can be a health problem because of lowered resistance to disease accompanied by fatigue and impaired body efficiency. This condition may be a symptom of or a predisposing factor in disease. Being underweight is especially serious in younger individuals, as underweight persons are more subject to tuberculosis and other opportunistic diseases. In children, it may result in retarded growth.

WHAT ARE THE CAUSES AND TREATMENT OF UNDERWEIGHT?

There are many reasons that an individual may weigh less than is desirable. For example, food intake that is insufficient for needs in quality and quantity (because of inadequate intake or poor absorption and utilization of food), wasting disease (e.g., cancer), increased metabolic rate (e.g., fevers, infection, hyperthyroidism, or burns), mental strain and worry, and excessive activity can all contribute to underweight.

An increase of 500 kilocalories a day in excess of need should result in a weight gain of 1 pound per week. An additional intake of two slices bread, 2 tablespoons of peanut butter or 2 ounces of cheese, and an extra two glasses of skim milk provides 500 kilocalories. If there is an adequate nutritional intake (at least the minimum number of recommended servings according to the Food Guide Pyramid), the additional kilocalories can appropriately come from added fats and sugars. Adding gravy, butter, mayonnaise, or heavy cream to foods can increase kilocalorie density of foods. Between-meal snacks such as milkshakes, puddings, and ice cream can also help promote weight gain. Treatment is aimed at developing appropriate food habits so that good nutritional status and weight gain can be maintained.

WHAT IS THE ROLE OF THE NURSE OR OTHER HEALTH CARE PROFESSIONAL IN PROMOTING HEALTHY WEIGHT AND PHYSICAL ACTIVITY?

Everyone, from the athlete to the older adult, needs access to reliable nutritional information. The Dietary Guidelines for Americans and the Food Guide Pyramid are excellent tools that the health professional can use effectively in teaching individuals to make good food choices for maintaining physical fitness. The registered dietitian is the health professional to consult for reliable nutritional information.

Sports nutrition myths are common, and the health professional has an important responsibility in dispelling misconceptions, such as the unwise belief that protein, vitamin, and mineral supplementation promotes better performance. The school nurse and physician play an important role in advising the coach, who must safeguard the health of students involved in various sports in which optimum performance is necessary.

The nurse or other health care professional can assist persons of all ages to identify appropriate weights for health and effective means to achieve changes in body composition. Female adolescents are particularly vulnerable to the media's representation of underweight models. The nurse or other health care professional can play a positive role in helping to modify unrealistic weight management in sports. There is much to be done to help our nation achieve weight and fitness goals that are positive and sound.

STUDY QUESTIONS AND ACTIVITIES

1. Who requires more kilocalories per kilogram of body weight, Anna Bernardo or her brother Joey? What factors have the greatest effect on energy needs?

2. Determine Anna Bernardo's body mass index (see Appendix 16). Is a weight goal of 100 pounds appropriate for her? How many kilocalories should she include daily to promote a sensible weight loss?

3. Two slices of whole-wheat bread contain 30 grams of carbohydrate and 6 grams of protein. How many kilocalories do the two slices contain? (NOTE: Count 1 gram of fat for each slice of whole-grain bread.)

4. How might you advise the Bernardo family to plan meals in order to meet the needs of all family members? Should separate meals be suggested? Why or why not?

5. Plan a 1200-kilocalorie diet pattern appropriate for weight loss and a 3000-kilocalorie diet to promote weight gain.

6. Class role-play: One student to play the school nurse, Mrs. Jones, and another to play Anna Bernardo. What should the nurse say when Anna asks where the diet plan is? How could the nurse discourage Anna from skipping meals to lose weight? How can the nurse advise Anna on a good weight goal and the means to attain it?

REFERENCES

American Dietetic Association: Position of The American Dietetic Association and The Canadian Dietetic Association: Nutrition for physical fitness and athletic performance for adults. J Am Diet Assoc, 1993; 93(6):691–695.

Baum JG, Clar HB, Sandler J: Preventing relapse in obesity through posttreatment maintenance systems: comparing the relative efficacy of two levels of therapist support. J Behav Med, 1991; 14(3):287–302.

Clark N: Nancy Clark's Sports Nutrition Guidebook. Champaign, IL, Leisure Press, 1990; pp 135–148.

Community Nutrition Institute: Science advisor dodges body weight controversy. Nutrition Week, September 1993; 23(34):3.

Cusin I, Rohner-Jeanrenaud F, Terrettaz J, Jeanrenaud B: Hyperinsulinemia and its impact on obesity and insulin resistance. Int J Obes Relat Metab Disord (England), December 1992; 16(Suppl 4):S1–11.

Czajka-Narins DM, Parham ES: Fear of fat: attitudes toward obesity. Nutrition Today, January/February 1990; pp 26–32.

Davis J, Sherer K: Applied Nutrition and Diet Therapy for Nurses, 2nd ed. Philadelphia, WB Saunders, 1994; p 588.

Goodrick GK, Foreyt JP: Why treatments for obesity don't last. J Am Diet Assoc, 1991; 91(10):1246–1247.

Grant JP: Handbook of Total Parenteral Nutrition, 2nd ed. Philadelphia, WB Saunders, 1992; p 16.

The Johns Hopkins Medical Letter, "Health After 50." January 1994; 5(11):8.

Lepke J: Super low-fat diets can't always keep big weight-loss promises. Environmental Nutrition, October 1993; 16(10):6.

Modan M, Halkin H, Almog S, et al.: Hyperinsulinemia. A link between hypertension obesity and glucose intolerance. J Clin Invest, 1985; 75(3):809–817.

National Academy of Sciences, National Research Council: Recommended Dietary Allowances, 10th ed. Washington, DC, 1989.

Pate RR: Physical activity in children and youth: relationship to obesity. Contemporary Nutrition, 1993; 18(2):1.

President's Council on Physical Fitness and Sports, 450 5 St. NW, Washington, DC 20201.

Telch CF, Agras WS, Rossiter EM, et al.: Group cognitive-behavioral treatment for the non-purging bulimic: an initial evaluation. J Consult Clin Psychol, 1990; 58:629–635.

U.S. Department of Health and Human Services: Surgeon General's Report on Nutrition and Health: Summary and Recommendations. Public Health Service, Publ. No. 88-50211. Washington DC, U.S. Government Printing Office, 1988.

University of California at Berkeley Wellness Letter: Nutrition and exercise: what your body needs, May 1993; p 4.

Wing RR: Behavioral treatment of severe obesity. Am J Clin Nutr, 1992; 55(2 Suppl):545S–551S.

CHAPTER 21

NUTRITION OF THE OLDER ADULT

CHAPTER TOPICS

CHAPTER INTRODUCTION
THE MEANING OF AGING
THE EFFECT OF AGING ON NUTRITIONAL STATUS
NUTRIENT NEEDS OF THE OLDER ADULT
COMMON CONDITIONS IN THE OLDER ADULT
FOOD-DRUG INTERACTIONS IN THE OLDER ADULT
THE ASSESSMENT OF NUTRITIONAL NEEDS IN THE OLDER ADULT
NUTRITION PROGRAMS FOR THE ELDERLY
INSTITUTIONAL MEAL SERVICE CONSIDERATIONS
FOOD SAFETY ISSUES FOR OLDER ADULTS
THE ROLE OF THE NURSE OR OTHER HEALTH CARE PROFESSIONAL IN PROMOTING HEALTH OF
THE OLDER ADULT

OBJECTIVES

After completing this chapter, you should be able to:
- Explain how physiological, economic, and social changes affect nutritional status
- Discuss how nutrient needs are modified in the aging process
- Explain how nutritional needs are identified in the elderly population
- Name and describe nutrition programs for the elderly
- Name some meal service and food safety considerations for older adults

TERMS TO IDENTIFY

Aging
Alzheimer's disease
Arthritis
Dementia
DETERMINE Checklist

Drug efficacy
Geriatrics
Gerontology
Kyphosis
Meals on Wheels

Nutrition Program for the
   Elderly
Nutrition Screening
   Initiative
Older Americans Act

Osteoporosis
Over-the-counter
   medications
Pernicious anemia

A FAMILY'S PERSPECTIVE
ON NUTRITION

R ita Bernardo was at the nursing home visiting her good friend Mabel Campbell. Mabel had built a farm herself, married, and now was in the nursing home at age 90 with Alzheimer's disease. How the neighbor kids missed her. She had always given them freshly baked cookies and they got to eat them in those amazing old rocking chairs that made you feel like you were going to tip over backward. But here Mabel was. She did not have the insurance coverage that would have allowed her to stay in her home. No, she had to sell her farm so that Medicaid would pay for her to be institutionalized. Away from her beloved farm. A sad irony to life. Rita came as often as she could to help Mabel eat. If the nursing staff did not assist, Mabel would forget to eat. But with help, she showed she still had a voracious appetite.

INTRODUCTION

The Bureau of the Census estimates that by the year 2000, the number of people 100 years of age and older will be approximately 100,000. The number of individuals 80 years and older will increase from 5.9 million to 26 million and those older than 55 years will compose one third of the population by the year 2050. About 30 years have been added to the average life expectancy since the turn of the century, when life expectancy was only 47 years. This extension of life expectancy has had and will continue to have a profound effect on our society and the health care system.

It is important to recognize the complexity of factors that influence elderly individuals in their selection of foods. These factors include income, household composition, cultural habits and customs, religion, ethnic background, and gender. It is also important for the health professional to realize that the process of aging diminishes the ability to ingest, digest, absorb, and metabolize nutrients in food. Thus, inadequate food choices are of particular concern in the elderly population, as it places them at increased risk of malnutrition and poor health.

FACT & FALLACY

FALLACY: Amino acid supplements will promote longevity.
FACT: The older adult's requirement for protein is essentially the same as that of a younger person, and there is no truth to the notion that amino acid supplements have any effect on the aging process. A wide variety of good protein sources are available, even for individuals who have poor dentition and sore gums. Eggs or egg whites, tuna, cottage cheese, peanut butter, and dried beans and peas are good substitutes for meat if chewing is difficult.

By keeping older adults at a good nutritional status, we can help them to maintain their health and independence, thereby lessening the demands on institutional care and improving their quality of life. The importance of good nutritional status in maintaining independence among the elderly cannot be overstated. Growing old need not be a burden on society, but increased attention to health is necessary.

WHAT IS MEANT BY GERONTOLOGY, GERIATRICS, AND AGING?

Gerontology is the study of the problems of aging in all its aspects (physiological, economic, and social). **Geriatrics** is the branch of medicine concerned with the treatment and prevention of diseases affecting the elderly population. **Aging** is a process in which the body's capacity to replace worn-out cells is reduced. It occurs at different rates in different individuals, but why aging occurs is unknown. The American Dietetic Association states:

> Aging refers to the normal, progressive, and irreversible biological changes that occur over the individual life span. Although the process occurs in all persons, for those over 65 years of age, it is often associated with significant changes in health and nutrition needs. About 85 per cent of older persons have one or more chronic, potentially debilitating diseases and could benefit from nutrition services, and up to half of older individuals have clinically identifiable nutrition problems requiring professional intervention. There are several unique characteristics of the older population that must be considered when nutritional status and planning intervention strategies are assessed: an increased susceptibility to chronic diseases such as osteoporosis, atherosclerosis, diabetes, hypertension, and cancer; poor dentition; age-related decreased organ function, which can adversely affect absorption, transportation, metabolism, and / or excretion of essential nutrients; increased use of prescription and over-the-counter medications; and alteration in psychological and social well-being and financial status, often causing diminished capability to shop and prepare meals (American Dietetic Association, 1991).

WHAT CHANGES OF AGING AFFECT NUTRITIONAL STATUS?

The older adult experiences social, physiological, and economic changes that affect nutrition, but careful consideration can resolve many of the associated concerns. A team approach is important.

Physical Changes

During the aging process, the basal metabolic rate slows and the amount of lean body mass (muscle tissue) is reduced. These changes, combined with a decrease in physical activity, result in a decrease in energy requirements and an increase in fatty tissue. Exercise needs to be part of daily activities. Even bedridden older adults can exercise (Fig. 21–1).

Perceptual changes may affect eating behavior. Taste may be altered because of a decrease in the number of taste buds that occurs as part of the aging process, or as an effect of disease states, nutritional deficiencies, or medications. A reduced ability to detect odors and impaired hearing and sight may reduce the enjoyment of the social aspects of eating. All of these perceptual changes may contribute to a lower intake of food.

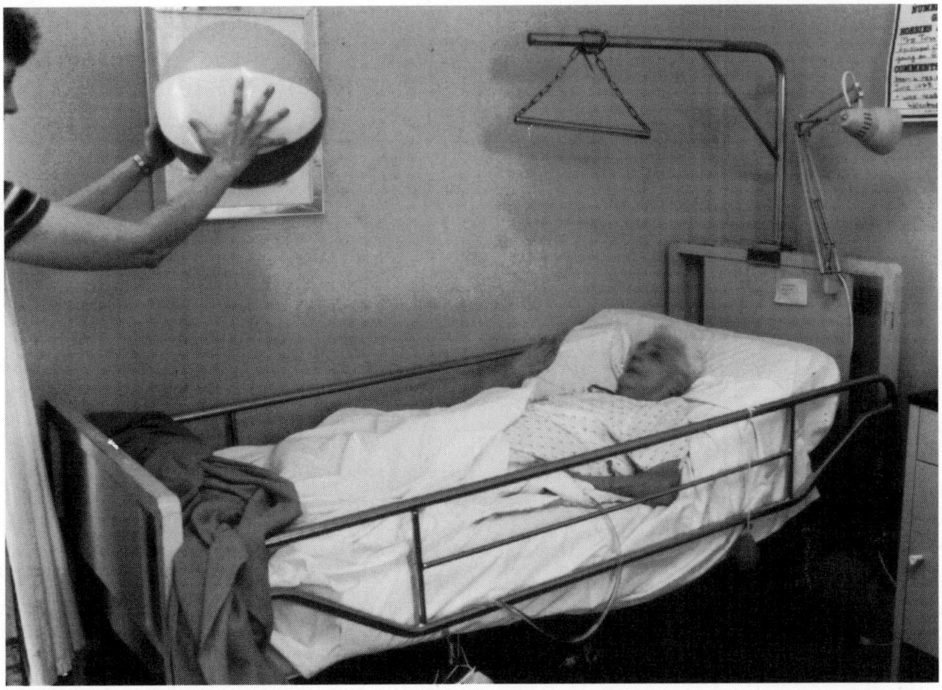

▲ FIGURE 21-1

Exercise is possible for even bedridden adults. (Courtesy of Cornell University Photography, Ithaca, NY.)

Loss of teeth is common in the elderly population. This condition may lead to altered food choices that may decrease the nutritive value of the diet.

If refined foodstuffs are eaten instead of raw fruits and vegetables, constipation may become a problem, since aging is accompanied by a decrease in the body's ability to move waste products through the gastrointestinal tract. Increasing the fiber content of the diet along with encouraging an adequate fluid intake and exercise will help control constipation. The use of mineral oil in treating constipation should be discouraged, since it reduces the absorption of the fat-soluble vitamins A, D, E, and K.

The kidneys also may not function as well as they do in younger individuals. This can result in nutrient loss because the kidneys are not able to conserve and reabsorb some nutrients. The buildup of toxins can also occur when the kidneys lose their ability to filter harmful substances. Since the sense of thirst diminishes with age, it is especially important to be aware of the need for fluids to promote the removal of wastes through the gastrointestinal tract and kidneys.

Decreases in body secretions occur with aging. For example, swallowing may become more difficult because of decreased saliva production, and pro-

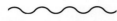

▲ T A B L E   2 1 - 1

DIETARY CONSIDERATIONS FOR PHYSIOLOGICAL, ECONOMIC, AND SOCIAL CHANGES AFFECTING THE OLDER ADULT

PROBLEM	COMMENT
Decreased sensation of smell, taste and sight; diminished appetite or eating ability	Adequate lighting should be provided. Foods should be colorful, well seasoned, and attractively served. Adequate mastication, oral hygiene, or smoking cessation may enhance taste perception. Serve bland food only when medically indicated.
Less efficient digestion	Four to 6 smaller meals are generally more acceptable. For total meal consumption, allow ample time in a pleasant environment.
Dental disease or lack of suitable dentures	Foods should be chopped, ground, or pureed only when the individual is unable to manage whole pieces (i.e., meats). However, some individuals can masticate whole pieces of meat with their gums. Proper oral hygiene should be encouraged.
Constipation	Sufficient fiber and fluids are necessary. Emphasize intake of raw and cooked fruits and vegetables; whole-grain breads and cereals. Encourage physical activity as tolerated, adequate rest and relaxation, regularity of meals and bowel habits. Discourage the use of mineral oil to avoid loss of fat-soluble vitamins.
Immobility	Immobility can result in constipation, obesity, decubitus ulcers, and loss of ability to shop for food (which could lead to poor nutrient consumption); may exacerbate osteoporosis by increasing urinary calcium.
Hearing impairment, memory loss, and short attention span	Receiving diet instructions or nutrition information can be problematic. Short, frequent sessions are preferred over long sessions. Effective communication skills, including clarity and volume of voice, are essential. Contact and instruct person or agency responsible for the individual's care.
Lactose intolerance; osteoporosis	The aged may be less tolerant of milk and milk products. Many persons find that they can tolerate milk in smaller amounts or milk products that have been fermented (e.g., buttermilk, yogurt, and cheese) or cooked (i.e., pudding, custard, cream soup, and sauces). Special emphasis should be given to other calcium-rich sources (e.g., hard cheeses, dark green, leafy vegetables) to reduce the risk of osteoporosis. Lactaid may be used to aid in the digestion of fresh milk.
Decreased tolerance to fat	Decrease amounts of fats added to or present in foods; avoid fried foods.
Decreased iron intake	Encourage intake of iron-rich foods in combination with high vitamin C foods, emphasizing economical sources (e.g., liver, iron-fortified cereals).
Low levels of other vitamins and minerals (e.g., folate, ascorbic acid, pyridoxine, vitamin A, and zinc)	Encourage intake of nutritionally adequate meals, with special consideration to protein and vitamin C–rich foods. Concentrated high-protein beverages and vitamin-mineral supplements may be needed to provide adequate nutrition.
Modified diets	The same nutritional concerns apply for geriatric persons as for younger adults. Ethnic, religious, social, and economic preferences should be given special consideration. Consider liberalizing the meal plan when oral intake is poor.
Arthritis	Less efficient manipulation will necessitate that food items be given in open or easy-to-open containers. Finger foods may be easily consumed. To alleviate discomfort from arthritis, ideal body weight should be maintained.

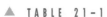

▲ TABLE 21-1

DIETARY CONSIDERATIONS FOR PHYSIOLOGICAL, ECONOMIC, AND SOCIAL CHANGES
AFFECTING THE OLDER ADULT *Continued*

PROBLEM	COMMENT
Economic limitations	Economical food buys (e.g., foods in season and on special sale) should be emphasized. Refer individual to available community programs (e.g., food stamps, food pantries).
Need for socialization	Institutionalized individuals should be encouraged to eat in a common dining room or discouraged from obtaining a private room. Social contact in a pleasant environment may stimulate the appetite. The noninstitutionalized individuals may benefit from community programs, such as home-delivered meals or congregate meals. Home-delivered meal programs may provide two meals a day (one hot and one cold) five times a week. Congregate meals provide at least one hot meal per day, five times a week. Both programs provide individuals with at least one third of the RDA. Home-delivered meals encourage independence, whereas congregate meals provide important social contacts.
Food faddism; misinformation	Available income may be spent on unnecessary vitamin-mineral supplements; provide counseling as needed.

From The Chicago Dietetic Association and The South Suburban Dietetic Association: Manual of Clinical Dietetics. 3rd ed. Chicago, The American Dietetic Association, 1988.

tein digestion is less efficient because of decreased hydrochloric acid secretion. The body's production of digestive enzymes is also decreased with aging.

Even though little is known about an elderly person's nutritional needs, meals should be planned according to the five food group system of the USDA's Food Guide Pyramid as discussed in Chapter 6. Six small meals a day are often more appropriate than three full-sized meals for someone with a small appetite. Breakfast is frequently the meal accepted best and can therefore be emphasized advantageously in menu planning. Beverages that are caffeine-free and alcohol-free can be counted as fluid and should be included with each meal and snack to prevent dehydration.

Economic Changes

For most individuals, advancing age eventually brings retirement from work. This usually results in a decrease in income, which may occur at a time when there is an increasing amount of money being spent for medical care. Consequently, less money may be available to buy food. Protein foods may be consumed in decreased amounts because they are expensive, require preparation, and may be difficult to chew and swallow. Excessive consumption of carbohydrate foods may occur because they are inexpensive, are easily stored without refrigeration, and are simple to prepare.

Social Changes

Losing a spouse, living alone or with a son's or daughter's family, and entering a nursing home are only a few of the social changes to which elderly persons may have to adapt. There is a loss of mobility and independence if physical impairments make driving a car or using public transportation difficult. Isolation from others will result unless there are friends or family on whom the elderly person can rely. The loss of independence that often accompanies these changes in social structure may reduce an elderly person's self-esteem. Such changes may cause the food intake of an elderly individual to suffer if he or she becomes depressed.

Grocery shopping may become more difficult for two reasons. Food labels and prices are hard to read because of visual impairment, and there is a growing trend toward larger supermarkets that require good mobility and physical stamina to traverse aisle after aisle. Transportation is also required.

Table 21–1 summarizes dietary considerations for these physiological, economic, and social changes affecting the older adult. Table 21–2 shows the effect of the physiological changes.

WHAT ARE THE NUTRIENT NEEDS OF THE OLDER ADULT?

The recommended dietary allowances (RDAs) of the Food and Nutrition Board of the National Academy of Sciences do not give any specific recommendation for the adult older than 51 years, as noted in the RDA table on

▲ TABLE 21-2

PHYSIOLOGICAL CHANGES IN THE ELDERLY

COMPONENT	FUNCTIONAL CHANGE	OUTCOME
Body composition	↓ Muscle mass	↑ Fat tissue in muscle size and strength
	↓ Basal metabolic rate	↓ Caloric requirements
	↓ Bone density	↑ Risk of osteoporosis
Perceptions	↓ Hearing	Feeling of isolation
		Reluctance to eat in public places or at large social affairs
	Slowing of adaptation to darkness	Need for brighter light to perform tasks
	↓ Number of taste buds	↓ Ability to taste salt, sweet
		↑ Ability to taste bitter and sour
	↓ Smell	↓ Threshold for odors
Gastrointestinal tract	↓ Motility	Constipation
	↓ Hydrochloric acid	↓ Efficiency of protein digestion
		More prone to food poisoning
	↓ Saliva production	Difficulty swallowing
Heart	↑ Blood pressure	↓ Ability to handle physical work and stress
	↓ Ability to use oxygen	
Lungs	↓ Capacity to oxygenate blood	↑ Fatigue
		↓ Capacity for exercise
Endocrine	↓ Number of secretory cells	↓ Blood hormone levels
	↓ Insulin production	↑ Blood sugar level
Kidney	↓ Renal blood flow	↓ Capacity for filtration and absorption

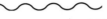

▲ TABLE 21-3

GENERAL RECOMMENDATIONS AND RATIONALE FOR NUTRIENT NEEDS OF THE OLDER ADULT

NUTRIENT	RECOMMENDATIONS	RATIONALE
Calories	51–75 years: reduce usual adult intake by 10%; >75 years: reduce usual adult intake by 20–25%	Necessary because of a decrease in basal metabolic rate, lean body mass, and physical activity
Protein	0.8 g/kg of ideal body weight or ≥12% of total kilocalories	Necessary for repletion of body proteins because of changes in body composition and protein metabolism
Fat	≤35% of total kilocalories (polyunsaturated fatty acids ≤10% of total kilocalories)	To decrease kilocalorie intake; to decrease risk of further atherosclerotic changes
Carbohydrates	To provide remaining kilocalories needed (approximately 50–55%), reduce intake of refined sugar and maintain or increase intake of complex carbohydrates	Refined sugar (sucrose) provides no nutritional value other than energy; complex carbohydrates often provide necessary vitamins, minerals, and dietary fiber
Calcium	≥800 to 1000 mg; 1500 mg may be needed for postmenopausal women	To prevent osteoporotic changes
Vitamins and other minerals	Nutrients should come from foods first; supplements may need to be medically prescribed	To maintain optimal nutritional status
Water	≥1 mL/kcal/day	To facilitate elimination, prevent dehydration

From The Chicago Dietetic Association and The South Suburban Dietetic Association: Manual of Clinical Dietetics. Chicago, The American Dietetic Association, 1988.

the inside front cover. Table 21–3 gives general recommendations and rationale for nutrient needs of the older adult.

Energy

According to the *Surgeon General's Report on Nutrition and Health* of 1988, until more is known, older Americans should consume sufficient nutrients and kilocalories and include levels of physical activity that maintain desirable weight, which may delay the onset of chronic disease. Because low-calorie diets may not supply sufficient nutrients, older adults should be advised to maintain at least moderate levels of activity to increase calorie needs (U.S. Department of Health and Human Services, 1988). We know that energy needs are lower for the older adult, since basal metabolism decreases gradually with aging. Food intake generally is lower, and the amount of lean body tissue decreases, whereas the amount of body fat increases.

Protein

Protein requirements do not decrease with age, and the RDA remains at 0.8 grams per kilogram of body weight. However, owing to the diminishing efficiency of protein utilization in the elderly, an increase to 1 gram per kilogram of body weight has been suggested (Chernoff, 1990). Also, with any age, protein requirements increase in response to certain physiological stresses such as infection, bone fractures, surgery, and burns.

Vitamins and Minerals

The RDA for vitamins and minerals is the same for the older adult as it is for the younger adult. However, because iron needs are decreased after menopause, women 51 years of age and older need 10 mg of iron per day compared with 15 mg of iron per day for younger women.

It is well known that exposure to sunlight increases the production of vitamin D in the skin, but persons who are confined to bed or who live in a cloudy climate cannot benefit and are at risk for deficiency of vitamin D, which then has an impact on calcium status. Drinking vitamin D–fortified milk is a good way to ensure adequate vitamin D and calcium. Lactose-free milk products are available and may be necessary because the digestive enzyme lactase can become diminished with advancing age.

The elderly do not appear to be at risk for vitamin-mineral toxicity when taking supplements at the RDA level but may be at increased risk when taking large doses because of decreased lean body mass and reduced kidney function. A review of the older adult's vitamin and mineral use by the health care professional can help identify potential toxic amounts of supplements.

Fluids

Fluids are frequently overlooked in the diets of the elderly. Young adults require an intake of 1 mL/kcal or 30 mL/kg of body weight. The elderly often lose their sense of thirst and may need to be encouraged to consume adequate fluids. It is particularly important for the elderly to meet their fluid needs to help prevent dehydration, which may result in constipation, increased body temperature, low blood pressure, mental confusion, and dental decay.

Fiber

Low intake of fiber is related to chronic disorders such as diverticulosis in older adults. The National Cancer Institute recommends consuming 20 to 30 grams of fiber per day, which is reflected in the USDA Food Guide Pyramid's minimum number of servings of fruits, vegetables, and whole grains.

WHAT CONDITIONS ARE COMMON IN THE OLDER ADULT?

Arthritis

There are two major forms of **arthritis:** osteoarthritis and rheumatoid arthritis. Many misconceptions exist concerning the role of nutrition in preventing and managing arthritis. Currently, nutrition plays no known role except for contributing to weight control which helps to decrease strain on the joints affected by osteoarthritis.

Rheumatoid arthritis is an inflammatory process that is currently best managed medically. Certain types of fat, such as fish oil, which can help reduce the inflammatory process, may play a part. However, the amount of fish oil needed for this effect may have other undesirable side effects and is currently not recommended. Control of blood sugar levels may also have an impact since low blood sugar levels, or the rise and fall in blood sugar levels after eating sweets, can trigger the production of histamine in some individuals. Although histamine production is related to allergies, there is no conclusive evidence that avoiding sugar will help control rheumatoid arthritis. Eating fewer sweets certainly will not cause any physical harm, however, and is part of weight management.

In the medical management of arthritis there are well documented nutritional implications. If large amounts of aspirin are used, vitamin C and folate intake needs to be increased. Steroid treatment increases the need for vitamins C and D, pyridoxine, folate, calcium, and phosphorus (Pronsky, 1993).

FACT & FALLACY

FALLACY: Arthritis can be cured by diet.
    FACT: At present, no known nutrient will help arthritis. The best approach nutritionally is the promotion of ideal body weight to put less strain on the weight-bearing joints.

Gout

Gout resembles arthritis and is characterized by pain in a single joint (often starting with the large toe), followed by complete remission. As the disease progresses, the attacks become more prolonged and more frequent. Eventually degenerative joint changes and deformity take place.

Obesity is frequently associated with gout, which is thought to be related to excessive eating, drinking, and lack of exercise. Food allergies may also precipitate an attack.

Alcohol is avoided in this condition, as are fatty foods, since they may inhibit excretion of urate and hinder weight control. Maintenance of sufficient fluid intake as well as ideal body weight is important. Rapid weight loss should be avoided.

It should be noted that drugs are usually more effective in lowering blood uric acid than are dietary modifications. Thus, dietary restrictions are usually no longer imposed.

Osteoporosis

Osteoporosis (porous bones) is a major health concern for the older adult and develops gradually over a lifetime. Osteoporosis greatly increases the risk of bone fractures such that activities of daily living may cause fractures. Age-related bone loss begins around the age of 35 to 40 years in both men and women, and approximately 24 million Americans are afflicted with this metabolic bone disorder. Osteoporosis is responsible for approximately 1.5 million bone fractures each year at a cost of 10 billion dollars (National Osteoporosis Foundation, 1991).

It has been noted that a woman may lose 20 to 30 per cent of her total skeleton during a 20-year period following menopause. Although the RDA for calcium is 800 mg, as much as 1500 mg of calcium daily may be needed to maintain calcium balance because of a reduced ability of the body to absorb this nutrient and because vitamin D synthesis in the skin is decreased in elderly individuals (Locniskar, 1988). A combination of weight-bearing exercises and estrogen replacement therapy may help prevent or slow age-related bone loss and reduce the risk of fractures in women. Men also develop osteoporosis but at a much lower rate owing to larger bone mass and more calcium through a higher intake of food.

FACT & FALLACY

FALLACY: Calcium-based antacid tablets should be taken to prevent osteoporosis.

FACT: Although this message is often advertised as an appropriate strategy to prevent osteoporosis, it is oversimplified and potentially harmful. It is known that individuals who have consumed adequate quantities of milk and milk products over their life span are less prone to the development of osteoporosis in their later years. However, it is still not clear whether the calcium in milk or other combinations of nutrients (such as magnesium) in the milk are of the most benefit. In addition, since antacids interfere with iron absorption (because of decreased hydrochloric acid secretion), the best approach is to eat or drink foods that are naturally rich in calcium and vitamin D, such as fortified milk. Moderate sun exposure will also help.

Pernicious Anemia

Individuals with **pernicious anemia** lack intrinsic factor and therefore cannot absorb dietary vitamin B_{12}, so vitamin B_{12} is given by injection. This condition increases in prevalence in the elderly but also can occur at any age when diseases of the gastrointestinal tract are involved.

Alzheimer's Disease and Dementia

Alzheimer's disease and **dementia** are diseases that progress in frequency and severity with age. Several problems occur with these conditions, including: forgetfulness and disorientation, pacing, inability to eat independently, weight gain or weight loss, dysphagia, food behavioral problems, constipation, and pouching. Owing to disorientation, a person with dementia needs to be reminded to chew and swallow. All of these problems may affect nutritional status. Interventions might include increasing kilocalories to prevent weight loss, increasing fluid intake for constipation, simplifying routines or requests, or offering finger foods to encourage feeding independence. Adaptive feeding devices may help (Consultant Dietitians in Health Care Facilities, 1992).

Pouching (retaining bits of food between the cheeks and gums) is sometimes observed, especially in nursing home patients. If the food retained in the mouth contains fermentable carbohydrate such as fruit, candy, or bread, acid production and plaque will occur, resulting in dental decay. Acidic foods such as oranges may cause erosion of tooth enamel if the food is pouched. Caregivers should inspect the mouth of persons known to pouch (Nutrition Focus, 1992).

WHAT ARE SOME CONCERNS RELATED TO FOOD-DRUG INTERACTIONS?

Approximately 30 per cent of all prescribed and **over-the-counter medications** (not prescribed) are used by persons over 65 years of age. Older persons often may take 3 to 7 separate drugs at any given time. Organ deterioration, underlying chronic diseases, dietary regimens, an unstable nutritional status, and other factors make the elderly particularly vulnerable to food and drug interactions. Quality of life and health may be affected as a result. Therefore, proper nutritional management is needed to avoid nutrient depletion and the reduction of **drug efficacy** (the ability of the drug to work) (Smith, 1990). Referral to a registered dietitian may be appropriate (see Chapter 7).

HOW IS THE OLDER ADULT'S NUTRITIONAL STATUS ASSESSED?

The nutrition assessment process is discussed in detail in Chapters 2 and 7, but a few important aspects about the older adult need to be mentioned. The nurse is often the first person to discover nutritional problems. In taking a diet history, it is important to note any type of food restrictions, ethnic or religious preferences, food aversions, and allergies. Also, certain signs of malnutrition may be noted during the physical examination. For example, low serum albumin is related to edema.

Factors such as bone loss and a shortening of the spinal column during later years indicate the need for current height measurement rather than relying on reported measurements from younger years. Height is frequently difficult to determine owing to **kyphosis** (hunched shoulders), although knee height can be used to estimate true height (see Appendix 17).

A calibrated balance beam scale is recommended for weighing ambulatory adults. A calibrated chair or bed scale may be used for those who are in wheelchairs or who are bedridden. Weights should be monitored weekly in the hospital and monthly in other health facilities, keeping in mind that fluid retention and dehydration can affect weight status.

What Is the Nutrition Screening Initiative and Its Role in Preventing Malnutrition in Older Adults?

Eighty-five per cent of the elderly suffer from chronic diseases that could benefit from dietary interventions. Unfortunately, the warning signs of poor nutritional health are often overlooked.

The **Nutrition Screening Initiative** began in 1990 as a 5-year, multifaceted effort to promote nutrition screening and better nutritional care of older adults. This effort is a project of the American Academy of Family Physicians, The American Dietetic Association, and the National Council on Aging. Many related organizations and health professionals continue to help guide the Initiative, which is aimed as a direct response to the call of the 1988 Surgeon General's Workshop on Health Promotion and Aging and the U.S. Department of Health and Human Services Report, Healthy People 2000, for increased nutrition screening (Nutrition Interventions Manual, 1992).

▲ TABLE 21-4

DETERMINE CHECKLIST

Disease

Any disease, illness, or chronic condition that causes changes in eating habits or makes eating difficult increases nutritional risk. Four of five adults have chronic diseases that are affected by diet. Confusion or memory loss that keeps getting worse is estimated to affect one of five or more of older adults. This can make it hard to remember what, when, or if food has been eaten. Feeling sad or depressed, which happens to about one in eight older adults, can cause big changes in appetite, digestion, energy level, weight, and well-being.

Eating Poorly

Eating too little and eating too much both lead to poor health. Eating the same foods day after day or not eating fruit, vegetables, and milk products daily will also cause poor nutritional health. One in five adults skips meals daily. Only 13 per cent of adults eat the minimum amount of fruit and vegetables needed. One in four adults drinks too much alcohol. Many health problems become worse if more than one or two alcoholic beverages are consumed daily.

Tooth Loss or Mouth Pain

A healthy mouth, teeth, and gums are needed to eat. Missing, loose, or rotten teeth or dentures that don't fit well or cause mouth sores make it hard to eat.

Economic Hardship

As many as 40 per cent of older Americans have incomes of less than $6,000 per year. Having less—or choosing to spend less—than $25 to $30 per week for food makes it very hard to procure adequate foods to stay healthy.

Reduced Social Contact

One third of all older people live alone. Being with people daily has a positive effect on morale, well-being, and eating habits.

Multiple Medicines

Many older Americans must take medicines for health problems. Almost half of older Americans take multiple medicines daily. Growing old may change the way we respond to drugs. The more medicines used, the greater the chance for side effects such as increased or decreased appetite, change in taste, constipation, weakness, drowsiness, diarrhea, and nausea. When taken in large doses, vitamins and minerals act like drugs and can cause harm. Doctors need to be alerted of all medications taken.

Involuntary Weight Loss or Gain

Losing or gaining a lot of weight when not trying to is an important sign that must not be ignored. Being overweight or underweight also increases the chance of poor health.

Needs Assistance in Self Care

Although most older people are able to eat, one in five has trouble walking, shopping, and buying and cooking food, especially as he or she gets older.

Elder Years Above Age 80

Most older people lead full and productive lives. But as age increases, risk of frailty and health problems increase. Older persons should check their nutritional health regularly.

Modified with permission by the Nutrition Screening Initiative, Washington, DC, a project of the American Academy of Family Physicians, the American Dietetic Association and the National Council on the Aging, Inc. and funded in part by a grant from Ross Laboratories, a division of Abbott Laboratories.

The Level I Screen of The Nutrition Screening Initiative is designed for social service and health professionals to identify older Americans who may need medical or nutritional attention. The Level II Screen provides more specific diagnostic information on nutritional status and is designed for use by health and medical professionals. A public awareness tool that older adults can use to assess their own nutritional risk is called the **DETER-MINE Checklist** (Table 21–4).

Many circumstances can negatively affect an elderly person's nutritional status, regardless of income. Warning signals include bereavement, physical or mental disabilities, and poor nutrition knowledge. Care providers can be taught to make observations in the home and then take appropriate steps to prevent the onset of a nutritional crisis. Practical actions can be simple, informal, and inexpensive. For example, one might provide transportation to social activities and assist in grocery shopping and the preparation of food. However, independence should be encouraged as much as possible in all activities, including eating, lest the individual lose the desire to eat and be further debilitated (Davies and Knutson, 1991).

WHAT NUTRITION PROGRAMS ARE AVAILABLE FOR THE OLDER ADULT?

The federal **Older Americans Act** provides the states with money to conduct nutrition programs for the elderly. Under this Title III legislation, a hot noon meal is served 5 days a week to elderly persons in senior centers. This funding also provides transportation for individuals who are otherwise unable to get to the center. Nutrition education, health services, and recreational activities are planned around meals. For homebound elderly persons, up to a week's worth of meals are prepared at the center and delivered. Each of the two daily meals provides one third of the RDA of nutrients. The Title IIIc program is commonly referred to as **The Nutrition Program for the Elderly.**

Meals on Wheels is a community-sponsored program that provides hot noon meals and cold evening meals to homebound elderly persons. The elderly person is charged for the meals based on ability to pay. This program is often operated by local hospitals.

The Food Stamp Program is available to low-income elderly individuals. In some states, food stamps can be used to pay for food provided by The Nutrition Program for the Elderly. Some older adults need to be persuaded that it is acceptable and appropriate for them to use food stamps owing to the negative media coverage over the past decade about the use of food stamps.

These nutrition programs have helped improve the nutritional status of the elderly population. Participation in these programs is enhanced by social work agencies that can direct the elderly population to the appropriate programs.

WHAT ARE INSTITUTIONAL MEAL SERVICE CONSIDERATIONS?

Mealtimes should be pleasant. Prompt and courteous service is a must. Elderly persons are likely to eat better and enjoy meals more when dining with others, and this habit should be promoted whenever possible.

The food will be more appealing if it is served at the proper temperature (i.e., hot foods hot and cold foods cold) and as soon after preparation as possible to maintain palatability. It may be necessary to cut meat into bite-sized pieces, butter bread, and open containers if the individual is unable to perform those tasks independently because of weakness or pain from arthritis, for example. Certain adaptive equipment may be needed to help maintain independence in feeding oneself. Plates and bowls may need to be stabilized with rubber pads (dycem mats) and suction cups. Soup may be more easily managed if poured into a cup. Foam-covered spoon and fork handles are useful for individuals who have lost some ability to handle silverware easily. See Chapter 18 for a description of various assistive eating devices.

Respect and dignity are important to the elderly. When serving a meal, address the person by the last name preceded by Mr. or Miss or Mrs. unless requested to do otherwise. Napkins and a damp cloth should be close at hand for wiping any spilled food from face or clothing. A vision- or hearing-impaired individual will appreciate patience and understanding. Food items and their location on the plate and at the place setting should be identified for a visually impaired person. For the visually impaired person who needs to be fed, it is vital that each bite of food be explained in advance to promote trust in the caregiver and to help the person distinguish the food being eaten.

WHAT ARE SOME FOOD SAFETY ISSUES FOR OLDER ADULTS?

Food preparation, shopping, and storing food can be very demanding jobs for many elderly persons living alone. The elderly are highly susceptible to food poisoning owing to declining immune systems. Tight budgets and ingrained feelings against waste cause many elderly people to store food longer than is safe. With declining vision and sense of taste, food spoilage may go undetected. Food preparation brings up safety concerns; for instance, an older adult may forget that the stove is turned on. Microwave ovens can be helpful in this regard. The health professional must be alert in identifying problems in household management.

WHAT IS THE ROLE OF THE NURSE OR OTHER HEALTH CARE PROFESSIONAL IN PROMOTING THE NUTRITIONAL HEALTH OF OLDER ADULTS?

Screening and identification of older adults who are at nutritional risk with referral to appropriate services is an important role for all health care professionals working with the population of older adults. Use of the tools developed by the Nutrition Screening Initiative is appropriate. Some practical interventions such as promoting a variety of foods from the Food Guide Pyramid; recommending seasonings such as herbs, spices, and lemon juice as alternative methods of flavoring to reduce salt and sugar intake; and advising on the importance of food safety to help prevent food poisoning are appropriate approaches for all health care professionals to take.

Since calorie needs are generally lower while nutrient needs remain high, the use of skim milk and lean meats and the limited use of sauces, gravies, fats, alcohol, and high-calorie desserts can be recommended for those individuals who are overweight. Low-calorie desserts can be encouraged as they enhance the nutritional value of the diet (e.g., canned fruits packed in their own juice, puddings and custard made with skim milk).

If chewing is a problem, tender, ground, or pureed meats; meat or fish loaves; and eggs may provide an acceptable solution. Stewed fruits may be better tolerated than raw ones. Regular foods can be chopped or ground, or even blended, providing a more appealing texture than baby foods. Adding meat to soups will also enhance the protein value of the diet. Breakfast-type foods are generally well accepted because they are easy to chew and swallow. When necessary, these breakfast-type meals can also be eaten at lunchtime and dinnertime, but they should include at least three of the food groups from the Food Guide Pyramid, for example, french toast with peach slices, or scrambled eggs made with mostly egg whites and served with lightly toasted whole-grain bread and a side dish of fruit.

STUDY QUESTIONS AND ACTIVITIES

1. Why is it necessary to understand the physiological changes that occur with aging?
2. Why are elderly individuals vulnerable to nutritional deficiencies?
3. How have the nutrition programs for elderly persons helped to improve their nutritional status?
4. Observe meal service at a local nursing home. How have the meals been modified to meet individual needs?
5. Take turns feeding a blindfolded classmate and then explain how a visually impaired adult reacts to such an experience. Pureed foods might also be tasted.
6. What dietary advice would be appropriate for an overweight widower who has hypertension and an elevated cholesterol level and relies on convenience foods?
7. What nutritional concerns might Mrs. Campbell from the opening case study have?

REFERENCES

American Dietetic Association: Position paper: Nutrition, aging, and the continuum of health care. J Am Diet Assoc. 1987; 87(3): 344–347.

Chernoff R: Physiologic aging and nutritional status. Nutr Clin Pract. 1990; 5:8–13.

Consultant Dietitians in Health Care Facilities (CDHCF), A Practice Group of The American Dietetic Association: Dining Skills: Practical Interventions for the Caregivers of the Eating-Disabled Older Adult, 1992.

Davies L, Knutson KC: Warning signals for malnutrition in the elderly. J Am Diet Assoc. 1991; 91(11):1413–1417.

Locniskar M: Nutrition and Health Symposium: The University of Texas at Austin, April 1988, summary report. Nutrition Today. 1988; 23(5):35.

National Osteoporosis Foundation. Physician Resource Manual on Osteoporosis. A Decision Making Guide, 2nd ed. Washington, DC, National Osteoporosis Foundation, 1991.

Nutrition Focus, Child Development & MR Center of the University of Washington, Seattle, 1992; July–Aug 7(4).

Nutrition Interventions Manual for Professionals: Caring for Older Americans. Nutrition

Screening Initiative, A Joint Effort of the American Academy of Family Physicians, The American Dietetic Association, and the National Council on Aging, Inc., Washington, DC: 1992.

Pronsky ZM: Powers and Moore's Food Medication Interactions, 8th ed., Published and distributed by Food-Medication Interactions, Pottstown, PA, 1993.

Smith CH: In Geriatric Nutrition, Morley, Glick, and Rubenstein (eds). New York, Raven Press, Ltd., 1990; p 371.

U.S. Department of Health and Human Services: Surgeon General's Report on Nutrition and Health, Summary and Recommendations. Public Health Service (Pub. No. 88-50211). Washington, DC, U.S. Government Printing Office, 1988.

NATIONAL AND INTERNATIONAL NUTRITION PROGRAMS AND CONCERNS

CHAPTER

22

OBJECTIVES

After completing this chapter you should be able to:
- Identify the basic focus of the various federal community nutrition programs for referral purposes
- Discuss the importance of controlling food quackery
- Identify appropriate uses of food additives
- Describe principles of home-based food sanitation
- Describe why public health professionals need to be advocates for consumer nutritional and health needs

TERMS TO IDENTIFY

Ambulatory care
Clostridium botulinum
Clostridium perfringens
Communicable disease
Economy Food Plan
Food additives
Food distribution system

Food fad
Food resource management
Food quack
Generally recognized as safe (GRAS) list
Holistic

Hospices
Palliative care
Paraprofessional
Poverty line
Salmonella
Staphylococcus aureus
Thrifty Food Plan

A FAMILY'S PERSPECTIVE ON NUTRITION

Maria Bernado sat by the window reflecting on the past 2 years as her growing 18-month-old son snuggled in her arms, nursing contentedly. She thought how she was going to miss moments like this when baby Tony stopped nursing altogether. She had continued to breast-feed even though she had returned to work long ago. She nursed Tony before and after work and more frequently on weekends. Expressing her milk at work over lunchtime had been easier than she had thought. And it made her feel good to watch her baby grow from her own milk. The La Leche League had been very helpful in promoting continued nursing. She would always be grateful for their help and planned to volunteer her time to help other women.

So much had happened these past 2 years, but they all had survived and all was looking better. Tony had his diabetes under good control and had lost about 25 pounds. He looked and felt great. It had almost been a blessing to have the diagnosis since he now took better care of his health. He had brought his cholesterol and triglyceride levels below 200 and his blood pressure was like a young man's, the doctor had said. And most importantly, he had stopped smoking. Finally! The nicotine patch had been a blessing. But the smoker's support group through the American Cancer Society had also helped.

Joey had been quite a scare. She felt a bit guilty for not having noticed the behaviors herself. Looking back she realized that he had been going to the bathroom right after meals for a long time. It had become such a pattern she hadn't even noticed it. And he had become so thin despite eating so much. She had just thought he was a growing boy who needed a lot of food. She would always be thankful that their dentist had called with his concerns. The school psychologist and nurse had been a big help following up on this issue with the wrestling coach. Hopefully other boys wouldn't make the same mistake. Joey wasn't out of the woods yet, but he was making good strides after seeing Doris DeLong, the social worker with the Employees' Assistance Program at Tony's work.

Anna was also doing much better now that her eating and exercise habits had improved. She seemed to have gained more self-confidence as she got her habits and weight gain under control. She might never be really thin, Maria thought, but at least she could be healthy and happy.

For all the headaches she may have caused, Nanna had truly been a blessing. Nanna even seemed pleased that both she and her son Antonio benefited from including fiber in their diet. A Bernardo trait, she had said. Now they made sure they both ate more whole grains and plenty of vegetables and dried beans. Since legumes were part of the typical family meals it had been quite easy to include more fiber. And when Nanna had been too ill with diverticulitis to cook, the temporary home-delivered meals from the Nutrition Program for the Elderly had been very helpful in her recovery.

Maria thought how grateful she was that her public health nurse, Betsy, had encouraged her to apply for the WIC program and food stamps during her pregnancy when she had to stop working. She wouldn't have applied on her own. After all, they weren't poor. They just didn't have the money to eat well while she had been laid up in bed.

All was going well, especially since she had returned to work and begun bringing home a paycheck again. And for the moment, she closed her eyes while thoroughly enjoying nursing her son and thought of even better days to come.

INTRODUCTION

Public health includes the promotion of nutrition in the community. Overconsumption of food can best be addressed through education. Inadequate nutrition, however, generally reflects an unfair **food distribution system** (the means by which food gets to the consumer from the producer) that is based on purchasing power. The extent of global hunger is appalling; thousands of people are dying from hunger-related conditions. Hunger in the United States is inexcusable, particularly when programs are in place that could provide adequate food access to all persons in need.

WHAT IS OUR NATION'S NUTRITIONAL STATUS?

National Food Consumption Survey

The U.S. Department of Agriculture (USDA) conducts a national food consumption survey approximately every 10 years. The survey that was carried out in 1977 and 1978 showed evidence of excessive intake of kilocalories, fat, cholesterol, sugar, salt, and alcohol. Generally, the intake of vitamin B_6 (pyridoxine), magnesium, iron, and zinc was shown to be below the Recommended Dietary Allowance (RDA) levels. Furthermore, elderly women were shown to have significantly low intake of calcium and vitamin B_6. On the other hand, data from this survey revealed that the diet of those with low incomes had improved since the previous USDA survey. This improvement was attributed to various food assistance programs.

Results of the 1987 National Food Consumption Survey (NFCS) indicate little positive change in dietary habits since the last survey (Wright et al., 1991). The intake of excessive fat, especially saturated fat, and inadequate intake of some vitamins and minerals from food sources continue despite major educational efforts. The challenge to alter Americans' eating habits in a positive way appears to demand more than educational messages.

Hunger in America

Hunger has always been and will always be with us, but the attempts to control its ravages have changed over the course of history. In this century, the Great Depression of the 1930s saw the establishment of soup kitchens and the Food Stamp Program. During the draft of World War II, poor nutritional status kept many young men from being admitted to the military service. In response to the observations of WWII, the School Lunch Program was expanded.

During the 1960s, the issue of domestic hunger received major attention and resulted in the expansion of food programs. But beginning in the 1980s and continuing into the 1990s, underconsumption was again becoming an acute problem. Many early advances of the 1960s to combat national hunger were being lost. This was due primarily to political reasons and a declining U.S. economy. Unemployment and underemployment (part-time work or low wages or both) increased the demand for public assistance. At the same time, beginning in the Reagan administration, these benefits were being decreased or eliminated for many families. The domestic hunger crisis continues, as reflected in the fact that an estimated 35 to 40 million Americans are eligible for food stamps but fewer than 27 million receive them (Community Nutrition Institute, 1993). And of the number of persons living in **poverty** (lacking the means to meet basic needs such as housing and food), 40 per cent are children (Mayer, 1990).

Many people find it difficult to accept the fact that a hunger problem exists in the United States, the "land of plenty," where agricultural production exists on a large scale. Some people may tend to think of welfare recipients as lazy. However, depending on family size, with a minimum hourly wage of $4.25, a family may fall within the category of poverty even if both parents work full-time (see Appendix 18). Community nutritionists, public health nurses, and other health care professionals working in the community have begun to recognize that educational strategies need to be complemented with legislative action to develop a more just food distribution system.

WHAT NATIONAL AGENCIES HELP TO IMPROVE NUTRITION?

Several federal programs give people access to food. In addition to federal programs, there are soup kitchens, food banks, and food pantries. These volunteer organizations depend on contributions as well as on local, state, and federal grants. These groups help feed the homeless, unemployed, working poor, and developmentally disabled in many states. A list of federal, state, and local governmental agencies, nongovernmental organizations, educational and industrial institutions, and private agencies interested in the nutritional welfare of the American family can be found in Table 22–1. Some other programs are as follows.

THE CHILD CARE FEEDING PROGRAM. This program promotes good nutrition through financial reimbursement. Those who qualify are licensed home day care providers and day care centers that serve nutritious meals.

THE EXPANDED FOOD AND NUTRITION EDUCATION PROGRAM (EFNEP). This program is offered by Cooperative Extension associations and is aimed primarily at the nutritional needs of low-income families. Local **paraprofessionals** (people who are trained by professionals) are trained in nutrition to provide free nutrition education at the homes of low-income families (Fig. 22–1). They focus on **food resource management** (strategies to control food costs) and other areas

▲ TABLE 22-1

STATE AND LOCAL AGENCIES AND NONGOVERNMENTAL ORGANIZATIONS THAT PROVIDE NUTRITIONAL SERVICES

GOVERNMENTAL

State and Local Levels

Department of Agriculture
State extension services
State experiment stations
State universities—Department of Food and Nutrition
Department of Welfare
Department of Health
Department of Education

NONGOVERNMENTAL

National Level

American Medical Association Council on Foods
National Academy of Sciences, National
  Research Council, Food and Nutrition Board
American Red Cross
Professional Organizations
  American Medical Association
  American Dietetic Association
  American Home Economics Association
  American Dental Association
  American Public Health Association
  American Heart Association
  American Nurses' Association
  American Institute of Nutrition

Funds and Foundations:
  Milbank Memorial Fund
  Nutrition Foundation
  Ford and Rockefeller Foundations
Metropolitan Life Insurance Company
Society of Nutrition Education
Industry sponsored:
  American Dry Milk Institute
  National Dairy Council
  Cereal Institute
  National Livestock and Meat Board

State and Local Levels

Educational agencies
Social agencies
Civic groups
United Community Services
Industry sponsored
American Red Cross
Infant welfare organizations
Church groups

relevant to nutrition, such as breast-feeding support for low-income mothers.

THE FOOD STAMP PROGRAM. This program provides food stamps that can be used to purchase food or seeds to grow food. The allotment is based on the **Thrifty Food Plan,** which is a meal plan designed to meet the lowest possible cost for nutritional adequacy. The Thrifty Food Plan, while beneficial, was not intended to serve long-term nutritional needs. Thus relying on food stamps solely to meet food and nutritional needs is an extreme challenge for even the best educated person.

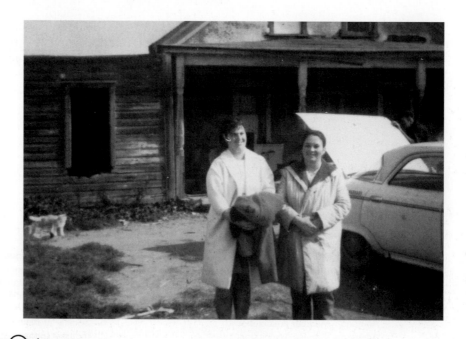

▲ F I G U R E   2 2 - 1

A Nutrition Teaching Assistant with EFNEP visits the home of a low-income family. (Courtesy of Cornell University Photography, Ithaca, NY.)

FACT & FALLACY

FALLACY: People would not experience hunger if they managed their food dollars properly.

FACT: This belief is disputed by an old but still relevant study by Peterkin and Hama that was based on the Nationwide Food Consumption Survey 1977–1978. The investigators found that, for the most part, food shopping practices of households with low food costs, those with low incomes, and those receiving food stamps were as good as or better than those of other households (Peterkin and Hama, 1983). In addition, they noted that although these low-income households generally had a higher nutrient return per dollar, they were still less likely to have adequate diets than were their fellow shoppers who spent more for food. This finding is related to the use of the Thrifty Food Plan (the plan that outlines typical menus) as the basis for the food stamp allotment. A more liberal food plan, such as the **Economy Food Plan** (the amount of money required for a monthly food stamp allotment that provides more flexibility in meeting nutritional needs), has been suggested by many nutritionists as a better way to ensure adequate nutritional intake by the impoverished population.

THE NUTRITION PROGRAM FOR THE ELDERLY. This program provides nutritious meals through congregate meal settings as well as home-delivered meals for homebound elderly individuals. Nutrition education and counseling on social service needs are provided. Meals on Wheels is a similar program that is often run out of hospitals.

PROJECT HEADSTART. This program is aimed at children 3 to 5 years old whose parents' income is below the poverty line. The program combines nutrition, social services, parent involvement, and health services within an educational setting. Nutritious meals and snacks are provided.

THE SCHOOL LUNCH AND BREAKFAST PROGRAM. This program provides nutritious foods at reduced cost for children whose families fall within 185 per cent of the poverty line (see Appendix 18). It further provides free meals for those below the poverty line. Government guidelines for school lunch patterns are provided in Appendix 19.

WOMEN, INFANTS, AND CHILDREN SUPPLEMENTAL NUTRITION PROGRAM (WIC). This program provides nutrition education and vouchers for prescribed supplemental foods. It is aimed at promoting the growth of the young child (Fig. 22–2). Women who are pregnant or breast-feeding, infants, and children up to the age of 5 years are eligible if the family income is within 185 per cent of the poverty line. Nutritional risk criteria such as low hematocrit, poor growth, frequent illness, or other qualifying medical condition are specified for enrollment in the WIC program. To further promote child welfare, single fathers, foster parents, or other guardians of children can receive WIC benefits for their children.

WHAT ARE SOME AMBULATORY CARE SERVICES OFFERING NUTRITION GUIDANCE?

Hospices

Ambulatory care (health care in a noninstitutional setting) is increasing as the costs of hospital-based care continue to rise. Two ambulatory programs are hospices and home health agencies.

Hospices offer supportive services for patients who are terminally ill and for their families. **Palliative** (noncurative) and supportive care is the general goal of hospices. The services may be in an institutional setting or based at home. The hospice movement is probably the best example of the change in attitude toward care of patients through a **holistic** approach (taking into account all aspects of a person's health, such as emotional and spiritual needs in addition to medical and nutritional needs).

In their services for terminally ill patients, emphasizing quality and not quantity of life, hospices have embraced the view espoused by Dr. Elizabeth Kubler-Ross that death is an integral part of the life stages. She was a pioneer in recognizing that terminally ill patients and their families go through stages of grief. These stages include denial, anger, and acceptance. Nutritional care may need to take into account the stage of grief that the family members are in. Nutritional goals promote maintaining comfort of

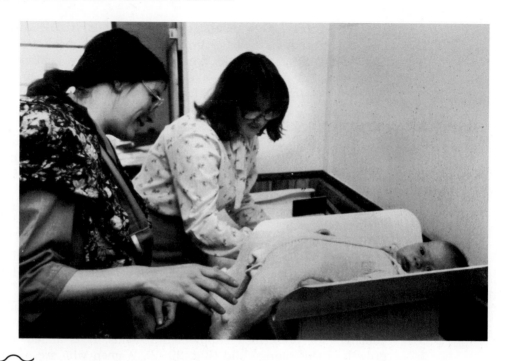

▲ FIGURE 22-2

Monitoring growth of an infant in the WIC program. (Courtesy of Cornell University Photography, Ithaca, NY.)

the patient over taking a curative approach. Therapeutic diet restrictions may become more lenient. Goals become more short-term, such as preventing dehydration or controlling constipation. If a family member is in denial, modifications to the patient's usual diet may not be accepted.

Appropriateness of Nutritional Support for the Terminally Ill

Nutritional support and other life-support measures for terminally ill patients can be viewed as either prolonging life or postponing death. The general philosophy of care for the terminally ill person is palliative care, promoting comfort versus treatment and cure. Thus, most dietary restrictions are lifted unless the comfort of the patient is jeopardized, such as in the case of dehydration or of a person with diabetes who may still benefit from controlled blood glucose levels, as physically the person will be expected to feel better under a controlled diet. Nutritional support for the person who is terminally ill generally focuses on oral feedings, but TPN or tube feedings cannot be ruled out. Each patient's case is unique and must be handled individually. The institution should have established, written guidelines for feeding the terminally ill patient. A registered dietitian can assist with the decision as to what form of nutrition intervention is appropriate, based on objective criteria.

Home Health
Agencies

Home health agencies are private programs that have nurses and some-times dietitians on staff to go to patients' homes. Nutritional care of the pa-tient is often provided by the attending nurse. Dietitians generally have limited roles in home health agencies because insurance policies usually do not cover the cost of dietitian services.

WHAT ARE SOME PUBLIC HEALTH CONCERNS THAT HAVE A BEARING ON NUTRITIONAL STATUS?

Food Sanitation

The health of a community depends on a safe food and water supply. Many agencies promote good sanitation practices in order to prevent disease and control **communicable disease** (disease that can spread from person to person, such as through water and food). These agencies are concerned with all aspects of food quality, including food preservation and food addi-tives, prevention of both natural and bacterial food poisoning, waterborne diseases, and the dangerous effects of pesticides and other toxic chemicals, such as the heavy metals lead and mercury. The U.S. Public Health Ser-vice, which is the principal health agency of the federal government, con-cerns itself with all factors affecting the health of people, including nutri-tion.

Food sanitation, although it appears at times unimportant to the general population, can be a matter of life or death, especially for the debilitated or acutely ill patient. Eating can be hazardous to one's health unless three general principles are adhered to: (1) clean, clean, clean; (2) when in doubt, throw it out; and (3) keep hot foods hot and cold foods cold.

Food Additives

The 1958 Food Additives Amendment was designed to protect the consumer. Because of this legislation, **food additives** (substances added to foods, gen-erally to make them safer to eat) used in processed food must be proved safe by industry before they can be incorporated into any food product. The **Generally Recognized As Safe (GRAS) list** is another approach used to control the safety of substances used in foods. Additives must meet strict guidelines for inclusion in the GRAS list. Examples of food additives in-clude the use of nitrites to prevent botulism in cured meat products. Ascor-bates and other ingredients are added to maintain quality in meat prod-ucts. Only minute quantities of these additives are used, usually in lower amounts than might exist naturally in many food products. The U.S. De-partment of Agriculture requires that additives meet the following require-ments:

1. They must be approved by the FDA and are limited to specific amounts.
2. They must meet a specific, justifiable need in the product.
3. They must not promote deception as to product freshness, quality, or weight.
4. They must be truthfully and properly listed on the product label.

Table 22–2 lists typical food additives. Table 22–3 lists food and nutrition–related responsibilities of federal agencies.

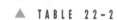

▲ **TABLE 22-2**

TYPICAL FOOD ADDITIVES, WHY AND WHERE USED

REASONS FOR USE	SUBSTANCE USED	FOODS
To Impart and Maintain Desired Consistency emulsifiers distribute tiny particles of one liquid in another to improve texture consistency, homogeneity, and quality; stabilizers and thickeners give smooth uniform texture, flavor, and desired consistency	Alginates, lecithin, mono- and diglycerides, agar-agar, methyl cellulose, sodium phosphates, carrageenan	Baked goods, cake mixes, salad dressings, frozen desserts, ice cream, chocolate milk, processed cheese
To Improve Nutritive Value medical and public health authorities endorse this use to eliminate and prevent certain diseases involving malnutrition; iodized salt has eliminated simple goiter; vitamin D in dairy products and infant foods has virtually eliminated rickets; niacin in bread, cornmeal, and cereals has eliminated pellagra in the southern states	Vitamin A, thiamine, niacin, riboflavin, ascorbic acid, vitamin D, iron, potassium iodide	Wheat flour, bread and biscuits, breakfast cereals, cornmeal, macaroni and noodle products, margarine, milk, iodized salt
To Enhance Flavor many spices and natural and synthetic flavors give us a desired variety of flavorful foods such as spice cake, gingerbread, and sausage	Cloves, ginger, citrus oils, amyl acetate, benzaldehyde	Ice cream, candy, gingerbread, spice cake, soft drinks, fruit-flavored gelatins, fruit-flavored toppings, sausage
To Provide Desired Texture leavening agents are used in the baking industry in cakes, biscuits, waffles, muffins, and other baked goods	Sodium bicarbonate, phosphates	Cakes, cookies, crackers
To Impart Tartness to Beverages	Citrus acid, lactic acid, phosphates, phosphoric acid	Soft drinks
To Maintain Appearance, Palatability, and Wholesomeness deterioration due to microbial growth or oxidation is delayed and food spoilage caused by mold, bacteria, and yeast is prevented or slowed by certain additives; antioxidants keep fats from turning rancid and certain fresh fruits from darkening during processing when cut and exposed to air	Propionic acid, sodium and calcium salts of propionic acid, ascorbic acid, butylated hydroxyanisole, butylated hydroxytoluene, benzoates	Bread, cheese, syrup, pie fillings, crackers, frozen and dried fruits, fruit juices, margarine, lard, shortening, potato chips, cake mixes
To Give Desired and Characteristic Color to increase acceptability and attractiveness by correcting objectionable natural variations	FDA-approved colors, such as annatto, carotene, cochineal, chlorophyll	Confections, bakery goods, soft drinks, cheeses, ice cream, jams, and jellies
Other Functions such as humectants to retain moisture in some foods and to keep others, including salts and powders, free flowing	Glycerine, magnesium carbonate	Coconut, table salt

From Chemical Manufacturers Association: Food Additives . . . Who Needs Them? Washington, DC, p 11.

Nutrition Misinformation

Food fads (a short-term, "quick-fix" diet or supplement) and nutritional quackery have multiplied as the science of nutrition has grown. A trained person can easily differentiate between accurate and unsound information. Unfortunately, the lay person is not always able to do this. In addition, the

FOOD AND NUTRITION-RELATED RESPONSIBILITIES OF FEDERAL AGENCIES

AGENCY	FUNCTION
Bureau of Alcohol, Tobacco and Firearms (BATF)	Regulation of alcoholic beverages
Consumer Product Safety Commission (CPSC)	Safety of food handling equipment
Department of Agriculture (USDA)	
Economics Research Service (ERS)	Analysis and reporting of food situation and outlook
Food and Nutrition Service (FNS)	Administration of the following programs: Food Stamp; School Lunch; Women, Infants and Children; and Donated Food
Food Safety and Inspection Service (FSIS)	Inspection and labeling of meat, poultry, and eggs; grading of all foods; controlling nitrite in cured meats and poultry
Human Nutrition Information Service (HNIS)	Food consumption standard tables for nutritive value of food, educational materials
Science and Education Administration (SEA)	Extension Service, Agricultural Research Service Cooperative State Research Service, National Agricultural Library
Department of Health and Human Services (HHS)	
Centers for Disease Control (CDC)	Analysis and reporting of incidence of food-borne diseases
Food and Drug Administration (FDA)	Food labeling, safety of food and food additives, inspection of food processing plants, control of food contaminants, food standards
National Institutes of Health (NIH)	Research related to diet and health
Environmental Protection Agency (EPA)	Standards for drinking water and water pollution, use of pesticides on food crops
Federal Trade Commission (FTC)	Food advertising, competition in food industry
National Marine Fisheries Service (NMFS)	Inspection, standards, and quality of seafood
Occupational Safety and Health Administration (OSHA)	Employee safety in food-processing plants

dramatic manner in which fads and fallacies are presented covers the falseness. Anything that is out of line with current scientific evidence can be considered misinformation.

The **food quack** of today has been likened to the patent medicine man of the past. The food quack uses scientific jargon to sell the product, be it a special food, special food preparation, special diet, regimen, a book, magazine, or reducing gadget. It is wise to be suspicious of any writer, lecturer, or TV speaker who makes claims contrary to accepted information. Be aware of (1) those who claim wholesome food is harmful or undesirable in some way; (2) those who use a scare technique in regard to health or claim to be a scientist or authority; and (3) those who claim association with an unheard-of organization or attack the FDA or medical, public health, or nutrition authorities. One should also be suspicious of any material that comes from an anonymous source.

Authorities on nutrition agree that more widespread and more effective dissemination of sound scientific information on nutrition is necessary to combat food and nutrition misinformation. The FDA has long been concerned about the promotion of food supplements as cure-alls for conditions requiring medical attention. Misleading promotion of food supplements violates federal law. It is carried on in the following ways:

1. So-called health food lecturers who claim, directly or indirectly, that the products they are promoting are of value in preventing and curing disease, when in fact they are ineffective for such purposes.
2. Door-to-door sales agents posing as experts on nutrition.
3. Pseudoscientific books and journals frequently recommending some particular food or food combination and often written by persons with little nutritional background or training. These materials may include advertisements for various products in which the publisher has a commercial interest.

Nutrition authorities agree that the best way to buy vitamins and minerals is in the packages provided by nature: whole-grain and enriched breads and cereals, vegetables, fruits, milk, eggs, meat, and fish. The normal American diet now includes such a variety of foods that most persons can hardly fail to have an ample supply of the essential food constituents if they choose foods wisely. The public should distrust any suggestion of self-medication with vitamins and minerals to cure diseases of the nerves, bones, blood, liver, kidneys, heart, or digestive system.

GENERAL POINTERS FOR PREPARING AND COOKING FOODS TO PREVENT FOOD POISONING

Lack of sanitation, insufficient cooking, and improper storage can allow bacteria in food to increase to dangerous levels. Some bacteria produce poisonous substances called toxins that cause illness when the food is eaten. To prevent food poisoning:

- Serve food soon after cooking or refrigerate promptly. Hot foods may be refrigerated if they do not raise the temperature of the refrigerator to greater than 45° F (7° C).
- Keep food in the refrigerator until served or reheated.
- Speed the cooling of leftovers by refrigerating them in shallow containers.
- Keep hot foods HOT (at temperatures greater than 140° F or 60° C) and cold foods COLD (less than 40° F or 4° C). Food may not be safe to eat if held more than 2 or 3 hours at temperatures between 60° F (15° C) and 125° F (52° C), the zone in which bacteria grow rapidly. Remember to count all time during preparation, storage, and serving.
- Thoroughly clean all dishes, utensils, and work surfaces with soap and water after each use. It is especially important to thoroughly clean equipment and work surfaces that have been used for raw food before you use them for cooked food. This prevents the cooked food from becoming contaminated with bacteria that may have been present in the raw food. Bacteria can be destroyed by rinsing utensils and work surfaces with chlorine laundry bleach in the proportion recommended on the package. Cutting

boards, meat grinders, blenders, and can openers particularly need this protection.

- Always wipe up spills with paper towels or other disposable material.
- Thoroughly cook meat to avoid *Escherichia coli* contamination.
- *If the odor or color of any food is poor or questionable, do not taste it. Throw it out. The food may be dangerous.*

How Does Personal Hygiene Affect Food Safety?

Anyone who has an infectious disease should not handle, prepare, or serve food. The bacteria in infected cuts or other skin infections may be the source of foodborne illness. Food handlers must always work with clean hands, clean hair, and clean fingernails and must wear clean clothing. Hands must be washed after using the toilet or assisting anyone using the toilet; after smoking or blowing the nose; after touching raw meat, poultry, or eggs; and before working with other food. Food should be mixed with clean utensils rather than with the hands; however, plastic gloves may be worn if it is easier to use the hands. Hands should be kept away from the mouth, nose, and hair. It is important to cover coughs and sneezes with disposable tissues. The same spoon should not be used more than once for tasting food while preparing, cooking, or serving.

What Are Some Types of Food Poisoning?

To understand the importance of food poisoning prevention, types of foodborne illnesses must be known. The more common ones are those caused by:

- *Salmonella*
- *Staphylococcus aureus* (also referred to as staph poisoning)
- *Clostridium botulinum* (causes botulism)
- *Clostridium perfringens*

Specific information on the causes, symptoms, and prevention of these bacterial foodborne illnesses is found in Table 22–4.

FACT & FALLACY

FALLACY: Adding an egg to a milkshake or making eggnog is a good idea for someone who is too ill to eat.

FACT: Raw eggs can contain salmonella (a type of bacteria), which can be deadly for a person who already has a weakened immune system. This is especially true of cracked or soiled eggs. Eggs should be used only in foods that are to be thoroughly cooked, such as baked goods or casseroles. Proper handling of foods with cooked eggs is also important. Set custards and puddings in ice water to cool quickly after their preparation. Then refrigerate promptly until serving time.

WHAT ARE WORLD PROBLEMS IN NUTRITION AND WHAT ARE THE INTERESTED AGENCIES?

In less developed countries, a large number of individuals are undernourished, malnourished, and hungry. The problem is greatest among women and children. People are hungry not only because there is not enough food but also because they are too poor to purchase the food that is available. Assessment of dietary intake, whether in a very precise way (Fig. 22–3) or through more informal means, is important. As much as half of the world's

▲ TABLE 22-4

BACTERIAL FOODBORNE ILLNESS: CAUSES, SYMPTOMS, AND PREVENTION

FOODS INVOLVED	SYMPTOMS	CHARACTERISTICS OF ILLNESS	PREVENTIVE MEASURES
Salmonellosis: *Salmonella*			
Bacteria widespread in nature, live and grow in intestinal tracts of human beings and animals. Foods involved: Poultry Red meats Eggs Dried foods Dairy products	Severe headache, followed by vomiting, diarrhea, abdominal cramps, fever. Infants, elderly, and persons with lower resistance are most susceptible. Severe infections cause high fever and may even cause death.	Transmitted by eating contaminated food or by contact with infected persons or carriers of the infection. Also transmitted by insects, rodents, and pets. *Onset:* Usually within 12 to 36 hours *Duration:* 2 to 7 days	Salmonellae are destroyed by heating the food to 140°F and holding for 10 minutes, or to higher temperature for less time (for instance, 155°F for a few seconds). Refrigeration at 40°F inhibits the multiplication of Salmonellae, but they remain alive in foods in the refrigerator or freezer and even in dried food.
Perfringens Poisoning: *Clostridium perfringens*			
Spore-forming bacteria that grow in the absence of oxygen. Temperatures reached in thorough cooking of most foods are sufficient to destroy vegetative cells, but heat-resistant spores can survive. Foods involved: Stews, soups, or gravies made from poultry or red meat	Nausea without vomiting, diarrhea, acute inflammation of stomach and intestines.	Transmitted by eating food contaminated with abnormally large numbers of bacteria. *Onset:* Usually within 8 to 20 hours *Duration:* May persist for 24 hours	To prevent growth of surviving bacteria in cooked meats, gravies, and meat casseroles that are to be eaten later, cool foods rapidly and refrigerate promptly at 40°F or below, or hold them above 140°F.
Staphylococcal Poisoning: *Staphylococcus aureus*			
Bacteria fairly resistant to heat. Bacteria growing in food produce a toxin that is extremely resistant to heat. Foods involved: Custards Egg salad Potato salad Chicken salad Macaroni salad Ham salad Salami Cheese	Vomiting, diarrhea, prostration, abdominal cramps. Generally mild and often attributed to other causes.	Transmitted by food handlers who carry the bacteria and by eating food containing the toxin. *Onset:* Usually within 3 to 8 hours *Duration:* 1 to 2 days	Growth of bacteria that produce toxin is inhibited by keeping hot foods above 140°F and cold foods at or above 40°F. Toxin is destroyed by boiling for several hours or heating the food in a pressure cooker at 240°F for 30 minutes.

▲ T A B L E   2 2 – 4

BACTERIAL FOODBORNE ILLNESS: CAUSES, SYMPTOMS, AND PREVENTION *Continued*

FOODS INVOLVED	SYMPTOMS	CHARACTERISTICS OF ILLNESS	PREVENTIVE MEASURES
Botulism: *Clostridium botulinum*			

Spore-forming organisms that grow and produce toxin in the absence of oxygen, such as in a sealed container.
Foods involved:
  Canned low-acid foods
  Smoked fish
	Double vision, inability to swallow, speech difficulty, progressive respiratory paralysis. Fatality rate is high, in the US about 65 per cent.	Transmitted by eating food containing the toxin.
		Onset: Usually within 12 to 36 hours or longer
		Duration: 3 to 6 days
			Bacterial spores in food are destroyed by high temperatures obtained only in the pressure canner.* More than 6 hours is needed to kill the spores at boiling temperature (212°F). The toxin is destroyed by boiling for 10 to 20 minutes; time required depends on type of food.

From U.S. Department of Agriculture: Keeping Food Safe to Eat—A Guide for Homemakers. Home and Garden Bulletin No. 162, Washington, DC.

* For processing times in home canning, see Home and Garden Bulletin No. 8, Home Canning of Fruits and Vegetables, and No. 106, Home Canning of Meat and Poultry. U.S. Department of Agriculture, Washington, DC.

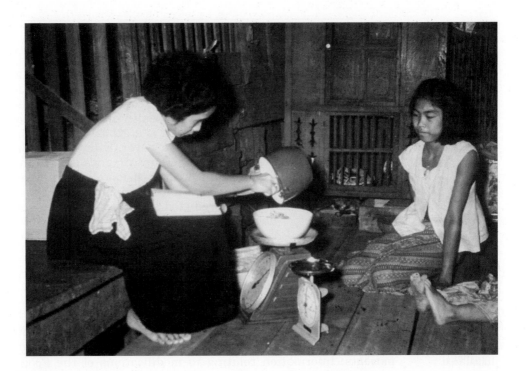

▲ F I G U R E   2 2 – 3

A Thai family's meal is weighed to assess dietary intake. Money to purchase food is often limited in less developed countries. (Courtesy of Cornell University Photography, Ithaca, NY.)

children may suffer some degree of malnutrition, temporary or permanent, that causes mental and physical developmental problems. Vitamin A deficiency is also a problem worldwide. Among impoverished countries, an estimated 5 million children show signs of moderate vitamin A deficiency and are therefore more vulnerable to infection and blindness. More than half a million children lose their sight every year (Bauernfeind, 1988).

The four basic ways of dealing with the international hunger problem are through (1) donation of food by various groups; (2) international efforts that direct the food to vulnerable groups, such as women and children; (3) promotion of agricultural production, food technology, and better use of the country's own food resources; and (4) economic assistance.

The United States has developed various programs and campaigns that assist developing countries in combating undernutrition. The U.S. Foreign Aid and Food for Peace programs and activities of the Agency for International Development are coordinated with United Nations agencies. The governments of many nations contribute to the organizations that distribute food or money for the purpose of improving nutritional standards. Some of these agencies are listed in Table 22–5.

FACT & FALLACY

FALLACY: The problem of world hunger cannot be solved.
FACT: The world is capable of growing enough food to end hunger if only every country had the political will. A country's level of wealth often dictates how well the people eat. Sri Lanka is a good example of how this need not be the case, however. Even though Sri Lanka is a poor country, the government's direct intervention with food distribution, provision of health care, and improvement in education has extended life expectancy far beyond its predicted ability (to about 70 years, with a reduction in infant mortality to 40 per 1000 live births as compared with 100 per 1000 for similar countries) (Anand and Kanbur, 1991).

WHAT IS THE ROLE OF THE NURSE OR OTHER HEALTH CARE PROFESSIONAL IN NATIONAL AND INTERNATIONAL NUTRITION PROGRAMS?

National Nutrition

Nurses or other health care professionals often provide nutrition education to a variety of groups such as pregnant women and diabetic or hypertensive patients. Information relating to modifications of the Food Guide Pyramid food groups, such as portion sizes and low-sodium, low-fat, or low-sugar alternatives is appropriate. Providing the patient with a rationale for making dietary changes that are in line with physiological needs particularly suits the nurse's skill level. Providing advice on low-cost food shopping is also ap-

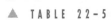

▲ TABLE 22-5

WORLD ORGANIZATIONS FOR BETTER NUTRITION

ORGANIZATION	PURPOSES
United Nations Food and Agriculture Organization (FAO)	Studies aspects of world food problems Raises nutrition standards by improving growth, distribution, and storage of food
World Health Organization (WHO)	Focus on worldwide health problems, including nutrition
United National Education, Scientific and Cultural Organization (UNESCO)	Improving the standard of living through science education and elimination of illiteracy
United Nations International Children's Emergency Fund (UNICEF)	Directs the distribution of milk to children worldwide through emergency relief, school feeding, and maternal-child health care centers
Oxford Famine Society (OXFAM-UK)	Donates money and services for agricultural development
CARE	Receives food from the Food for Peace Program for relief activities
World Bank	Sponsors international projects through agricultural and nutritional divisions

propriate (Table 22–6). Consultation should be made with a registered dietitian and physician regarding individual diet needs that go beyond basic nutrition, particularly when good nutrition may be jeopardized.

A health care team approach can help promote good nutritional status. The nurse or other health professional can help combat potentially dangerous nutrition myths and fads by providing correct information and assisting the public in recognizing false nutritional health claims. On a larger scale, the health care professional can help raise society's health consciousness by

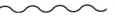

▲ TABLE 22-6

MONEY-SAVING FOOD SHOPPING SKILLS

- Use less tender cuts of meat, which are less expensive. To tenderize, cook slowly with moisture (such as in stews) or grind, cube, or pound the meat. Marinating in an acid such as lemon or tomato juice also helps to tenderize meat.
- Extend meat, poultry, and fish by making casseroles using legumes (dried beans), pasta, rice, or potatoes.
- Include meatless meals once or twice a week using legumes, eggs, cheese, or peanut butter in its place for protein.
- Buy in bulk whenever possible and freeze as needed.
- Study unit pricing to determine the best buy per pound or ounce.
- Take advantage of specials and use coupons.
- Try lower-priced, "generic" store brands, which are often of similar quality to more expensive brands.
- Plan meals to include leftovers.
- Shop for low-cost foods within each food group.
- Use food labels to compare nutritional value for cost to get your money's worth.

documenting the health needs of persons such as those with low incomes and those who are homeless. This documentation is necessary in order to justify equitable allocation of resources with legislators and other policy-makers.

It is important for the nurse or other health care professional to be aware of programs for referral purposes and direct care. Ambulatory care in particular is a growing means of health care, with the nurse often being called upon to help patients cope with therapeutic diets and to help prevent the effects of poor food sanitation on the debilitated patient.

International Nutrition

Solving international nutrition concerns is a more complex issue. The health care professional should be aware of programs that can be effectively promoted, such as taking vitamin A tablets to prevent blindness. Food programs meant to help should be closely examined. For example, providing dried milk powder to populations at risk of lactose intolerance is counterproductive. Attempts to solve world hunger must be undertaken in a way that empowers rather than creates dependency. Individuals can have an impact on world hunger by contacting political leaders to express concern. Efforts by credible international agencies such as the Agency for International Development and the United Nations (see previous discussion) can be supported. For Americans, eating less meat contributes, if only in a small way: It takes about 4 pounds of grain to produce 1 pound of meat; grain grown to feed cattle could be redirected to feed the world's hungry.

STUDY QUESTIONS AND ACTIVITIES

1. What community programs helped the Bernardo family in the opening chapter case study?
2. How has legislation had an impact on public health in relation to food and nutrition issues?
3. What existing programs promote good nutrition?
4. What are the signs of a food faddist?
5. Visit or call your local health department. Learn about any nutrition activities that are conducted under the auspices of the department.
6. Identify other organizations in your area that focus on the promotion of nutrition. Describe who they are and what their programs cover.
7. How much income would the Bernardo's have to have yearly to keep them above the poverty level? Above 175 per cent of the poverty level? Compute the hourly wage needed to make this income.
8. Contact your legislator through a letter or a phone call to express your support for legislation on a public health issue.

9. Have a student volunteer swab the inside of a home refrigerator using a cotton-tipped swab. Rub the swab on a Petri dish. Observe bacterial growth in class.

10. How might you assist a low-income individual who has hypertension and who needs to rely on donated canned foods?

REFERENCES

Anand S, Kanbur SMR: Public policy and basic needs provision: intervention and achievement in Sri Lanka. In Dreze J, Sen A: The Political Economy of Hunger. Clarendon Press: Oxford, 1991; pp 59–90.

Bauernfeind JC: Vitamin A deficiency: a staggering problem of health and sight. Nutrition Today, March/April, 1988; p 34.

Community Nutrition Institute: Food stamp program points to deep fissures in American economy. Nutrition Week, February 5, 1993; 23(6):2.

Mayer J: Nutritional problems in the United States: then and now two decades later. Nutrition Today, January/February, 1990; p 18.

Peterkin BB, Hama MY: Food shopping skills of the rich and the poor. Family Economics Rev. 1983; 3:8.

Wright HS, Guthrie HA, Wang MQ, Bernardo V: The 1987–88 Nationwide Food Consumption Survey: an update on the nutrient intake of respondents. Nutrition Today, May/June, 1991; p 27.

American Dental Association
211 East Chicago Avenue
Chicago, IL 60611

American Diabetes Association
18 East 48th Street
New York, NY 10017
Diabetes Forecast (bimonthly)

American Dietetic Association (ADA)
216 West Jackson Boulevard
Suite 800
Chicago, IL 60606-6995
Journal of the American Diabetes Association (monthly)

American Heart Association (AHA)
7320 Greenville Avenue
Dallas, TX 75231

American Home Economics Association (AHEA)
2010 Massachusetts Avenue, NW
Washington, DC 20036
Journal of Home Economics (five times a year)

American Institute of Nutrition (AIN)
9650 Rockville Pike
Bethesda, MD 20014
Journal of Nutrition (monthly)

American Medical Association (AMA)
535 North Dearborn Street
Chicago, IL 60610
Journal of the American Medical Association (weekly)

American Public Health Association (APHA)
1015 16th Street, NW
Washington, DC 20005
American Journal of Public Health (monthly)
The Nation's Health (monthly newspaper)

American Society of Clinical Nutrition, Inc. (ASCN)
9650 Rockville Pike
Bethesda, MD 20014
The American Journal of Clinical Nutrition (monthly)

American Society for Parenteral and Enteral Nutrition (ASPEN)
6110 Executive Boulevard, Suite 810
Rockville, MD 20852
Journal of Parenteral and Enteral Nutrition (bimonthly)
ASPEN Update (monthly newsletter)

Food and Drug Administration (FDA)
Consumer Information
Public Documents Distribution Center
Pueblo, CO 81009

Food and Nutrition Board (FNB) of National Research Council (NRC)
2101 Constitution Avenue, NW
Washington, DC 20418

National Dairy Council
6300 North River Road
Rosemont, IL 60018
Dairy Council Digest (bimonthly newsletter)

Nutrition Foundation, Inc.
888 17th Street, NW
Washington, DC 20006
Nutrition Reviews (monthly)

Nutrition Today
703 Giddings Avenue
Annapolis, MD 21401
Nutrition Today (bimonthly)

Society for Nutrition Education (SNE)
2140 Shattuck Avenue, Suite 1110
Berkeley, CA 94704
Journal of Nutrition Education (quarterly)

US Department of Agriculture
Institute of Home Economics
Washington, DC 20250
List of publications available from Office of Information

US Department of Health and Human Services
Washington, DC 20204
List of publications available from Office of Information

Appendix 2 Nutrition Materials

Free or inexpensive nutrition materials and product information are available by writing to the following addresses:

American Institute of Baking
  400 East Ontario Street
  Chicago, IL 60611

Armour Food Companies
  ConAgra Center
  One Central Park Plaza
  Omaha, NE 61802

Borden, Inc.
  Consumer Products Division
  108 East Broad Street
  Columbus, OH 43215

California Raisin Advisory Board
  P.O. Box 5335
  Fresno, CA 93755

Campbell Soup Company
  Consumer Products Division
  Camden, NJ 08101

Carnation Company
  Specialty Foods Division
  5045 Wilshire Boulevard
  Los Angeles, CA 90036

Del Monte Corporation
  Consumer and Education Services
  Box 3757
  San Francisco, CA 94119

Evaporated Milk Association
  288 North La Salle Avenue
  Chicago, IL 60601

Florida Citrus Commission
  Box 148
  Lakeland, FL 33802

General Foods Corporation
  250 North Street
  White Plains, NY 10625

General Mills, Inc.
  9200 Wayzata Boulevard
  Minneapolis, MN 55440

Kellogg Company
  235 Porter Street
  Battle Creek, MI 49016

Kraft, Inc.
  Consumer Products Division
  43rd Street below Woodland Avenue
  Philadelphia, PA 19104

LactAid, Inc.
  P.O. Box 111
  Pleasantville, NJ 08232

McDonald's Corporation
  Consumer Products Division
  McDonald's Plaza
  Oakbrook, IL 60521

Mead Johnson Nutritional Division
  Evansville, IN 47721

Metropolitan Life Insurance Co.
  Health and Welfare Division
  1 Madison Avenue
  New York, NY 10010

Nabisco Brands, Inc.
  Consumer Products Division
  Nabisco Brands Plaza
  Route #10
  Parsipany, NJ 07054

National Livestock and Meat Board
  Nutrition Research Department
  444 North Michigan Avenue
  Chicago, IL 60611

Peanut Association
  342 Madison Avenue
  New York, NY 10017

Poultry and Egg National Board
  250 West 57th Street
  New York, NY 10010

Potato Board
  1385 South Colorado Boulevard
  Denver, CO 80222

The Quaker Oats Company
  Consumer Products Division
  Merchandise Mart Plaza
  Chicago, IL 60654

Ralston-Purina Company
  Checkerboard Square
  St. Louis, MO 63164

Ross Laboratories
Columbus, OH 43216

Sandoz Nutrition Corporation
5320 West 23rd Street
P.O. Box 370
Minneapolis, MN 55440

Sunkist Growers
P.O. Box 2706, Terminal Annex
Los Angeles, CA 90054

Wheat Flour Institute
309 West Jackson Boulevard
Chicago, IL 60606

Appendix 3 Metric Conversions and Equivalents

EQUIVALENTS

1 oz = 30 g (approximate)
1 lb = 454 g
1 g = 1 mL
1 kg = 2.2 lb
1 tsp = 5 mL
1 tbsp = 15 mL
1 c. = 16 tbsp = 240 mL
1 L = 1000 mL
1 mg = 1000 µg

METRIC MEASUREMENT CONVERSIONS

SYMBOL	WHEN YOU KNOW	MULTIPLY BY	TO FIND	SYMBOL
Length				
in	inches	2.54	centimeters	cm
ft	feet	30	centimeters	cm
yd	yards	0.9	meters	m
mi	miles	1.6	kilometers	km
mm	millimeters	0.04	inches	in
cm	centimeters	0.4	inches	in
m	meters	3.3	feet	ft
m	meters	1.1	yards	yd
km	kilometers	0.6	miles	mi
Mass (Weight)				
oz	ounces	28	grams	g
lb	pounds	0.45	kilograms	kg
g	grams	0.035	ounce	oz
kg	kilograms	2.2	pounds	lb
	stones (British)	14	pounds	lb
Volume				
tsp	teaspoons	5	milliliters	mL
tbsp	tablespoons	15	milliliters	mL
fl oz	fluid ounces	30	milliliters	mL
c.	cups	0.24	liters	L
pt	pints	0.47	liters	L
qt	quarts	0.95	liters	L
gal (US)	gallons (US)	3.8	liters	L
gal (Imp)	gallons (Imperial)	4.5	liters	L
ft^3	cubic feet	0.028	cubic meters	m^3
yd^3	cubic yards	0.76	cubic meters	m^3
mL	milliliters	0.03	fluid ounces	fl oz
L	liters	2.1	pints	pt
L	liters	1.06	quarts	qt

**METRIC
MEASUREMENT
CONVERSIONS**

SYMBOL	WHEN YOU KNOW	MULTIPLY BY	TO FIND	SYMBOL
Volume				
L	liters	0.26	gallons (US)	gal (US)
L	liters	0.22	gallons (Imperial)	gal (Imp)

Temperature

$° C = (° F - 32) \times .555$

$° F = (° C \times 1.8) + 32$

BURGER KING

NUTRITIONAL INFORMATION CHART

	Serving Size (g)	Calories	Calories From Fat	Protein (g)	Carbo-hydrates (g)
BURGERS					
WHOPPER® SANDWICH	270	630	342	27	44
WHOPPER® WITH CHEESE SANDWICH	294	720	414	32	46
DOUBLE WHOPPER® SANDWICH	351	860	495	46	44
DOUBLE WHOPPER® WITH CHEESE SANDWICH	375	950	567	51	46
CHEESEBURGER	115	300	126	16	28
WHOPPER JR.® WITH CHEESE	145	380	198	16	29
HAMBURGER	103	260	90	14	28
WHOPPER JR.®	133	330	171	14	28
BACON DOUBLE CHEESEBURGER	149	470	252	30	26
BACON DOUBLE CHEESEBURGER DELUXE	185	570	342	32	26
DOUBLE CHEESEBURGER	161	450	225	27	29
SANDWICH/SIDE ORDERS					
BK BROILER® CHICKEN SANDWICH	154	280	90	20	29
CHICKEN SANDWICH	229	700	378	27	54
BK BIG FISH SANDWICH	255	710	387	24	58
BUTTERFLY SHRIMP	116	300	153	15	21
CHICKEN TENDERS™ (6 piece)	90	236	117	16	14
CHEF SALAD†	273	178	81	17	7
CHUNKY CHICKEN SALAD†	258	142	36	20	8
GARDEN SALAD†	223	95	45	6	8
DINNER SALAD/SIDE SALAD†	99	20	0	1	4
DINNER ROLL	25	80	18	3	13
BAKED POTATO	200	210	0	5	48
FRENCH FRIES (MEDIUM, SALTED)	116	372	180	5	43
ONION RINGS	97	339	171	5	38
POPCORN (AS SERVED)	28	130	54	3	17
DUTCH APPLE PIE	113	308	135	3	39
SNICKERS® ICE CREAM BAR	57	220	126	5	20
DRINKS					
VANILLA SHAKE (MEDIUM)	284	310	54	9	53
CHOCOLATE SHAKE (MEDIUM)	284	320	63	9	54
CHOCOLATE SHAKE (MEDIUM, SYRUP ADDED)	312	400	81	10	68
STRAWBERRY SHAKE (MEDIUM, SYRUP ADDED)	312	370	54	10	67
COCA-COLA® CLASSIC (MEDIUM)	22 (FL OZ)	264	0	0	70
DIET COKE® (MEDIUM)	22 (FL OZ)	1	0	0	0
SPRITE® (MEDIUM)	22 (FL OZ)	264	0	0	66
ORANGE JUICE	183	82	0	1	20
COFFEE	244	2	0	0	0
MILK - 2% LOW FAT	244	121	45	8	12
BREAKFAST					
CROISSAN'WICH® WITH BACON, EGG AND CHEESE	118	353	207	16	19
CROISSAN'WICH® WITH SAUSAGE, EGG AND CHEESE	159	534	360	21	22
CROISSAN'WICH® WITH HAM, EGG AND CHEESE	144	351	198	19	20
BREAKFAST BUDDY™ WITH SAUSAGE, EGG AND CHEESE	84	255	144	11	15
FRENCH TOAST STICKS	141	440	243	4	60
HASH BROWNS	71	213	108	2	25
MINI MUFFINS - BLUEBERRY #	95	292	126	4	37

| FAT (g)** | | | | | | | | | | |
Total	Saturated fatty acids	Mono-unsaturated fatty acids	Poly-Unsaturated fatty acids	Cholesterol (mg)	Sodium (mg)	% USDRA Protein	% USDRA Calcium	% USDRA Iron	% USDRA Vitamin A	% USDRA Vitamin C
38	11	13	13	90	880	40	8	30	10	20
46	16	16	13	115	1190	50	20	30	20	20
55	19	22	13	170	950	70	8	40	10	20
63	23	24	13	195	1260	80	25	40	20	20
14	6	6	1	45	660	25	10	15	6	4
22	7	8	7	50	660	25	10	15	8	8
10	4	5	1	30	500	20	2	15	2	4
19	5	6	7	40	500	20	4	15	4	8
28	13	12	2	100	800	45	20	20	8	*
38	15	14	7	110	990	50	20	20	10	4
25	12	10	2	90	840	40	20	20	10	4
10	2	4	4	50	770	30	4	10	2	6
42	8	16	18	60	1440	40	8	20	*	*
43	8	14	20	60	1110	35	8	20	2	2
17	5	11	2	105	610	25	15	6	0	4
13	3	8	2	38	541	25	*	4	2	*
9	4	3	1	103	568	26	16	9	95	25
4	1	1	1	49	443	31	4	7	92	34
5	3	1	0	15	125	9	15	6	100	58
0	0	0	0	0	10	0	0	2	90	15
2	0	1	1	0	140	4	1	5	*	*
0	0	0	0	0	15	8	2	15	0	50
20	5	12	2	0	238	8	*	7	*	5
19	5	12	2	0	628	7	11	3	15	*
6	3	2	1	15	540	4	0	2	0	0
15	3	8	4	0	228	4	*	6	*	8
14	7	5	2	15	65	6	6	2	2	*
6	4	2	0	20	230	15	30	*	6	6
7	5	2	0	20	230	10	20	10	4	*
9	5	2	0	20	350	15	30	2	6	6
6	4	2	0	20	240	15	30	*	6	6
0	0	0	0	0	@	*	*	*	*	*
0	0	0	0	0	@	*	*	*	*	*
0	0	0	0	0	@	*	*	*	*	*
0	0	0	0	0	2	*	*	*	3	119
0	0	0	0	0	122	13	30	*	10	4
5	3	1	0	18	122	13	30	*	10	4
23	8	12	2	230	780	24	14	10	10	*
40	14	21	4	258	985	32	15	16	10	*
22	7	11	2	236	1373	29	14	12	10	*
16	6	8	2	127	492	17	8	10	5	*
27	7	14	5	0	490	6	6	15	*	*
12	3	8	1	0	318	3	*	2	12	9
14	3	4	8	72	244	7	4	7	*	*

NUTRITIONAL INFORMATION CHART (con't)

		Serving Size (g)	Calories	Calories from fat	Protein (g)	Carbo-hydrates (g)
CONDIMENTS	**SANDWICH CONDIMENTS/TOPPINGS:**					
	PROCESSED AMERICAN CHEESE	25	92	63	5	1
	CREAM CHEESE	28	98	90	2	1
	LETTUCE	21	3	0	0	0
	TOMATO	28	6	0	0	1
	ONION	14	5	0	0	1
	PICKLES	14	1	0	0	0
	KETCHUP	14	17	0	0	4
	MUSTARD	3	2	0	0	0
	MAYONNAISE	28	210	207	0	1
	TARTAR SAUCE	28	175	171	0	0
	BK BROILER® SAUCE	11	37	36	0	1
	LAND O' LAKES® WHIPPED CLASSIC BLEND	10	65	63	0	0
	SOUR CREAM	28	60	54	1	1
	COCKTAIL SAUCE	21	20	0	0	4
	BULL'S EYE® BARBECUE SAUCE	14	22	0	0	5
	BACON BITS	3	16	9	1	0
	CROUTONS	7	31	9	1	5
	BURGER KING SALAD DRESSINGS:					
	THOUSAND ISLAND DRESSING	30	145	117	1	8
	FRENCH DRESSING	30	145	99	0	12
	RANCH DRESSING	30	175	162	1	2
	BLEU CHEESE DRESSING	30	150	144	1	1
	REDUCED CALORIE LIGHT ITALIAN DRESSING	30	15	9	0	3
	DIPPING SAUCES:					
	A.M. EXPRESS® DIP	28	84	0	0	21
	HONEY DIPPING SAUCE	28	91	0	0	23
	RANCH DIPPING SAUCE	28	171	162	0	2
	BARBECUE DIPPING SAUCE	28	36	0	0	9
	SWEET & SOUR DIPPING SAUCE	28	45	0	0	11

Total	FAT (g)** Saturated fatty acids	Mono-unsaturated fatty acids	Poly-unsaturated fatty acids	Cholesterol (mg)	Sodium (mg)	% USDRA Protein	% USDRA Calcium	% USDRA Iron	% USDRA Vitamin A	% USDRA Vitamin C
7	5	2	0	25	312	8	14	* *	8	*
10	5	4	-	28	86	4	2	*	7	*
0	0	0	0	0	2	*	* *	*	*	*
0	0	0	0	0	3	*	*	*	4	9
0	0	0	0	0	0	*	*	*	*	*
0	0	0	0	0	119	*	*	*	*	*
0	0	0	0	0	183	*	*	*	5	8
0	0	0	0	0	34	*	*	*	*	*
23	3	5	14	20	160	*	*	*	*	*
19	3	4	12	15	220	*	*	*	*	*
4	1	1	2	5	74	*	*	*	*	*
7	N/A	N/A	N/A	0	74	0	0	0	8	0
6	4	2	0	15	15	0	2	0	4	0
0	0	0	0	0	260	0	0	0	4	2
0	0	0	0	0	47	*	*	*	*	*
1	-	1	-	5	-	*	*	*	*	*
1	-	-	-	-	90	*	*	*	*	*
13	3	3	7	18	202	*	*	*	32	*
11	2	5	4	0	200	*	*	*	15	*
18	3	4	11	10	158	*	*	*	*	*
16	3	4	8	29	256	2	*	*	*	*
1	0	0	0	0	355	*	*	*	*	*
0	0	0	0	0	18	*	*	*	*	*
0	0	0	0	0	12	*	*	*	*	*
18	3	4	10	0	208	*	*	*	*	*
0	0	0	0	0	397	*	*	*	3	4
0	0	0	0	0	52	*	*	*	*	*

†=Without Dressing @=Depends on the water supply *=Contains less than 2% of the U.S.R.D.A. **="Total fats" are mixtures of triglycerides (glycerol and fatty acids) and other substances and therfore, may slightly exceed the sum of fatty acids. -=Data negligible #=May not be available in all restaurants

SANDWICH CONTENTS:
WHOPPER® Sandwich - 100% beef patty, sesame seed bun, tomato, lettuce, mayonnaise, ketchup, pickles, onion.
WHOPPER® with Cheese Sandwich - 100% beef patty, sesame seed bun, cheese, tomato, lettuce, mayonnaise, ketchup, pickles, onion.
Double WHOPPER® Sandwich - 100% beef patties, sesame bun, tomato, lettuce, mayonnaise, ketchup, pickles, onion.
Double WHOPPER® Sandwich with Cheese - 100% beef patties, sesame bun, cheese, tomato, lettuce, mayonnaise, ketchup, pickles, onion.

Cheeseburger - 100% beef patty, sesame seed bun, cheese, ketchup, pickles, mustard.
WHOPPER Jr.® with Cheese - 100% beef patty, sesame seed bun, cheese, tomato, lettuce, mayonnaise, ketchup, pickles.
Hamburger - 100% beef patty, sesame seed bun, ketchup, pickles, mustard.
WHOPPER Jr.® - 100% beef patty, sesame seed bun, tomato, lettuce, mayonnaise, ketchup, pickles.
Bacon Double Cheeseburger - 100% beef patties, sesame seed bun, bacon, cheese.
Bacon Double Cheeseburger Deluxe - 100% beef patties, sesame seed bun, bacon, cheese, tomato, lettuce, mayonnaise.

Double Cheeseburger - 100% beef patties, sesame seed bun, cheese, ketchup, pickles, mustard.
BK BROILER® Chicken Sandwich - broiled chicken patty, oat bran bun, lettuce, tomato, BK BROILER® sauce.
Chicken Sandwich - breaded chicken patty, specialty bun, lettuce, mayonnaise.
BK BIG FISH - breaded fish filet, sesame seed bun, lettuce, tartar sauce.
BREAKFAST BUDDY - Buddies bun, sausage, egg and cheese.

McDONALD'S

NUTRITION FACTS

Amount Per Serving

	Calories	Calories from Fat	Total Fat (g)	Saturated Fat (g)	Cholesterol (mg)	Sodium (mg)	Food Exchanges
SANDWICHES/FRENCH FRIES							
Hamburger	255	80	9	3	35	490	2 starch, 1 medium fat meat, 1 fat
Cheeseburger	305	115	13	5	50	725	2 starch, 1½ medium fat meat, 1 fat
Quarter Pounder	410	180	20	8	85	645	2 starch, 3 medium fat meat, 1 fat
Quarter Pounder with Cheese	510	250	28	11	115	1110	2 starch, 3½ medium fat meat, 2 fat
McLean Deluxe	320	90	10	4	60	670	2 starch, 3 lean meat
McLean Deluxe with Cheese	370	125	14	5	75	890	2 starch, 3 lean meat, 1 fat
Big Mac	500	235	26	9	100	890	3 starch, 3 medium fat meat, 2 fat
Filet-O-Fish	370	160	18	4	50	730	2½ starch, 1 medium fat meat, 2 fat
McChicken Sandwich	470	225	25	5	60	830	2½ starch, 2 medium fat meat, 3 fat
Chicken Fajita	190	70	8	2	35	310	1 starch, 1 lean meat, 1 fat
Small French Fries	220	110	12	2.5	0	110	2 starch, 2 fat
Medium French Fries	320	155	17	3.5	0	150	2½ starch, 3 fat
Large French Fries	400	200	22	5	0	200	3 starch, 4 fat
CHICKEN McNUGGETS/SAUCES							
Chicken McNuggets (6 piece)	270	135	15	3.5	55	580	1 starch, 2 medium fat meat, 1 fat
Hot Mustard Sauce	70	30	3.5	0.5	5	250	½ fruit, ½ fat
Barbeque Sauce	50	5	0.5	0	0	340	1 fruit
Sweet 'N Sour Sauce	60	0	0	0	0	190	1 fruit
Honey*	45	0	0	0	0	0	1 fruit
SALADS/SALAD DRESSINGS							
Chef Salad	170	80	9	4	110	400	1 vegetable, 2 medium fat meat
Chunky Chicken Salad	150	35	4	1	80	230	1 vegetable, 3 lean meat
Garden Salad	50	20	2	0.5	65	70	1 vegetable
Side Salad	30	10	1	0.5	30	35	1 vegetable
Croutons	50	20	2	0.5	0	140	½ starch
Bacon Bits	15	10	1	0.5	1	95	Free
Bleu Cheese (2.5 oz pkt)	250	180	20	5	35	750	5 fat
Ranch (2 oz pkt)	220	180	20	4	20	520	5 fat
1000 Island (2.5 oz pkt)	225	135	15	5	40	500	5 fat
Lite Vinaigrette (2 oz pkt)	50	20	2	0.5	0	240	1 fat
Red French Reduced Calorie (2 oz pkt)	160	70	8	1	0	460	1 starch, 2 fat
BREAKFAST							
Egg McMuffin	280	100	11	4	235	710	2 starch, 2 medium fat meat
Sausage McMuffin	345	180	20	7	60	770	2 starch, 1½ medium fat meat, 2 fat
Sausage McMuffin with Egg	430	225	25	8	270	920	2 starch, 2½ medium fat meat, 2 fat
English Muffin	170	35	4	1	0	285	2 starch, 1 fat
Sausage Biscuit	420	250	28	8	45	1040	2 starch, 1 medium fat meat, 4 fat
Sausage Biscuit with Egg	505	300	33	10	260	1210	2 starch, 2 medium fat meat, 4 fat
Bacon, Egg & Cheese Biscuit	440	235	26	8	240	1215	2 starch, 2 medium fat meat, 3 fat
Biscuit	260	115	13	3	1	730	2 starch, 2 fat

The following trademarks used herein are owned by McDonald's Corporation: Quarter Pounder, McLean Deluxe, Big Mac, Filet-O-Fish, McChicken, Chicken McNuggets, Egg McMuffin, Sausage McMuffin, McDonaldland.

	Calories	Calories from Fat	Total Fat (g)	Saturated Fat (g)	Cholesterol (mg)	Sodium (mg)	Food Exchanges
BREAKFAST (continued)							
Sausage	160	135	15	5	45	310	1 high fat meat, 1½ fat
Scrambled Eggs (2)	140	90	10	3	425	290	2 medium fat meat
Hash Browns	130	65	7	1	0	330	1 starch, 1½ fat
Hotcakes (Plain)	245	35	4	1	10	570	3 starch, 1 fat
Hotcakes (Margarine & Syrup*)	435	110	12	2	10	685	3 starch, 2 fat, 2 fruit
Breakfast Burrito	280	155	17	4	135	580	1 starch, 2 medium fat meat, 1 fat
Cheerios*	80	10	1	0	0	210	1 starch
Wheaties*	90	10	1	0	0	220	1 starch
MUFFINS/DANISH							
Apple Bran Muffin	180	0	0	0	0	200	2½ starch
Apple Danish*	390	155	17	4	25	370	3½ starch, 3 fat
Iced Cheese Danish*	390	190	21	6	45	420	3 starch, 4 fat
Cinnamon Raisin Danish*	440	190	21	5	35	430	3½ starch, 4 fat
Raspberry Danish*	410	145	16	3	25	310	4 starch, 3 fat
DESSERTS/SHAKES							
Vanilla Lowfat Frozen Yogurt Cone	110	10	1	0.5	5	80	1½ starch
Strawberry Lowfat Frozen Yogurt Sundae*	210	10	1	0.5	5	95	2 starch, 1 fruit
Hot Fudge Lowfat Frozen Yogurt Sundae*	240	25	3	2	5	170	2 starch, 1 fruit, ½ fat
Hot Caramel Lowfat Frozen Yogurt Sundae*	270	25	3	1.5	15	180	2 starch, 1½ fruit, ½ fat
Baked Apple Pie*	280	135	15	2	0	90	1 starch, 1 fruit, 3 fat
McDonaldland Cookies*	290	80	9	1	0	300	3 starch, 2 fat
Chocolaty Chip Cookies*	330	135	15	4	5	280	2½ starch, 3 fat
Vanilla Shake*	310	45	5	3	25	170	3½ starch, 1 fat
Chocolate Shake*	350	55	6	4	25	240	4 starch, 1 fat
Strawberry Shake*	340	45	5	3	25	170	4 starch, 1 fat
BEVERAGES							
1% Lowfat Milk, 8 fl oz	110	20	2	1.5	10	130	1 lowfat milk
Orange Juice, 6 fl oz	80	0	0	0	0	20	1 fruit
Grapefruit Juice, 6 fl oz	70	0	0	0	0	20	1 fruit
Apple Juice, 6 fl oz	80	0	0	0	0	10	1 fruit
Coca-Cola Classic,** 16 oz (small)	145	0	0	0	0	15	3 fruit
diet Coke,** 16 oz (small)	1	0	0	0	0	20	Free
Sprite,** 16 oz (small)	140	0	0	0	0	35	3 fruit
Hi-C* Orange Drink,* 16 oz (small)	160	0	0	0	0	35	3 fruit

Soft drink analysis is based on finished drinks with ice. Sizes include child (12 oz), small (16 oz), medium (21 oz), and large (32 oz).

*Menu items that contain moderate to high amounts of sugar (to assist persons with diabetes).

Nutrition analysis was obtained from Hazleton Laboratories America, Inc., combined with data from the USDA and McDonald's suppliers. Food exchanges were calculated by certified diabetes educator Marion J. Franz, M.S., R.D., director of nutrition at the International Diabetes Center. Exchange calculations are based on *Exchange Lists for Meal Planning*, 1986, American Diabetes Association, Inc., The American Dietetic Association.

If you have any questions about McDonald's and nutrition, please contact McDonald's Nutrition Information Center, McDonald's Corporation, Oak Brook, IL 60521, or call 708-575-FOOD.

NUTRITIONAL INFORMATION

This nutrition and ingredient guide was created to help you make informed meal choices when visiting Wendy's so you can plan a balanced diet. This is a complete ingredient list and nutritional analysis of Wendy's main menu items.

The nutrition analysis is provided for many menu items, such as baked potatoes, chili and prepared salads. For made-to-order items, such as your favorite sandwich or salad from our salad bar, you can calculate nutrition information by adding the components.

For example, to find the calories for a Single with ketchup, onion and tomato, add the total calories for each sandwich component: ¼ lb. hamburger patty (190), sandwich bun (160), ketchup (10), onion (0) and tomato (5) for a total of 365 calories. You can calculate your favorite salad the same way. (Note: Your totals may differ slightly from those listed. Wendy's calculations follow the federal regulations regarding the rounding of nutritional data).

WENDY'S

SANDWICHES

	Serving Size	Weight (g)	Calories	Calories from Fat	Total Fat (g)	Saturated (g)	Cholesterol (mg)	Sodium (mg)	Total Carbohydrates (g)	Dietary Fiber (g)	Sugars (g)	Protein (g)	Vitamin A	Vitamin C	Calcium	Iron
Plain Single	1 ea.	133	350	140	15	6	70	510	31	2	5	24	0	0	10	30
Single with everything	1 ea.	219	440	200	23	7	75	860	36	3	9	26	4	10	10	30
Big Bacon Classic	1 ea.	287	640	330	36	13	110	1500	44	3	11	37	10	25	25	35
Jr. Hamburger	1 ea.	117	270	80	9	3	35	600	34	2	7	15	2	2	10	20
Jr. Cheeseburger	1 ea.	129	320	120	13	5	45	770	34	2	7	18	4	2	15	20
Jr. Bacon Cheeseburger	1 ea.	170	440	230	25	8	65	870	33	2	7	22	6	15	20	25
Jr. Cheeseburger Deluxe	1 ea.	179	390	180	20	7	50	820	36	3	8	18	8	10	20	20
Hamburger, Kids' Meal	1 ea.	111	270	80	9	3	35	600	33	2	7	15	2	2	10	20
Cheeseburger, Kids' Meal	1 ea.	123	310	120	13	5	45	770	33	2	7	18	4	2	15	20
Grilled Chicken Sandwich	1 ea.	177	290	60	7	1.5	55	720	35	2	8	24	2	10	10	15
Breaded Chicken Sandwich	1 ea.	208	450	180	20	4	60	740	43	2	6	26	2	10	10	80
Chicken Club Sandwich	1 ea.	220	520	230	25	6	75	990	44	2	6	30	2	15	10	80
SANDWICH COMPONENTS																
¼ lb. Hamburger Patty	1 ea.	74	190	110	12	5	70	220	0	0	0	19	0	0	0	20
Jr. Hamburger Patty	1 ea.	37	90	60	6	2.5	35	110	0	0	0	10	0	0	0	10
Grilled Chicken Fillet	1 pc.	70	100	20	2.5	0.5	50	380	0	0	0	19	0	0	0	2
Breaded Chicken Fillet	1 pc.	99	220	90	10	2	55	400	11	0	0	21	0	0	0	70
Kaiser Bun	1 ea.	67	190	30	3	0.5	0	340	36	2	6	6	0	0	10	10
Sandwich Bun	1 ea.	56	160	25	2.5	0.5	0	280	29	2	5	5	0	0	8	10
American Cheese	1 sl.	18	70	50	6	4	15	260	0	0	0	4	6	0	10	0
American Cheese, Jr.	1 sl.	12	45	35	4	2.5	10	170	0	0	0	3	4	0	8	0
Bacon	1 sl.	6	30	20	2.5	1	5	125	0	0	0	2	0	2	0	0
Ketchup	1 t.	7	10	0	0	0	0	95	2	0	2	0	2	2	0	0
Lettuce	1 leaf	15	0	0	0	0	0	0	0	0	0	0	0	0	0	0
Mayonnaise	1½ t.	9	70	60	7	1	5	45	0	0	0	0	0	0	0	0
Mustard	½ t.	5	0	0	0	0	0	65	0	0	0	0	0	0	0	0
Onion	4 rings	13	0	0	0	0	0	0	1	0	1	0	0	2	0	0
Pickles	4 sl.	11	0	0	0	0	0	140	0	0	0	0	0	0	0	0
Red. Cal. Honey Mustard	1 t.	7	25	15	1.5	0	0	45	2	0	2	0	0	0	0	0
Tomatoes	1 sl.	26	5	0	0	0	0	0	1	0	1	0	2	8	0	0

SANDWICH CONTENTS

PLAIN SINGLE: ¼- lb. Patty, Sandwich Bun.
SINGLE WITH EVERYTHING: ¼-lb. Patty, Mayonnaise, Ketchup, Mustard, Pickles, Onion, Tomato, Lettuce, Sandwich Bun.
BIG BACON CLASSIC: ¼-lb. Patty, American Cheese Slice, Bacon, Mayonnaise, Ketchup, Pickles, Onion, Tomato, Lettuce, Kaiser Bun.
JR. HAMBURGER: 2 oz. Patty, Ketchup, Mustard, Pickles, Onion, Sandwich Bun.
JR. CHEESEBURGER: 2 oz. Patty, American Cheese Slice, Ketchup, Mustard, Pickles, Onion, Sandwich Bun.
JR. BACON CHEESEBURGER: 2 oz. Patty, American Cheese Slice, Bacon, Mayonnaise, Tomato, Lettuce, Sandwich Bun.
JR. CHEESEBURGER DELUXE: 2 oz. Patty, American Cheese Slice, Mayonnaise, Ketchup, Mustard, Pickles, Onion, Tomato, Lettuce, Sandwich Bun.
KIDS' MEAL HAMBURGER: 2 oz. Patty, Ketchup, Mustard, Pickles, Sandwich Bun.
KIDS' MEAL CHEESEBURGER: 2 oz. Patty, American Cheese Slice, Ketchup, Mustard, Pickles, Sandwich Bun.
GRILLED CHICKEN SANDWICH: Grilled Chicken Fillet, Honey Mustard Sauce, Tomato, Lettuce, Sandwich Bun.
BREADED CHICKEN SANDWICH: Breaded Chicken Fillet, Mayonnaise, Tomato, Lettuce, Sandwich Bun.
CHICKEN CLUB SANDWICH: Breaded Chicken FIllet, Mayonnaise, Tomato, Lettuce, Bacon, Sandwich Bun.

POTATOES, CHILI & NUGGETS

	Serving Size	Weight (g)	Calories	Calories from Fat	Total Fat (g)**	Saturated (g)	Cholesterol (mg)	Sodium (mg)	Total Carbohydrates (g)	Dietary Fiber (g)	Sugars (g)	Protein (g)	Vitamin A	Vitamin C	Calcium	Iron
FRENCH FRIES																
Small	3.2 oz.	91	240	100	12	2.5	0	150	33	3	0	3	0	10	2	4
Medium	4.8 oz.	136	360	160	17	4	0	220	50	4	0	5	0	15	2	6
Biggie	6.0 oz.	170	450	190	22	5	0	280	62	6	0	6	0	20	2	8
BAKED POTATO																
Plain	10 oz.	284	310	0	0	0	0	25	71	7	5	7	0	60	2	20
Bacon & Cheese	1 ea.	380	530	160	18	4	20	1280	77	7	5	17	10	60	8	25
Broccoli & Cheese	1 ea.	411	460	120	14	2.5	0	440	79	9	5	9	25	110	10	25
Cheese	1 ea.	383	560	200	23	8	30	610	77	7	5	14	20	60	30	20
Chili & Cheese	1 ea.	139	610	220	24	9	45	700	82	9	5	21	20	70	30	35
Sour Cream & Chives	1 ea.	314	380	60	6	4	15	40	74	8	6	8	20	80	8	25
Sour Cream	1 pkt.	28	60	50	6	4	10	15	1	0	1	0	6	0	4	0
Whipped Margarine	1 pkt.	14	60	50	5	1	0	105	0	0	0	0	15	0	0	0
Small	8 oz.	227	190	60	6	2.5	40	670	20	5	N/A	19	10	10	8	30
Large	12 oz.	340	290	90	9	4	60	1000	31	7	N/A	28	15	20	10	45
Cheddar Cheese, shredded	2 T.	17	70	50	6	3	15	110	1	0	0	4	4	0	10	0
Saltine Crackers	2 ea.	6	25	5	0.5	0	0	80	4	0	0	0	0	0	0	2
CHICKEN NUGGETS																
6 piece	6	94	280	180	20	5	50	600	12	0	N/A	14	0	0	2	4
Barbeque Sauce	1 pkt.	28	50	0	0		0	100	11	N/A	N/A	1	6	0	0	4
Honey	1 pkt.	14	45	0	0	0	0	0	12	0	12	0	0	0	0	0
Sweet & Sour Sauce	1 pkt.	28	45	0	0	0	0	55	11	N/A	N/A	0	0	0	0	2
Sweet Mustard Sauce	1 pkt.	28	50	10	1	0	0	140	9	N/A	N/A	1	0	0	0	0

DESSERTS, BEVERAGES

	Serving Size	Weight (g)	Calories	Calories from Fat	Total Fat (g)**	Saturated (g)	Cholesterol (mg)	Sodium (mg)	Total Carbohydrates (g)	Dietary Fiber (g)	Sugars (g)	Protein (g)	Vitamin A	Vitamin C	Calcium	Iron
DESSERTS																
Chocolate Chip Cookie	1 ea.	64	280	120	13	4	15	260	39	1	N/A	3	2	0	2	8
Frosty Dairy Dessert, small	12 oz.	243	340	90	10	5	40	200	57	3	47	9	8	0	30	6
Medium	16 oz.	324	460	120	13	7	55	260	76	4	63	12	10	0	40	6
Large	20 oz.	405	570	150	17	9	70	330	95	5	79	15	10	0	50	8
BEVERAGES																
Cola, small	8 oz.	227	90	0	0	0	0	10	24	0	24	0	0	0	0	0
Diet Cola, small	8 oz.	227	0	0	0	0	0	20	0	0	0	0	0	0	0	0
Lemon-Lime Soft Drink, sm.	8 oz.	227	90	0	0	0	0	25	24	0	24	0	0	0	0	0
Lemonade, small	8 oz.	227	90	0	0	0	0	5	24	0	21	0	0	15	0	2
Coffee	6 oz.	170	0	0	0	0	0	0	1	0	1	0	0	0	0	0
Decaffeinated Coffee	6 oz.	170	0	0	0	0	0	0	1	0	1	0	0	0	0	0
Hot Chocolate	6 oz.	170	9	10	1	0.5	0	120	19	2	N/A	3	0	0	8	2
Tea, Hot	6 oz.	170	0	0	0	0	0	0	0	0	0	0	0	0	0	0
Tea, Iced	6 oz.	170	0	0	0	0	0	0	0	0	0	0	0	0	0	0
Milk, 2%	8 oz.	227	110	40	4	2.5	15	115	11	0	11	8	15	4	30	0

To determine nutritional information for a Kids' size soft drink, multiply by .7; medium soft drink, multiply by 1.2; Biggie soft drink, multiply by 2. Soft drink serving size reflects the amount of liquid in a 16 oz. beverage cup.

GARDEN SPOT® SALAD BAR

	Serving Size	Weight (g)	Calories	Calories from Fat	Total Fat (g)**	Saturated (g)	Cholesterol (mg)	Sodium (mg)	Total Carbohydrates (g)	Dietary Fiber (g)	Sugars (g)	Protein (g)	Vitamin A	Vitamin C	Calcium	Iron
Applesauce	2 T.	39	30	0	0	0	0	0	7	0	7	0	0	0	0	0
Bacon Bits	2 T.	15	40	15	1.5	0.5	5	540	1	0	0	6	0	0	0	0
Broccoli	¼ C.	14	0	0	0	0	0	0	1	0	0	0	4	20	0	0
Cantaloupe, sliced	1 pc.	45	15	0	0	0	0	0	4	0	3	0	15	30	0	0
Carrots	¼ C.	16	5	0	0	0	0	5	2	0	1	0	45	2	0	0
Cauliflower	¼ C.	16	0	0	0	0	0	0	1	0	0	0	0	10	0	0
Cheddar Chips	2 T.	12	70	40	4	1	0	200	5	0	0	1	0	0	2	2
Cheese, shredded (imitation)	2 T.	17	50	40	4	1	0	230	1	0	1	3	2	0	10	0
Chicken Salad	2 T.	35	70	45	5	1	0	135	2	0	N/A	4	0	2	0	2
Chives	1 T.	1	0	0	0	0	0	0	1	0	0	0	6	10	0	2
Chow Mein Noodles	¼ C.	7	35	20	2	0	0	30	4	0	0	0	0	0	0	2
Cole Slaw	2 T.	36	45	25	3	0	5	65	5	1	4	0	0	45	2	2
Cottage Cheese	2 T.	31	30	15	1.5	1	5	125	1	0	1	4	2	0	2	0
Croutons	2 T.	6	30	10	1	0	0	75	4	0	N/A	0	0	0	0	0
Cucumbers	2 sl.	15	0	0	0	0	0	0	0	0	0	0	0	2	0	0
Eggs, hard cooked	2 T.	26	40	25	3	1	110	30	0	0	0	3	4	0	2	2
Green Peas	2 T.	21	15	0	0	0	0	25	3	1	1	1	2	6	0	2
Green Peppers	2 pc.	8	0	0	0	0	0	0	1	0	0	0	0	10	0	0
Honeydew Melon, sliced	1 pc.	52	20	0	0	0	0	5	5	0	4	0	0	20	0	0
Jalapeno Peppers	1 T.	11	0	0	0	0	0	160	1	0	0	0	2	2	0	2
Lettuce (Iceberg/Romaine)	1 C.	75	10	0	0	0	0	5	2	1	0	0	6	10	2	2
Mushrooms	¼ C.	14	0	0	0	0	0	0	1	0	0	0	0	0	0	0
Olives, Black	2 T.	14	15	15	1.5	0	0	120	1	0	0	0	0	0	2	2
Orange, sectioned	1 pc.	31	10	0	0	0	0	0	5	1	N/A	0	0	35	2	2
Pasta Salad	2 T.	35	25	0	0	0	0	75	3	1	0	0	20	0	0	0
Peaches, sliced	1 pc.	29	15	0	0	0	0	0	4	0	4	0	2	2	0	0
Pepperoni, sliced	6 sl.	6	30	25	3	1	5	70	0	0	0	1	2	0	0	0
Pineapple, chunked	4 pc.	32	20	0	0	0	0	0	5	0	5	0	0	6	0	0
Potato Salad	2 T.	36	80	60	7	2.5	5	180	5	0	0	0	0	6	0	0
Pudding, Chocolate	¼ C.	50	70	30	3	0.5	0	60	10	0	8	0	0	0	10	2
Pudding, Vanilla	¼ C.	50	70	30	3	0.5	0	60	10	0	9	0	0	0	10	2
Red Onions	3 rings	13	0	0	0	0	0	0	1	0	1	0	0	2	0	0
Seafood Salad	¼ C.	37	70	40	4	0.5	0	300	5	0	N/A	3	0	2	15	2
Sesame Breadstick	1 ea.	3	15	0	0	0	0	20	2	0	0	0	0	0	0	0
Strawberries	1 ea.	25	10	0	0	0	0	0	2	1	1	0	0	25	0	0
Strawberry Banana Dessert	¼ C.	47	30	0	0	0	0	0	8	1	5	0	0	20	0	2
Sunflower Seeds & Raisins	2 T.	16	80	45	5	0.5	0	0	5	1	3	0	0	2	2	2
Tomato, wedged	1 pc.	26	5	0	0	0	0	0	1	0	1	0	2	8	0	0
Turkey Ham, diced	2 T.	22	50	35	4	1	25	280	0	0	0	3	0	0	2	2
Watermelon, wedged	1 pc.	62	20	0	0	0	0	0	4	0	4	0	2	10	0	0

SALAD/SUPERBAR

	Serving Size	Weight (g)	Calories	Calories from Fat	Total Fat (g) **	Saturated (g)	Cholesterol (mg)	Sodium (mg)	Total Carbohydrates (g)	Dietary Fiber (g)	Sugars (g)	Protein (g)	Vitamin A	Vitamin C	Calcium	Iron
Salad Dressings †																
Blue Cheese	2 T.	28	180	170	19	3	15	180	1	0	0	1	0	0	2	0
Blue Cheese, Red. Cal, Red. Fat	2 T.	28	70	60	7	1.5	15	260	2	0	1	0	0	0	2	0
Celery Seed	2 T.	28	100	60	7	1	10	220	10	0	8	0	0	0	0	2
French	2 T.	28	120	90	11	1.5	0	300	7	0	6	0	4	2	0	0
French, Fat Free	2 T.	28	35	0	0	0	0	180	8	0	7	0	0	0	0	0
French, Sweet Red	2 T.	28	130	90	10	1.5	0	250	10	0	8	0	2	2	0	0
Italian Caesar	2 T.	28	150	150	16	2.5	15	230	0	0	0	0	0	0	2	0
Italian, Golden	2 T.	28	90	60	7	1	0	450	6	0	5	0	0	0	0	0
Italian, Red. Cal., Red. Fat	2 T.	28	40	30	3	0.5	0	330	3	0	2	0	0	2	0	2
Hidden Valley® Ranch	2 T.	28	90	90	10	1.5	10	210	1	0	0	0	0	0	2	0
Salad Oil	1 T.	14	130	130	14	2	0	0	0	0	0	0	0	0	0	0
Thousand Island	2 T.	28	130	120	13	2	10	160	4	0	2	0	2	2	0	0
Wine Vinegar	1 T.	14	0	0	0	0	0	0	0	0	0	0	0	0	0	0
FRESH SALADS TO GO (without dressing)																
Caesar Side Salad	1 ea.	89	110	50	5	2	15	580	7	2	0	9	20	25	10	6
Deluxe Garden Salad	1 ea.	271	110	50	6	1	0	320	10	4	4	7	60	60	20	8
Grilled Chicken Salad	1 ea.	338	200	70	8	1.5	50	690	10	4	4	25	60	60	20	10
Side Salad	1 ea.	155	60	25	3	0.5	0	160	5	2	2	4	30	30	10	4
Taco Salad	1 ea.	510	580	270	30	11	75	1060	51	11	2	33	35	50	45	45
Soft Breadstick	1 ea.	44	130	30	3	0.5	5	250	24	1	N/A	4	0	0	4	8
SUPERBAR (where available)																
Alfredo Sauce	¼ C.	40	30	10	1.5	0	0	250	4	0	N/A	0	0	0	4	0
Cheese Sauce	¼ C.	35	25	10	1	0	0	190	3	N/A	N/A	0	0	0	4	0
Macaroni & Cheese	½ C.	92	130	60	6	2.5	5	320	14	0	N/A	4	0	0	4	4
Parmesan Cheese, grated	2 T.	16	70	45	5	3	15	220	1	0	0	6	4	0	20	0
Picanté Sauce	2 T.	29	10	0	0	0	0	260	2	0	0	0	2	2	0	0
Refried Beans	¼ C.	54	80	30	3	1	0	300	14	5	0	4	0	0	2	8
Red Peppers, Crushed	1 T.	5	15	5	1	0	0	0	3	1	1	0	45	6	0	2
Rice, Spanish	¼ C.	50	60	10	1	0	0	390	11	1	N/A	1	4	0	4	8
Rotini	½ C.	55	90	15	2	0	0	N/A	15	1	N/A	3	0	0	0	4
Sour Topping	2 T.	28	60	50	5	5	0	30	2	0	2	0	0	0	0	0
Spaghetti Sauce	¼ C.	44	30	0	0	0	0	340	6	0	N/A	0	0	0	2	0
Spaghetti Meat Sauce	¼ C.	41	45	10	1.5	0.5	5	230	6	1	N/A	3	2	2	0	2
Taco Chips	8 ea.	25	120	60	7	1	0	90	14	2	0	2	0	0	4	2
Taco Meat	2 T.	38	80	40	4	1	15	200	2	N/A	N/A	7	0	0	2	8
Taco Sauce	2 T.	22	10	0	0	0	0	110	2	0	N/A	0	2	2	0	2
Taco Shells	1 ea.	11	60	35	4	0.5	0	15	6	1	0	1	0	0	0	10
Tortilla, Flour	1 ea.	35	110	25	2.5	0.5	0	210	18	1	1	3	0	0	6	6

† 2 T. = 1 ladle = 1 oz.
Packets = 2 oz. except Italian Caesar = 1.5 oz.

Symbol Key
**   total fats are comprised of many substances other than those listed
N/A   information not available

Appendix 5 Nutritive Value of the Edible Part of Food*

(Tr indicates nutrient present in trace amount.)

Item No.	Foods, approximate measures, units, and weight (weight of edible portion only)			Water	Food energy	Pro-tein	Fat	Fatty acids		
								Satu-rated	Mono-unsatu-rated	Poly-unsatu-rated
	Beverages		Grams	Per-cent	Cal-ories	Grams	Grams	Grams	Grams	Grams
	Alcoholic:									
	Beer:									
1	Regular-----------------------	12 fl oz--------	360	92	150	1	0	0.0	0.0	0.0
2	Light-------------------------	12 fl oz--------	355	95	95	1	0	0.0	0.0	0.0
	Gin, rum, vodka, whiskey:									
3	80-proof----------------------	1-1/2 fl oz-----	42	67	95	0	0	0.0	0.0	0.0
4	86-proof----------------------	1-1/2 fl oz-----	42	64	105	0	0	0.0	0.0	0.0
5	90-proof----------------------	1-1/2 fl oz-----	42	62	110	0	0	0.0	0.0	0.0
	Wines:									
6	Dessert-----------------------	3-1/2 fl oz-----	103	77	140	Tr	0	0.0	0.0	0.0
	Table:									
7	Red--------------------------	3-1/2 fl oz-----	102	88	75	Tr	0	0.0	0.0	0.0
8	White------------------------	3-1/2 fl oz-----	102	87	80	Tr	0	0.0	0.0	0.0
	Carbonated:[2]									
9	Club soda---------------------	12 fl oz--------	355	100	0	0	0	0.0	0.0	0.0
	Cola type:									
10	Regular-----------------------	12 fl oz--------	369	89	160	0	0	0.0	0.0	0.0
11	Diet, artificially sweetened	12 fl oz--------	355	100	Tr	0	0	0.0	0.0	0.0
12	Ginger ale---------------------	12 fl oz--------	366	91	125	0	0	0.0	0.0	0.0
13	Grape-------------------------	12 fl oz--------	372	88	180	0	0	0.0	0.0	0.0
14	Lemon-lime--------------------	12 fl oz--------	372	89	155	0	0	0.0	0.0	0.0
15	Orange------------------------	12 fl oz--------	372	88	180	0	0	0.0	0.0	0.0
16	Pepper type-------------------	12 fl oz--------	369	89	160	0	0	0.0	0.0	0.0
17	Root beer---------------------	12 fl oz--------	370	89	165	0	0	0.0	0.0	0.0
	Cocoa and chocolate-flavored beverages. See Dairy Products (items 95-98).									
	Coffee:									
18	Brewed------------------------	6 fl oz---------	180	100	Tr	Tr	Tr	Tr	Tr	Tr
19	Instant, prepared (2 tsp powder plus 6 fl oz water)----------	6 fl oz---------	182	99	Tr	Tr	Tr	Tr	Tr	Tr
	Fruit drinks, noncarbonated:									
	Canned:									
20	Fruit punch drink------------	6 fl oz---------	190	88	85	Tr	0	0.0	0.0	0.0
21	Grape drink------------------	6 fl oz---------	187	86	100	Tr	0	0.0	0.0	0.0
22	Pineapple-grapefruit juice drink---------------------	6 fl oz---------	187	87	90	Tr	Tr	Tr	Tr	Tr
	Frozen:									
	Lemonade concentrate:									
23	Undiluted------------------	6-fl-oz can-----	219	49	425	Tr	Tr	Tr	Tr	¹r
24	Diluted with 4-1/3 parts water by volume----------	6 fl oz---------	185	89	80	Tr	Tr	Tr	Tr	Tr
	Limeade concentrate:									
25	Undiluted------------------	6-fl-oz can-----	218	50	410	Tr	Tr	Tr	Tr	Tr
26	Diluted with 4-1/3 parts water by volume----------	6 fl oz---------	185	89	75	Tr	Tr	Tr	Tr	Tr
	Fruit juices. See type under Fruits and Fruit Juices.									
	Milk beverages. See Dairy Products (items 92-105).									
	Tea:									
27	Brewed------------------------	8 fl oz---------	240	100	Tr	Tr	Tr	Tr	Tr	Tr
	Instant, powder, prepared:									
28	Unsweetened (1 tsp powder plus 8 fl oz water)--------	8 fl oz---------	241	100	Tr	Tr	Tr	Tr	Tr	Tr
29	Sweetened (3 tsp powder plus 8 fl oz water)-------------	8 fl oz---------	262	91	85	Tr	Tr	Tr	Tr	Tr

[1]Value not determined.
[2]Mineral content varies depending on water source.

Nutrients in Indicated Quantity

Cho-les-terol	Carbo-hydrate	Calcium	Phos-phorus	Iron	Potas-sium	Sodium	Vitamin A value (IU)	Vitamin A value (RE)	Thiamin	Ribo-flavin	Niacin	Ascorbic acid	Item No.
Milli-grams	Grams	Milli-grams	Milli-grams	Milli-grams	Milli-grams	Milli-grams	Inter-national units	Retinol equiva-lents	Milli-grams	Milli-grams	Milli-grams	Milli-grams	
0	13	14	50	0.1	115	18	0	0	0.02	0.09	1.8	0	1
0	5	14	43	0.1	64	11	0	0	0.03	0.11	1.4	0	2
0	Tr	Tr	Tr	Tr	1	Tr	0	0	Tr	Tr	Tr	0	3
0	Tr	Tr	Tr	Tr	1	Tr	0	0	Tr	Tr	Tr	0	4
0	Tr	Tr	Tr	Tr	1	Tr	0	0	Tr	Tr	Tr	0	5
0	8	8	9	0.2	95	9	(^{1})	(^{1})	0.01	0.02	0.2	0	6
0	3	8	18	0.4	113	5	(^{1})	(^{1})	0.00	0.03	0.1	0	7
0	3	9	14	0.3	83	5	(^{1})	(^{1})	0.00	0.01	0.1	0	8
0	0	18	0	Tr	0	78	0	0	0.00	0.00	0.0	0	9
0	41	11	52	0.2	7	18	0	0	0.00	0.00	0.0	0	10
0	Tr	14	39	0.2	7	[3]32	0	0	0.00	0.00	0.0	0	11
0	32	11	0	0.1	4	29	0	0	0.00	0.00	0.0	0	12
0	46	15	0	0.4	4	48	0	0	0.00	0.00	0.0	0	13
0	39	7	0	0.4	4	33	0	0	0.00	0.00	0.0	0	14
0	46	15	4	0.3	7	52	0	0	0.00	0.00	0.0	0	15
0	41	11	41	0.1	4	37	0	0	0.00	0.00	0.0	0	16
0	42	15	0	0.2	4	48	0	0	0.00	0.00	0.0	0	17
0	Tr	4	2	Tr	124	2	0	0	0.00	0.02	0.4	0	18
0	1	2	6	0.1	71	Tr	0	0	0.00	0.03	0.6	0	19
0	22	15	2	0.4	48	15	20	2	0.03	0.04	Tr	[4]61	20
0	26	2	2	0.3	9	11	Tr	Tr	0.01	0.01	Tr	[4]64	21
0	23	13	7	0.9	97	24	60	6	0.06	0.04	0.5	[4]110	22
0	112	9	13	0.4	153	4	40	4	0.04	0.07	0.7	66	23
0	21	2	2	0.1	30	1	10	1	0.01	0.02	0.2	13	24
0	108	11	13	0.2	129	Tr	Tr	Tr	0.02	0.02	0.2	26	25
0	20	2	2	Tr	24	Tr	Tr	Tr	Tr	Tr	Tr	4	26
0	Tr	0	2	Tr	36	1	0	0	0.00	0.03	Tr	0	27
0	1	1	4	Tr	61	1	0	0	0.00	0.02	0.1	0	28
0	22	1	3	Tr	49	Tr	0	0	0.00	0.04	0.1	0	29

[3]Blend of aspartame and saccharin; if only sodium saccharin is used, sodium is 75 mg; if only aspartame is used, sodium is 23 mg.
[4]With added ascorbic acid.

Nutritive Value of the Edible Part of Food (Continued)
(Tr indicates nutrient present in trace amount.)

Item No.	Foods, approximate measures, units, and weight (weight of edible portion only)		Water	Food energy	Pro-tein	Fat	Fatty acids		
							Satu-rated	Mono-unsatu-rated	Poly-unsatu-rated
	Dairy Products	Grams	Per-cent	Cal-ories	Grams	Grams	Grams	Grams	Grams
	Butter. See Fats and Oils (items 128-130).								
	Cheese:								
	Natural:								
30	Blue----------------------- 1 oz------------	28	42	100	6	8	5.3	2.2	0.2
31	Camembert (3 wedges per 4-oz container)---------------- 1 wedge---------	38	52	115	8	9	5.8	2.7	0.3
	Cheddar:								
32	Cut pieces----------------- 1 oz------------	28	37	115	7	9	6.0	2.7	0.3
33	1 in³-----------	17	37	70	4	6	3.6	1.6	0.2
34	Shredded------------------- 1 cup-----------	113	37	455	28	37	23.8	10.6	1.1
	Cottage (curd not pressed down):								
	Creamed (cottage cheese, 4% fat):								
35	Large curd--------------- 1 cup-----------	225	79	235	28	10	6.4	2.9	0.3
36	Small curd--------------- 1 cup-----------	210	79	215	26	9	6.0	2.7	0.3
37	With fruit-------------- 1 cup-----------	226	72	280	22	8	4.9	2.2	0.2
38	Lowfat (2%)-------------- 1 cup-----------	226	79	205	31	4	2.8	1.2	0.1
39	Uncreamed (cottage cheese dry curd, less than 1/2% fat)--------------------- 1 cup-----------	145	80	125	25	1	0.4	0.2	Tr
40	Cream----------------------- 1 oz------------	28	54	100	2	10	6.2	2.8	0.4
41	Feta------------------------ 1 oz------------	28	55	75	4	6	4.2	1.3	0.2
	Mozzarella, made with:								
42	Whole milk---------------- 1 oz------------	28	54	80	6	6	3.7	1.9	0.2
43	Part skim milk (low moisture)---------------- 1 oz------------	28	49	80	8	5	3.1	1.4	0.1
44	Muenster-------------------- 1 oz------------	28	42	105	7	9	5.4	2.5	0.2
	Parmesan, grated:								
45	Cup, not pressed down------ 1 cup-----------	100	18	455	42	30	19.1	8.7	0.7
46	Tablespoon---------------- 1 tbsp----------	5	18	25	2	2	1.0	0.4	Tr
47	Ounce--------------------- 1 oz------------	28	18	130	12	9	5.4	2.5	0.2
48	Provolone------------------ 1 oz------------	28	41	100	7	8	4.8	2.1	0.2
	Ricotta, made with:								
49	Whole milk---------------- 1 cup-----------	246	72	430	28	32	20.4	8.9	0.9
50	Part skim milk------------ 1 cup-----------	246	74	340	28	19	12.1	5.7	0.6
51	Swiss----------------------- 1 oz------------	28	37	105	8	8	5.0	2.1	0.3
	Pasteurized process cheese:								
52	American-------------------- 1 oz------------	28	39	105	6	9	5.6	2.5	0.3
53	Swiss----------------------- 1 oz------------	28	42	95	7	7	4.5	2.0	0.2
54	Pasteurized process cheese food, American -------------- 1 oz------------	28	43	95	6	7	4.4	2.0	0.2
55	Pasteurized process cheese spread, American------------- 1 oz------------	28	48	80	5	6	3.8	1.8	0.2
	Cream, sweet:								
56	Half-and-half (cream and milk) 1 cup-----------	242	81	315	7	28	17.3	8.0	1.0
57	1 tbsp----------	15	81	20	Tr	2	1.1	0.5	0.1
58	Light, coffee, or table-------- 1 cup-----------	240	74	470	6	46	28.8	13.4	1.7
59	1 tbsp----------	15	74	30	Tr	3	1.8	0.8	0.1
	Whipping, unwhipped (volume about double when whipped):								
60	Light----------------------- 1 cup-----------	239	64	700	5	74	46.2	21.7	2.1
61	1 tbsp----------	15	64	45	Tr	5	2.9	1.4	0.1
62	Heavy----------------------- 1 cup-----------	238	58	820	5	88	54.8	25.4	3.3
63	1 tbsp----------	15	58	50	Tr	6	3.5	1.6	0.2
64	Whipped topping, (pressurized) 1 cup-----------	60	61	155	2	13	8.3	3.9	0.5
65	1 tbsp----------	3	61	10	Tr	1	0.4	0.2	Tr
66	Cream, sour----------------------- 1 cup-----------	230	71	495	7	48	30.0	13.9	1.8
67	1 tbsp----------	12	71	25	Tr	3	1.6	0.7	0.1

Nutrients in Indicated Quantity

Cho-les-terol	Carbo-hydrate	Calcium	Phos-phorus	Iron	Potas-sium	Sodium	Vitamin A value (IU)	Vitamin A value (RE)	Thiamin	Ribo-flavin	Niacin	Ascorbic acid	Item No.
Milli-grams	Grams	Milli-grams	Milli-grams	Milli-grams	Milli-grams	Milli-grams	Inter-national units	Retinol equiva-lents	Milli-grams	Milli-grams	Milli-grams	Milli-grams	
21	1	150	110	0.1	73	396	200	65	0.01	0.11	0.3	0	30
27	Tr	147	132	0.1	71	320	350	96	0.01	0.19	0.2	0	31
30	Tr	204	145	0.2	28	176	300	86	0.01	0.11	Tr	0	32
18	Tr	123	87	0.1	17	105	180	52	Tr	0.06	Tr	0	33
119	1	815	579	0.8	111	701	1,200	342	0.03	0.42	0.1	0	34
34	6	135	297	0.3	190	911	370	108	0.05	0.37	0.3	Tr	35
31	6	126	277	0.3	177	850	340	101	0.04	0.34	0.3	Tr	36
25	30	108	236	0.2	151	915	280	81	0.04	0.29	0.2	Tr	37
19	8	155	340	0.4	217	918	160	45	0.05	0.42	0.3	Tr	38
10	3	46	151	0.3	47	19	40	12	0.04	0.21	0.2	0	39
31	1	23	30	0.3	34	84	400	124	Tr	0.06	Tr	0	40
25	1	140	96	0.2	18	316	130	36	0.04	0.24	0.3	0	41
22	1	147	105	0.1	19	106	220	68	Tr	0.07	Tr	0	42
15	1	207	149	0.1	27	150	180	54	0.01	0.10	Tr	0	43
27	Tr	203	133	0.1	38	178	320	90	Tr	0.09	Tr	0	44
79	4	1,376	807	1.0	107	1,861	700	173	0.05	0.39	0.3	0	45
4	Tr	69	40	Tr	5	93	40	9	Tr	0.02	Tr	0	46
22	1	390	229	0.3	30	528	200	49	0.01	0.11	0.1	0	47
20	1	214	141	0.1	39	248	230	75	0.01	0.09	Tr	0	48
124	7	509	389	0.9	257	207	1,210	330	0.03	0.48	0.3	0	49
76	13	669	449	1.1	307	307	1,060	278	0.05	0.46	0.2	0	50
26	1	272	171	Tr	31	74	240	72	0.01	0.10	Tr	0	51
27	Tr	174	211	0.1	46	406	340	82	0.01	0.10	Tr	0	52
24	1	219	216	0.2	61	388	230	65	Tr	0.08	Tr	0	53
18	2	163	130	0.2	79	337	260	62	0.01	0.13	Tr	0	54
16	2	159	202	0.1	69	381	220	54	0.01	0.12	Tr	0	55
89	10	254	230	0.2	314	98	1,050	259	0.08	0.36	0.2	2	56
6	1	16	14	Tr	19	6	70	16	0.01	0.02	Tr	Tr	57
159	9	231	192	0.1	292	95	1,730	437	0.08	0.36	0.1	2	58
10	1	14	12	Tr	18	6	110	27	Tr	0.02	Tr	Tr	59
265	7	166	146	0.1	231	82	2,690	705	0.06	0.30	0.1	1	60
17	Tr	10	9	Tr	15	5	170	44	Tr	0.02	Tr	Tr	61
326	7	154	149	0.1	179	89	3,500	1,002	0.05	0.26	0.1	1	62
21	Tr	10	9	Tr	11	6	220	63	Tr	0.02	Tr	Tr	63
46	7	61	54	Tr	88	78	550	124	0.02	0.04	Tr	0	64
2	Tr	3	3	Tr	4	4	30	6	Tr	Tr	Tr	0	65
102	10	268	195	0.1	331	123	1,820	448	0.08	0.34	0.2	2	66
5	1	14	10	Tr	17	6	90	23	Tr	0.02	Tr	Tr	67

Nutritive Value of the Edible Part of Food (Continued)
(Tr indicates nutrient present in trace amount.)

Item No.	Foods, approximate measures, units, and weight (weight of edible portion only)			Water	Food energy	Pro-tein	Fat	Fatty acids		
								Satu-rated	Mono-unsatu-rated	Poly-unsatu-rated
			Grams	Per-cent	Cal-ories	Grams	Grams	Grams	Grams	Grams
	Dairy Products—Con.									
	Cream products, imitation (made with vegetable fat):									
	Sweet:									
	Creamers:									
68	Liquid (frozen)------------	1 tbsp----------	15	77	20	Tr	1	1.4	Tr	Tr
69	Powdered-------------------	1 tsp----------	2	2	10	Tr	1	0.7	Tr	Tr
	Whipped topping:									
70	Frozen---------------------	1 cup----------	75	50	240	1	19	16.3	1.2	0.4
71		1 tbsp----------	4	50	15	Tr	1	0.9	0.1	Tr
	Powdered, made with whole milk---------------------									
72		1 cup----------	80	67	150	3	10	8.5	0.7	0.2
73		1 tbsp----------	4	67	10	Tr	Tr	0.4	Tr	Tr
74	Pressurized----------------	1 cup----------	70	60	185	1	16	13.2	1.3	0.2
75		1 tbsp----------	4	60	10	Tr	1	0.8	0.1	Tr
76	Sour dressing (filled cream type product, nonbutterfat)--	1 cup----------	235	75	415	8	39	31.2	4.6	1.1
77		1 tbsp----------	12	75	20	Tr	2	1.6	0.2	0.1
	Ice cream. See Milk desserts, frozen (items 106-111).									
	Ice milk. See Milk desserts, frozen (items 112-114).									
	Milk:									
	Fluid:									
78	Whole (3.3% fat)-------------	1 cup----------	244	88	150	8	8	5.1	2.4	0.3
	Lowfat (2%):									
79	No milk solids added-------	1 cup----------	244	89	120	8	5	2.9	1.4	0.2
80	Milk solids added, label claim less than 10 g of protein per cup----------	1 cup----------	245	89	125	9	5	2.9	1.4	0.2
	Lowfat (1%):									
81	No milk solids added-------	1 cup----------	244	90	100	8	3	1.6	0.7	0.1
82	Milk solids added, label claim less than 10 g of protein per cup----------	1 cup----------	245	90	105	9	2	1.5	0.7	0.1
	Nonfat (skim):									
83	No milk solids added-------	1 cup----------	245	91	85	8	Tr	0.3	0.1	Tr
84	Milk solids added, label claim less than 10 g of protein per cup----------	1 cup----------	245	90	90	9	1	0.4	0.2	Tr
85	Buttermilk------------------	1 cup----------	245	90	100	8	2	1.3	0.6	0.1
	Canned:									
86	Condensed, sweetened---------	1 cup----------	306	27	980	24	27	16.8	7.4	1.0
	Evaporated:									
87	Whole milk-----------------	1 cup----------	252	74	340	17	19	11.6	5.9	0.6
88	Skim milk------------------	1 cup----------	255	79	200	19	1	0.3	0.2	Tr
	Dried:									
89	Buttermilk------------------	1 cup----------	120	3	465	41	7	4.3	2.0	0.3
	Nonfat, instant									
90	Envelope, 3.2 oz, net wt.[6]	1 envelope------	91	4	325	32	1	0.4	0.2	Tr
91	Cup------------------------	1 cup----------	68	4	245	24	Tr	0.3	0.1	Tr
	Milk beverages:									
	Chocolate milk (commercial):									
92	Regular---------------------	1 cup----------	250	82	210	8	8	5.3	2.5	0.3
93	Lowfat (2%)-----------------	1 cup----------	250	84	180	8	5	3.1	1.5	0.2
94	Lowfat (1%)-----------------	1 cup----------	250	85	160	8	3	1.5	0.8	0.1

[5] Vitamin A value is largely from beta-carotene used for coloring.
[6] Yields 1 qt of fluid milk when reconstituted according to package directions.

							Nutrients in Indicated Quantity						
Cho-les-terol	Carbo-hydrate	Calcium	Phos-phorus	Iron	Potas-sium	Sodium	Vitamin A value		Thiamin	Ribo-flavin	Niacin	Ascorbic acid	Item No.
							(IU)	(RE)					
Milli-grams	Grams	Milli-grams	Milli-grams	Milli-grams	Milli-grams	Milli-grams	Inter-national units	Retinol equiva-lents	Milli-grams	Milli-grams	Milli-grams	Milli-grams	
0	2	1	10	Tr	29	12	[5]10	[5]1	0.00	0.00	0.0	0	68
0	1	Tr	8	Tr	16	4	Tr	Tr	0.00	Tr	0.0	0	69
0	17	5	6	0.1	14	19	[5]650	[5]65	0.00	0.00	0.0	0	70
0	1	Tr	Tr	Tr	1	1	[5]30	[5]3	0.00	0.00	0.0	0	71
8	13	72	69	Tr	121	53	[5]290	[5]39	0.02	0.09	Tr	1	72
Tr	1	4	3	Tr	6	3	[5]10	[5]2	Tr	Tr	Tr	Tr	73
0	11	4	13	Tr	13	43	[5]330	[5]33	0.00	0.00	0.0	0	74
0	1	Tr	1	Tr	1	2	[5]20	[5]2	0.00	0.00	0.0	0	75
13	11	266	205	0.1	380	113	20	5	0.09	0.38	0.2	2	76
1	1	14	10	Tr	19	6	Tr	Tr	Tr	0.02	Tr	Tr	77
33	11	291	228	0.1	370	120	310	76	0.09	0.40	0.2	2	78
18	12	297	232	0.1	377	122	500	139	0.10	0.40	0.2	2	79
18	12	313	245	0.1	397	128	500	140	0.10	0.42	0.2	2	80
10	12	300	235	0.1	381	123	500	144	0.10	0.41	0.2	2	81
10	12	313	245	0.1	397	128	500	145	0.10	0.42	0.2	2	82
4	12	302	247	0.1	406	126	500	149	0.09	0.34	0.2	2	83
5	12	316	255	0.1	418	130	500	149	0.10	0.43	0.2	2	84
9	12	285	219	0.1	371	257	80	20	0.08	0.38	0.1	2	85
104	166	868	775	0.6	1,136	389	1,000	248	0.28	1.27	0.6	8	86
74	25	657	510	0.5	764	267	610	136	0.12	0.80	0.5	5	87
9	29	738	497	0.7	845	293	1,000	298	0.11	0.79	0.4	3	88
83	59	1,421	1,119	0.4	1,910	621	260	65	0.47	1.89	1.1	7	89
17	47	1,120	896	0.3	1,552	499	[7]2,160	[7]646	0.38	1.59	0.8	5	90
12	35	837	670	0.2	1,160	373	[7]1,610	[7]483	0.28	1.19	0.6	4	91
31	26	280	251	0.6	417	149	300	73	0.09	0.41	0.3	2	92
17	26	284	254	0.6	422	151	500	143	0.09	0.41	0.3	2	93
7	26	287	256	0.6	425	152	500	148	0.10	0.42	0.3	2	94

[7]With added vitamin A.

Nutritive Value of the Edible Part of Food (Continued)

(Tr indicates nutrient present in trace amount.)

Item No.	Foods, approximate measures, units, and weight (weight of edible portion only)		Water	Food energy	Pro-tein	Fat	Fatty acids		
							Satu-rated	Mono-unsatu-rated	Poly-unsatu-rated
		Grams	Per-cent	Cal-ories	Grams	Grams	Grams	Grams	Grams
	Dairy Products—Con.								
	Milk beverages:								
	Cocoa and chocolate-flavored beverages:								
95	Powder containing nonfat dry milk----------------------	1 oz------------	28	1	100	3	1	0.6	0.3	Tr
96	Prepared (6 oz water plus 1 oz powder)-------------	1 serving-------	206	86	100	3	1	0.6	0.3	Tr
97	Powder without nonfat dry milk---------------------	3/4 oz----------	21	1	75	1	1	0.3	0.2	Tr
98	Prepared (8 oz whole milk plus 3/4 oz powder)------	1 serving-------	265	81	225	9	9	5.4	2.5	0.3
99	Eggnog (commercial)------------	1 cup-----------	254	74	340	10	19	11.3	5.7	0.9
	Malted milk:								
	Chocolate:								
100	Powder---------------------	3/4 oz ---------	21	2	85	1	1	0.5	0.3	0.1
101	Prepared (8 oz whole milk plus 3/4 oz powder)----	1 serving-------	265	81	235	9	9	5.5	2.7	0.4
	Natural:								
102	Powder---------------------	3/4 oz----------	21	3	85	3	2	0.9	0.5	0.3
103	Prepared (8 oz whole milk plus 3/4 oz powder)----	1 serving-------	265	81	235	11	10	6.0	2.9	0.6
	Shakes, thick:								
104	Chocolate--------------------	10-oz container	283	72	335	9	8	4.8	2.2	0.3
105	Vanilla---------------------	10-oz container	283	74	315	11	9	5.3	2.5	0.3
	Milk desserts, frozen:								
	Ice cream, vanilla:								
	Regular (about 11% fat):								
106	Hardened-------------------	1/2 gal---------	1,064	61	2,155	38	115	71.3	33.1	4.3
107		1 cup-----------	133	61	270	5	14	8.9	4.1	0.5
108		3 fl oz---------	50	61	100	2	5	3.4	1.6	0.2
109	Soft serve (frozen custard)	1 cup-----------	173	60	375	7	23	13.5	6.7	1.0
110	Rich (about 16% fat), hardened-------------------	1/2 gal---------	1,188	59	2,805	33	190	118.3	54.9	7.1
111		1 cup-----------	148	59	350	4	24	14.7	6.8	0.9
	Ice milk, vanilla:								
112	Hardened (about 4% fat)------	1/2 gal---------	1,048	69	1,470	41	45	28.1	13.0	1.7
113		1 cup-----------	131	69	185	5	6	3.5	1.6	0.2
114	Soft serve (about 3% fat)----	1 cup-----------	175	70	225	8	5	2.9	1.3	0.2
115	Sherbet (about 2% fat)--------	1/2 gal---------	1,542	66	2,160	17	31	19.0	8.8	1.1
116		1 cup-----------	193	66	270	2	4	2.4	1.1	0.1
	Yogurt:								
	With added milk solids:								
	Made with lowfat milk:								
117	Fruit-flavored[8]------------	8-oz container--	227	74	230	10	2	1.6	0.7	0.1
118	Plain---------------------	8-oz container--	227	85	145	12	4	2.3	1.0	0.1
119	Made with nonfat milk--------	8-oz container--	227	85	125	13	Tr	0.3	0.1	Tr
	Without added milk solids:								
120	Made with whole milk---------	8-oz container--	227	88	140	8	7	4.8	2.0	0.2
	Eggs								
	Eggs, large (24 oz per dozen):								
	Raw:								
121	Whole, without shell---------	1 egg-----------	50	75	80	6	6	1.7	2.2	0.7
122	White-----------------------	1 white---------	33	88	15	3	Tr	0.0	0.0	0.0
123	Yolk------------------------	1 yolk----------	17	49	65	3	6	1.7	2.2	0.7
	Cooked:								
124	Fried in butter-------------	1 egg-----------	46	68	95	6	7	2.7	2.7	0.8
125	Hard-cooked, shell removed---	1 egg-----------	50	75	80	6	6	1.7	2.2	0.7
126	Poached---------------------	1 egg-----------	50	74	80	6	6	1.7	2.2	0.7
127	Scrambled (milk added) in butter. Also omelet--------	1 egg-----------	64	73	110	7	8	3.2	2.9	0.8

[8]Carbohydrate content varies widely because of amount of sugar added and amount and solids content of added flavoring. Consult the label if more precise values for carbohydrate and calories are needed.

Nutrients in Indicated Quantity

Cho-les-terol	Carbo-hydrate	Calcium	Phos-phorus	Iron	Potas-sium	Sodium	Vitamin A value (IU)	Vitamin A value (RE)	Thiamin	Ribo-flavin	Niacin	Ascorbic acid	Item No.
Milli-grams	Grams	Milli-grams	Milli-grams	Milli-grams	Milli-grams	Milli-grams	Inter-national units	Retinol equiva-lents	Milli-grams	Milli-grams	Milli-grams	Milli-grams	
1	22	90	88	0.3	223	139	Tr	Tr	0.03	0.17	0.2	Tr	95
1	22	90	88	0.3	223	139	Tr	Tr	0.03	0.17	0.2	Tr	96
0	19	7	26	0.7	136	56	Tr	Tr	Tr	0.03	0.1	Tr	97
33	30	298	254	0.9	508	176	310	76	0.10	0.43	0.3	3	98
149	34	330	278	0.5	420	138	890	203	0.09	0.48	0.3	4	99
1	18	13	37	0.4	130	49	20	5	0.04	0.04	0.4	0	100
34	29	304	265	0.5	500	168	330	80	0.14	0.43	0.7	2	101
4	15	56	79	0.2	159	96	70	17	0.11	0.14	1.1	0	102
37	27	347	307	0.3	529	215	380	93	0.20	0.54	1.3	2	103
30	60	374	357	0.9	634	314	240	59	0.13	0.63	0.4	0	104
33	50	413	326	0.3	517	270	320	79	0.08	0.55	0.4	0	105
476	254	1,406	1,075	1.0	2,052	929	4,340	1,064	0.42	2.63	1.1	6	106
59	32	176	134	0.1	257	116	540	133	0.05	0.33	0.1	1	107
22	12	66	51	Tr	96	44	200	50	0.02	0.12	0.1	Tr	108
153	38	236	199	0.4	338	153	790	199	0.08	0.45	0.2	1	109
703	256	1,213	927	0.8	1,771	868	7,200	1,758	0.36	2.27	0.9	5	110
88	32	151	115	0.1	221	108	900	219	0.04	0.28	0.1	1	111
146	232	1,409	1,035	1.5	2,117	836	1,710	419	0.61	2.78	0.9	6	112
18	29	176	129	0.2	265	105	210	52	0.08	0.35	0.1	1	113
13	38	274	202	0.3	412	163	175	44	0.12	0.54	0.2	1	114
113	469	827	594	2.5	1,585	706	1,480	308	0.26	0.71	1.0	31	115
14	59	103	74	0.3	198	88	190	39	0.03	0.09	0.1	4	116
10	43	345	271	0.2	442	133	100	25	0.08	0.40	0.2	1	117
14	16	415	326	0.2	531	159	150	36	0.10	0.49	0.3	2	118
4	17	452	355	0.2	579	174	20	5	0.11	0.53	0.3	2	119
29	11	274	215	0.1	351	105	280	68	0.07	0.32	0.2	1	120
274	1	28	90	1.0	65	69	260	78	0.04	0.15	Tr	0	121
0	Tr	4	4	Tr	45	50	0	0	Tr	0.09	Tr	0	122
272	Tr	26	86	0.9	15	8	310	94	0.04	0.07	Tr	0	123
278	1	29	91	1.1	66	162	320	94	0.04	0.14	Tr	0	124
274	1	28	90	1.0	65	69	260	78	0.04	0.14	Tr	0	125
273	1	28	90	1.0	65	146	260	78	0.03	0.13	Tr	0	126
282	2	54	109	1.0	97	176	350	102	0.04	0.18	Tr	Tr	127

Nutritive Value of the Edible Part of Food (Continued)

(Tr indicates nutrient present in trace amount.)

Item No.	Foods, approximate measures, units, and weight (weight of edible portion only)			Water	Food energy	Pro-tein	Fat	Fatty acids		
								Satu-rated	Mono-unsatu-rated	Poly-unsatu-rated
			Grams	Per-cent	Cal-ories	Grams	Grams	Grams	Grams	Grams
	Fats and Oils									
	Butter (4 sticks per lb):									
128	Stick-------------------------	1/2 cup---------	113	16	810	1	92	57.1	26.4	3.4
129	Tablespoon (1/8 stick)---------	1 tbsp----------	14	16	100	Tr	11	7.1	3.3	0.4
130	Pat (1 in square, 1/3 in high; 90 per lb)------------	1 pat-----------	5	16	35	Tr	4	2.5	1.2	0.2
131	Fats, cooking (vegetable shortenings)------------------	1 cup-----------	205	0	1,810	0	205	51.3	91.2	53.5
132		1 tbsp----------	13	0	115	0	13	3.3	5.8	3.4
133	Lard---------------------------	1 cup-----------	205	0	1,850	0	205	80.4	92.5	23.0
134		1 tbsp----------	13	0	115	0	13	5.1	5.9	1.5
	Margarine:									
135	Imitation (about 40% fat), soft	8-oz container--	227	58	785	1	88	17.5	35.6	31.3
136		1 tbsp----------	14	58	50	Tr	5	1.1	2.2	1.9
	Regular (about 80% fat): Hard (4 sticks per lb):									
137	Stick----------------------	1/2 cup---------	113	16	810	1	91	17.9	40.5	28.7
138	Tablespoon (1/8 stick)-----	1 tbsp----------	14	16	100	Tr	11	2.2	5.0	3.6
139	Pat (1 in square, 1/3 in high; 90 per lb)---------	1 pat-----------	5	16	35	Tr	4	0.8	1.8	1.3
140	Soft-----------------------	8-oz container--	227	16	1,625	2	183	31.3	64.7	78.5
141		1 tbsp----------	14	16	100	Tr	11	1.9	4.0	4.8
	Spread (about 60% fat): Hard (4 sticks per lb):									
142	Stick----------------------	1/2 cup---------	113	37	610	1	69	15.9	29.4	20.5
143	Tablespoon (1/8 stick)-----	1 tbsp----------	14	37	75	Tr	9	2.0	3.6	2.5
144	Pat (1 in square, 1/3 in high; 90 per lb)---------	1 pat-----------	5	37	25	Tr	3	0.7	1.3	0.9
145	Soft-----------------------	8-oz container--	227	37	1,225	1	138	29.1	71.5	31.3
146		1 tbsp----------	14	37	75	Tr	9	1.8	4.4	1.9
	Oils, salad or cooking:									
147	Corn-----------------------	1 cup-----------	218	0	1,925	0	218	27.7	52.8	128.0
148		1 tbsp----------	14	0	125	0	14	1.8	3.4	8.2
149	Olive----------------------	1 cup-----------	216	0	1,910	0	216	29.2	159.2	18.1
150		1 tbsp----------	14	0	125	0	14	1.9	10.3	1.2
151	Peanut---------------------	1 cup-----------	216	0	1,910	0	216	36.5	99.8	69.1
152		1 tbsp----------	14	0	125	0	14	2.4	6.5	4.5
153	Safflower------------------	1 cup-----------	218	0	1,925	0	218	19.8	26.4	162.4
154		1 tbsp----------	14	0	125	0	14	1.3	1.7	10.4
155	Soybean oil, hydrogenated (partially hardened)---------	1 cup-----------	218	0	1,925	0	218	32.5	93.7	82.0
156		1 tbsp----------	14	0	125	0	14	2.1	6.0	5.3
157	Soybean-cottonseed oil blend, hydrogenated-----------------	1 cup-----------	218	0	1,925	0	218	39.2	64.3	104.9
158		1 tbsp----------	14	0	125	0	14	2.5	4.1	6.7
159	Sunflower------------------	1 cup-----------	218	0	1,925	0	218	22.5	42.5	143.2
160		1 tbsp----------	14	0	125	0	14	1.4	2.7	9.2
	Salad dressings: Commercial:									
161	Blue cheese----------------	1 tbsp----------	15	32	75	1	8	1.5	1.8	4.2
	French:									
162	Regular-----------------	1 tbsp----------	16	35	85	Tr	9	1.4	4.0	3.5
163	Low calorie-------------	1 tbsp----------	16	75	25	Tr	2	0.2	0.3	1.0
	Italian:									
164	Regular-----------------	1 tbsp----------	15	34	80	Tr	9	1.3	3.7	3.2
165	Low calorie-------------	1 tbsp----------	15	86	5	Tr	Tr	Tr	Tr	Tr
	Mayonnaise:									
166	Regular-----------------	1 tbsp----------	14	15	100	Tr	11	1.7	3.2	5.8
167	Imitation--------------	1 tbsp----------	15	63	35	Tr	3	0.5	0.7	1.6
168	Mayonnaise type-------------	1 tbsp----------	15	40	60	Tr	5	0.7	1.4	2.7
169	Tartar sauce---------------	1 tbsp----------	14	34	75	Tr	8	1.2	2.6	3.9
	Thousand island:									
170	Regular-----------------	1 tbsp----------	16	46	60	Tr	6	1.0	1.3	3.2
171	Low calorie-------------	1 tbsp----------	15	69	25	Tr	2	0.2	0.4	0.9

[9] For salted butter; unsalted butter contains 12 mg sodium per stick, 2 mg per tbsp, or 1 mg per pat.
[10] Values for vitamin A are year-round average.

| | | | | | | | Nutrients in Indicated Quantity | | | | | | |

Cholesterol	Carbohydrate	Calcium	Phosphorus	Iron	Potassium	Sodium	Vitamin A value		Thiamin	Riboflavin	Niacin	Ascorbic acid	Item No.
							(IU)	(RE)					
Milligrams	Grams	Milligrams	Milligrams	Milligrams	Milligrams	Milligrams	International units	Retinol equivalents	Milligrams	Milligrams	Milligrams	Milligrams	
247	Tr	27	26	0.2	29	[9]933	[10]3,460	[10]852	0.01	0.04	Tr	0	128
31	Tr	3	3	Tr	4	[9]116	[10]430	[10]106	Tr	Tr	Tr	0	129
11	Tr	1	1	Tr	1	[9]41	[10]150	[10]38	Tr	Tr	Tr	0	130
0	0	0	0	0.0	0	0	0	0	0.00	0.00	0.0	0	131
0	0	0	0	0.0	0	0	0	0	0.00	0.00	0.0	0	132
195	0	0	0	0.0	0	0	0	0	0.00	0.00	0.0	0	133
12	0	0	0	0.0	0	0	0	0	0.00	0.00	0.0	0	134
0	1	40	31	0.0	57	[11]2,178	[12]7,510	[12]2,254	0.01	0.05	Tr	Tr	135
0	Tr	2	2	0.0	4	[11]134	[12]460	[12]139	Tr	Tr	Tr	Tr	136
0	1	34	26	0.1	48	[11]1,066	[12]3,740	[12]1,122	0.01	0.04	Tr	Tr	137
0	Tr	4	3	Tr	6	[11]132	[12]460	[12]139	Tr	0.01	Tr	Tr	138
0	Tr	1	1	Tr	2	[11]47	[12]170	[12]50	Tr	Tr	Tr	Tr	139
0	1	60	46	0.0	86	[11]2,449	[12]7,510	[12]2,254	0.02	0.07	Tr	Tr	140
0	Tr	4	3	0.0	5	[11]151	[12]460	[12]139	Tr	Tr	Tr	Tr	141
0	0	24	18	0.0	34	[11]1,123	[12]3,740	[12]1,122	0.01	0.03	Tr	Tr	142
0	0	3	2	0.0	4	[11]139	[12]460	[12]139	Tr	Tr	Tr	Tr	143
0	0	1	1	0.0	1	[11]50	[12]170	[12]50	Tr	Tr	Tr	Tr	144
0	0	47	37	0.0	68	[11]2,256	[12]7,510	[12]2,254	0.02	0.06	Tr	Tr	145
0	0	3	2	0.0	4	[11]139	[12]460	[12]139	Tr	Tr	Tr	Tr	146
0	0	0	0	0.0	0	0	0	0	0.00	0.00	0.0	0	147
0	0	0	0	0.0	0	0	0	0	0.00	0.00	0.0	0	148
0	0	0	0	0.0	0	0	0	0	0.00	0.00	0.0	0	149
0	0	0	0	0.0	0	0	0	0	0.00	0.00	0.0	0	150
0	0	0	0	0.0	0	0	0	0	0.00	0.00	0.0	0	151
0	0	0	0	0.0	0	0	0	0	0.00	0.00	0.0	0	152
0	0	0	0	0.0	0	0	0	0	0.00	0.00	0.0	0	153
0	0	0	0	0.0	0	0	0	0	0.00	0.00	0.0	0	154
0	0	0	0	0.0	0	0	0	0	0.00	0.00	0.0	0	155
0	0	0	0	0.0	0	0	0	0	0.00	0.00	0.0	0	156
0	0	0	0	0.0	0	0	0	0	0.00	0.00	0.0	0	157
0	0	0	0	0.0	0	0	0	0	0.00	0.00	0.0	0	158
0	0	0	0	0.0	0	0	0	0	0.00	0.00	0.0	0	159
0	0	0	0	0.0	0	0	0	0	0.00	0.00	0.0	0	160
3	1	12	11	Tr	6	164	30	10	Tr	0.02	Tr	Tr	161
0	1	2	1	Tr	2	188	Tr	Tr	Tr	Tr	Tr	Tr	162
0	2	6	5	Tr	3	306	Tr	Tr	Tr	Tr	Tr	Tr	163
0	1	1	1	Tr	5	162	30	3	Tr	Tr	Tr	Tr	164
0	2	1	1	Tr	4	136	Tr	Tr	Tr	Tr	Tr	Tr	165
8	Tr	3	4	0.1	5	80	40	12	0.00	0.00	Tr	0	166
4	2	Tr	Tr	0.0	2	75	0	0	0.00	0.00	0.0	0	167
4	4	2	4	Tr	1	107	30	13	Tr	Tr	Tr	0	168
4	1	3	4	0.1	11	182	30	9	Tr	Tr	0.0	Tr	169
4	2	2	3	0.1	18	112	50	15	Tr	Tr	Tr	0	170
2	2	2	3	0.1	17	150	50	14	Tr	Tr	Tr	0	171

[11]For salted margarine.
[12]Based on average vitamin A content of fortified margarine. Federal specifications for fortified margarine require a minimum of 15,000 IU per pound.

Nutritive Value of the Edible Part of Food (Continued)

(Tr indicates nutrient present in trace amount.)

Item No.	Foods, approximate measures, units, and weight (weight of edible portion only)		Water	Food energy	Pro-tein	Fat	Fatty acids		
							Satu-rated	Mono-unsatu-rated	Poly-unsatu-rated
		Grams	Per-cent	Cal-ories	Grams	Grams	Grams	Grams	Grams
	Fats and Oils—Con.								
	Salad dressings:								
	Prepared from home recipe:								
172	Cooked type[13] ----------------	1 tbsp----------	16	69	25	1	2	0.5	0.6	0.3
173	Vinegar and oil--------------	1 tbsp----------	16	47	70	0	8	1.5	2.4	3.9
	Fish and Shellfish								
	Clams:								
174	Raw, meat only-----------------	3 oz------------	85	82	65	11	1	0.3	0.3	0.3
175	Canned, drained solids---------	3 oz------------	85	77	85	13	2	0.5	0.5	0.4
176	Crabmeat, canned----------------	1 cup----------	135	77	135	23	3	0.5	0.8	1.4
177	Fish sticks, frozen, reheated, (stick, 4 by 1 by 1/2 in)------	1 fish stick----	28	52	70	6	3	0.8	1.4	0.8
	Flounder or Sole, baked, with lemon juice:								
178	With butter--------------------	3 oz------------	85	73	120	16	6	3.2	1.5	0.5
179	With margarine-----------------	3 oz------------	85	73	120	16	6	1.2	2.3	1.9
180	Without added fat--------------	3 oz------------	85	78	80	17	1	0.3	0.2	0.4
181	Haddock, breaded, fried[14] --------	3 oz------------	85	61	175	17	9	2.4	3.9	2.4
182	Halibut, broiled, with butter and lemon juice---------------	3 oz------------	85	67	140	20	6	3.3	1.6	0.7
183	Herring, pickled----------------	3 oz------------	85	59	190	17	13	4.3	4.6	3.1
184	Ocean perch, breaded, fried[14] ----	1 fillet--------	85	59	185	16	11	2.6	4.6	2.8
	Oysters:								
185	Raw, meat only (13-19 medium Selects)----------------------	1 cup----------	240	85	160	20	4	1.4	0.5	1.4
186	Breaded, fried[14] ---------------	1 oyster--------	45	65	90	5	5	1.4	2.1	1.4
	Salmon:								
187	Canned (pink), solids and liquid----------------------	3 oz------------	85	71	120	17	5	0.9	1.5	2.1
188	Baked (red)--------------------	3 oz------------	85	67	140	21	5	1.2	2.4	1.4
189	Smoked-------------------------	3 oz------------	85	59	150	18	8	2.6	3.9	0.7
190	Sardines, Atlantic, canned in oil, drained solids------------	3 oz------------	85	62	175	20	9	2.1	3.7	2.9
191	Scallops, breaded, frozen, reheated----------------------	6 scallops------	90	59	195	15	10	2.5	4.1	2.5
	Shrimp:								
192	Canned, drained solids---------	3 oz------------	85	70	100	21	1	0.2	0.2	0.4
193	French fried (7 medium)[16] ------	3 oz------------	85	55	200	16	10	2.5	4.1	2.6
194	Trout, broiled, with butter and lemon juice-------------------	3 oz------------	85	63	175	21	9	4.1	2.9	1.6
	Tuna, canned, drained solids:								
195	Oil pack, chunk light----------	3 oz------------	85	61	165	24	7	1.4	1.9	3.1
196	Water pack, solid white--------	3 oz------------	85	63	135	30	1	0.3	0.2	0.3
197	Tuna salad[17] ---------------------	1 cup----------	205	63	375	33	19	3.3	4.9	9.2
	Fruits and Fruit Juices								
	Apples:								
	Raw:								
	Unpeeled, without cores:								
198	2-3/4-in diam. (about 3 per lb with cores)-----------	1 apple---------	138	84	80	Tr	Tr	0.1	Tr	0.1
199	3-1/4-in diam. (about 2 per lb with cores)-----------	1 apple---------	212	84	125	Tr	1	0.1	Tr	0.2
200	Peeled, sliced----------------	1 cup----------	110	84	65	Tr	Tr	0.1	Tr	0.1
201	Dried, sulfured----------------	10 rings--------	64	32	155	1	Tr	Tr	Tr	0.1
202	Apple juice, bottled or canned[19]	1 cup----------	248	88	115	Tr	Tr	Tr	Tr	0.1
	Applesauce, canned:								
203	Sweetened--------------------	1 cup----------	255	80	195	Tr	Tr	0.1	Tr	0.1
204	Unsweetened------------------	1 cup----------	244	88	105	Tr	Tr	Tr	Tr	Tr

[13] Fatty acid values apply to product made with regular margarine.
[14] Dipped in egg, milk, and breadcrumbs; fried in vegetable shortening.
[15] If bones are discarded, value for calcium will be greatly reduced.
[16] Dipped in egg, breadcrumbs, and flour; fried in vegetable shortening.

Nutrients in Indicated Quantity

Cholesterol	Carbohydrate	Calcium	Phosphorus	Iron	Potassium	Sodium	Vitamin A value		Thiamin	Riboflavin	Niacin	Ascorbic acid	Item No.
							(IU)	(RE)					
Milligrams	Grams	Milligrams	Milligrams	Milligrams	Milligrams	Milligrams	International units	Retinol equivalents	Milligrams	Milligrams	Milligrams	Milligrams	
9	2	13	14	0.1	19	117	70	20	0.01	0.02	Tr	Tr	172
0	Tr	0	0	0.0	1	Tr	0	0	0.00	0.00	0.0	0	173
43	2	59	138	2.6	154	102	90	26	0.09	0.15	1.1	9	174
54	2	47	116	3.5	119	102	90	26	0.01	0.09	0.9	3	175
135	1	61	246	1.1	149	1,350	50	14	0.11	0.11	2.6	0	176
26	4	11	58	0.3	94	53	20	5	0.03	0.05	0.6	0	177
68	Tr	13	187	0.3	272	145	210	54	0.05	0.08	1.6	1	178
55	Tr	14	187	0.3	273	151	230	69	0.05	0.08	1.6	1	179
59	Tr	13	197	0.3	286	101	30	10	0.05	0.08	1.7	1	180
75	7	34	183	1.0	270	123	70	20	0.06	0.10	2.9	0	181
62	Tr	14	206	0.7	441	103	610	174	0.06	0.07	7.7	1	182
85	0	29	128	0.9	85	850	110	33	0.04	0.18	2.8	0	183
66	7	31	191	1.2	241	138	70	20	0.10	0.11	2.0	0	184
120	8	226	343	15.6	290	175	740	223	0.34	0.43	6.0	24	185
35	5	49	73	3.0	64	70	150	44	0.07	0.10	1.3	4	186
34	0	[15]167	243	0.7	307	443	60	18	0.03	0.15	6.8	0	187
60	0	26	269	0.5	305	55	290	87	0.18	0.14	5.5	0	188
51	0	12	208	0.8	327	1,700	260	77	0.17	0.17	6.8	0	189
85	0	[15]371	424	2.6	349	425	190	56	0.03	0.17	4.6	0	190
70	10	39	203	2.0	369	298	70	21	0.11	0.11	1.6	0	191
128	1	98	224	1.4	104	1,955	50	15	0.01	0.03	1.5	0	192
168	11	61	154	2.0	189	384	90	26	0.06	0.09	2.8	0	193
71	Tr	26	259	1.0	297	122	230	60	0.07	0.07	2.3	1	194
55	0	7	199	1.6	298	303	70	20	0.04	0.09	10.1	0	195
48	0	17	202	0.6	255	468	110	32	0.03	0.10	13.4	0	196
80	19	31	281	2.5	531	877	230	53	0.06	0.14	13.3	6	197
0	21	10	10	0.2	159	Tr	70	7	0.02	0.02	0.1	8	198
0	32	15	15	0.4	244	Tr	110	11	0.04	0.03	0.2	12	199
0	16	4	8	0.1	124	Tr	50	5	0.02	0.01	0.1	4	200
0	42	9	24	0.9	288	[18]56	0	0	0.00	0.10	0.6	2	201
0	29	17	17	0.9	295	7	Tr	Tr	0.05	0.04	0.2	[20]2	202
0	51	10	18	0.9	156	8	30	3	0.03	0.07	0.5	[20]4	203
0	28	7	17	0.3	183	5	70	7	0.03	0.06	0.5	[20]3	204

[17] Made with drained chunk light tuna, celery, onion, pickle relish, and mayonnaise-type salad dressing.
[18] Sodium bisulfite used to preserve color; unsulfited product would contain less sodium.
[19] Also applies to pasteurized apple cider.
[20] Without added ascorbic acid. For value with added ascorbic acid, refer to label.

Nutritive Value of the Edible Part of Food (Continued)

(Tr indicates nutrient present in trace amount.)

Item No.	Foods, approximate measures, units, and weight (weight of edible portion only)			Water	Food energy	Pro-tein	Fat	Fatty acids		
								Satu-rated	Mono-unsatu-rated	Poly-unsatu-rated
			Grams	Per-cent	Cal-ories	Grams	Grams	Grams	Grams	Grams
	Fruits and Fruit Juices—Con.									
	Apricots:									
205	Raw, without pits (about 12 per lb with pits)----------------	3 apricots------	106	86	50	1	Tr	Tr	0.2	0.1
	Canned (fruit and liquid):									
206	Heavy syrup pack------------	1 cup-----------	258	78	215	1	Tr	Tr	0.1	Tr
207		3 halves--------	85	78	70	Tr	Tr	Tr	Tr	Tr
208	Juice pack------------------	1 cup-----------	248	87	120	2	Tr	Tr	Tr	Tr
209		3 halves--------	84	87	40	1	Tr	Tr	Tr	Tr
	Dried:									
210	Uncooked (28 large or 37 medium halves per cup)-----	1 cup-----------	130	31	310	5	1	Tr	0.3	0.1
211	Cooked, unsweetened, fruit and liquid----------------	1 cup-----------	250	76	210	3	Tr	Tr	0.2	0.1
212	Apricot nectar, canned-------	1 cup-----------	251	85	140	1	Tr	Tr	0.1	Tr
	Avocados, raw, whole, without skin and seed:									
213	California (about 2 per lb with skin and seed)---------------	1 avocado-------	173	73	305	4	30	4.5	19.4	3.5
214	Florida (about 1 per lb with skin and seed)---------------	1 avocado-------	304	80	340	5	27	5.3	14.8	4.5
	Bananas, raw, without peel:									
215	Whole (about 2-1/2 per lb with peel)------------------------	1 banana--------	114	74	105	1	1	0.2	Tr	0.1
216	Sliced-----------------------	1 cup-----------	150	74	140	2	1	0.3	0.1	0.1
217	Blackberries, raw-------------	1 cup-----------	144	86	75	1	1	0.2	0.1	0.1
	Blueberries:									
218	Raw--------------------------	1 cup----------	145	85	80	1	1	Tr	0.1	0.3
219	Frozen, sweetened-------------	10-oz container	284	77	230	1	Tr	Tr	0.1	0.2
220		1 cup-----------	230	77	185	1	Tr	Tr	Tr	0.1
	Cantaloup. See Melons (item 251).									
	Cherries:									
221	Sour, red, pitted, canned, water pack------------------	1 cup-----------	244	90	90	2	Tr	0.1	0.1	0.1
222	Sweet, raw, without pits and stems------------------------	10 cherries-----	68	81	50	1	1	0.1	0.2	0.2
223	Cranberry juice cocktail, bottled, sweetened-------------	1 cup-----------	253	85	145	Tr	Tr	Tr	Tr	0.1
224	Cranberry sauce, sweetened, canned, strained--------------	1 cup-----------	277	61	420	1	Tr	Tr	0.1	0.2
	Dates:									
225	Whole, without pits------------	10 dates--------	83	23	230	2	Tr	0.1	0.1	Tr
226	Chopped-----------------------	1 cup-----------	178	23	490	4	1	0.3	0.2	Tr
227	Figs, dried----------------------	10 figs---------	187	28	475	6	2	0.4	0.5	1.0
	Fruit cocktail, canned, fruit and liquid:									
228	Heavy syrup pack---------------	1 cup-----------	255	80	185	1	Tr	Tr	Tr	0.1
229	Juice pack----------------------	1 cup-----------	248	87	115	1	Tr	Tr	Tr	Tr
	Grapefruit:									
230	Raw, without peel, membrane and seeds (3-3/4-in diam., 1 lb 1 oz, whole, with refuse)----	1/2 grapefruit--	120	91	40	1	Tr	Tr	Tr	Tr
231	Canned, sections with syrup----	1 cup-----------	254	84	150	1	Tr	Tr	Tr	0.1
	Grapefruit juice:									
232	Raw---------------------------	1 cup-----------	247	90	95	1	Tr	Tr	Tr	0.1
	Canned:									
233	Unsweetened-------------------	1 cup-----------	247	90	95	1	Tr	Tr	Tr	0.1
234	Sweetened---------------------	1 cup-----------	250	87	115	1	Tr	Tr	Tr	0.1
	Frozen concentrate, unsweetened									
235	Undiluted---------------------	6-fl-oz can-----	207	62	300	4	1	0.1	0.1	0.2
236	Diluted with 3 parts water by volume---------------------	1 cup-----------	247	89	100	1	Tr	Tr	Tr	0.1

[20] Without added ascorbic acid. For value with added ascorbic acid, refer to label.
[21] With added ascorbic acid.

Nutrients in Indicated Quantity

Cho-les-terol	Carbo-hydrate	Calcium	Phos-phorus	Iron	Potas-sium	Sodium	Vitamin A value		Thiamin	Ribo-flavin	Niacin	Ascorbic acid	Item No.
							(IU)	(RE)					
Milli-grams	Grams	Milli-grams	Milli-grams	Milli-grams	Milli-grams	Milli-grams	Inter-national units	Retinol equiva-lents	Milli-grams	Milli-grams	Milli-grams	Milli-grams	
0	12	15	20	0.6	314	1	2,770	277	0.03	0.04	0.6	11	205
0	55	23	31	0.8	361	10	3,170	317	0.05	0.06	1.0	8	206
0	18	8	10	0.3	119	3	1,050	105	0.02	0.02	0.3	3	207
0	31	30	50	0.7	409	10	4,190	419	0.04	0.05	0.9	12	208
0	10	10	17	0.3	139	3	1,420	142	0.02	0.02	0.3	4	209
0	80	59	152	6.1	1,791	13	9,410	941	0.01	0.20	3.9	3	210
0	55	40	103	4.2	1,222	8	5,910	591	0.02	0.08	2.4	4	211
0	36	18	23	1.0	286	8	3,300	330	0.02	0.04	0.7	[20]2	212
0	12	19	73	2.0	1,097	21	1,060	106	0.19	0.21	3.3	14	213
0	27	33	119	1.6	1,484	15	1,860	186	0.33	0.37	5.8	24	214
0	27	7	23	0.4	451	1	90	9	0.05	0.11	0.6	10	215
0	35	9	30	0.5	594	2	120	12	0.07	0.15	0.8	14	216
0	18	46	30	0.8	282	Tr	240	24	0.04	0.06	0.6	30	217
0	20	9	15	0.2	129	9	150	15	0.07	0.07	0.5	19	218
0	62	17	20	1.1	170	3	120	12	0.06	0.15	0.7	3	219
0	50	14	16	0.9	138	2	100	10	0.05	0.12	0.6	2	220
0	22	27	24	3.3	239	17	1,840	184	0.04	0.10	0.4	5	221
0	11	10	13	0.3	152	Tr	150	15	0.03	0.04	0.3	5	222
0	38	8	3	0.4	61	10	10	1	0.01	0.04	0.1	[21]108	223
0	108	11	17	0.6	72	80	60	6	0.04	0.06	0.3	6	224
0	61	27	33	1.0	541	2	40	4	0.07	0.08	1.8	0	225
0	131	57	71	2.0	1,161	5	90	9	0.16	0.18	3.9	0	226
0	122	269	127	4.2	1,331	21	250	25	0.13	0.16	1.3	1	227
0	48	15	28	0.7	224	15	520	52	0.05	0.05	1.0	5	228
0	29	20	35	0.5	236	10	760	76	0.03	0.04	1.0	7	229
0	10	14	10	0.1	167	Tr	[22]10	[22]1	0.04	0.02	0.3	41	230
0	39	36	25	1.0	328	5	Tr	Tr	0.10	0.05	0.6	54	231
0	23	22	37	0.5	400	2	20	2	0.10	0.05	0.5	94	232
0	22	17	27	0.5	378	2	20	2	0.10	0.05	0.6	72	233
0	28	20	28	0.9	405	5	20	2	0.10	0.06	0.8	67	234
0	72	56	101	1.0	1,002	6	60	6	0.30	0.16	1.6	248	235
0	24	20	35	0.3	336	2	20	2	0.10	0.05	0.5	83	236

[22]For white grapefruit; pink grapefruit have about 310 IU or 31 RE.

Nutritive Value of the Edible Part of Food (Continued)

(Tr indicates nutrient present in trace amount.)

Item No.	Foods, approximate measures, units, and weight (weight of edible portion only)			Water	Food energy	Pro-tein	Fat	Fatty acids		
								Satu-rated	Mono-unsatu-rated	Poly-unsatu-rated
			Grams	Per-cent	Cal-ories	Grams	Grams	Grams	Grams	Grams
	Fruits and Fruit Juices—Con.									
	Grapes, European type (adherent skin), raw:									
237	Thompson Seedless	10 grapes	50	81	35	Tr	Tr	0.1	Tr	0.1
238	Tokay and Emperor, seeded types	10 grapes	57	81	40	Tr	Tr	0.1	Tr	0.1
	Grape juice:									
239	Canned or bottled	1 cup	253	84	155	1	Tr	0.1	Tr	0.1
	Frozen concentrate, sweetened:									
240	Undiluted	6-fl-oz can	216	54	385	1	1	0.2	Tr	0.2
241	Diluted with 3 parts water by volume	1 cup	250	87	125	Tr	Tr	0.1	Tr	0.1
242	Kiwifruit, raw, without skin (about 5 per lb with skin)	1 kiwifruit	76	83	45	1	Tr	Tr	0.1	0.1
243	Lemons, raw, without peel and seeds (about 4 per lb with peel and seeds)	1 lemon	58	89	15	1	Tr	Tr	Tr	0.1
	Lemon juice:									
244	Raw	1 cup	244	91	60	1	Tr	Tr	Tr	Tr
245	Canned or bottled, unsweetened	1 cup	244	92	50	1	1	0.1	Tr	0.2
246		1 tbsp	15	92	5	Tr	Tr	Tr	Tr	Tr
247	Frozen, single-strength, unsweetened	6-fl-oz can	244	92	55	1	1	0.1	Tr	0.2
	Lime juice:									
248	Raw	1 cup	246	90	65	1	Tr	Tr	Tr	0.1
249	Canned, unsweetened	1 cup	246	93	50	1	1	0.1	0.1	0.2
250	Mangos, raw, without skin and seed (about 1-1/2 per lb with skin and seed)	1 mango	207	82	135	1	1	0.1	0.2	0.1
	Melons, raw, without rind and cavity contents:									
251	Cantaloup, orange-fleshed (5-in diam., 2-1/3 lb, whole, with rind and cavity contents)	1/2 melon	267	90	95	2	1	0.1	0.1	0.3
252	Honeydew (6-1/2-in diam., 5-1/4 lb, whole, with rind and cavity contents)	1/10 melon	129	90	45	1	Tr	Tr	Tr	0.1
253	Nectarines, raw, without pits (about 3 per lb with pits)	1 nectarine	136	86	65	1	1	0.1	0.2	0.3
	Oranges, raw:									
254	Whole, without peel and seeds (2-5/8-in diam., about 2-1/2 per lb, with peel and seeds)	1 orange	131	87	60	1	Tr	Tr	Tr	Tr
255	Sections without membranes	1 cup	180	87	85	2	Tr	Tr	Tr	Tr
	Orange juice:									
256	Raw, all varieties	1 cup	248	88	110	2	Tr	0.1	0.1	0.1
257	Canned, unsweetened	1 cup	249	89	105	1	Tr	Tr	0.1	0.1
258	Chilled	1 cup	249	88	110	2	1	0.1	0.1	0.2
	Frozen concentrate:									
259	Undiluted	6-fl-oz can	213	58	340	5	Tr	0.1	0.1	0.1
260	Diluted with 3 parts water by volume	1 cup	249	88	110	2	Tr	Tr	Tr	Tr
261	Orange and grapefruit juice, canned	1 cup	247	89	105	1	Tr	Tr	Tr	Tr
262	Papayas, raw, 1/2-in cubes	1 cup	140	86	65	1	Tr	0.1	0.1	Tr
	Peaches:									
	Raw:									
263	Whole, 2-1/2-in diam., peeled, pitted (about 4 per lb with peels and pits)	1 peach	87	88	35	1	Tr	Tr	Tr	Tr
264	Sliced	1 cup	170	88	75	1	Tr	Tr	0.1	0.1
	Canned, fruit and liquid:									
265	Heavy syrup pack	1 cup	256	79	190	1	Tr	Tr	0.1	0.1
266		1 half	81	79	60	Tr	Tr	Tr	Tr	Tr
267	Juice pack	1 cup	248	87	110	2	Tr	Tr	Tr	Tr
268		1 half	77	87	35	Tr	Tr	Tr	Tr	Tr

[20]Without added ascorbic acid. For value with added ascorbic acid, refer to label.
[21]With added ascorbic acid.

						Nutrients in Indicated Quantity							
Cho-les-terol	Carbo-hydrate	Calcium	Phos-phorus	Iron	Potas-sium	Sodium	Vitamin A value		Thiamin	Ribo-flavin	Niacin	Ascorbic acid	Item No.
							(IU)	(RE)					
Milli-grams	Grams	Milli-grams	Milli-grams	Milli-grams	Milli-grams	Milli-grams	Inter-national units	Retinol equiva-lents	Milli-grams	Milli-grams	Milli-grams	Milli-grams	
0	9	6	7	0.1	93	1	40	4	0.05	0.03	0.2	5	237
0	10	6	7	0.1	105	1	40	4	0.05	0.03	0.2	6	238
0	38	23	28	0.6	334	8	20	2	0.07	0.09	0.7	[20]Tr	239
0	96	28	32	0.8	160	15	60	6	0.11	0.20	0.9	[21]179	240
0	32	10	10	0.3	53	5	20	2	0.04	0.07	0.3	[21]60	241
0	11	20	30	0.3	252	4	130	13	0.02	0.04	0.4	74	242
0	5	15	9	0.3	80	1	20	2	0.02	0.01	0.1	31	243
0	21	17	15	0.1	303	2	50	5	0.07	0.02	0.2	112	244
0	16	27	22	0.3	249	[23]51	40	4	0.10	0.02	0.5	61	245
0	1	2	1	Tr	15	[23]3	Tr	Tr	0.01	Tr	Tr	4	246
0	16	20	20	0.3	217	2	30	3	0.14	0.03	0.3	77	247
0	22	22	17	0.1	268	2	20	2	0.05	0.02	0.2	72	248
0	16	30	25	0.6	185	[23]39	40	4	0.08	0.01	0.4	16	249
0	35	21	23	0.3	323	4	8,060	806	0.12	0.12	1.2	57	250
0	22	29	45	0.6	825	24	8,610	861	0.10	0.06	1.5	113	251
0	12	8	13	0.1	350	13	50	5	0.10	0.02	0.8	32	252
0	16	7	22	0.2	288	Tr	1,000	100	0.02	0.06	1.3	7	253
0	15	52	18	0.1	237	Tr	270	27	0.11	0.05	0.4	70	254
0	21	72	25	0.2	326	Tr	370	37	0.16	0.07	0.5	96	255
0	26	27	42	0.5	496	2	500	50	0.22	0.07	1.0	124	256
0	25	20	35	1.1	436	5	440	44	0.15	0.07	0.8	86	257
0	25	25	27	0.4	473	2	190	19	0.28	0.05	0.7	82	258
0	81	68	121	0.7	1,436	6	590	59	0.60	0.14	1.5	294	259
0	27	22	40	0.2	473	2	190	19	0.20	0.04	0.5	97	260
0	25	20	35	1.1	390	7	290	29	0.14	0.07	0.8	72	261
0	17	35	12	0.3	247	9	400	40	0.04	0.04	0.5	92	262
0	10	4	10	0.1	171	Tr	470	47	0.01	0.04	0.9	6	263
0	19	9	20	0.2	335	Tr	910	91	0.03	0.07	1.7	11	264
0	51	8	28	0.7	236	15	850	85	0.03	0.06	1.6	7	265
0	16	2	9	0.2	75	5	270	27	0.01	0.02	0.5	2	266
0	29	15	42	0.7	317	10	940	94	0.02	0.04	1.4	9	267
0	9	5	13	0.2	99	3	290	29	0.01	0.01	0.4	3	268

[23]Sodium benzoate and sodium bisulfite added as preservatives.

Nutritive Value of the Edible Part of Food (Continued)
(Tr indicates nutrient present in trace amount.)

Item No.	Foods, approximate measures, units, and weight (weight of edible portion only)		Grams	Water Per-cent	Food energy Cal-ories	Pro-tein Grams	Fat Grams	Fatty acids		
								Satu-rated Grams	Mono-unsatu-rated Grams	Poly-unsatu-rated Grams
	Fruits and Fruit Juices—Con.									
	Peaches:									
	Dried:									
269	Uncooked---------------------	1 cup-----------	160	32	380	6	1	0.1	0.4	0.6
270	Cooked, unsweetened, fruit and liquid-----------------	1 cup-----------	258	78	200	3	1	0.1	0.2	0.3
271	Frozen, sliced, sweetened------	10-oz container	284	75	265	2	Tr	Tr	0.1	0.2
272		1 cup-----------	250	75	235	2	Tr	Tr	0.1	0.2
	Pears:									
	Raw, with skin, cored:									
273	Bartlett, 2-1/2-in diam. (about 2-1/2 per lb with cores and stems)-----------	1 pear----------	166	84	100	1	1	Tr	0.1	0.2
274	Bosc, 2-1/2-in diam. (about 3 per lb with cores and stems)-------------------	1 pear----------	141	84	85	1	1	Tr	0.1	0.1
275	D'Anjou, 3-in diam. (about 2 per lb with cores and stems)-------------------	1 pear----------	200	84	120	1	1	Tr	0.2	0.2
	Canned, fruit and liquid:									
276	Heavy syrup pack-------------	1 cup-----------	255	80	190	1	Tr	Tr	0.1	0.1
277		1 half----------	79	80	60	Tr	Tr	Tr	Tr	Tr
278	Juice pack-------------------	1 cup-----------	248	86	125	1	Tr	Tr	Tr	Tr
279		1 half----------	77	86	40	Tr	Tr	Tr	Tr	Tr
	Pineapple:									
280	Raw, diced--------------------	1 cup-----------	155	87	75	1	1	Tr	0.1	0.2
	Canned, fruit and liquid:									
	Heavy syrup pack:									
281	Crushed, chunks, tidbits---	1 cup-----------	255	79	200	1	Tr	Tr	Tr	0.1
282	Slices--------------------	1 slice--------	58	79	45	Tr	Tr	Tr	Tr	Tr
	Juice pack:									
283	Chunks or tidbits----------	1 cup-----------	250	84	150	1	Tr	Tr	Tr	0.1
284	Slices--------------------	1 slice--------	58	84	35	Tr	Tr	Tr	Tr	Tr
285	Pineapple juice, unsweetened, canned------------------------	1 cup-----------	250	86	140	1	Tr	Tr	Tr	0.1
	Plantains, without peel:									
286	Raw--------------------------	1 plantain------	179	65	220	2	1	0.3	0.1	0.1
287	Cooked, boiled, sliced--------	1 cup-----------	154	67	180	1	Tr	0.1	Tr	0.1
	Plums, without pits:									
	Raw:									
288	2-1/8-in diam. (about 6-1/2 per lb with pits)--------	1 plum----------	66	85	35	1	Tr	Tr	0.3	0.1
289	1-1/2-in diam. (about 15 per lb with pits)-------------	1 plum----------	28	85	15	Tr	Tr	Tr	0.1	Tr
	Canned, purple, fruit and liquid:									
290	Heavy syrup pack-------------	1 cup-----------	258	76	230	1	Tr	Tr	0.2	0.1
291		3 plums--------	133	76	120	Tr	Tr	Tr	0.1	Tr
292	Juice pack-------------------	1 cup-----------	252	84	145	1	Tr	Tr	Tr	Tr
293		3 plums--------	95	84	55	Tr	Tr	Tr	Tr	Tr
	Prunes, dried:									
294	Uncooked----------------------	4 extra large or 5 large prunes	49	32	115	1	Tr	Tr	0.2	0.1
295	Cooked, unsweetened, fruit and liquid----------------------	1 cup-----------	212	70	225	2	Tr	Tr	0.3	0.1
296	Prune juice, canned or bottled---	1 cup-----------	256	81	180	2	Tr	Tr	0.1	Tr
	Raisins, seedless:									
297	Cup, not pressed down----------	1 cup-----------	145	15	435	5	1	0.2	Tr	0.2
298	Packet, 1/2 oz (1-1/2 tbsp)----	1 packet--------	14	15	40	Tr	Tr	Tr	Tr	Tr
	Raspberries:									
299	Raw--------------------------	1 cup-----------	123	87	60	1	1	Tr	0.1	0.4
300	Frozen, sweetened-------------	10-oz container	284	73	295	2	Tr	Tr	Tr	0.3
301		1 cup-----------	250	73	255	2	Tr	Tr	Tr	0.2

[21] With added ascorbic acid.

Nutrients in Indicated Quantity

Cho-les-terol	Carbo-hydrate	Calcium	Phos-phorus	Iron	Potas-sium	Sodium	Vitamin A value (IU)	Vitamin A value (RE)	Thiamin	Ribo-flavin	Niacin	Ascorbic acid	Item No.
Milli-grams	Grams	Milli-grams	Milli-grams	Milli-grams	Milli-grams	Milli-grams	Inter-national units	Retinol equiva-lents	Milli-grams	Milli-grams	Milli-grams	Milli-grams	
0	98	45	190	6.5	1,594	11	3,460	346	Tr	0.34	7.0	8	269
0	51	23	98	3.4	826	5	510	51	0.01	0.05	3.9	10	270
0	68	9	31	1.1	369	17	810	81	0.04	0.10	1.9	[21]268	271
0	60	8	28	0.9	325	15	710	71	0.03	0.09	1.6	[21]236	272
0	25	18	18	0.4	208	Tr	30	3	0.03	0.07	0.2	7	273
0	21	16	16	0.4	176	Tr	30	3	0.03	0.06	0.1	6	274
0	30	22	22	0.5	250	Tr	40	4	0.04	0.08	0.2	8	275
0	49	13	18	0.6	166	13	10	1	0.03	0.06	0.6	3	276
0	15	4	6	0.2	51	4	Tr	Tr	0.01	0.02	0.2	1	277
0	32	22	30	0.7	238	10	10	1	0.03	0.03	0.5	4	278
0	10	7	9	0.2	74	3	Tr	Tr	0.01	0.01	0.2	1	279
0	19	11	11	0.6	175	2	40	4	0.14	0.06	0.7	24	280
0	52	36	18	1.0	265	3	40	4	0.23	0.06	0.7	19	281
0	12	8	4	0.2	60	1	10	1	0.05	0.01	0.2	4	282
0	39	35	15	0.7	305	3	100	10	0.24	0.05	0.7	24	283
0	9	8	3	0.2	71	1	20	2	0.06	0.01	0.2	6	284
0	34	43	20	0.7	335	3	10	1	0.14	0.06	0.6	27	285
0	57	5	61	1.1	893	7	2,020	202	0.09	0.10	1.2	33	286
0	48	3	43	0.9	716	8	1,400	140	0.07	0.08	1.2	17	287
0	9	3	7	0.1	114	Tr	210	21	0.03	0.06	0.3	6	288
0	4	1	3	Tr	48	Tr	90	9	0.01	0.03	0.1	3	289
0	60	23	34	2.2	235	49	670	67	0.04	0.10	0.8	1	290
0	31	12	17	1.1	121	25	340	34	0.02	0.05	0.4	1	291
0	38	25	38	0.9	388	3	2,540	254	0.06	0.15	1.2	7	292
0	14	10	14	0.3	146	1	960	96	0.02	0.06	0.4	3	293
0	31	25	39	1.2	365	2	970	97	0.04	0.08	1.0	2	294
0	60	49	74	2.4	708	4	650	65	0.05	0.21	1.5	6	295
0	45	31	64	3.0	707	10	10	1	0.04	0.18	2.0	10	296
0	115	71	141	3.0	1,089	17	10	1	0.23	0.13	1.2	5	297
0	11	7	14	0.3	105	2	Tr	Tr	0.02	0.01	0.1	Tr	298
0	14	27	15	0.7	187	Tr	160	16	0.04	0.11	1.1	31	299
0	74	43	48	1.8	324	3	170	17	0.05	0.13	0.7	47	300
0	65	38	43	1.6	285	3	150	15	0.05	0.11	0.6	41	301

Nutritive Value of the Edible Part of Food (Continued)

(Tr indicates nutrient present in trace amount.)

Item No.	Foods, approximate measures, units, and weight (weight of edible portion only)			Water	Food energy	Pro- tein	Fat	Fatty acids		
								Satu- rated	Mono- unsatu- rated	Poly- unsatu- rated
			Grams	Per- cent	Cal- ories	Grams	Grams	Grams	Grams	Grams
	Fruits and Fruit Juices—Con.									
302	Rhubarb, cooked, added sugar-----	1 cup-----------	240	68	280	1	Tr	Tr	Tr	0.1
	Strawberries:									
303	Raw, capped, whole-------------	1 cup-----------	149	92	45	1	1	Tr	0.1	0.3
304	Frozen, sweetened, sliced------	10-oz container	284	73	275	2	Tr	Tr	0.1	0.2
305		1 cup-----------	255	73	245	1	Tr	Tr	Tr	0.2
	Tangerines:									
306	Raw, without peel and seeds (2-3/8-in diam., about 4 per lb, with peel and seeds)-----	1 tangerine-----	84	88	35	1	Tr	Tr	Tr	Tr
307	Canned, light syrup, fruit and liquid----------------------	1 cup-----------	252	83	155	1	Tr	Tr	Tr	0.1
308	Tangerine juice, canned, sweet- ened------------------------	1 cup-----------	249	87	125	1	Tr	Tr	Tr	0.1
	Watermelon, raw, without rind and seeds:									
309	Piece (4 by 8 in wedge with rind and seeds; 1/16 of 32-2/3-lb melon, 10 by 16 in)	1 piece---------	482	92	155	3	2	0.3	0.2	1.0
310	Diced-------------------------	1 cup-----------	160	92	50	1	1	0.1	0.1	0.3
	Grain Products									
311	Bagels, plain or water, enriched, 3-1/2-in diam.[24] ---------------	1 bagel---------	68	29	200	7	2	0.3	0.5	0.7
312	Barley, pearled, light, uncooked	1 cup-----------	200	11	700	16	2	0.3	0.2	0.9
	Biscuits, baking powder, 2-in diam. (enriched flour, vege- table shortening):									
313	From home recipe---------------	1 biscuit-------	28	28	100	2	5	1.2	2.0	1.3
314	From mix-----------------------	1 biscuit-------	28	29	95	2	3	0.8	1.4	0.9
315	From refrigerated dough--------	1 biscuit-------	20	30	65	1	2	0.6	0.9	0.6
	Breadcrumbs, enriched:									
316	Dry, grated--------------------	1 cup-----------	100	7	390	13	5	1.5	1.6	1.0
	Soft. See White bread (item 351).									
	Breads:									
317	Boston brown bread, canned, slice, 3-1/4 in by 1/2 in[25]--	1 slice---------	45	45	95	2	1	0.3	0.1	0.1
	Cracked-wheat bread (3/4 en- riched wheat flour, 1/4 cracked wheat flour):[25]									
318	Loaf, 1 lb--------------------	1 loaf----------	454	35	1,190	42	16	3.1	4.3	5.7
319	Slice (18 per loaf)----------	1 slice---------	25	35	65	2	1	0.2	0.2	0.3
320	Toasted---------------------	1 slice---------	21	26	65	2	1	0.2	0.2	0.3
	French or vienna bread, en- riched:[25]									
321	Loaf, 1 lb-------------------	1 loaf----------	454	34	1,270	43	18	3.8	5.7	5.9
	Slice:									
322	French, 5 by 2-1/2 by 1 in	1 slice---------	35	34	100	3	1	0.3	0.4	0.5
323	Vienna, 4-3/4 by 4 by 1/2 in---------------------	1 slice---------	25	34	70	2	1	0.2	0.3	0.3
	Italian bread, enriched:									
324	Loaf, 1 lb-------------------	1 loaf----------	454	32	1,255	41	4	0.6	0.3	1.6
325	Slice, 4-1/2 by 3-1/4 by 3/4 in---------------------	1 slice---------	30	32	85	3	Tr	Tr	Tr	0.1
	Mixed grain bread, enriched:[25]									
326	Loaf, 1 lb-------------------	1 loaf----------	454	37	1,165	45	17	3.2	4.1	6.5
327	Slice (18 per loaf)----------	1 slice---------	25	37	65	2	1	0.2	0.2	0.4
328	Toasted---------------------	1 slice---------	23	27	65	2	1	0.2	0.2	0.4

[24] Egg bagels have 44 mg cholesterol and 22 IU or 7 RE vitamin A per bagel.
[25] Made with vegetable shortening.

							Nutrients in Indicated Quantity						
Cho-les-terol	Carbo-hydrate	Calcium	Phos-phorus	Iron	Potas-sium	Sodium	Vitamin A value		Thiamin	Ribo-flavin	Niacin	Ascorbic acid	Item No.
							(IU)	(RE)					
Milli-grams	Grams	Milli-grams	Milli-grams	Milli-grams	Milli-grams	Milli-grams	Inter-national units	Retinol equiva-lents	Milli-grams	Milli-grams	Milli-grams	Milli-grams	
0	75	348	19	0.5	230	2	170	17	0.04	0.06	0.5	8	302
0	10	21	28	0.6	247	1	40	4	0.03	0.10	0.3	84	303
0	74	31	37	1.7	278	9	70	7	0.05	0.14	1.1	118	304
0	66	28	33	1.5	250	8	60	6	0.04	0.13	1.0	106	305
0	9	12	8	0.1	132	1	770	77	0.09	0.02	0.1	26	306
0	41	18	25	0.9	197	15	2,120	212	0.13	0.11	1.1	50	307
0	30	45	35	0.5	443	2	1,050	105	0.15	0.05	0.2	55	308
0	35	39	43	0.8	559	10	1,760	176	0.39	0.10	1.0	46	309
0	11	13	14	0.3	186	3	590	59	0.13	0.03	0.3	15	310
0	38	29	46	1.8	50	245	0	0	0.26	0.20	2.4	0	311
0	158	32	378	4.2	320	6	0	0	0.24	0.10	6.2	0	312
Tr	13	47	36	0.7	32	195	10	3	0.08	0.08	0.8	Tr	313
Tr	14	58	128	0.7	56	262	20	4	0.12	0.11	0.8	Tr	314
1	10	4	79	0.5	18	249	0	0	0.08	0.05	0.7	0	315
5	73	122	141	4.1	152	736	0	0	0.35	0.35	4.8	0	316
3	21	41	72	0.9	131	113	[26]0	[26] 0	0.06	0.04	0.7	0	317
0	227	295	581	12.1	608	1,966	Tr	Tr	1.73	1.73	15.3	Tr	318
0	12	16	32	0.7	34	106	Tr	Tr	0.10	0.09	0.8	Tr	319
0	12	16	32	0.7	34	106	Tr	Tr	0.07	0.09	0.8	Tr	320
0	230	499	386	14.0	409	2,633	Tr	Tr	2.09	1.59	18.2	Tr	321
0	18	39	30	1.1	32	203	Tr	Tr	0.16	0.12	1.4	Tr	322
0	13	28	21	0.8	23	145	Tr	Tr	0.12	0.09	1.0	Tr	323
0	256	77	350	12.7	336	2,656	0	0	1.80	1.10	15.0	0	324
0	17	5	23	0.8	22	176	0	0	0.12	0.07	1.0	0	325
0	212	472	962	14.8	990	1,870	Tr	Tr	1.77	1.73	18.9	Tr	326
0	12	27	55	0.8	56	106	Tr	Tr	0.10	0.10	1.1	Tr	327
0	12	27	55	0.8	56	106	Tr	Tr	0.08	0.10	1.1	Tr	328

[26] Made with white cornmeal. If made with yellow cornmeal, value is 32 IU or 3 RE.

Nutritive Value of the Edible Part of Food (Continued)

(Tr indicates nutrient present in trace amount.)

Item No.	Foods, approximate measures, units, and weight (weight of edible portion only)			Water	Food energy	Pro- tein	Fat	Fatty acids		
								Satu- rated	Mono- unsatu- rated	Poly- unsatu- rated
	Grain Products—Con.		Grams	Per- cent	Cal- ories	Grams	Grams	Grams	Grams	Grams
	Breads:									
	Oatmeal bread, enriched:[25]									
329	Loaf, 1 lb--------------------	1 loaf----------	454	37	1,145	38	20	3.7	7.1	8.2
330	Slice (18 per loaf)----------	1 slice---------	25	37	65	2	1	0.2	0.4	0.5
331	Toasted--------------------	1 slice---------	23	30	65	2	1	0.2	0.4	0.5
332	Pita bread, enriched, white, 6-1/2-in diam.---------------	1 pita----------	60	31	165	6	1	0.1	0.1	0.4
	Pumpernickel (2/3 rye flour, 1/3 enriched wheat flour):[25]									
333	Loaf, 1 lb--------------------	1 loaf----------	454	37	1,160	42	16	2.6	3.6	6.4
334	Slice, 5 by 4 by 3/8 in------	1 slice---------	32	37	80	3	1	0.2	0.3	0.5
335	Toasted--------------------	1 slice---------	29	28	80	3	1	0.2	0.3	0.5
	Raisin bread, enriched:[25]									
336	Loaf, 1 lb--------------------	1 loaf----------	454	33	1,260	37	18	4.1	6.5	6.7
337	Slice (18 per loaf)----------	1 slice---------	25	33	65	2	1	0.2	0.3	0.4
338	Toasted--------------------	1 slice---------	21	24	65	2	1	0.2	0.3	0.4
	Rye bread, light (2/3 enriched wheat flour, 1/3 rye flour):[25]									
339	Loaf, 1 lb--------------------	1 loaf----------	454	37	1,190	38	17	3.3	5.2	5.5
340	Slice, 4-3/4 by 3-3/4 by 7/16 in-------------------	1 slice---------	25	37	65	2	1	0.2	0.3	0.3
341	Toasted--------------------	1 slice---------	22	28	65	2	1	0.2	0.3	0.3
	Wheat bread, enriched:[25]									
342	Loaf, 1 lb--------------------	1 loaf----------	454	37	1,160	43	19	3.9	7.3	4.5
343	Slice (18 per loaf)----------	1 slice---------	25	37	65	2	1	0.2	0.4	0.3
344	Toasted--------------------	1 slice---------	23	28	65	3	1	0.2	0.4	0.3
	White bread, enriched:[25]									
345	Loaf, 1 lb--------------------	1 loaf----------	454	37	1,210	38	18	5.6	6.5	4.2
346	Slice (18 per loaf)--------	1 slice---------	25	37	65	2	1	0.3	0.4	0.2
347	Toasted------------------	1 slice---------	22	28	65	2	1	0.3	0.4	0.2
348	Slice (22 per loaf)--------	1 slice---------	20	37	55	2	1	0.2	0.3	0.2
349	Toasted------------------	1 slice---------	17	28	55	2	1	0.2	0.3	0.2
350	Cubes----------------------	1 cup----------	30	37	80	2	1	0.4	0.4	0.3
351	Crumbs, soft----------------	1 cup----------	45	37	120	4	2	0.6	0.6	0.4
	Whole-wheat bread:[25]									
352	Loaf, 1 lb--------------------	1 loaf----------	454	38	1,110	44	20	5.8	6.8	5.2
353	Slice (16 per loaf)----------	1 slice---------	28	38	70	3	1	0.4	0.4	0.3
354	Toasted--------------------	1 slice---------	25	29	70	3	1	0.4	0.4	0.3
	Bread stuffing (from enriched bread), prepared from mix:									
355	Dry type--------------------	1 cup----------	140	33	500	9	31	6.1	13.3	9.6
356	Moist type--------------------	1 cup----------	203	61	420	9	26	5.3	11.3	8.0
	Breakfast cereals:									
	Hot type, cooked:									
	Corn (hominy) grits:									
357	Regular and quick, enriched	1 cup----------	242	85	145	3	Tr	Tr	0.1	0.2
358	Instant, plain-------------	1 pkt----------	137	85	80	2	Tr	Tr	Tr	0.1
	Cream of Wheat®:									
359	Regular, quick, instant----	1 cup----------	244	86	140	4	Tr	0.1	Tr	0.2
360	Mix'n Eat, plain----------	1 pkt----------	142	82	100	3	Tr	Tr	Tr	0.1
361	Malt-O-Meal® ---------------	1 cup----------	240	88	120	4	Tr	Tr	Tr	0.1
	Oatmeal or rolled oats:									
362	Regular, quick, instant, nonfortified-------------	1 cup----------	234	85	145	6	2	0.4	0.8	1.0
	Instant, fortified:									
363	Plain--------------------	1 pkt----------	177	86	105	4	2	0.3	0.6	0.7
364	Flavored----------------	1 pkt----------	164	76	160	5	2	0.3	0.7	0.8

[25] Made with vegetable shortening.
[27] Nutrient added.
[28] Cooked without salt. If salt is added according to label recommendations, sodium content is 540 mg.
[29] For white corn grits. Cooked yellow grits contain 145 IU or 14 RE.
[30] Value based on label declaration for added nutrients.

Nutrients in Indicated Quantity

Cho-les-terol	Carbo-hydrate	Calcium	Phos-phorus	Iron	Potas-sium	Sodium	Vitamin A value (IU)	Vitamin A value (RE)	Thiamin	Ribo-flavin	Niacin	Ascorbic acid	Item No.
Milli-grams	Grams	Milli-grams	Milli-grams	Milli-grams	Milli-grams	Milli-grams	Inter-national units	Retinol equiva-lents	Milli-grams	Milli-grams	Milli-grams	Milli-grams	
0	212	267	563	12.0	707	2,231	0	0	2.09	1.20	15.4	0	329
0	12	15	31	0.7	39	124	0	0	0.12	0.07	0.9	0	330
0	12	15	31	0.7	39	124	0	0	0.09	0.07	0.9	0	331
0	33	49	60	1.4	71	339	0	0	0.27	0.12	2.2	0	332
0	218	322	990	12.4	1,966	2,461	0	0	1.54	2.36	15.0	0	333
0	16	23	71	0.9	141	177	0	0	0.11	0.17	1.1	0	334
0	16	23	71	0.9	141	177	0	0	0.09	0.17	1.1	0	335
0	239	463	395	14.1	1,058	1,657	Tr	Tr	1.50	2.81	18.6	Tr	336
0	13	25	22	0.8	59	92	Tr	Tr	0.08	0.15	1.0	Tr	337
0	13	25	22	0.8	59	92	Tr	Tr	0.06	0.15	1.0	Tr	338
0	218	363	658	12.3	926	3,164	0	0	1.86	1.45	15.0	0	339
0	12	20	36	0.7	51	175	0	0	0.10	0.08	0.8	0	340
0	12	20	36	0.7	51	175	0	0	0.08	0.08	0.8	0	341
0	213	572	835	15.8	627	2,447	Tr	Tr	2.09	1.45	20.5	Tr	342
0	12	32	47	0.9	35	138	Tr	Tr	0.12	0.08	1.2	Tr	343
0	12	32	47	0.9	35	138	Tr	Tr	0.10	0.08	1.2	Tr	344
0	222	572	490	12.9	508	2,334	Tr	Tr	2.13	1.41	17.0	Tr	345
0	12	32	27	0.7	28	129	Tr	Tr	0.12	0.08	0.9	Tr	346
0	12	32	27	0.7	28	129	Tr	Tr	0.09	0.08	0.9	Tr	347
0	10	25	21	0.6	22	101	Tr	Tr	0.09	0.06	0.7	Tr	348
0	10	25	21	0.6	22	101	Tr	Tr	0.07	0.06	0.7	Tr	349
0	15	38	32	0.9	34	154	Tr	Tr	0.14	0.09	1.1	Tr	350
0	22	57	49	1.3	50	231	Tr	Tr	0.21	0.14	1.7	Tr	351
0	206	327	1,180	15.5	799	2,887	Tr	Tr	1.59	0.95	17.4	Tr	352
0	13	20	74	1.0	50	180	Tr	Tr	0.10	0.06	1.1	Tr	353
0	13	20	74	1.0	50	180	Tr	Tr	0.08	0.06	1.1	Tr	354
0	50	92	136	2.2	126	1,254	910	273	0.17	0.20	2.5	0	355
67	40	81	134	2.0	118	1,023	850	256	0.10	0.18	1.6	0	356
0	31	0	29	[27]1.5	53	[28]0	[29]0	[29]0	[27]0.24	[27]0.15	[27]2.0	0	357
0	18	7	16	[27]1.0	29	343	0	0	[27]0.18	[27]0.08	[27]1.3	0	358
0	29	[30]54	[31]43	[30]10.9	46	[31,32]5	0	0	[30]0.24	[30]0.07	[30]1.5	0	359
0	21	[30]20	[30]20	[30]8.1	38	241	[30]1,250	[30]376	[30]0.43	[30]0.28	[30]5.0	0	360
0	26	5	[30]24	[30]9.6	31	[33]2	0	0	[30]0.48	[30]0.24	[30]5.8	0	361
0	25	19	178	1.6	131	[34]2	40	4	0.26	0.05	0.3	0	362
0	18	[27]163	133	[27]6.3	99	[27]285	[27]1,510	[27]453	[27]0.53	[27]0.28	[27]5.5	0	363
0	31	[27]168	148	[27]6.7	137	[27]254	[27]1,530	[27]460	[27]0.53	[27]0.38	[27]5.9	Tr	364

[31] For regular and instant cereal. For quick cereal, phosphorus is 102 mg and sodium is 142 mg.
[32] Cooked without salt. If salt is added according to label recommendations, sodium content is 390 mg.
[33] Cooked without salt. If salt is added according to label recommendations, sodium content is 324 mg.
[34] Cooked without salt. If salt is added according to label recommendations, sodium content is 374 mg.

Nutritive Value of the Edible Part of Food (Continued)

(Tr indicates nutrient present in trace amount.)

Item No.	Foods, approximate measures, units, and weight (weight of edible portion only)			Water	Food energy	Pro-tein	Fat	Fatty acids		
								Satu-rated	Mono-unsatu-rated	Poly-unsatu-rated
			Grams	Per-cent	Cal-ories	Grams	Grams	Grams	Grams	Grams
	Grain Products—Con.									
	Breakfast cereals:									
	Ready to eat:									
365	All-Bran® (about 1/3 cup)----	1 oz-----------	28	3	70	4	1	0.1	0.1	0.3
366	Cap'n Crunch® (about 3/4 cup)	1 oz-----------	28	3	120	1	3	1.7	0.3	0.4
367	Cheerios® (about 1-1/4 cup)--	1 oz-----------	28	5	110	4	2	0.3	0.6	0.7
	Corn Flakes (about 1-1/4 cup):									
368	Kellogg's® -----------------	1 oz-----------	28	3	110	2	Tr	Tr	Tr	Tr
369	Toasties® -----------------	1 oz-----------	28	3	110	2	Tr	Tr	Tr	Tr
	40% Bran Flakes:									
370	Kellogg's® (about 3/4 cup)	1 oz-----------	28	3	90	4	1	0.1	0.1	0.3
371	Post® (about 2/3 cup)------	1 oz-----------	28	3	90	3	Tr	0.1	0.1	0.2
372	Froot Loops® (about 1 cup)---	1 oz-----------	28	3	110	2	1	0.2	0.1	0.1
373	Golden Grahams® (about 3/4 cup)-----------------------	1 oz-----------	28	2	110	2	1	0.7	0.1	0.2
374	Grape-Nuts® (about 1/4 cup)--	1 oz-----------	28	3	100	3	Tr	Tr	Tr	0.1
375	Honey Nut Cheerios® (about 3/4 cup)-------------------	1 oz-----------	28	3	105	3	1	0.1	0.3	0.3
376	Lucky Charms® (about 1 cup)--	1 oz-----------	28	3	110	3	1	0.2	0.4	0.4
377	Nature Valley® Granola (about 1/3 cup)-------------------	1 oz-----------	28	4	125	3	5	3.3	0.7	0.7
378	100% Natural Cereal (about 1/4 cup)-------------------	1 oz-----------	28	2	135	3	6	4.1	1.2	0.5
379	Product 19® (about 3/4 cup)--	1 oz-----------	28	3	110	3	Tr	Tr	Tr	0.1
	Raisin Bran:									
380	Kellogg's® (about 3/4 cup)	1 oz-----------	28	8	90	3	1	0.1	0.1	0.3
381	Post® (about 1/2 cup)------	1 oz-----------	28	9	85	3	1	0.1	0.1	0.3
382	Rice Krispies® (about 1 cup)	1 oz-----------	28	2	110	2	Tr	Tr	Tr	0.1
383	Shredded Wheat (about 2/3 cup)-----------------------	1 oz-----------	28	5	100	3	1	0.1	0.1	0.3
384	Special K® (about 1-1/3 cup)	1 oz-----------	28	2	110	6	Tr	Tr	Tr	Tr
385	Super Sugar Crisp® (about 7/8 cup)-----------------------	1 oz-----------	28	2	105	2	Tr	Tr	Tr	0.1
386	Sugar Frosted Flakes, Kellogg's® (about 3/4 cup)	1 oz-----------	28	3	110	1	Tr	Tr	Tr	Tr
387	Sugar Smacks® (about 3/4 cup)	1 oz-----------	28	3	105	2	1	0.1	0.1	0.2
388	Total® (about 1 cup)---------	1 oz-----------	28	4	100	3	1	0.1	0.1	0.3
389	Trix® (about 1 cup)----------	1 oz-----------	28	3	110	2	Tr	0.2	0.1	0.1
390	Wheaties® (about 1 cup)------	1 oz-----------	28	5	100	3	Tr	0.1	Tr	0.2
391	Buckwheat flour, light, sifted---	1 cup-----------	98	12	340	6	1	0.2	0.4	0.4
392	Bulgur, uncooked-----------------	1 cup-----------	170	10	600	19	3	1.2	0.3	1.2
	Cakes prepared from cake mixes with enriched flour:[35]									
	Angelfood:									
393	Whole cake, 9-3/4-in diam. tube cake------------------	1 cake----------	635	38	1,510	38	2	0.4	0.2	1.0
394	Piece, 1/12 of cake----------	1 piece---------	53	38	125	3	Tr	Tr	Tr	0.1
	Coffeecake, crumb:									
395	Whole cake, 7-3/4 by 5-5/8 by 1-1/4 in---------------	1 cake----------	430	30	1,385	27	41	11.8	16.7	9.6
396	Piece, 1/6 of cake----------	1 piece---------	72	30	230	5	7	2.0	2.8	1.6
	Devil's food with chocolate frosting:									
397	Whole, 2-layer cake, 8- or 9-in diam.------------------	1 cake----------	1,107	24	3,755	49	136	55.6	51.4	19.7
398	Piece, 1/16 of cake----------	1 piece---------	69	24	235	3	8	3.5	3.2	1.2
399	Cupcake, 2-1/2-in diam.-------	1 cupcake-------	35	24	120	2	4	1.8	1.6	0.6
	Gingerbread:									
400	Whole cake, 8 in square------	1 cake----------	570	37	1,575	18	39	9.6	16.4	10.5
401	Piece, 1/9 of cake----------	1 piece---------	63	37	175	2	4	1.1	1.8	1.2

[27] Nutrient added.
[30] Value based on label declaration for added nutrients.

Nutrients in Indicated Quantity

Cho-les-terol	Carbo-hydrate	Calcium	Phos-phorus	Iron	Potas-sium	Sodium	Vitamin A value (IU)	Vitamin A value (RE)	Thiamin	Ribo-flavin	Niacin	Ascorbic acid	Item No.
Milli-grams	Grams	Milli-grams	Milli-grams	Milli-grams	Milli-grams	Milli-grams	Inter-national units	Retinol equiva-lents	Milli-grams	Milli-grams	Milli-grams	Milli-grams	
0	21	23	264	[30]4.5	350	320	[30]1,250	[30]375	[30]0.37	[30]0.43	[30]5.0	[30]15	365
0	23	5	36	[27]7.5	37	213	40	[30]4	[27]0.50	[27]0.55	[27]6.6	0	366
0	20	48	134	[30]4.5	101	307	[30]1,250	[30]375	[30]0.37	[30]0.43	[30]5.0	[30]15	367
0	24	1	18	[30]1.8	26	351	[30]1,250	[30]375	[30]0.37	[30]0.43	[30]5.0	[30]15	368
0	24	1	12	[27]0.7	33	297	[30]1,250	[30]375	[30]0.37	[30]0.43	[30]5.0	0	369
0	22	14	139	[30]8.1	180	264	[30]1,250	[30]375	[30]0.37	[30]0.43	[30]5.0	0	370
0	22	12	179	[30]4.5	151	260	[30]1,250	[30]375	[30]0.37	[30]0.43	[30]5.0	0	371
0	25	3	24	[30]4.5	26	145	[30]1,250	[30]375	[30]0.37	[30]0.43	[30]5.0	[30]15	372
Tr	24	17	41	[30]4.5	63	346	[30]1,250	[30]375	[30]0.37	[30]0.43	[30]5.0	[30]15	373
0	23	11	71	1.2	95	197	[30]1,250	[30]375	[30]0.37	[30]0.43	[30]5.0	0	374
0	23	20	105	[30]4.5	99	257	[30]1,250	[30]375	[30]0.37	[30]0.43	[30]5.0	[30]15	375
0	23	32	79	[30]4.5	59	201	[30]1,250	[30]375	[30]0.37	[30]0.43	[30]5.0	[30]15	376
0	19	18	89	0.9	98	58	20	2	0.10	0.05	0.2	0	377
Tr	18	49	104	0.8	140	12	20	2	0.09	0.15	0.6	0	378
0	24	3	40	[30]18.0	44	325	[30]5,000	[30]1,501	[30]1.50	[30]1.70	[30]20.0	[30]60	379
0	21	10	105	[30]3.5	147	207	[30]960	[30]288	[30]0.28	[30]0.34	[30]3.9	0	380
0	21	13	119	[30]4.5	175	185	[30]1,250	[30]375	[30]0.37	[30]0.43	[30]5.0	0	381
0	25	4	34	[30]1.8	29	340	[30]1,250	[30]375	[30]0.37	[30]0.43	[30]5.0	[30]15	382
0	23	11	100	1.2	102	3	0	0	0.07	0.08	1.5	0	383
Tr	21	8	55	[30]4.5	49	265	[30]1,250	[30]375	[30]0.37	[30]0.43	[30]5.0	[30]15	384
0	26	6	52	[30]1.8	105	25	[30]1,250	[30]375	[30]0.37	[30]0.43	[30]5.0	0	385
0	26	1	21	[30]1.8	18	230	[30]1,250	[30]375	[30]0.37	[30]0.43	[30]5.0	[30]15	386
0	25	3	31	[30]1.8	42	75	[30]1,250	[30]375	[30]0.37	[30]0.43	[30]5.0	[30]15	387
0	22	48	118	[30]18.0	106	352	[30]5,000	[30]1,501	[30]1.50	[30]1.70	[30]20.0	[30]60	388
0	25	6	19	[30]4.5	27	181	[30]1,250	[30]375	[30]0.37	[30]0.43	[30]5.0	[30]15	389
0	23	43	98	[30]4.5	106	354	[30]1,250	[30]375	[30]0.37	[30]0.43	[30]5.0	[30]15	390
0	78	11	86	1.0	314	2	0	0	0.08	0.04	0.4	0	391
0	129	49	575	9.5	389	7	0	0	0.48	0.24	7.7	0	392
0	342	527	1,086	2.7	845	3,226	0	0	0.32	1.27	1.6	0	393
0	29	44	91	0.2	71	269	0	0	0.03	0.11	0.1	0	394
279	225	262	748	7.3	469	1,853	690	194	0.82	0.90	7.7	1	395
47	38	44	125	1.2	78	310	120	32	0.14	0.15	1.3	Tr	396
598	645	653	1,162	22.1	1,439	2,900	1,660	498	1.11	1.66	10.0	1	397
37	40	41	72	1.4	90	181	100	31	0.07	0.10	0.6	Tr	398
19	20	21	37	0.7	46	92	50	16	0.04	0.05	0.3	Tr	399
6	291	513	570	10.8	1,562	1,733	0	0	0.86	1.03	7.4	1	400
1	32	57	63	1.2	173	192	0	0	0.09	0.11	0.8	Tr	401

[35] Excepting angelfood cake, cakes were made from mixes containing vegetable shortening and frostings were made with margarine.

Nutritive Value of the Edible Part of Food (Continued)

(Tr indicates nutrient present in trace amount.)

Item No.	Foods, approximate measures, units, and weight (weight of edible portion only)			Water	Food energy	Pro-tein	Fat	Fatty acids		
								Satu-rated	Mono-unsatu-rated	Poly-unsatu-rated
			Grams	Per-cent	Cal-ories	Grams	Grams	Grams	Grams	Grams

Grain Products—Con.

	Cakes prepared from cake mixes with enriched flour: [35]									
	Yellow with chocolate frosting:									
402	Whole, 2-layer cake, 8- or 9-in diam.	1 cake	1,108	26	3,735	45	125	47.8	48.8	21.8
403	Piece, 1/16 of cake	1 piece	69	26	235	3	8	3.0	3.0	1.4
	Cakes prepared from home recipes using enriched flour:									
	Carrot, with cream cheese frosting: [36]									
404	Whole cake, 10-in diam. tube cake	1 cake	1,536	23	6,175	63	328	66.0	135.2	107.5
405	Piece, 1/16 of cake	1 piece	96	23	385	4	21	4.1	8.4	6.7
	Fruitcake, dark: [36]									
406	Whole cake, 7-1/2-in diam., 2-1/4-in high tube cake	1 cake	1,361	18	5,185	74	228	47.6	113.0	51.7
407	Piece, 1/32 of cake, 2/3-in arc	1 piece	43	18	165	2	7	1.5	3.6	1.6
	Plain sheet cake: [37]									
	Without frosting:									
408	Whole cake, 9-in square	1 cake	777	25	2,830	35	108	29.5	45.1	25.6
409	Piece, 1/9 of cake	1 piece	86	25	315	4	12	3.3	5.0	2.8
	With uncooked white frosting:									
410	Whole cake, 9-in square	1 cake	1,096	21	4,020	37	129	41.6	50.4	26.3
411	Piece, 1/9 of cake	1 piece	121	21	445	4	14	4.6	5.6	2.9
	Pound: [38]									
412	Loaf, 8-1/2 by 3-1/2 by 3-1/4 in	1 loaf	514	22	2,025	33	94	21.1	40.9	26.7
413	Slice, 1/17 of loaf	1 slice	30	22	120	2	5	1.2	2.4	1.6
	Cakes, commercial, made with en-riched flour:									
	Pound:									
414	Loaf, 8-1/2 by 3-1/2 by 3 in	1 loaf	500	24	1,935	26	94	52.0	30.0	4.0
415	Slice, 1/17 of loaf	1 slice	29	24	110	2	5	3.0	1.7	0.2
	Snack cakes:									
416	Devil's food with creme filling (2 small cakes per pkg)	1 small cake	28	20	105	1	4	1.7	1.5	0.6
417	Sponge with creme filling (2 small cakes per pkg)	1 small cake	42	19	155	1	5	2.3	2.1	0.5
	White with white frosting:									
418	Whole, 2-layer cake, 8- or 9-in diam.	1 cake	1,140	24	4,170	43	148	33.1	61.6	42.2
419	Piece, 1/16 of cake	1 piece	71	24	260	3	9	2.1	3.8	2.6
	Yellow with chocolate frosting:									
420	Whole, 2-layer cake, 8- or 9-in diam.	1 cake	1,108	23	3,895	40	175	92.0	58.7	10.0
421	Piece, 1/16 of cake	1 piece	69	23	245	2	11	5.7	3.7	0.6
	Cheesecake:									
422	Whole cake, 9-in diam.	1 cake	1,110	46	3,350	60	213	119.9	65.5	14.4
423	Piece, 1/12 of cake	1 piece	92	46	280	5	18	9.9	5.4	1.2
	Cookies made with enriched flour:									
	Brownies with nuts:									
424	Commercial, with frosting, 1-1/2 by 1-3/4 by 7/8 in	1 brownie	25	13	100	1	4	1.6	2.0	0.6
425	From home recipe, 1-3/4 by 1-3/4 by 7/8 in [36]	1 brownie	20	10	95	1	6	1.4	2.8	1.2
	Chocolate chip:									
426	Commercial, 2-1/4-in diam., 3/8 in thick	4 cookies	42	4	180	2	9	2.9	3.1	2.6

[35] Excepting angelfood cake, cakes were made from mixes containing vegetable shortening and frostings were made with margarine.
[36] Made with vegetable oil.

| | | | | | | | Nutrients in Indicated Quantity | | | | | | |

Cho-les-terol	Carbo-hydrate	Calcium	Phos-phorus	Iron	Potas-sium	Sodium	Vitamin A value (IU)	Vitamin A value (RE)	Thiamin	Ribo-flavin	Niacin	Ascorbic acid	Item No.
Milli-grams	Grams	Milli-grams	Milli-grams	Milli-grams	Milli-grams	Milli-grams	Inter-national units	Retinol equiva-lents	Milli-grams	Milli-grams	Milli-grams	Milli-grams	
576	638	1,008	2,017	15.5	1,208	2,515	1,550	465	1.22	1.66	11.1	1	402
36	40	63	126	1.0	75	157	100	29	0.08	0.10	0.7	Tr	403
1183	775	707	998	21.0	1,720	4,470	2,240	246	1.83	1.97	14.7	23	404
74	48	44	62	1.3	108	279	140	15	0.11	0.12	0.9	1	405
640	783	1,293	1,592	37.6	6,138	2,123	1,720	422	2.41	2.55	17.0	504	406
20	25	41	50	1.2	194	67	50	13	0.08	0.08	0.5	16	407
552	434	497	793	11.7	614	2,331	1,320	373	1.24	1.40	10.1	2	408
61	48	55	88	1.3	68	258	150	41	0.14	0.15	1.1	Tr	409
636	694	548	822	11.0	669	2,488	2,190	647	1.21	1.42	9.9	2	410
70	77	61	91	1.2	74	275	240	71	0.13	0.16	1.1	Tr	411
555	265	339	473	9.3	483	1,645	3,470	1,033	0.93	1.08	7.8	1	412
32	15	20	28	0.5	28	96	200	60	0.05	0.06	0.5	Tr	413
1100	257	146	517	8.0	443	1,857	2,820	715	0.96	1.12	8.1	0	414
64	15	8	30	0.5	26	108	160	41	0.06	0.06	0.5	0	415
15	17	21	26	1.0	34	105	20	4	0.06	0.09	0.7	0	416
7	27	14	44	0.6	37	155	30	9	0.07	0.06	0.6	0	417
46	670	536	1,585	15.5	832	2,827	640	194	3.19	2.05	27.6	0	418
3	42	33	99	1.0	52	176	40	12	0.20	0.13	1.7	0	419
609	620	366	1,884	19.9	1,972	3,080	1,850	488	0.78	2.22	10.0	0	420
38	39	23	117	1.2	123	192	120	30	0.05	0.14	0.6	0	421
2053	317	622	977	5.3	1,088	2,464	2,820	833	0.33	1.44	5.1	56	422
170	26	52	81	0.4	90	204	230	69	0.03	0.12	0.4	5	423
14	16	13	26	0.6	50	59	70	18	0.08	0.07	0.3	Tr	424
18	11	9	26	0.4	35	51	20	6	0.05	0.05	0.3	Tr	425
5	28	13	41	0.8	68	140	50	15	0.10	0.23	1.0	Tr	426

[37]Cake made with vegetable shortening; frosting with margarine.
[38]Made with margarine.

Nutritive Value of the Edible Part of Food (Continued)

(Tr indicates nutrient present in trace amount.)

Item No.	Foods, approximate measures, units, and weight (weight of edible portion only)		Water	Food energy	Pro-tein	Fat	Fatty acids		
							Satu-rated	Mono-unsatu-rated	Poly-unsatu-rated
		Grams	Per-cent	Cal-ories	Grams	Grams	Grams	Grams	Grams
	Grain Products—Con.								
	Cookies made with enriched flour:								
	Chocolate chip:								
427	From home recipe, 2-1/3-in diam.[25]	4 cookies	40	3	185	2	11	3.9	4.3	2.0
428	From refrigerated dough, 2-1/4-in diam., 3/8 in thick	4 cookies	48	5	225	2	11	4.0	4.4	2.0
429	Fig bars, square, 1-5/8 by 1-5/8 by 3/8 in or rectangu-lar, 1-1/2 by 1-3/4 by 1/2 in	4 cookies	56	12	210	2	4	1.0	1.5	1.0
430	Oatmeal with raisins, 2-5/8-in diam., 1/4 in thick	4 cookies	52	4	245	3	10	2.5	4.5	2.8
431	Peanut butter cookie, from home recipe, 2-5/8-in diam.[25]	4 cookies	48	3	245	4	14	4.0	5.8	2.8
432	Sandwich type (chocolate or vanilla), 1-3/4-in diam., 3/8 in thick	4 cookies	40	2	195	2	8	2.0	3.6	2.2
	Shortbread:								
433	Commercial	4 small cookies	32	6	155	2	8	2.9	3.0	1.1
434	From home recipe [38]	2 large cookies	28	3	145	2	8	1.3	2.7	3.4
435	Sugar cookie, from refrigerated dough, 2-1/2-in diam., 1/4 in thick	4 cookies	48	4	235	2	12	2.3	5.0	3.6
436	Vanilla wafers, 1-3/4-in diam., 1/4 in thick	10 cookies	40	4	185	2	7	1.8	3.0	1.8
437	Corn chips	1-oz package	28	1	155	2	9	1.4	2.4	3.7
	Cornmeal:								
438	Whole-ground, unbolted, dry form	1 cup	122	12	435	11	5	0.5	1.1	2.5
439	Bolted (nearly whole-grain), dry form	1 cup	122	12	440	11	4	0.5	0.9	2.2
	Degermed, enriched:								
440	Dry form	1 cup	138	12	500	11	2	0.2	0.4	0.9
441	Cooked	1 cup	240	88	120	3	Tr	Tr	0.1	0.2
	Crackers:[39]								
	Cheese:								
442	Plain, 1 in square	10 crackers	10	4	50	1	3	0.9	1.2	0.3
443	Sandwich type (peanut butter)	1 sandwich	8	3	40	1	2	0.4	0.8	0.3
444	Graham, plain, 2-1/2 in square	2 crackers	14	5	60	1	1	0.4	0.6	0.4
445	Melba toast, plain	1 piece	5	4	20	1	Tr	0.1	0.1	0.1
446	Rye wafers, whole-grain, 1-7/8 by 3-1/2 in	2 wafers	14	5	55	1	1	0.3	0.4	0.3
447	Saltines [40]	4 crackers	12	4	50	1	1	0.5	0.4	0.2
448	Snack-type, standard	1 round cracker	3	3	15	Tr	1	0.2	0.4	0.1
449	Wheat, thin	4 crackers	8	3	35	1	1	0.5	0.5	0.4
450	Whole-wheat wafers	2 crackers	8	4	35	1	2	0.5	0.6	0.4
451	Croissants, made with enriched flour, 4-1/2 by 4 by 1-3/4 in	1 croissant	57	22	235	5	12	3.5	6.7	1.4
	Danish pastry, made with enriched flour:								
	Plain without fruit or nuts:								
452	Packaged ring, 12 oz	1 ring	340	27	1,305	21	71	21.8	28.6	15.6
453	Round piece, about 4-1/4-in diam., 1 in high	1 pastry	57	27	220	4	12	3.6	4.8	2.6
454	Ounce	1 oz	28	27	110	2	6	1.8	2.4	1.3
455	Fruit, round piece	1 pastry	65	30	235	4	13	3.9	5.2	2.9
	Doughnuts, made with enriched flour:								
456	Cake type, plain, 3-1/4-in diam., 1 in high	1 doughnut	50	21	210	3	12	2.8	5.0	3.0
457	Yeast-leavened, glazed, 3-3/4-in diam., 1-1/4 in high	1 doughnut	60	27	235	4	13	5.2	5.5	0.9
458	English muffins, plain, enriched	1 muffin	57	42	140	5	1	0.3	0.2	0.3
459	Toasted	1 muffin	50	29	140	5	1	0.3	0.2	0.3

[25]Made with vegetable shortening.
[38]Made with margarine.

							Nutrients in Indicated Quantity							
Cho-les-terol	Carbo-hydrate	Calcium	Phos-phorus	Iron	Potas-sium	Sodium	Vitamin A value		Thiamin	Ribo-flavin	Niacin	Ascorbic acid	Item No.
							(IU)	(RE)					
Milli-grams	Grams	Milli-grams	Milli-grams	Milli-grams	Milli-grams	Milli-grams	Inter-national units	Retinol equiva-lents	Milli-grams	Milli-grams	Milli-grams	Milli-grams	
18	26	13	34	1.0	82	82	20	5	0.06	0.06	0.6	0	427
22	32	13	34	1.0	62	173	30	8	0.06	0.10	0.9	0	428
27	42	40	34	1.4	162	180	60	6	0.08	0.07	0.7	Tr	429
2	36	18	58	1.1	90	148	40	12	0.09	0.08	1.0	0	430
22	28	21	60	1.1	110	142	20	5	0.07	0.07	1.9	0	431
0	29	12	40	1.4	66	189	0	0	0.09	0.07	0.8	0	432
27	20	13	39	0.8	38	123	30	8	0.10	0.09	0.9	0	433
0	17	6	31	0.6	18	125	300	89	0.08	0.06	0.7	Tr	434
29	31	50	91	0.9	33	261	40	11	0.09	0.06	1.1	0	435
25	29	16	36	0.8	50	150	50	14	0.07	0.10	1.0	0	436
0	16	35	52	0.5	52	233	110	11	0.04	0.05	0.4	1	437
0	90	24	312	2.2	346	1	620	62	0.46	0.13	2.4	0	438
0	91	21	272	2.2	303	1	590	59	0.37	0.10	2.3	0	439
0	108	8	137	5.9	166	1	610	61	0.61	0.36	4.8	0	440
0	26	2	34	1.4	38	0	140	14	0.14	0.10	1.2	0	441
6	6	11	17	0.3	17	112	20	5	0.05	0.04	0.4	0	442
1	5	7	25	0.3	17	90	Tr	Tr	0.04	0.03	0.6	0	443
0	11	6	20	0.4	36	86	0	0	0.02	0.03	0.6	0	444
0	4	6	10	0.1	11	44	0	0	0.01	0.01	0.1	0	445
0	10	7	44	0.5	65	115	0	0	0.06	0.03	0.5	0	446
4	9	3	12	0.5	17	165	0	0	0.06	0.05	0.6	0	447
0	2	3	6	0.1	4	30	Tr	Tr	0.01	0.01	0.1	0	448
0	5	3	15	0.3	17	69	Tr	Tr	0.04	0.03	0.4	0	449
0	5	3	22	0.2	31	59	0	0	0.02	0.03	0.4	0	450
13	27	20	64	2.1	68	452	50	13	0.17	0.13	1.3	0	451
292	152	360	347	6.5	316	1,302	360	99	0.95	1.02	8.5	Tr	452
49	26	60	58	1.1	53	218	60	17	0.16	0.17	1.4	Tr	453
24	13	30	29	0.5	26	109	30	8	0.08	0.09	0.7	Tr	454
56	28	17	80	1.3	57	233	40	11	0.16	0.14	1.4	Tr	455
20	24	22	111	1.0	58	192	20	5	0.12	0.12	1.1	Tr	456
21	26	17	55	1.4	64	222	Tr	Tr	0.28	0.12	1.8	0	457
0	27	96	67	1.7	331	378	0	0	0.26	0.19	2.2	0	458
0	27	96	67	1.7	331	378	0	0	0.23	0.19	2.2	0	459

[39]Crackers made with enriched flour except for rye wafers and whole-wheat wafers.
[40]Made with lard.

Nutritive Value of the Edible Part of Food (Continued)

(Tr indicates nutrient present in trace amount.)

Item No.	Foods, approximate measures, units, and weight (weight of edible portion only)		Water	Food energy	Pro-tein	Fat	Fatty acids		
							Satu-rated	Mono-unsatu-rated	Poly-unsatu-rated
		Grams	Per-cent	Cal-ories	Grams	Grams	Grams	Grams	Grams
	Grain Products—Con.								
460	French toast, from home recipe---	1 slice--------	65	53	155	6	7	1.6	2.0	1.6
	Macaroni, enriched, cooked (cut lengths, elbows, shells):									
461	Firm stage (hot)--------------	1 cup----------	130	64	190	7	1	0.1	0.1	0.3
	Tender stage:									
462	Cold-------------------------	1 cup----------	105	72	115	4	Tr	0.1	0.1	0.2
463	Hot--------------------------	1 cup----------	140	72	155	5	1	0.1	0.1	0.2
	Muffins made with enriched flour, 2-1/2-in diam., 1-1/2 in high:									
	From home recipe:									
464	Blueberry [25]-------------------	1 muffin--------	45	37	135	3	5	1.5	2.1	1.2
465	Bran [36]-----------------------	1 muffin--------	45	35	125	3	6	1.4	1.6	2.3
466	Corn (enriched, degermed cornmeal and flour) [25]------	1 muffin--------	45	33	145	3	5	1.5	2.2	1.4
	From commercial mix (egg and water added):									
467	Blueberry--------------------	1 muffin--------	45	33	140	3	5	1.4	2.0	1.2
468	Bran------------------------	1 muffin--------	45	28	140	3	4	1.3	1.6	1.0
469	Corn------------------------	1 muffin--------	45	30	145	3	6	1.7	2.3	1.4
470	Noodles (egg noodles), enriched, cooked-----------------------	1 cup----------	160	70	200	7	2	0.5	0.6	0.6
471	Noodles, chow mein, canned------	1 cup----------	45	11	220	6	11	2.1	7.3	0.4
	Pancakes, 4-in diam.:									
472	Buckwheat, from mix (with buck-wheat and enriched flours), egg and milk added-----------	1 pancake-------	27	58	55	2	2	0.9	0.9	0.5
	Plain:									
473	From home recipe using enriched flour-------------	1 pancake-------	27	50	60	2	2	0.5	0.8	0.5
474	From mix (with enriched flour), egg, milk, and oil added--------------------	1 pancake-------	27	54	60	2	2	0.5	0.9	0.5
	Piecrust, made with enriched flour and vegetable shorten-ing, baked:									
475	From home recipe, 9-in diam.---	1 pie shell-----	180	15	900	11	60	14.8	25.9	15.7
476	From mix, 9-in diam.-----------	Piecrust for 2-crust pie-----	320	19	1,485	20	93	22.7	41.0	25.0
	Pies, piecrust made with enriched flour, vegetable shortening, 9-in diam.:									
	Apple:									
477	Whole-----------------------	1 pie----------	945	48	2,420	21	105	27.4	44.4	26.5
478	Piece, 1/6 of pie------------	1 piece--------	158	48	405	3	18	4.6	7.4	4.4
	Blueberry:									
479	Whole-----------------------	1 pie----------	945	51	2,285	23	102	25.5	44.4	27.4
480	Piece, 1/6 of pie------------	1 piece--------	158	51	380	4	17	4.3	7.4	4.6
	Cherry:									
481	Whole-----------------------	1 pie----------	945	47	2,465	25	107	28.4	46.3	27.4
482	Piece, 1/6 of pie------------	1 piece--------	158	47	410	4	18	4.7	7.7	4.6
	Creme:									
483	Whole-----------------------	1 pie----------	910	43	2,710	20	139	90.1	23.7	6.4
484	Piece, 1/6 of pie------------	1 piece--------	152	43	455	3	23	15.0	4.0	1.1
	Custard:									
485	Whole-----------------------	1 pie----------	910	58	1,985	56	101	33.7	40.0	19.1
486	Piece, 1/6 of pie------------	1 piece--------	152	58	330	9	17	5.6	6.7	3.2
	Lemon meringue:									
487	Whole-----------------------	1 pie----------	840	47	2,140	31	86	26.0	34.4	17.6
488	Piece, 1/6 of pie------------	1 piece--------	140	47	355	5	14	4.3	5.7	2.9
	Peach:									
489	Whole-----------------------	1 pie----------	945	48	2,410	24	101	24.6	43.5	26.5
490	Piece, 1/6 of pie------------	1 piece--------	158	48	405	4	17	4.1	7.3	4.4

[25] Made with vegetable shortening.

							Vitamin A value						
Cho-les-terol	Carbo-hydrate	Calcium	Phos-phorus	Iron	Potas-sium	Sodium	(IU)	(RE)	Thiamin	Ribo-flavin	Niacin	Ascorbic acid	Item No.
Milli-grams	Grams	Milli-grams	Milli-grams	Milli-grams	Milli-grams	Milli-grams	Inter-national units	Retinol equiva-lents	Milli-grams	Milli-grams	Milli-grams	Milli-grams	
112	17	72	85	1.3	86	257	110	32	0.12	0.16	1.0	Tr	460
0	39	14	85	2.1	103	1	0	0	0.23	0.13	1.8	0	461
0	24	8	53	1.3	64	1	0	0	0.15	0.08	1.2	0	462
0	32	11	70	1.7	85	1	0	0	0.20	0.11	1.5	0	463
19	20	54	46	0.9	47	198	40	9	0.10	0.11	0.9	1	464
24	19	60	125	1.4	99	189	230	30	0.11	0.13	1.3	3	465
23	21	66	59	0.9	57	169	80	15	0.11	0.11	0.9	Tr	466
45	22	15	90	0.9	54	225	50	11	0.10	0.17	1.1	Tr	467
28	24	27	182	1.7	50	385	100	14	0.08	0.12	1.9	0	468
42	22	30	128	1.3	31	291	90	16	0.09	0.09	0.8	Tr	469
50	37	16	94	2.6	70	3	110	34	0.22	0.13	1.9	0	470
5	26	14	41	0.4	33	450	0	0	0.05	0.03	0.6	0	471
20	6	59	91	0.4	66	125	60	17	0.04	0.05	0.2	Tr	472
16	9	27	38	0.5	33	115	30	10	0.06	0.07	0.5	Tr	473
16	8	36	71	0.7	43	160	30	7	0.09	0.12	0.8	Tr	474
0	79	25	90	4.5	90	1,100	0	0	0.54	0.40	5.0	0	475
0	141	131	272	9.3	179	2,602	0	0	1.06	0.80	9.9	0	476
0	360	76	208	9.5	756	2,844	280	28	1.04	0.76	9.5	9	477
0	60	13	35	1.6	126	476	50	5	0.17	0.13	1.6	2	478
0	330	104	217	12.3	945	2,533	850	85	1.04	0.85	10.4	38	479
0	55	17	36	2.1	158	423	140	14	0.17	0.14	1.7	6	480
0	363	132	236	9.5	992	2,873	4,160	416	1.13	0.85	9.5	0	481
0	61	22	40	1.6	166	480	700	70	0.19	0.14	1.6	0	482
46	351	273	919	6.8	796	2,207	1,250	391	0.36	0.89	6.4	0	483
8	59	46	154	1.1	133	369	210	65	0.06	0.15	1.1	0	484
1010	213	874	1,028	9.1	1,247	2,612	2,090	573	0.82	1.91	5.5	0	485
169	36	146	172	1.5	208	436	350	96	0.14	0.32	0.9	0	486
857	317	118	412	8.4	420	2,369	1,430	395	0.59	0.84	5.0	25	487
143	53	20	69	1.4	70	395	240	66	0.10	0.14	0.8	4	488
0	361	95	274	11.3	1,408	2,533	6,900	690	1.04	0.95	14.2	28	489
0	60	16	46	1.9	235	423	1,150	115	0.17	0.16	2.4	5	490

[36] Made with vegetable oil.

Nutritive Value of the Edible Part of Food (Continued)
(Tr indicates nutrient present in trace amount.)

Item No.	Foods, approximate measures, units, and weight (weight of edible portion only)			Water	Food energy	Pro-tein	Fat	Fatty acids		
								Satu-rated	Mono-unsatu-rated	Poly-unsatu-rated
			Grams	Per-cent	Cal-ories	Grams	Grams	Grams	Grams	Grams
	Grain Products—Con.									
	Pies, piecrust made with enriched flour, vegetable shortening, 9-inch diam.:									
	Pecan:									
491	Whole------------------------	1 pie------------	825	20	3,450	42	189	28.1	101.5	47.0
492	Piece, 1/6 of pie------------	1 piece---------	138	20	575	7	32	4.7	17.0	7.9
	Pumpkin:									
493	Whole------------------------	1 pie------------	910	59	1,920	36	102	38.2	40.0	18.2
494	Piece, 1/6 of pie------------	1 piece---------	152	59	320	6	17	6.4	6.7	3.0
	Pies, fried:									
495	Apple-------------------------	1 pie------------	85	43	255	2	14	5.8	6.6	0.6
496	Cherry------------------------	1 pie-----------	85	42	250	2	14	5.8	6.7	0.6
	Popcorn, popped:									
497	Air-popped, unsalted----------	1 cup-----------	8	4	30	1	Tr	Tr	0.1	0.2
498	Popped in vegetable oil, salted	1 cup-----------	11	3	55	1	3	0.5	1.4	1.2
499	Sugar syrup coated------------	1 cup-----------	35	4	135	2	1	0.1	0.3	0.6
	Pretzels, made with enriched flour:									
500	Stick, 2-1/4 in long----------	10 pretzels-----	3	3	10	Tr	Tr	Tr	Tr	Tr
501	Twisted, dutch, 2-3/4 by 2-5/8 in-------------------------	1 pretzel-------	16	3	65	2	1	0.1	0.2	0.2
502	Twisted, thin, 3-1/4 by 2-1/4 by 1/4 in--------------------	10 pretzels-----	60	3	240	6	2	0.4	0.8	0.6
	Rice:									
503	Brown, cooked, served hot------	1 cup-----------	195	70	230	5	1	0.3	0.3	0.4
	White, enriched:									
	Commercial varieties, all types:									
504	Raw--------------------------	1 cup-----------	185	12	670	12	1	0.2	0.2	0.3
505	Cooked, served hot---------	1 cup-----------	205	73	225	4	Tr	0.1	0.1	0.1
506	Instant, ready-to-serve, hot	1 cup-----------	165	73	180	4	0	0.1	0.1	0.1
	Parboiled:									
507	Raw--------------------------	1 cup-----------	185	10	685	14	1	0.1	0.1	0.2
508	Cooked, served hot---------	1 cup-----------	175	73	185	4	Tr	Tr	Tr	0.1
	Rolls, enriched:									
	Commercial:									
509	Dinner, 2-1/2-in diam., 2 in high-----------------------	1 roll----------	28	32	85	2	2	0.5	0.8	0.6
510	Frankfurter and hamburger (8 per 11-1/2-oz pkg.)--------	1 roll----------	40	34	115	3	2	0.5	0.8	0.6
511	Hard, 3-3/4-in diam., 2 in high-----------------------	1 roll----------	50	25	155	5	2	0.4	0.5	0.6
512	Hoagie or submarine, 11-1/2 by 3 by 2-1/2 in-----------	1 roll----------	135	31	400	11	8	1.8	3.0	2.2
	From home recipe:									
513	Dinner, 2-1/2-in diam., 2 in high-----------------------	1 roll----------	35	26	120	3	3	0.8	1.2	0.9
	Spaghetti, enriched, cooked:									
514	Firm stage, "al dente," served hot-------------------------	1 cup-----------	130	64	190	7	1	0.1	0.1	0.3
515	Tender stage, served hot-------	1 cup-----------	140	73	155	5	1	0.1	0.1	0.2
516	Toaster pastries------------------	1 pastry--------	54	13	210	2	6	1.7	3.6	0.4
517	Tortillas, corn------------------	1 tortilla------	30	45	65	2	1	0.1	0.3	0.6
	Waffles, made with enriched flour, 7-in diam.:									
518	From home recipe--------------	1 waffle--------	75	37	245	7	13	4.0	4.9	2.6
519	From mix, egg and milk added---	1 waffle--------	75	42	205	7	8	2.7	2.9	1.5
	Wheat flours:									
	All-purpose or family flour, enriched:									
520	Sifted, spooned--------------	1 cup-----------	115	12	420	12	1	0.2	0.1	0.5
521	Unsifted, spooned------------	1 cup-----------	125	12	455	13	1	0.2	0.1	0.5
522	Cake or pastry flour, enriched, sifted, spooned--------------	1 cup-----------	96	12	350	7	1	0.1	0.1	0.3
523	Self-rising, enriched, unsifted, spooned-----------	1 cup-----------	125	12	440	12	1	0.2	0.1	0.5
524	Whole-wheat, from hard wheats, stirred----------------------	1 cup-----------	120	12	400	16	2	0.3	0.3	1.1

							Vitamin A value						Item
Cho-les-terol	Carbo-hydrate	Calcium	Phos-phorus	Iron	Potas-sium	Sodium	(IU)	(RE)	Thiamin	Ribo-flavin	Niacin	Ascorbic acid	No.
Milli-grams	Grams	Milli-grams	Milli-grams	Milli-grams	Milli-grams	Milli-grams	Inter-national units	Retinol equiva-lents	Milli-grams	Milli-grams	Milli-grams	Milli-grams	
569	423	388	850	27.2	1,015	1,823	1,320	322	1.82	0.99	6.6	0	491
95	71	65	142	4.6	170	305	220	54	0.30	0.17	1.1	0	492
655	223	464	628	8.2	1,456	1,947	22,480	2,493	0.82	1.27	7.3	0	493
109	37	78	105	1.4	243	325	3,750	416	0.14	0.21	1.2	0	494
14	31	12	34	0.9	42	326	30	3	0.09	0.06	1.0	1	495
13	32	11	41	0.7	61	371	190	19	0.06	0.06	0.6	1	496
0	6	1	22	0.2	20	Tr	10	1	0.03	0.01	0.2	0	497
0	6	3	31	0.3	19	86	20	2	0.01	0.02	0.1	0	498
0	30	2	47	0.5	90	Tr	30	3	0.13	0.02	0.4	0	499
0	2	1	3	0.1	3	48	0	0	0.01	0.01	0.1	0	500
0	13	4	15	0.3	16	258	0	0	0.05	0.04	0.7	0	501
0	48	16	55	1.2	61	966	0	0	0.19	0.15	2.6	0	502
0	50	23	142	1.0	137	0	0	0	0.18	0.04	2.7	0	503
0	149	44	174	5.4	170	9	0	0	0.81	0.06	6.5	0	504
0	50	21	57	1.8	57	0	0	0	0.23	0.02	2.1	0	505
0	40	5	31	1.3	0	0	0	0	0.21	0.02	1.7	0	506
0	150	111	370	5.4	278	17	0	0	0.81	0.07	6.5	0	507
0	41	33	100	1.4	75	0	0	0	0.19	0.02	2.1	0	508
Tr	14	33	44	0.8	36	155	Tr	Tr	0.14	0.09	1.1	Tr	509
Tr	20	54	44	1.2	56	241	Tr	Tr	0.20	0.13	1.6	Tr	510
Tr	30	24	46	1.4	49	313	0	0	0.20	0.12	1.7	0	511
Tr	72	100	115	3.8	128	683	0	0	0.54	0.33	4.5	0	512
12	20	16	36	1.1	41	98	30	8	0.12	0.12	1.2	0	513
0	39	14	85	2.0	103	1	0	0	0.23	0.13	1.8	0	514
0	32	11	70	1.7	85	1	0	0	0.20	0.11	1.5	0	515
0	38	104	104	2.2	91	248	520	52	0.17	0.18	2.3	4	516
0	13	42	55	0.6	43	1	80	8	0.05	0.03	0.4	0	517
102	26	154	135	1.5	129	445	140	39	0.18	0.24	1.5	Tr	518
59	27	179	257	1.2	146	515	170	49	0.14	0.23	0.9	Tr	519
0	88	18	100	5.1	109	2	0	0	0.73	0.46	6.1	0	520
0	95	20	109	5.5	119	3	0	0	0.80	0.50	6.6	0	521
0	76	16	70	4.2	91	2	0	0	0.58	0.38	5.1	0	522
0	93	331	583	5.5	113	1,349	0	0	0.80	0.50	6.6	0	523
0	85	49	446	5.2	444	4	0	0	0.66	0.14	5.2	0	524

Nutrients in Indicated Quantity

Nutritive Value of the Edible Part of Food (Continued)

(Tr indicates nutrient present in trace amount.)

Item No.	Foods, approximate measures, units, and weight (weight of edible portion only)			Water	Food energy	Pro-tein	Fat	Fatty acids		
								Satu-rated	Mono-unsatu-rated	Poly-unsatu-rated
	Legumes, Nuts, and Seeds		Grams	Per-cent	Cal-ories	Grams	Grams	Grams	Grams	Grams
	Almonds, shelled:									
525	Slivered, packed	1 cup	135	4	795	27	70	6.7	45.8	14.8
526	Whole	1 oz	28	4	165	6	15	1.4	9.6	3.1
	Beans, dry:									
	Cooked, drained:									
527	Black	1 cup	171	66	225	15	1	0.1	0.1	0.5
528	Great Northern	1 cup	180	69	210	14	1	0.1	0.1	0.6
529	Lima	1 cup	190	64	260	16	1	0.2	0.1	0.5
530	Pea (navy)	1 cup	190	69	225	15	1	0.1	0.1	0.7
531	Pinto	1 cup	180	65	265	15	1	0.1	0.1	0.5
	Canned, solids and liquid:									
	White with:									
532	Frankfurters (sliced)	1 cup	255	71	365	19	18	7.4	8.8	0.7
533	Pork and tomato sauce	1 cup	255	71	310	16	7	2.4	2.7	0.7
534	Pork and sweet sauce	1 cup	255	66	385	16	12	4.3	4.9	1.2
535	Red kidney	1 cup	255	76	230	15	1	0.1	0.1	0.6
536	Black-eyed peas, dry, cooked (with residual cooking liquid)	1 cup	250	80	190	13	1	0.2	Tr	0.3
537	Brazil nuts, shelled	1 oz	28	3	185	4	19	4.6	6.5	6.8
538	Carob flour	1 cup	140	3	255	6	Tr	Tr	0.1	0.1
	Cashew nuts, salted:									
539	Dry roasted	1 cup	137	2	785	21	63	12.5	37.4	10.7
540		1 oz	28	2	165	4	13	2.6	7.7	2.2
541	Roasted in oil	1 cup	130	4	750	21	63	12.4	36.9	10.6
542		1 oz	28	4	165	5	14	2.7	8.1	2.3
543	Chestnuts, European (Italian), roasted, shelled	1 cup	143	40	350	5	3	0.6	1.1	1.2
544	Chickpeas, cooked, drained	1 cup	163	60	270	15	4	0.4	0.9	1.9
	Coconut:									
	Raw:									
545	Piece, about 2 by 2 by 1/2 in	1 piece	45	47	160	1	15	13.4	0.6	0.2
546	Shredded or grated	1 cup	80	47	285	3	27	23.8	1.1	0.3
547	Dried, sweetened, shredded	1 cup	93	13	470	3	33	29.3	1.4	0.4
548	Filberts (hazelnuts), chopped	1 cup	115	5	725	15	72	5.3	56.5	6.9
549		1 oz	28	5	180	4	18	1.3	13.9	1.7
550	Lentils, dry, cooked	1 cup	200	72	215	16	1	0.1	0.2	0.5
551	Macadamia nuts, roasted in oil, salted	1 cup	134	2	960	10	103	15.4	80.9	1.8
552		1 oz	28	2	205	2	22	3.2	17.1	0.4
	Mixed nuts, with peanuts, salted:									
553	Dry roasted	1 oz	28	2	170	5	15	2.0	8.9	3.1
554	Roasted in oil	1 oz	28	2	175	5	16	2.5	9.0	3.8
555	Peanuts, roasted in oil, salted	1 cup	145	2	840	39	71	9.9	35.5	22.6
556		1 oz	28	2	165	8	14	1.9	6.9	4.4
557	Peanut butter	1 tbsp	16	1	95	5	8	1.4	4.0	2.5
558	Peas, split, dry, cooked	1 cup	200	70	230	16	1	0.1	0.1	0.3
559	Pecans, halves	1 cup	108	5	720	8	73	5.9	45.5	18.1
560		1 oz	28	5	190	2	19	1.5	12.0	4.7
561	Pine nuts (pinyons), shelled	1 oz	28	6	160	3	17	2.7	6.5	7.3
562	Pistachio nuts, dried, shelled	1 oz	28	4	165	6	14	1.7	9.3	2.1
563	Pumpkin and squash kernels, dry, hulled	1 oz	28	7	155	7	13	2.5	4.0	5.9
564	Refried beans, canned	1 cup	290	72	295	18	3	0.4	0.6	1.4
565	Sesame seeds, dry, hulled	1 tbsp	8	5	45	2	4	0.6	1.7	1.9
566	Soybeans, dry, cooked, drained	1 cup	180	71	235	20	10	1.3	1.9	5.3
	Soy products:									
567	Miso	1 cup	276	53	470	29	13	1.8	2.6	7.3
568	Tofu, piece 2-1/2 by 2-3/4 by 1 in	1 piece	120	85	85	9	5	0.7	1.0	2.9
569	Sunflower seeds, dry, hulled	1 oz	28	5	160	6	14	1.5	2.7	9.3
570	Tahini	1 tbsp	15	3	90	3	8	1.1	3.0	3.5

[41]Cashews without salt contain 21 mg sodium per cup or 4 mg per oz.
[42]Cashews without salt contain 22 mg sodium per cup or 5 mg per oz.
[43]Macadamia nuts without salt contain 9 mg sodium per cup or 2 mg per oz.

Nutrients in Indicated Quantity

Cholesterol	Carbohydrate	Calcium	Phosphorus	Iron	Potassium	Sodium	Vitamin A value		Thiamin	Riboflavin	Niacin	Ascorbic acid	Item No.
							(IU)	(RE)					
Milligrams	Grams	Milligrams	Milligrams	Milligrams	Milligrams	Milligrams	International units	Retinol equivalents	Milligrams	Milligrams	Milligrams	Milligrams	
0	28	359	702	4.9	988	15	0	0	0.28	1.05	4.5	1	525
0	6	75	147	1.0	208	3	0	0	0.06	0.22	1.0	Tr	526
0	41	47	239	2.9	608	1	Tr	Tr	0.43	0.05	0.9	0	527
0	38	90	266	4.9	749	13	0	0	0.25	0.13	1.3	0	528
0	49	55	293	5.9	1,163	4	0	0	0.25	0.11	1.3	0	529
0	40	95	281	5.1	790	13	0	0	0.27	0.13	1.3	0	530
0	49	86	296	5.4	882	3	Tr	Tr	0.33	0.16	0.7	0	531
30	32	94	303	4.8	668	1,374	330	33	0.18	0.15	3.3	Tr	532
10	48	138	235	4.6	536	1,181	330	33	0.20	0.08	1.5	5	533
10	54	161	291	5.9	536	969	330	33	0.15	0.10	1.3	5	534
0	42	74	278	4.6	673	968	10	1	0.13	0.10	1.5	0	535
0	35	43	238	3.3	573	20	30	3	0.40	0.10	1.0	0	536
0	4	50	170	1.0	170	1	Tr	Tr	0.28	0.03	0.5	Tr	537
0	126	390	102	5.7	1,275	24	Tr	Tr	0.07	0.07	2.2	Tr	538
0	45	62	671	8.2	774	[41]877	0	0	0.27	0.27	1.9	0	539
0	9	13	139	1.7	160	[41]181	0	0	0.06	0.06	0.4	0	540
0	37	53	554	5.3	689	[42]814	0	0	0.55	0.23	2.3	0	541
0	8	12	121	1.2	150	[42]177	0	0	0.12	0.05	0.5	0	542
0	76	41	153	1.3	847	3	30	3	0.35	0.25	1.9	37	543
0	45	80	273	4.9	475	11	Tr	Tr	0.18	0.09	0.9	0	544
0	7	6	51	1.1	160	9	0	0	0.03	0.01	0.2	1	545
0	12	11	90	1.9	285	16	0	0	0.05	0.02	0.4	3	546
0	44	14	99	1.8	313	244	0	0	0.03	0.02	0.4	1	547
0	18	216	359	3.8	512	3	80	8	0.58	0.13	1.3	1	548
0	4	53	88	0.9	126	1	20	2	0.14	0.03	0.3	Tr	549
0	38	50	238	4.2	498	26	40	4	0.14	0.12	1.2	0	550
0	17	60	268	2.4	441	[43]348	10	1	0.29	0.15	2.7	0	551
0	4	13	57	0.5	93	[43]74	Tr	Tr	0.06	0.03	0.6	0	552
0	7	20	123	1.0	169	[44]190	Tr	Tr	0.06	0.06	1.3	0	553
0	6	31	131	0.9	165	[44]185	10	1	0.14	0.06	1.4	Tr	554
0	27	125	734	2.8	1,019	[45]626	0	0	0.42	0.15	21.5	0	555
0	5	24	143	0.5	199	[45]122	0	0	0.08	0.03	4.2	0	556
0	3	5	60	0.3	110	75	0	0	0.02	0.02	2.2	0	557
0	42	22	178	3.4	592	26	80	8	0.30	0.18	1.8	0	558
0	20	39	314	2.3	423	1	140	14	0.92	0.14	1.0	2	559
0	5	10	83	0.6	111	Tr	40	4	0.24	0.04	0.3	1	560
0	5	2	10	0.9	178	20	10	1	0.35	0.06	1.2	1	561
0	7	38	143	1.9	310	2	70	7	0.23	0.05	0.3	Tr	562
0	5	12	333	4.2	229	5	110	11	0.06	0.09	0.5	Tr	563
0	51	141	245	5.1	1,141	1,228	0	0	0.14	0.16	1.4	17	564
0	1	11	62	0.6	33	3	10	1	0.06	0.01	0.4	0	565
0	19	131	322	4.9	972	4	50	5	0.38	0.16	1.1	0	566
0	65	188	853	4.7	922	8,142	110	11	0.17	0.28	0.8	0	567
0	3	108	151	2.3	50	8	0	0	0.07	0.04	0.1	0	568
0	5	33	200	1.9	195	1	10	1	0.65	0.07	1.3	Tr	569
0	3	21	119	0.7	69	5	10	1	0.24	0.02	0.8	1	570

[44]Mixed nuts without salt contain 3 mg sodium per oz.
[45]Peanuts without salt contain 22 mg sodium per cup or 4 mg per oz.

Nutritive Value of the Edible Part of Food (Continued)

(Tr indicates nutrient present in trace amount.)

Item No.	Foods, approximate measures, units, and weight (weight of edible portion only)			Water	Food energy	Pro-tein	Fat	Fatty acids		
								Satu-rated	Mono-unsatu-rated	Poly-unsatu-rated
			Grams	Per-cent	Cal-ories	Grams	Grams	Grams	Grams	Grams
	Legumes, Nuts, and Seeds—Con.									
	Walnuts:									
571	Black, chopped-----------------	1 cup----------	125	4	760	30	71	4.5	15.9	46.9
572		1 oz-----------	28	4	170	7	16	1.0	3.6	10.6
573	English or Persian, pieces or chips----------------------	1 cup----------	120	4	770	17	74	6.7	17.0	47.0
574		1 oz-----------	28	4	180	4	18	1.6	4.0	11.1
	Meat and Meat Products									
	Beef, cooked:[46]									
	Cuts braised, simmered, or pot roasted:									
	Relatively fat such as chuck blade:									
575	Lean and fat, piece, 2-1/2 by 2-1/2 by 3/4 in-------	3 oz-----------	85	43	325	22	26	10.8	11.7	0.9
576	Lean only from item 575----	2.2 oz---------	62	53	170	19	9	3.9	4.2	0.3
	Relatively lean, such as bottom round:									
577	Lean and fat, piece, 4-1/8 by 2-1/4 by 1/2 in-------	3 oz-----------	85	54	220	25	13	4.8	5.7	0.5
578	Lean only from item 577----	2.8 oz---------	78	57	175	25	8	2.7	3.4	0.3
	Ground beef, broiled, patty, 3 by 5/8 in:									
579	Lean------------------------	3 oz-----------	85	56	230	21	16	6.2	6.9	0.6
580	Regular---------------------	3 oz-----------	85	54	245	20	18	6.9	7.7	0.7
581	Heart, lean, braised-----------	3 oz-----------	85	65	150	24	5	1.2	0.8	1.6
582	Liver, fried, slice, 6-1/2 by 2-3/8 by 3/8 in[47]-----------	3 oz-----------	85	56	185	23	7	2.5	3.6	1.3
	Roast, oven cooked, no liquid added:									
	Relatively fat, such as rib:									
583	Lean and fat, 2 pieces, 4-1/8 by 2-1/4 by 1/4 in	3 oz-----------	85	46	315	19	26	10.8	11.4	0.9
584	Lean only from item 583----	2.2 oz---------	61	57	150	17	9	3.6	3.7	0.3
	Relatively lean, such as eye of round:									
585	Lean and fat, 2 pieces, 2-1/2 by 2-1/2 by 3/8 in	3 oz-----------	85	57	205	23	12	4.9	5.4	0.5
586	Lean only from item 585----	2.6 oz---------	75	63	135	22	5	1.9	2.1	0.2
	Steak:									
	Sirloin, broiled:									
587	Lean and fat, piece, 2-1/2 by 2-1/2 by 3/4 in	3 oz-----------	85	53	240	23	15	6.4	6.9	0.6
588	Lean only from item 587----	2.5 oz---------	72	59	150	22	6	2.6	2.8	0.3
589	Beef, canned, corned------------	3 oz-----------	85	59	185	22	10	4.2	4.9	0.4
590	Beef, dried, chipped-------------	2.5 oz---------	72	48	145	24	4	1.8	2.0	0.2
	Lamb, cooked:									
	Chops, (3 per lb with bone):									
	Arm, braised:									
591	Lean and fat---------------	2.2 oz---------	63	44	220	20	15	6.9	6.0	0.9
592	Lean only from item 591----	1.7 oz---------	48	49	135	17	7	2.9	2.6	0.4
	Loin, broiled:									
593	Lean and fat---------------	2.8 oz---------	80	54	235	22	16	7.3	6.4	1.0
594	Lean only from item 593----	2.3 oz---------	64	61	140	19	6	2.6	2.4	0.4
	Leg, roasted:									
595	Lean and fat, 2 pieces, 4-1/8 by 2-1/4 by 1/4 in---------	3 oz-----------	85	59	205	22	13	5.6	4.9	0.8
596	Lean only from item 595------	2.6 oz---------	73	64	140	20	6	2.4	2.2	0.4
	Rib, roasted:									
597	Lean and fat, 3 pieces, 2-1/2 by 2-1/2 by 1/4 in---------	3 oz-----------	85	47	315	18	26	12.1	10.6	1.5
598	Lean only from item 597------	2 oz-----------	57	60	130	15	7	3.2	3.0	0.5

[46]Outer layer of fat was removed to within approximately 1/2 inch of the lean. Deposits of fat within the cut were not removed.
[47]Fried in vegetable shortening.

Nutrients in Indicated Quantity

| Cholesterol | Carbohydrate | Calcium | Phosphorus | Iron | Potassium | Sodium | Vitamin A value | | Thiamin | Riboflavin | Niacin | Ascorbic acid | Item No. |
							(IU)	(RE)					
Milligrams	Grams	Milligrams	Milligrams	Milligrams	Milligrams	Milligrams	International units	Retinol equivalents	Milligrams	Milligrams	Milligrams	Milligrams	
0	15	73	580	3.8	655	1	370	37	0.27	0.14	0.9	Tr	571
0	3	16	132	0.9	149	Tr	80	8	0.06	0.03	0.2	Tr	572
0	22	113	380	2.9	602	12	150	15	0.46	0.18	1.3	4	573
0	5	27	90	0.7	142	3	40	4	0.11	0.04	0.3	1	574
87	0	11	163	2.5	163	53	Tr	Tr	0.06	0.19	2.0	0	575
66	0	8	146	2.3	163	44	Tr	Tr	0.05	0.17	1.7	0	576
81	0	5	217	2.8	248	43	Tr	Tr	0.06	0.21	3.3	0	577
75	0	4	212	2.7	240	40	Tr	Tr	0.06	0.20	3.0	0	578
74	0	9	134	1.8	256	65	Tr	Tr	0.04	0.18	4.4	0	579
76	0	9	144	2.1	248	70	Tr	Tr	0.03	0.16	4.9	0	580
164	0	5	213	6.4	198	54	Tr	Tr	0.12	1.31	3.4	5	581
410	7	9	392	5.3	309	90	[48]30,690	[48]9,120	0.18	3.52	12.3	23	582
72	0	8	145	2.0	246	54	Tr	Tr	0.06	0.16	3.1	0	583
49	0	5	127	1.7	218	45	Tr	Tr	0.05	0.13	2.7	0	584
62	0	5	177	1.6	308	50	Tr	Tr	0.07	0.14	3.0	0	585
52	0	3	170	1.5	297	46	Tr	Tr	0.07	0.13	2.8	0	586
77	0	9	186	2.6	306	53	Tr	Tr	0.10	0.23	3.3	0	587
64	0	8	176	2.4	290	48	Tr	Tr	0.09	0.22	3.1	0	588
80	0	17	90	3.7	51	802	Tr	Tr	0.02	0.20	2.9	0	589
46	0	14	287	2.3	142	3,053	Tr	Tr	0.05	0.23	2.7	0	590
77	0	16	132	1.5	195	46	Tr	Tr	0.04	0.16	4.4	0	591
59	0	12	111	1.3	162	36	Tr	Tr	0.03	0.13	3.0	0	592
78	0	16	162	1.4	272	62	Tr	Tr	0.09	0.21	5.5	0	593
60	0	12	145	1.3	241	54	Tr	Tr	0.08	0.18	4.4	0	594
78	0	8	162	1.7	273	57	Tr	Tr	0.09	0.24	5.5	0	595
65	0	6	150	1.5	247	50	Tr	Tr	0.08	0.20	4.6	0	596
77	0	19	139	1.4	224	60	Tr	Tr	0.08	0.18	5.5	0	597
50	0	12	111	1.0	179	46	Tr	Tr	0.05	0.13	3.5	0	598

[48] Value varies widely.

Nutritive Value of the Edible Part of Food (Continued)

(Tr indicates nutrient present in trace amount.)

Item No.	Foods, approximate measures, units, and weight (weight of edible portion only)			Water	Food energy	Pro-tein	Fat	Fatty acids		
								Satu-rated	Mono-unsatu-rated	Poly-unsatu-rated
	Meat and Meat Products—Con.		Grams	Per-cent	Cal-ories	Grams	Grams	Grams	Grams	Grams
	Pork, cured, cooked:									
	Bacon:									
599	Regular----------------------	3 medium slices	19	13	110	6	9	3.3	4.5	1.1
600	Canadian-style---------------	2 slices--------	46	62	85	11	4	1.3	1.9	0.4
	Ham, light cure, roasted:									
601	Lean and fat, 2 pieces, 4-1/4 by 2-1/4 by 1/4 in---------	3 oz------------	85	58	205	18	14	5.1	6.7	1.5
602	Lean only from item 601------	2.4 oz----------	68	66	105	17	4	1.3	1.7	0.4
603	Ham, canned, roasted, 2 pieces, 4-1/8 by 2-1/4 by 1/4 in-----	3 oz------------	85	67	140	18	7	2.4	3.5	0.8
	Luncheon meat:									
604	Canned, spiced or unspiced, slice, 3 by 2 by 1/2 in----	2 slices--------	42	52	140	5	13	4.5	6.0	1.5
605	Chopped ham (8 slices per 6 oz pkg)--------------------	2 slices--------	42	64	95	7	7	2.4	3.4	0.9
	Cooked ham (8 slices per 8-oz pkg):									
606	Regular------------------	2 slices--------	57	65	105	10	6	1.9	2.8	0.7
607	Extra lean--------------	2 slices--------	57	71	75	11	3	0.9	1.3	0.3
	Pork, fresh, cooked:									
	Chop, loin (cut 3 per lb with bone):									
	Broiled:									
608	Lean and fat--------------	3.1 oz----------	87	50	275	24	19	7.0	8.8	2.2
609	Lean only from item 608----	2.5 oz----------	72	57	165	23	8	2.6	3.4	0.9
	Pan fried:									
610	Lean and fat--------------	3.1 oz----------	89	45	335	21	27	9.8	12.5	3.1
611	Lean only from item 610----	2.4 oz----------	67	54	180	19	11	3.7	4.8	1.3
	Ham (leg), roasted:									
612	Lean and fat, piece, 2-1/2 by 2-1/2 by 3/4 in------------	3 oz------------	85	53	250	21	18	6.4	8.1	2.0
613	Lean only from item 612------	2.5 oz----------	72	60	160	20	8	2.7	3.6	1.0
	Rib, roasted:									
614	Lean and fat, piece, 2-1/2 by 3/4 in---------------------	3 oz------------	85	51	270	21	20	7.2	9.2	2.3
615	Lean only from item 614------	2.5 oz----------	71	57	175	20	10	3.4	4.4	1.2
	Shoulder cut, braised:									
616	Lean and fat, 3 pieces, 2-1/2 by 2-1/2 by 1/4 in---------	3 oz------------	85	47	295	23	22	7.9	10.0	2.4
617	Lean only from item 616------	2.4 oz----------	67	54	165	22	8	2.8	3.7	1.0
	Sausages (See also Luncheon meats, items 604-607):									
618	Bologna, slice (8 per 8-oz pkg)	2 slices--------	57	54	180	7	16	6.1	7.6	1.4
619	Braunschweiger, slice (6 per 6-oz pkg)--------------------	2 slices--------	57	48	205	8	18	6.2	8.5	2.1
620	Brown and serve (10-11 per 8-oz pkg), browned-----------	1 link----------	13	45	50	2	5	1.7	2.2	0.5
621	Frankfurter (10 per 1-lb pkg), cooked (reheated)------------	1 frankfurter---	45	54	145	5	13	4.8	6.2	1.2
622	Pork link (16 per 1-lb pkg), cooked[50] --------------------	1 link----------	13	45	50	3	4	1.4	1.8	0.5
	Salami:									
623	Cooked type, slice (8 per 8-oz pkg)------------------	2 slices--------	57	60	145	8	11	4.6	5.2	1.2
624	Dry type, slice (12 per 4-oz pkg)----------------------	2 slices--------	20	35	85	5	7	2.4	3.4	0.6
625	Sandwich spread (pork, beef)---	1 tbsp----------	15	60	35	1	3	0.9	1.1	0.4
626	Vienna sausage (7 per 4-oz can)	1 sausage-------	16	60	45	2	4	1.5	2.0	0.3
	Veal, medium fat, cooked, bone removed:									
627	Cutlet, 4-1/8 by 2-1/4 by 1/2 in, braised or broiled-------	3 oz------------	85	60	185	23	9	4.1	4.1	0.6
628	Rib, 2 pieces, 4-1/8 by 2-1/4 by 1/4 in, roasted-----------	3 oz------------	85	55	230	23	14	6.0	6.0	1.0

[49] Contains added sodium ascorbate. If sodium ascorbate is not added, ascorbic acid content is negligible.

Nutrients in Indicated Quantity

Cholesterol	Carbohydrate	Calcium	Phosphorus	Iron	Potassium	Sodium	Vitamin A value (IU)	Vitamin A value (RE)	Thiamin	Riboflavin	Niacin	Ascorbic acid	Item No.
Milligrams	Grams	Milligrams	Milligrams	Milligrams	Milligrams	Milligrams	International units	Retinol equivalents	Milligrams	Milligrams	Milligrams	Milligrams	
16	Tr	2	64	0.3	92	303	0	0	0.13	0.05	1.4	6	599
27	1	5	136	0.4	179	711	0	0	0.38	0.09	3.2	10	600
53	0	6	182	0.7	243	1,009	0	0	0.51	0.19	3.8	0	601
37	0	5	154	0.6	215	902	0	0	0.46	0.17	3.4	0	602
35	Tr	6	188	0.9	298	908	0	0	0.82	0.21	4.3	[49]19	603
26	1	3	34	0.3	90	541	0	0	0.15	0.08	1.3	Tr	604
21	0	3	65	0.3	134	576	0	0	0.27	0.09	1.6	[49]8	605
32	2	4	141	0.6	189	751	0	0	0.49	0.14	3.0	[49]16	606
27	1	4	124	0.4	200	815	0	0	0.53	0.13	2.8	[49]15	607
84	0	3	184	0.7	312	61	10	3	0.87	0.24	4.3	Tr	608
71	0	4	176	0.7	302	56	10	1	0.83	0.22	4.0	Tr	609
92	0	4	190	0.7	323	64	10	3	0.91	0.24	4.6	Tr	610
72	0	3	178	0.7	305	57	10	1	0.84	0.22	4.0	Tr	611
79	0	5	210	0.9	280	50	10	2	0.54	0.27	3.9	Tr	612
68	0	5	202	0.8	269	46	10	1	0.50	0.25	3.6	Tr	613
69	0	9	190	0.8	313	37	10	3	0.50	0.24	4.2	Tr	614
56	0	8	182	0.7	300	33	10	2	0.45	0.22	3.8	Tr	615
93	0	6	162	1.4	286	75	10	3	0.46	0.26	4.4	Tr	616
76	0	5	151	1.3	271	68	10	1	0.40	0.24	4.0	Tr	617
31	2	7	52	0.9	103	581	0	0	0.10	0.08	1.5	[49]12	618
89	2	5	96	5.3	113	652	8,010	2,405	0.14	0.87	4.8	[49]6	619
9	Tr	1	14	0.1	25	105	0	0	0.05	0.02	0.4	0	620
23	1	5	39	0.5	75	504	0	0	0.09	0.05	1.2	[49]12	621
11	Tr	4	24	0.2	47	168	0	0	0.10	0.03	0.6	Tr	622
37	1	7	66	1.5	113	607	0	0	0.14	0.21	2.0	[49]7	623
16	1	2	28	0.3	76	372	0	0	0.12	0.06	1.0	[49]5	624
6	2	2	9	0.1	17	152	10	1	0.03	0.02	0.3	0	625
8	Tr	2	8	0.1	16	152	0	0	0.01	0.02	0.3	0	626
109	0	9	196	0.8	258	56	Tr	Tr	0.06	0.21	4.6	0	627
109	0	10	211	0.7	259	57	Tr	Tr	0.11	0.26	6.6	0	628

¹One patty (8 per pound) of bulk sausage is equivalent to 2 links.

Nutritive Value of the Edible Part of Food (Continued)

(Tr indicates nutrient present in trace amount.)

Item No.	Foods, approximate measures, units, and weight (weight of edible portion only)			Water	Food energy	Pro-tein	Fat	Fatty acids		
								Satu-rated	Mono-unsatu-rated	Poly-unsatu-rated
	Mixed Dishes and Fast Foods		Grams	Per-cent	Cal-ories	Grams	Grams	Grams	Grams	Grams
	Mixed dishes:									
629	Beef and vegetable stew, from home recipe-----------------	1 cup----------	245	82	220	16	11	4.4	4.5	0.5
630	Beef potpie, from home recipe, baked, piece, 1/3 of 9-in diam. pie[51] ------------------	1 piece---------	210	55	515	21	30	7.9	12.9	7.4
631	Chicken a la king, cooked, from home recipe------------	1 cup----------	245	68	470	27	34	12.9	13.4	6.2
632	Chicken and noodles, cooked, from home recipe------------	1 cup----------	240	71	365	22	18	5.1	7.1	3.9
	Chicken chow mein:									
633	Canned----------------------	1 cup----------	250	89	95	7	Tr	0.1	0.1	0.8
634	From home recipe-----------	1 cup----------	250	78	255	31	10	4.1	4.9	3.5
635	Chicken potpie, from home recipe, baked, piece, 1/3 of 9-in diam. pie[51] -------------	1 piece---------	232	57	545	23	31	10.3	15.5	6.6
636	Chili con carne with beans, canned---------------------	1 cup----------	255	72	340	19	16	5.8	7.2	1.0
637	Chop suey with beef and pork, from home recipe-----------	1 cup----------	250	75	300	26	17	4.3	7.4	4.2
	Macaroni (enriched) and cheese:									
638	Canned[52] ----------------------	1 cup----------	240	80	230	9	10	4.7	2.9	1.3
639	From home recipe[38] -----------	1 cup----------	200	58	430	17	22	9.8	7.4	3.6
640	Quiche Lorraine, 1/8 of 8-in diam. quiche[51] ---------------	1 slice---------	176	47	600	13	48	23.2	17.8	4.1
	Spaghetti (enriched) in tomato sauce with cheese:									
641	Canned-----------------------	1 cup----------	250	80	190	6	2	0.4	0.4	0.5
642	From home recipe-------------	1 cup----------	250	77	260	9	9	3.0	3.6	1.2
	Spaghetti (enriched) with meat-balls and tomato sauce:									
643	Canned-----------------------	1 cup----------	250	78	260	12	10	2.4	3.9	3.1
644	From home recipe-------------	1 cup----------	248	70	330	19	12	3.9	4.4	2.2
	Fast food entrees:									
	Cheeseburger:									
645	Regular----------------------	1 sandwich------	112	46	300	15	15	7.3	5.6	1.0
646	4 oz patty-------------------	1 sandwich------	194	46	525	30	31	15.1	12.2	1.4
	Chicken, fried. See Poultry and Poultry Products (items 656-659).									
647	Enchilada---------------------	1 enchilada-----	230	72	235	20	16	7.7	6.7	0.6
648	English muffin, egg, cheese, and bacon--------------------	1 sandwich------	138	49	360	18	18	8.0	8.0	0.7
	Fish sandwich:									
649	Regular, with cheese---------	1 sandwich------	140	43	420	16	23	6.3	6.9	7.7
650	Large, without cheese--------	1 sandwich------	170	48	470	18	27	6.3	8.7	9.5
	Hamburger:									
651	Regular----------------------	1 sandwich------	98	46	245	12	11	4.4	5.3	0.5
652	4 oz patty-------------------	1 sandwich------	174	50	445	25	21	7.1	11.7	0.6
653	Pizza, cheese, 1/8 of 15-in diam. pizza[51] ---------------	1 slice---------	120	46	290	15	9	4.1	2.6	1.3
654	Roast beef sandwich------------	1 sandwich------	150	52	345	22	13	3.5	6.9	1.8
655	Taco-------------------------	1 taco---------	81	55	195	9	11	4.1	5.5	0.8

[38] Made with margarine.
[51] Crust made with vegetable shortening and enriched flour.

							Vitamin A value						
Cho-les-terol	Carbo-hydrate	Calcium	Phos-phorus	Iron	Potas-sium	Sodium	(IU)	(RE)	Thiamin	Ribo-flavin	Niacin	Ascorbic acid	Item No.
Milli-grams	Grams	Milli-grams	Milli-grams	Milli-grams	Milli-grams	Milli-grams	Inter-national units	Retinol equiva-lents	Milli-grams	Milli-grams	Milli-grams	Milli-grams	
71	15	29	184	2.9	613	292	5,690	568	0.15	0.17	4.7	17	629
42	39	29	149	3.8	334	596	4,220	517	0.29	0.29	4.8	6	630
221	12	127	358	2.5	404	760	1,130	272	0.10	0.42	5.4	12	631
103	26	26	247	2.2	149	600	430	130	0.05	0.17	4.3	Tr	632
8	18	45	85	1.3	418	725	150	28	0.05	0.10	1.0	13	633
75	10	58	293	2.5	473	718	280	50	0.08	0.23	4.3	10	634
56	42	70	232	3.0	343	594	7,220	735	0.32	0.32	4.9	5	635
28	31	82	321	4.3	594	1,354	150	15	0.08	0.18	3.3	8	636
68	13	60	248	4.8	425	1,053	600	60	0.28	0.38	5.0	33	637
24	26	199	182	1.0	139	730	260	72	0.12	0.24	1.0	Tr	638
44	40	362	322	1.8	240	1,086	860	232	0.20	0.40	1.8	1	639
285	29	211	276	1.0	283	653	1,640	454	0.11	0.32	Tr	Tr	640
3	39	40	88	2.8	303	955	930	120	0.35	0.28	4.5	10	641
8	37	80	135	2.3	408	955	1,080	140	0.25	0.18	2.3	13	642
23	29	53	113	3.3	245	1,220	1,000	100	0.15	0.18	2.3	5	643
89	39	124	236	3.7	665	1,009	1,590	159	0.25	0.30	4.0	22	644
44	28	135	174	2.3	219	672	340	65	0.26	0.24	3.7	1	645
104	40	236	320	4.5	407	1,224	670	128	0.33	0.48	7.4	3	646
19	24	97	198	3.3	653	1,332	2,720	352	0.18	0.26	Tr	Tr	647
213	31	197	290	3.1	201	832	650	160	0.46	0.50	3.7	1	648
56	39	132	223	1.8	274	667	160	25	0.32	0.26	3.3	2	649
91	41	61	246	2.2	375	621	110	15	0.35	0.23	3.5	1	650
32	28	56	107	2.2	202	463	80	14	0.23	0.24	3.8	1	651
71	38	75	225	4.8	404	763	160	28	0.38	0.38	7.8	1	652
56	39	220	216	1.6	230	699	750	106	0.34	0.29	4.2	2	653
55	34	60	222	4.0	338	757	240	32	0.40	0.33	6.0	2	654
21	15	109	134	1.2	263	456	420	57	0.09	0.07	1.4	1	655

[52]Made with corn oil.

Nutritive Value of the Edible Part of Food (Continued)

(Tr indicates nutrient present in trace amount.)

Item No.	Foods, approximate measures, units, and weight (weight of edible portion only)			Water	Food energy	Pro-tein	Fat	Fatty acids		
								Satu-rated	Mono-unsatu-rated	Poly-unsatu-rated
			Grams	Per-cent	Cal-ories	Grams	Grams	Grams	Grams	Grams
	Poultry and Poultry Products									
	Chicken:									
	Fried, flesh, with skin:[53]									
	Batter dipped:									
656	Breast, 1/2 breast (5.6 oz with bones)--------------	4.9 oz----------	140	52	365	35	18	4.9	7.6	4.3
657	Drumstick (3.4 oz with bones)-------------------	2.5 oz----------	72	53	195	16	11	3.0	4.6	2.7
	Flour coated:									
658	Breast, 1/2 breast (4.2 oz with bones)--------------	3.5 oz----------	98	57	220	31	9	2.4	3.4	1.9
659	Drumstick (2.6 oz with bones)-------------------	1.7 oz----------	49	57	120	13	7	1.8	2.7	1.6
	Roasted, flesh only:									
660	Breast, 1/2 breast (4.2 oz with bones and skin)-------	3.0 oz----------	86	65	140	27	3	0.9	1.1	0.7
661	Drumstick, (2.9 oz with bones and skin)------------------	1.6 oz----------	44	67	75	12	2	0.7	0.8	0.6
662	Stewed, flesh only, light and dark meat, chopped or diced--	1 cup----------	140	67	250	38	9	2.6	3.3	2.2
663	Chicken liver, cooked------------	1 liver--------	20	68	30	5	1	0.4	0.3	0.2
664	Duck, roasted, flesh only--------	1/2 duck--------	221	64	445	52	25	9.2	8.2	3.2
	Turkey, roasted, flesh only:									
665	Dark meat, piece, 2-1/2 by 1-5/8 by 1/4 in--------------	4 pieces--------	85	63	160	24	6	2.1	1.4	1.8
666	Light meat, piece, 4 by 2 by 1/4 in----------------------	2 pieces--------	85	66	135	25	3	0.9	0.5	0.7
	Light and dark meat:									
667	Chopped or diced----------	1 cup----------	140	65	240	41	7	2.3	1.4	2.0
668	Pieces (1 slice white meat, 4 by 2 by 1/4 in and 2 slices dark meat, 2-1/2 by 1-5/8 by 1/4 in)--------	3 pieces--------	85	65	145	25	4	1.4	0.9	1.2
	Poultry food products:									
	Chicken:									
669	Canned, boneless-------------	5 oz------------	142	69	235	31	11	3.1	4.5	2.5
670	Frankfurter (10 per 1-lb pkg)	1 frankfurter---	45	58	115	6	9	2.5	3.8	1.8
671	Roll, light (6 slices per 6 oz pkg)--------------------	2 slices--------	57	69	90	11	4	1.1	1.7	0.9
	Turkey:									
672	Gravy and turkey, frozen-----	5-oz package----	142	85	95	8	4	1.2	1.4	0.7
673	Ham, cured turkey thigh meat (8 slices per 8-oz pkg)----	2 slices--------	57	71	75	11	3	1.0	0.7	0.9
674	Loaf, breast meat (8 slices per 6-oz pkg)--------------	2 slices--------	42	72	45	10	1	0.2	0.2	0.1
675	Patties, breaded, battered, fried (2.25 oz)-----------	1 patty---------	64	50	180	9	12	3.0	4.8	3.0
676	Roast, boneless, frozen, sea-soned, light and dark meat, cooked--------------------	3 oz------------	85	68	130	18	5	1.6	1.0	1.4
	Soups, Sauces, and Gravies									
	Soups:									
	Canned, condensed:									
	Prepared with equal volume of milk:									
677	Clam chowder, New England--	1 cup----------	248	85	165	9	7	3.0	2.3	1.1
678	Cream of chicken----------	1 cup----------	248	85	190	7	11	4.6	4.5	1.6
679	Cream of mushroom----------	1 cup----------	248	85	205	6	14	5.1	3.0	4.6
680	Tomato--------------------	1 cup----------	248	85	160	6	6	2.9	1.6	1.1

[53] Fried in vegetable shortening.

Nutrients in Indicated Quantity

Cho-les-terol	Carbo-hydrate	Calcium	Phos-phorus	Iron	Potas-sium	Sodium	Vitamin A value		Thiamin	Ribo-flavin	Niacin	Ascorbic acid	Item No.
							(IU)	(RE)					
Milli-grams	Grams	Milli-grams	Milli-grams	Milli-grams	Milli-grams	Milli-grams	Inter-national units	Retinol equiva-lents	Milli-grams	Milli-grams	Milli-grams	Milli-grams	
119	13	28	259	1.8	281	385	90	28	0.16	0.20	14.7	0	656
62	6	12	106	1.0	134	194	60	19	0.08	0.15	3.7	0	657
87	2	16	228	1.2	254	74	50	15	0.08	0.13	13.5	0	658
44	1	6	86	0.7	112	44	40	12	0.04	0.11	3.0	0	659
73	0	13	196	0.9	220	64	20	5	0.06	0.10	11.8	0	660
41	0	5	81	0.6	108	42	30	8	0.03	0.10	2.7	0	661
116	0	20	210	1.6	252	98	70	21	0.07	0.23	8.6	0	662
126	Tr	3	62	1.7	28	10	3,270	983	0.03	0.35	0.9	3	663
197	0	27	449	6.0	557	144	170	51	0.57	1.04	11.3	0	664
72	0	27	173	2.0	246	67	0	0	0.05	0.21	3.1	0	665
59	0	16	186	1.1	259	54	0	0	0.05	0.11	5.8	0	666
106	0	35	298	2.5	417	98	0	0	0.09	0.25	7.6	0	667
65	0	21	181	1.5	253	60	0	0	0.05	0.15	4.6	0	668
88	0	20	158	2.2	196	714	170	48	0.02	0.18	9.0	3	669
45	3	43	48	0.9	38	616	60	17	0.03	0.05	1.4	0	670
28	1	24	89	0.6	129	331	50	14	0.04	0.07	3.0	0	671
26	7	20	115	1.3	87	787	60	18	0.03	0.18	2.6	0	672
32	Tr	6	108	1.6	184	565	0	0	0.03	0.14	2.0	0	673
17	0	3	97	0.2	118	608	0	0	0.02	0.05	3.5	[54]0	674
40	10	9	173	1.4	176	512	20	7	0.06	0.12	1.5	0	675
45	3	4	207	1.4	253	578	0	0	0.04	0.14	5.3	0	676
22	17	186	156	1.5	300	992	160	40	0.07	0.24	1.0	3	677
27	15	181	151	0.7	273	1,047	710	94	0.07	0.26	0.9	1	678
20	15	179	156	0.6	270	1,076	150	37	0.08	0.28	0.9	2	679
17	22	159	149	1.8	449	932	850	109	0.13	0.25	1.5	68	680

[54]If sodium ascorbate is added, product contains 11 mg ascorbic acid.

Nutritive Value of the Edible Part of Food (Continued)

(Tr indicates nutrient present in trace amount.)

Item No.	Foods, approximate measures, units, and weight (weight of edible portion only)		Water	Food energy	Pro-tein	Fat	Fatty acids		
							Satu-rated	Mono-unsatu-rated	Poly-unsatu-rated
		Grams	Per-cent	Cal-ories	Grams	Grams	Grams	Grams	Grams
	Soups, Sauces, and Gravies—Con.								
	Soups:								
	Canned, condensed:								
	Prepared with equal volume of water:								
681	Bean with bacon----------- 1 cup-----------	253	84	170	8	6	1.5	2.2	1.8
682	Beef broth, bouillon, consomme---------------- 1 cup-----------	240	98	15	3	1	0.3	0.2	Tr
683	Beef noodle------------ 1 cup-----------	244	92	85	5	3	1.1	1.2	0.5
684	Chicken noodle----------- 1 cup-----------	241	92	75	4	2	0.7	1.1	0.6
685	Chicken rice-------------- 1 cup-----------	241	94	60	4	2	0.5	0.9	0.4
686	Clam chowder, Manhattan---- 1 cup-----------	244	90	80	4	2	0.4	0.4	1.3
687	Cream of chicken---------- 1 cup-----------	244	91	115	3	7	2.1	3.3	1.5
688	Cream of mushroom--------- 1 cup-----------	244	90	130	2	9	2.4	1.7	4.2
689	Minestrone--------------- 1 cup-----------	241	91	80	4	3	0.6	0.7	1.1
690	Pea, green--------------- 1 cup-----------	250	83	165	9	3	1.4	1.0	0.4
691	Tomato------------------ 1 cup-----------	244	90	85	2	2	0.4	0.4	1.0
692	Vegetable beef----------- 1 cup-----------	244	92	80	6	2	0.9	0.8	0.1
693	Vegetarian-------------- 1 cup-----------	241	92	70	2	2	0.3	0.8	0.7
	Dehydrated:								
	Unprepared:								
694	Bouillon------------- 1 pkt-----------	6	3	15	1	1	0.3	0.2	Tr
695	Onion---------------- 1 pkt-----------	7	4	20	1	Tr	0.1	0.2	Tr
	Prepared with water:								
696	Chicken noodle------------ 1 pkt (6-fl-oz)	188	94	40	2	1	0.2	0.4	0.3
697	Onion-------------------- 1 pkt (6-fl-oz)	184	96	20	1	Tr	0.1	0.2	0.1
698	Tomato vegetable---------- 1 pkt (6-fl-oz)	189	94	40	1	1	0.3	0.2	0.1
	Sauces:								
	From dry mix:								
699	Cheese, prepared with milk--- 1 cup-----------	279	77	305	16	17	9.3	5.3	1.6
700	Hollandaise, prepared with water-------------------- 1 cup-----------	259	84	240	5	20	11.6	5.9	0.9
701	White sauce, prepared with milk--------------------- 1 cup-----------	264	81	240	10	13	6.4	4.7	1.7
	From home recipe:								
702	White sauce, medium[55]-------- 1 cup-----------	250	73	395	10	30	9.1	11.9	7.2
	Ready to serve:								
703	Barbecue--------------------- 1 tbsp----------	16	81	10	Tr	Tr	Tr	0.1	0.1
704	Soy------------------------- 1 tbsp----------	18	68	10	2	0	0.0	0.0	0.0
	Gravies:								
	Canned:								
705	Beef----------------------- 1 cup-----------	233	87	125	9	5	2.7	2.3	0.2
706	Chicken-------------------- 1 cup-----------	238	85	190	5	14	3.4	6.1	3.6
707	Mushroom------------------- 1 cup-----------	238	89	120	3	6	1.0	2.8	2.4
	From dry mix:								
708	Brown---------------------- 1 cup-----------	261	91	80	3	2	0.9	0.8	0.1
709	Chicken-------------------- 1 cup-----------	260	91	85	3	2	0.5	0.9	0.4
	Sugars and Sweets								
	Candy:								
710	Caramels, plain or chocolate--- 1 oz-----------	28	8	115	1	3	2.2	0.3	0.1
	Chocolate:								
711	Milk, plain------------------- 1 oz-----------	28	1	145	2	9	5.4	3.0	0.3
712	Milk, with almonds----------- 1 oz-----------	28	2	150	3	10	4.8	4.1	0.7
713	Milk, with peanuts----------- 1 oz-----------	28	1	155	4	11	4.2	3.5	1.5
714	Milk, with rice cereal------- 1 oz-----------	28	2	140	2	7	4.4	2.5	0.2
715	Semisweet, small pieces (60 per oz)-------------------- 1 cup or 6 oz---	170	1	860	7	61	36.2	19.9	1.9
716	Sweet (dark)---------------- 1 oz-----------	28	1	150	1	10	5.9	3.3	0.3
717	Fondant, uncoated (mints, candy corn, other)------------------ 1 oz-----------	28	3	105	Tr	0	0.0	0.0	0.0
718	Fudge, chocolate, plain-------- 1 oz-----------	28	8	115	1	3	2.1	1.0	0.1
719	Gum drops--------------------- 1 oz-----------	28	12	100	Tr	Tr	Tr	Tr	0.1

[55] Made with enriched flour, margarine, and whole milk.

Nutrients in Indicated Quantity

Cho-les-terol	Carbo-hydrate	Calcium	Phos-phorus	Iron	Potas-sium	Sodium	Vitamin A value		Thiamin	Ribo-flavin	Niacin	Ascorbic acid	Item No.
							(IU)	(RE)					
Milli-grams	Grams	Milli-grams	Milli-grams	Milli-grams	Milli-grams	Milli-grams	Inter-national units	Retinol equiva-lents	Milli-grams	Milli-grams	Milli-grams	Milli-grams	
3	23	81	132	2.0	402	951	890	89	0.09	0.03	0.6	2	681
Tr	Tr	14	31	0.4	130	782	0	0	Tr	0.05	1.9	0	682
5	9	15	46	1.1	100	952	630	63	0.07	0.06	1.1	Tr	683
7	9	17	36	0.8	55	1,106	710	71	0.05	0.06	1.4	Tr	684
7	7	17	22	0.7	101	815	660	66	0.02	0.02	1.1	Tr	685
2	12	34	59	1.9	261	1,808	920	92	0.06	0.05	1.3	3	686
10	9	34	37	0.6	88	986	560	56	0.03	0.06	0.8	Tr	687
2	9	46	49	0.5	100	1,032	0	0	0.05	0.09	0.7	1	688
2	11	34	55	0.9	313	911	2,340	234	0.05	0.04	0.9	1	689
0	27	28	125	2.0	190	988	200	20	0.11	0.07	1.2	2	690
0	17	12	34	1.8	264	871	690	69	0.09	0.05	1.4	65	691
5	10	17	41	1.1	173	956	1,890	189	0.04	0.05	1.0	2	692
0	12	22	34	1.1	210	822	3,010	301	0.05	0.05	0.9	1	693
1	1	4	19	0.1	27	1,019	Tr	Tr	Tr	0.01	0.3	0	694
Tr	4	10	23	0.1	47	627	Tr	Tr	0.02	0.04	0.4	Tr	695
2	6	24	24	0.4	23	957	50	5	0.05	0.04	0.7	Tr	696
0	4	9	22	0.1	48	635	Tr	Tr	0.02	0.04	0.4	Tr	697
0	8	6	23	0.5	78	856	140	14	0.04	0.03	0.6	5	698
53	23	569	438	0.3	552	1,565	390	117	0.15	0.56	0.3	2	699
52	14	124	127	0.9	124	1,564	730	220	0.05	0.18	0.1	Tr	700
34	21	425	256	0.3	444	797	310	92	0.08	0.45	0.5	3	701
32	24	292	238	0.9	381	888	1,190	340	0.15	0.43	0.8	2	702
0	2	3	3	0.1	28	130	140	14	Tr	Tr	0.1	1	703
0	2	3	38	0.5	64	1,029	0	0	0.01	0.02	0.6	0	704
7	11	14	70	1.6	189	117	0	0	0.07	0.08	1.5	0	705
5	13	48	69	1.1	259	1,373	880	264	0.04	0.10	1.1	0	706
0	13	17	36	1.6	252	1,357	0	0	0.08	0.15	1.6	0	707
2	14	66	47	0.2	61	1,147	0	0	0.04	0.09	0.9	0	708
3	14	39	47	0.3	62	1,134	0	0	0.05	0.15	0.8	3	709
1	22	42	35	0.4	54	64	Tr	Tr	0.01	0.05	0.1	Tr	710
6	16	50	61	0.4	96	23	30	10	0.02	0.10	0.1	Tr	711
5	15	65	77	0.5	125	23	30	8	0.02	0.12	0.2	Tr	712
5	13	49	83	0.4	138	19	30	8	0.07	0.07	1.4	Tr	713
6	18	48	57	0.2	100	46	30	8	0.01	0.08	0.1	Tr	714
0	97	51	178	5.8	593	24	30	3	0.10	0.14	0.9	Tr	715
0	16	7	41	0.6	86	5	10	1	0.01	0.04	0.1	Tr	716
0	27	2	Tr	0.1	1	57	0	0	Tr	Tr	Tr	0	717
1	21	22	24	0.3	42	54	Tr	Tr	0.01	0.03	0.1	Tr	718
0	25	2	Tr	0.1	1	10	0	0	0.00	Tr	Tr	0	719

Nutritive Value of the Edible Part of Food (Continued)

(Tr indicates nutrient present in trace amount.)

Item No.	Foods, approximate measures, units, and weight (weight of edible portion only)		Water	Food energy	Pro-tein	Fat	Fatty acids		
							Satu-rated	Mono-unsatu-rated	Poly-unsatu-rated
		Grams	Per-cent	Cal-ories	Grams	Grams	Grams	Grams	Grams
	Sugars and Sweets—Con.								
	Candy:								
720	Hard----------------------- 1 oz------------	28	1	110	0	0	0.0	0.0	0.0
721	Jelly beans-------------------- 1 oz------------	28	6	105	Tr	Tr	Tr	Tr	0.1
722	Marshmallows------------------ 1 oz-----------	28	17	90	1	0	0.0	0.0	0.0
723	Custard, baked---------------- 1 cup-----------	265	77	305	14	15	6.8	5.4	0.7
724	Gelatin dessert prepared with gelatin dessert powder and water----------------------- 1/2 cup---------	120	84	70	2	0	0.0	0.0	0.0
725	Honey, strained or extracted----- 1 cup-----------	339	17	1,030	1	0	0.0	0.0	0.0
726	1 tbsp----------	21	17	65	Tr	0	0.0	0.0	0.0
727	Jams and preserves-------------- 1 tbsp----------	20	29	55	Tr	Tr	0.0	Tr	Tr
728	1 packet--------	14	29	40	Tr	Tr	0.0	Tr	Tr
729	Jellies----------------------- 1 tbsp----------	18	28	50	Tr	Tr	Tr	Tr	Tr
730	1 packet--------	14	28	40	Tr	Tr	Tr	Tr	Tr
731	Popsicle, 3-fl-oz size----------- 1 popsicle------	95	80	70	0	0	0.0	0.0	0.0
	Puddings:								
	Canned:								
732	Chocolate-------------------- 5-oz can--------	142	68	205	3	11	9.5	0.5	0.1
733	Tapioca---------------------- 5-oz can--------	142	74	160	3	5	4.8	Tr	Tr
734	Vanilla---------------------- 5-oz can--------	142	69	220	2	10	9.5	0.2	0.1
	Dry mix, prepared with whole milk:								
	Chocolate:								
735	Instant-------------------- 1/2 cup--------	130	71	155	4	4	2.3	1.1	0.2
736	Regular (cooked)------------ 1/2 cup--------	130	73	150	4	4	2.4	1.1	0.1
737	Rice------------------------- 1/2 cup--------	132	73	155	4	4	2.3	1.1	0.1
738	Tapioca---------------------- 1/2 cup--------	130	75	145	4	4	2.3	1.1	0.1
	Vanilla:								
739	Instant-------------------- 1/2 cup--------	130	73	150	4	4	2.2	1.1	0.2
740	Regular (cooked)------------ 1/2 cup--------	130	74	145	4	4	2.3	1.0	0.1
	Sugars:								
741	Brown, pressed down----------- 1 cup----------	220	2	820	0	0	0.0	0.0	0.0
	White:								
742	Granulated------------------- 1 cup-----------	200	1	770	0	0	0.0	0.0	0.0
743	1 tbsp-----------	12	1	45	0	0	0.0	0.0	0.0
744	1 packet--------	6	1	25	0	0	0.0	0.0	0.0
745	Powdered, sifted, spooned into cup------------------ 1 cup----------	100	1	385	0	0	0.0	0.0	0.0
	Syrups:								
	Chocolate-flavored syrup or topping:								
746	Thin type-------------------- 2 tbsp----------	38	37	85	1	Tr	0.2	0.1	0.1
747	Fudge type------------------- 2 tbsp----------	38	25	125	2	5	3.1	1.7	0.2
748	Molasses, cane, blackstrap----- 2 tbsp----------	40	24	85	0	0	0.0	0.0	0.0
749	Table syrup (corn and maple)--- 2 tbsp----------	42	25	122	0	0	0.0	0.0	0.0
	Vegetables and Vegetable Products								
750	Alfalfa seeds, sprouted, raw----- 1 cup----------	33	91	10	1	Tr	Tr	Tr	0.1
751	Artichokes, globe or French, cooked, drained--------------- 1 artichoke-----	120	87	55	3	Tr	Tr	Tr	0.1
	Asparagus, green:								
	Cooked, drained:								
	From raw:								
752	Cuts and tips-------------- 1 cup-----------	180	92	45	5	1	0.1	Tr	0.2
753	Spears, 1/2-in diam. at base------------------ 4 spears--------	60	92	15	2	Tr	Tr	Tr	0.1
	From frozen:								
754	Cuts and tips-------------- 1 cup-----------	180	91	50	5	1	0.2	Tr	0.3
755	Spears, 1/2-in diam. at base-------------------- 4 spears--------	60	91	15	2	Tr	0.1	Tr	0.1
756	Canned, spears, 1/2-in diam. at base------------------- 4 spears--------	80	95	10	1	Tr	Tr	Tr	0.1
757	Bamboo shoots, canned, drained--- 1 cup-----------	131	94	25	2	1	0.1	Tr	0.2

[56] For regular pack; special dietary pack contains 3 mg sodium.

Nutrients in Indicated Quantity

Cholesterol	Carbohydrate	Calcium	Phosphorus	Iron	Potassium	Sodium	Vitamin A value		Thiamin	Riboflavin	Niacin	Ascorbic acid	Item No.
							(IU)	(RE)					
Milligrams	Grams	Milligrams	Milligrams	Milligrams	Milligrams	Milligrams	International units	Retinol equivalents	Milligrams	Milligrams	Milligrams	Milligrams	
0	28	Tr	2	0.1	1	7	0	0	0.10	0.00	0.0	0	720
0	26	1	1	0.3	11	7	0	0	0.00	Tr	Tr	0	721
0	23	1	2	0.5	2	25	0	0	0.00	Tr	Tr	0	722
278	29	297	310	1.1	387	209	530	146	0.11	0.50	0.3	1	723
0	17	2	23	Tr	Tr	55	0	0	0.00	0.00	0.0	0	724
0	279	17	20	1.7	173	17	0	0	0.02	0.14	1.0	3	725
0	17	1	1	0.1	11	1	0	0	Tr	0.01	0.1	Tr	726
0	14	4	2	0.2	18	2	Tr	Tr	Tr	0.01	Tr	Tr	727
0	10	3	1	0.1	12	2	Tr	Tr	Tr	Tr	Tr	Tr	728
0	13	2	Tr	0.1	16	5	Tr	Tr	Tr	0.01	Tr	1	729
0	10	1	Tr	Tr	13	4	Tr	Tr	Tr	Tr	Tr	1	730
0	18	0	0	Tr	4	11	0	0	0.00	0.00	0.0	0	731
1	30	74	117	1.2	254	285	100	31	0.04	0.17	0.6	Tr	732
Tr	28	119	113	0.3	212	252	Tr	Tr	0.03	0.14	0.4	Tr	733
1	33	79	94	0.2	155	305	Tr	Tr	0.03	0.12	0.6	Tr	734
14	27	130	329	0.3	176	440	130	33	0.04	0.18	0.1	1	735
15	25	146	120	0.2	190	167	140	34	0.05	0.20	0.1	1	736
15	27	133	110	0.5	165	140	140	33	0.10	0.18	0.6	1	737
15	25	131	103	0.1	167	152	140	34	0.04	0.18	0.1	1	738
15	27	129	273	0.1	164	375	140	33	0.04	0.17	0.1	1	739
15	25	132	102	0.1	166	178	140	34	0.04	0.18	0.1	1	740
0	212	187	56	4.8	757	97	0	0	0.02	0.07	0.2	0	741
0	199	3	Tr	0.1	7	5	0	0	0.00	0.00	0.0	0	742
0	12	Tr	Tr	Tr	Tr	Tr	0	0	0.00	0.00	0.0	0	743
0	6	Tr	Tr	Tr	Tr	Tr	0	0	0.00	0.00	0.0	0	744
0	100	1	Tr	Tr	4	2	0	0	0.00	0.00	0.0	0	745
0	22	6	49	0.8	85	36	Tr	Tr	Tr	0.02	0.1	0	746
0	21	38	60	0.5	82	42	40	13	0.02	0.08	0.1	0	747
0	22	274	34	10.1	1,171	38	0	0	0.04	0.08	0.8	0	748
0	32	1	4	Tr	7	19	0	0	0.00	0.00	0.0	0	749
0	1	11	23	0.3	26	2	50	5	0.03	0.04	0.2	3	750
0	12	47	72	1.6	316	79	170	17	0.07	0.06	0.7	9	751
0	8	43	110	1.2	558	7	1,490	149	0.18	0.22	1.9	49	752
0	3	14	37	0.4	186	2	500	50	0.06	0.07	0.6	16	753
0	9	41	99	1.2	392	7	1,470	147	0.12	0.19	1.9	44	754
0	3	14	33	0.4	131	2	490	49	0.04	0.06	0.6	15	755
0	2	11	30	0.5	122	[56]278	380	38	0.04	0.07	0.7	13	756
0	4	10	33	0.4	105	9	10	1	0.03	0.03	0.2	1	757

Nutritive Value of the Edible Part of Food (Continued)

(Tr indicates nutrient present in trace amount.)

Item No.	Foods, approximate measures, units, and weight (weight of edible portion only)		Water	Food energy	Pro- tein	Fat	Fatty acids		
							Satu- rated	Mono- unsatu- rated	Poly- unsatu- rated
	Vegetables and Vegetable Products—Con.	Grams	Per- cent	Cal- ories	Grams	Grams	Grams	Grams	Grams
	Beans:								
	Lima, immature seeds, frozen, cooked, drained:								
758	Thick-seeded types (Ford- hooks)-------------------- 1 cup-----------	170	74	170	10	1	0.1	Tr	0.3
759	Thin-seeded types (baby limas)-------------------- 1 cup-----------	180	72	190	12	1	0.1	Tr	0.3
	Snap:								
	Cooked, drained:								
760	From raw (cut and French style)-------------------- 1 cup-----------	125	89	45	2	Tr	0.1	Tr	0.2
761	From frozen (cut)---------- 1 cup-----------	135	92	35	2	Tr	Tr	Tr	0.1
762	Canned, drained solids (cut) 1 cup-----------	135	93	25	2	Tr	Tr	Tr	0.1
	Beans, mature. See Beans, dry (items 527-535) and Black-eyed peas, dry (item 536).								
	Bean sprouts (mung):								
763	Raw------------------------ 1 cup-----------	104	90	30	3	Tr	Tr	Tr	0.1
764	Cooked, drained---------------- 1 cup-----------	124	93	25	3	Tr	Tr	Tr	Tr
	Beets:								
	Cooked, drained:								
765	Diced or sliced------------- 1 cup-----------	170	91	55	2	Tr	Tr	Tr	Tr
766	Whole beets, 2-in diam.------- 2 beets---------	100	91	30	1	Tr	Tr	Tr	Tr
767	Canned, drained solids, diced or sliced------------------- 1 cup-----------	170	91	55	2	Tr	Tr	Tr	0.1
768	Beet greens, leaves and stems, cooked, drained--------------- 1 cup-----------	144	89	40	4	Tr	Tr	0.1	0.1
	Black-eyed peas, immature seeds, cooked and drained:								
769	From raw---------------------- 1 cup-----------	165	72	180	13	1	0.3	0.1	0.6
770	From frozen------------------- 1 cup-----------	170	66	225	14	1	0.3	0.1	0.5
	Broccoli:								
771	Raw------------------------- 1 spear---------	151	91	40	4	1	0.1	Tr	0.3
	Cooked, drained:								
	From raw:								
772	Spear, medium-------------- 1 spear---------	180	90	50	5	1	0.1	Tr	0.2
773	Spears, cut into 1/2-in pieces------------------- 1 cup-----------	155	90	45	5	Tr	0.1	Tr	0.2
	From frozen:								
774	Piece, 4-1/2 to 5 in long-- 1 piece---------	30	91	10	1	Tr	Tr	Tr	Tr
775	Chopped-------------------- 1 cup-----------	185	91	50	6	Tr	Tr	Tr	0.1
	Brussels sprouts, cooked, drained:								
776	From raw, 7-8 sprouts, 1-1/4 to 1-1/2-in diam.------------ 1 cup-----------	155	87	60	4	1	0.2	0.1	0.4
777	From frozen------------------- 1 cup-----------	155	87	65	6	1	0.1	Tr	0.3
	Cabbage, common varieties:								
778	Raw, coarsely shredded or sliced---------------------- 1 cup-----------	70	93	15	1	Tr	Tr	Tr	0.1
779	Cooked, drained-------------- 1 cup-----------	150	94	30	1	Tr	Tr	Tr	0.2
	Cabbage, Chinese:								
780	Pak-choi, cooked, drained------ 1 cup-----------	170	96	20	3	Tr	Tr	Tr	0.1
781	Pe-tsai, raw, 1-in pieces------ 1 cup-----------	76	94	10	1	Tr	Tr	Tr	0.1
782	Cabbage, red, raw, coarsely shredded or sliced------------- 1 cup-----------	70	92	20	1	Tr	Tr	Tr	0.1
783	Cabbage, savoy, raw, coarsely shredded or sliced------------- 1 cup-----------	70	91	20	1	Tr	Tr	Tr	Tr

[57] For green varieties; yellow varieties contain 101 IU or 10 RE.
[58] For green varieties; yellow varieties contain 151 IU or 15 RE.
[59] For regular pack; special dietary pack contains 3 mg sodium.

Cho-les-terol	Carbo-hydrate	Calcium	Phos-phorus	Iron	Potas-sium	Sodium	Vitamin A value (IU)	Vitamin A value (RE)	Thiamin	Ribo-flavin	Niacin	Ascorbic acid	Item No.
Milli-grams	Grams	Milli-grams	Milli-grams	Milli-grams	Milli-grams	Milli-grams	Inter-national units	Retinol equiva-lents	Milli-grams	Milli-grams	Milli-grams	Milli-grams	
0	32	37	107	2.3	694	90	320	32	0.13	0.10	1.8	22	758
0	35	50	202	3.5	740	52	300	30	0.13	0.10	1.4	10	759
0	10	58	49	1.6	374	4	[57]830	[57]83	0.09	0.12	0.8	12	760
0	8	61	32	1.1	151	18	[58]710	[58]71	0.06	0.10	0.6	11	761
0	6	35	26	1.2	147	[59]339	[60]470	[60]47	0.02	0.08	0.3	6	762
0	6	14	56	0.9	155	6	20	2	0.09	0.13	0.8	14	763
0	5	15	35	0.8	125	12	20	2	0.06	0.13	1.0	14	764
0	11	19	53	1.1	530	83	20	2	0.05	0.02	0.5	9	765
0	7	11	31	0.6	312	49	10	1	0.03	0.01	0.3	6	766
0	12	26	29	3.1	252	[61]466	20	2	0.02	0.07	0.3	7	767
0	8	164	59	2.7	1,309	347	7,340	734	0.17	0.42	0.7	36	768
0	30	46	196	2.4	693	7	1,050	105	0.11	0.18	1.8	3	769
0	40	39	207	3.6	638	9	130	13	0.44	0.11	1.2	4	770
0	8	72	100	1.3	491	41	2,330	233	0.10	0.18	1.0	141	771
0	10	205	86	2.1	293	20	2,540	254	0.15	0.37	1.4	113	772
0	9	177	74	1.8	253	17	2,180	218	0.13	0.32	1.2	97	773
0	2	15	17	0.2	54	7	570	57	0.02	0.02	0.1	12	774
0	10	94	102	1.1	333	44	3,500	350	0.10	0.15	0.8	74	775
0	13	56	87	1.9	491	33	1,110	111	0.17	0.12	0.9	96	776
0	13	37	84	1.1	504	36	910	91	0.16	0.18	0.8	71	777
0	4	33	16	0.4	172	13	90	9	0.04	0.02	0.2	33	778
0	7	50	38	0.6	308	29	130	13	0.09	0.08	0.3	36	779
0	3	158	49	1.8	631	58	4,370	437	0.05	0.11	0.7	44	780
0	2	59	22	0.2	181	7	910	91	0.03	0.04	0.3	21	781
0	4	36	29	0.3	144	8	30	3	0.04	0.02	0.2	40	782
0	4	25	29	0.3	161	20	700	70	0.05	0.02	0.2	22	783

[60] For green varieties; yellow varieties contain 142 IU or 14 RE.
[61] For regular pack; special dietary pack contains 78 mg sodium.

Nutritive Value of the Edible Part of Food (Continued)

(Tr indicates nutrient present in trace amount.)

Item No.	Foods, approximate measures, units, and weight (weight of edible portion only)			Water	Food energy	Pro-tein	Fat	Fatty acids		
								Satu-rated	Mono-unsatu-rated	Poly-unsatu-rated
	Vegetables and Vegetable Products—Con.		Grams	Per-cent	Cal-ories	Grams	Grams	Grams	Grams	Grams
	Carrots:									
	Raw, without crowns and tips, scraped:									
784	Whole, 7-1/2 by 1-1/8 in, or strips, 2-1/2 to 3 in long	1 carrot or 18 strips--------	72	88	30	1	Tr	Tr	Tr	0.1
785	Grated----------------------	1 cup-----------	110	88	45	1	Tr	Tr	Tr	0.1
	Cooked, sliced, drained:									
786	From raw--------------------	1 cup-----------	156	87	70	2	Tr	0.1	Tr	0.1
787	From frozen-----------------	1 cup-----------	146	90	55	2	Tr	Tr	Tr	0.1
788	Canned, sliced, drained solids	1 cup-----------	146	93	35	1	Tr	0.1	Tr	0.1
	Cauliflower:									
789	Raw, (flowerets)-------------	1 cup-----------	100	92	25	2	Tr	Tr	Tr	0.1
	Cooked, drained:									
790	From raw (flowerets)---------	1 cup-----------	125	93	30	2	Tr	Tr	Tr	0.1
791	From frozen (flowerets)------	1 cup-----------	180	94	35	3	Tr	0.1	Tr	0.2
	Celery, pascal type, raw:									
792	Stalk, large outer, 8 by 1-1/2 in (at root end)-------------	1 stalk---------	40	95	5	Tr	Tr	Tr	Tr	Tr
793	Pieces, diced----------------	1 cup-----------	120	95	20	1	Tr	Tr	Tr	0.1
	Collards, cooked, drained:									
794	From raw (leaves without stems)	1 cup-----------	190	96	25	2	Tr	0.1	Tr	0.2
795	From frozen (chopped)----------	1 cup-----------	170	88	60	5	1	0.1	0.1	0.4
	Corn, sweet:									
	Cooked, drained:									
796	From raw, ear 5 by 1-3/4 in--	1 ear-----------	77	70	85	3	1	0.2	0.3	0.5
	From frozen:									
797	Ear, trimmed to about 3-1/2 in long-----------------	1 ear-----------	63	73	60	2	Tr	0.1	0.1	0.2
798	Kernels---------------------	1 cup-----------	165	76	135	5	Tr	Tr	Tr	0.1
	Canned:									
799	Cream style-----------------	1 cup-----------	256	79	185	4	1	0.2	0.3	0.5
800	Whole kernel, vacuum pack----	1 cup-----------	210	77	165	5	1	0.2	0.3	0.5
	Cowpeas. See Black-eyed peas, immature (items 769,770), mature (item 536).									
801	Cucumber, with peel, slices, 1/8 in thick (large, 2-1/8-in diam.; small, 1-3/4-in diam.)--	6 large or 8 small slices	28	96	5	Tr	Tr	Tr	Tr	Tr
802	Dandelion greens, cooked, drained	1 cup-----------	105	90	35	2	1	0.1	Tr	0.3
803	Eggplant, cooked, steamed--------	1 cup-----------	96	92	25	1	Tr	Tr	Tr	0.1
804	Endive, curly (including esca-role), raw, small pieces-------	1 cup-----------	50	94	10	1	Tr	Tr	Tr	Tr
805	Jerusalem-artichoke, raw, sliced	1 cup-----------	150	78	115	3	Tr	0.0	Tr	Tr
	Kale, cooked, drained:									
806	From raw, chopped--------------	1 cup-----------	130	91	40	2	1	0.1	Tr	0.3
807	From frozen, chopped----------	1 cup-----------	130	91	40	4	1	0.1	Tr	0.3
808	Kohlrabi, thickened bulb-like stems, cooked, drained, diced--	1 cup-----------	165	90	50	3	Tr	Tr	Tr	0.1
	Lettuce, raw:									
	Butterhead, as Boston types:									
809	Head, 5-in diam-------------	1 head----------	163	96	20	2	Tr	Tr	Tr	0.2
810	Leaves----------------------	1 outer or 2 inner leaves--	15	96	Tr	Tr	Tr	Tr	Tr	Tr
	Crisphead, as iceberg:									
811	Head, 6-in diam-------------	1 head----------	539	96	70	5	1	0.1	Tr	0.5
812	Wedge, 1/4 of head----------	1 wedge---------	135	96	20	1	Tr	Tr	Tr	0.1
813	Pieces, chopped or shredded--	1 cup-----------	55	96	5	1	Tr	Tr	Tr	0.1
814	Looseleaf (bunching varieties including romaine or cos), chopped or shredded pieces---	1 cup-----------	56	94	10	1	Tr	Tr	Tr	0.1

[62] For regular pack; special dietary pack contains 61 mg sodium.
[63] For yellow varieties; white varieties contain only a trace of vitamin A.

Nutrients in Indicated Quantity

Cho-les-terol	Carbo-hydrate	Calcium	Phos-phorus	Iron	Potas-sium	Sodium	Vitamin A value (IU)	Vitamin A value (RE)	Thiamin	Ribo-flavin	Niacin	Ascorbic acid	Item No.
Milli-grams	Grams	Milli-grams	Milli-grams	Milli-grams	Milli-grams	Milli-grams	Inter-national units	Retinol equiva-lents	Milli-grams	Milli-grams	Milli-grams	Milli-grams	
0	7	19	32	0.4	233	25	20,250	2,025	0.07	0.04	0.7	7	784
0	11	30	48	0.6	355	39	30,940	3,094	0.11	0.06	1.0	10	785
0	16	48	47	1.0	354	103	38,300	3,830	0.05	0.09	0.8	4	786
0	12	41	38	0.7	231	86	25,850	2,585	0.04	0.05	0.6	4	787
0	8	37	35	0.9	261	[62]352	20,110	2,011	0.03	0.04	0.8	4	788
0	5	29	46	0.6	355	15	20	2	0.08	0.06	0.6	72	789
0	6	34	44	0.5	404	8	20	2	0.08	0.07	0.7	69	790
0	7	31	43	0.7	250	32	40	4	0.07	0.10	0.6	56	791
0	1	14	10	0.2	114	35	50	5	0.01	0.01	0.1	3	792
0	4	43	31	0.6	341	106	150	15	0.04	0.04	0.4	8	793
0	5	148	19	0.8	177	36	4,220	422	0.03	0.08	0.4	19	794
0	12	357	46	1.9	427	85	10,170	1,017	0.08	0.20	1.1	45	795
0	19	2	79	0.5	192	13	[63]170	[63]17	0.17	0.06	1.2	5	796
0	14	2	47	0.4	158	3	[63]130	[63]13	0.11	0.04	1.0	3	797
0	34	3	78	0.5	229	8	[63]410	[63]41	0.11	0.12	2.1	4	798
0	46	8	131	1.0	343	[64]730	[63]250	[63]25	0.06	0.14	2.5	12	799
0	41	11	134	0.9	391	[65]571	[63]510	[63]51	0.09	0.15	2.5	17	800
0	1	4	5	0.1	42	1	10	1	0.01	0.01	0.1	1	801
0	7	147	44	1.9	244	46	12,290	1,229	0.14	0.18	0.5	19	802
0	6	6	21	0.3	238	3	60	6	0.07	0.02	0.6	1	803
0	2	26	14	0.4	157	11	1,030	103	0.04	0.04	0.2	3	804
0	26	21	117	5.1	644	6	30	3	0.30	0.09	2.0	6	805
0	7	94	36	1.2	296	30	9,620	962	0.07	0.09	0.7	53	806
0	7	179	36	1.2	417	20	8,260	826	0.06	0.15	0.9	33	807
0	11	41	74	0.7	561	35	60	6	0.07	0.03	0.6	89	808
0	4	52	38	0.5	419	8	1,580	158	0.10	0.10	0.5	13	809
0	Tr	5	3	Tr	39	1	150	15	0.01	0.01	Tr	1	810
0	11	102	108	2.7	852	49	1,780	178	0.25	0.16	1.0	21	811
0	3	26	27	0.7	213	12	450	45	0.06	0.04	0.3	5	812
0	1	10	11	0.3	87	5	180	18	0.03	0.02	0.1	2	813
0	2	38	14	0.8	148	5	1,060	106	0.03	0.04	0.2	10	814

[64] For regular pack; special dietary pack contains 8 mg sodium.
[65] For regular pack; special dietary pack contains 6 mg sodium.

Nutritive Value of the Edible Part of Food (Continued)

(Tr indicates nutrient present in trace amount.)

Item No.	Foods, approximate measures, units, and weight (weight of edible portion only)			Water	Food energy	Pro-tein	Fat	Fatty acids		
								Satu-rated	Mono-unsatu-rated	Poly-unsatu-rated
			Grams	Per-cent	Cal-ories	Grams	Grams	Grams	Grams	Grams
	Vegetables and Vegetable Products—Con.									
	Mushrooms:									
815	Raw, sliced or chopped	1 cup	70	92	20	1	Tr	Tr	Tr	0.1
816	Cooked, drained	1 cup	156	91	40	3	1	0.1	Tr	0.3
817	Canned, drained solids	1 cup	156	91	35	3	Tr	0.1	Tr	0.2
818	Mustard greens, without stems and									
	midribs, cooked, drained	1 cup	140	94	20	3	Tr	Tr	0.2	0.1
819	Okra pods, 3 by 5/8 in, cooked	8 pods	85	90	25	2	Tr	Tr	Tr	Tr
	Onions:									
	Raw:									
820	Chopped	1 cup	160	91	55	2	Tr	0.1	0.1	0.2
821	Sliced	1 cup	115	91	40	1	Tr	0.1	Tr	0.1
822	Cooked (whole or sliced),									
	drained	1 cup	210	92	60	2	Tr	0.1	Tr	0.1
823	Onions, spring, raw, bulb (3/8-in diam.) and white portion of top	6 onions	30	92	10	1	Tr	Tr	Tr	Tr
824	Onion rings, breaded, par-fried, frozen, prepared	2 rings	20	29	80	1	5	1.7	2.2	1.0
	Parsley:									
825	Raw	10 sprigs	10	88	5	Tr	Tr	Tr	Tr	Tr
826	Freeze-dried	1 tbsp	0.4	2	Tr	Tr	Tr	Tr	Tr	Tr
827	Parsnips, cooked (diced or 2 in lengths), drained	1 cup	156	78	125	2	Tr	0.1	0.2	0.1
828	Peas, edible pod, cooked, drained	1 cup	160	89	65	5	Tr	0.1	Tr	0.2
	Peas, green:									
829	Canned, drained solids	1 cup	170	82	115	8	1	0.1	0.1	0.3
830	Frozen, cooked, drained	1 cup	160	80	125	8	Tr	0.1	Tr	0.2
	Peppers:									
831	Hot chili, raw	1 pepper	45	88	20	1	Tr	Tr	Tr	Tr
	Sweet (about 5 per lb, whole), stem and seeds removed:									
832	Raw	1 pepper	74	93	20	1	Tr	Tr	Tr	0.2
833	Cooked, drained	1 pepper	73	95	15	Tr	Tr	Tr	Tr	0.1
	Potatoes, cooked:									
	Baked (about 2 per lb, raw):									
834	With skin	1 potato	202	71	220	5	Tr	0.1	Tr	0.1
835	Flesh only	1 potato	156	75	145	3	Tr	Tr	Tr	0.1
	Boiled (about 3 per lb, raw):									
836	Peeled after boiling	1 potato	136	77	120	3	Tr	Tr	Tr	0.1
837	Peeled before boiling	1 potato	135	77	115	2	Tr	Tr	Tr	0.1
	French fried, strip, 2 to 3-1/2 in long, frozen:									
838	Oven heated	10 strips	50	53	110	2	4	2.1	1.8	0.3
839	Fried in vegetable oil	10 strips	50	38	160	2	8	2.5	1.6	3.8
	Potato products, prepared:									
	Au gratin:									
840	From dry mix	1 cup	245	79	230	6	10	6.3	2.9	0.3
841	From home recipe	1 cup	245	74	325	12	19	11.6	5.3	0.7
842	Hashed brown, from frozen	1 cup	156	56	340	5	18	7.0	8.0	2.1
	Mashed:									
	From home recipe:									
843	Milk added	1 cup	210	78	160	4	1	0.7	0.3	0.1
844	Milk and margarine added	1 cup	210	76	225	4	9	2.2	3.7	2.5
845	From dehydrated flakes (without milk), water, milk, butter, and salt added	1 cup	210	76	235	4	12	7.2	3.3	0.5
846	Potato salad, made with mayonnaise	1 cup	250	76	360	7	21	3.6	6.2	9.3
	Scalloped:									
847	From dry mix	1 cup	245	79	230	5	11	6.5	3.0	0.5
848	From home recipe	1 cup	245	81	210	7	9	5.5	2.5	0.4

[66] For regular pack; special dietary pack contains 3 mg sodium.
[67] For red peppers; green peppers contain 350 IU or 35 RE.
[68] For green peppers; red peppers contain 4,220 IU or 422 RE.

Nutrients in Indicated Quantity

Cho-les-terol	Carbo-hydrate	Calcium	Phos-phorus	Iron	Potas-sium	Sodium	Vitamin A value		Thiamin	Ribo-flavin	Niacin	Ascorbic acid	Item No.
							(IU)	(RE)					
Milli-grams	Grams	Milli-grams	Milli-grams	Milli-grams	Milli-grams	Milli-grams	Inter-national units	Retinol equiva-lents	Milli-grams	Milli-grams	Milli-grams	Milli-grams	
0	3	4	73	0.9	259	3	0	0	0.07	0.31	2.9	2	815
0	8	9	136	2.7	555	3	0	0	0.11	0.47	7.0	6	816
0	8	17	103	1.2	201	663	0	0	0.13	0.03	2.5	0	817
0	3	104	57	1.0	283	22	4,240	424	0.06	0.09	0.6	35	818
0	6	54	48	0.4	274	4	490	49	0.11	0.05	0.7	14	819
0	12	40	46	0.6	248	3	0	0	0.10	0.02	0.2	13	820
0	8	29	33	0.4	178	2	0	0	0.07	0.01	0.1	10	821
0	13	57	48	0.4	319	17	0	0	0.09	0.02	0.2	12	822
0	2	18	10	0.6	77	1	1,500	150	0.02	0.04	0.1	14	823
0	8	6	16	0.3	26	75	50	5	0.06	0.03	0.7	Tr	824
0	1	13	4	0.6	54	4	520	52	0.01	0.01	0.1	9	825
0	Tr	1	2	0.2	25	2	250	25	Tr	0.01	Tr	1	826
0	30	58	108	0.9	573	16	0	0	0.13	0.08	1.1	20	827
0	11	67	88	3.2	384	6	210	21	0.20	0.12	0.9	77	828
0	21	34	114	1.6	294	[66]372	1,310	131	0.21	0.13	1.2	16	829
0	23	38	144	2.5	269	139	1,070	107	0.45	0.16	2.4	16	830
0	4	8	21	0.5	153	3	[67]4,840	[67]484	0.04	0.04	0.4	109	831
0	4	4	16	0.9	144	2	[68]390	[68]39	0.06	0.04	0.4	[69]95	832
0	3	3	11	0.6	94	1	[70]280	[70]28	0.04	0.03	0.3	[71]81	833
0	51	20	115	2.7	844	16	0	0	0.22	0.07	3.3	26	834
0	34	8	78	0.5	610	8	0	0	0.16	0.03	2.2	20	835
0	27	7	60	0.4	515	5	0	0	0.14	0.03	2.0	18	836
0	27	11	54	0.4	443	7	0	0	0.13	0.03	1.8	10	837
0	17	5	43	0.7	229	16	0	0	0.06	0.02	1.2	5	838
0	20	10	47	0.4	366	108	0	0	0.09	0.01	1.6	5	839
12	31	203	233	0.8	537	1,076	520	76	0.05	0.20	2.3	8	840
56	28	292	277	1.6	970	1,061	650	93	0.16	0.28	2.4	24	841
0	44	23	112	2.4	680	53	0	0	0.17	0.03	3.8	10	842
4	37	55	101	0.6	628	636	40	12	0.18	0.08	2.3	14	843
4	35	55	97	0.5	607	620	360	42	0.18	0.08	2.3	13	844
29	32	103	118	0.5	489	697	380	44	0.23	0.11	1.4	20	845
170	28	48	130	1.6	635	1,323	520	83	0.19	0.15	2.2	25	846
27	31	88	137	0.9	497	835	360	51	0.05	0.14	2.5	8	847
29	26	140	154	1.4	926	821	330	47	0.17	0.23	2.6	26	848

[69]For green peppers; red peppers contain 141 mg ascorbic acid.
[70]For green peppers; red peppers contain 2,740 IU or 274 RE.
[71]For green peppers; red peppers contain 121 mg ascorbic acid.

Nutritive Value of the Edible Part of Food (Continued)

(Tr indicates nutrient present in trace amount.)

Item No.	Foods, approximate measures, units, and weight (weight of edible portion only)		Water	Food energy	Pro- tein	Fat	Fatty acids		
							Satu- rated	Mono- unsatu- rated	Poly- unsatu- rated
	Vegetables and Vegetable Products—Con.	Grams	Per- cent	Cal- ories	Grams	Grams	Grams	Grams	Grams
849	Potato chips--------------------	10 chips--------	20	3	105	1	7	1.8	1.2	3.6
	Pumpkin:									
850	Cooked from raw, mashed--------	1 cup-----------	245	94	50	2	Tr	0.1	Tr	Tr
851	Canned-------------------------	1 cup-----------	245	90	85	3	1	0.4	0.1	Tr
852	Radishes, raw, stem ends, rootlets cut off---------------	4 radishes------	18	95	5	Tr	Tr	Tr	Tr	Tr
853	Sauerkraut, canned, solids and liquid-------------------------	1 cup-----------	236	93	45	2	Tr	0.1	Tr	0.1
	Seaweed:									
854	Kelp, raw----------------------	1 oz------------	28	82	10	Tr	Tr	0.1	Tr	Tr
855	Spirulina, dried---------------	1 oz------------	28	5	80	16	2	0.8	0.2	0.6
	Southern peas. See Black-eyed peas, immature (items 769,770), mature (item 536).									
	Spinach:									
856	Raw, chopped-------------------	1 cup-----------	55	92	10	2	Tr	Tr	Tr	0.1
	Cooked, drained:									
857	From raw----------------------	1 cup-----------	180	91	40	5	Tr	0.1	Tr	0.2
858	From frozen (leaf)-----------	1 cup-----------	190	90	55	6	Tr	0.1	Tr	0.2
859	Canned, drained solids---------	1 cup-----------	214	92	50	6	1	0.2	Tr	0.4
860	Spinach souffle----------------	1 cup-----------	136	74	220	11	18	7.1	6.8	3.1
	Squash, cooked:									
861	Summer (all varieties), sliced, drained----------------------	1 cup-----------	180	94	35	2	1	0.1	Tr	0.2
862	Winter (all varieties), baked, cubes-------------------------	1 cup-----------	205	89	80	2	1	0.3	0.1	0.5
	Sunchoke. See Jerusalem-arti- choke (item 805).									
	Sweetpotatoes:									
	Cooked (raw, 5 by 2 in; about 2-1/2 per lb):									
863	Baked in skin, peeled--------	1 potato--------	114	73	115	2	Tr	Tr	Tr	0.1
864	Boiled, without skin--------	1 potato--------	151	73	160	2	Tr	0.1	Tr	0.2
865	Candied, 2-1/2 by 2-in piece---	1 piece---------	105	67	145	1	3	1.4	0.7	0.2
	Canned:									
866	Solid pack (mashed)----------	1 cup-----------	255	74	260	5	1	0.1	Tr	0.2
867	Vacuum pack, piece 2-3/4 by 1 in----------------------	1 piece---------	40	76	35	1	Tr	Tr	Tr	Tr
	Tomatoes:									
868	Raw, 2-3/5-in diam. (3 per 12 oz pkg.)--------------------	1 tomato--------	123	94	25	1	Tr	Tr	Tr	0.1
869	Canned, solids and liquid------	1 cup-----------	240	94	50	2	1	0.1	0.1	0.2
870	Tomato juice, canned-----------	1 cup-----------	244	94	40	2	Tr	Tr	Tr	0.1
	Tomato products, canned:									
871	Paste--------------------------	1 cup-----------	262	74	220	10	2	0.3	0.4	0.9
872	Puree--------------------------	1 cup-----------	250	87	105	4	Tr	Tr	Tr	0.1
873	Sauce--------------------------	1 cup-----------	245	89	75	3	Tr	0.1	0.1	0.2
874	Turnips, cooked, diced---------	1 cup-----------	156	94	30	1	Tr	Tr	Tr	0.1
	Turnip greens, cooked, drained:									
875	From raw (leaves and stems)----	1 cup-----------	144	93	30	2	Tr	0.1	Tr	0.1
876	From frozen (chopped)----------	1 cup-----------	164	90	50	5	1	0.2	Tr	0.3
877	Vegetable juice cocktail, canned	1 cup-----------	242	94	45	2	Tr	Tr	Tr	0.1
	Vegetables, mixed:									
878	Canned, drained solids---------	1 cup-----------	163	87	75	4	Tr	0.1	Tr	0.2
879	Frozen, cooked, drained--------	1 cup-----------	182	83	105	5	Tr	0.1	Tr	0.1
880	Waterchestnuts, canned---------	1 cup-----------	140	86	70	1	Tr	Tr	Tr	Tr

[1] Value not determined.
[72] With added salt; if none is added, sodium content is 58 mg.
[73] For regular pack; special dietary pack contains 31 mg sodium.
[74] With added salt; if none is added, sodium content is 24 mg.

							Nutrients in Indicated Quantity						
Cho-les-terol	Carbo-hydrate	Calcium	Phos-phorus	Iron	Potas-sium	Sodium	Vitamin A value		Thiamin	Ribo-flavin	Niacin	Ascorbic acid	Item No.
							(IU)	(RE)					
Milli-grams	Grams	Milli-grams	Milli-grams	Milli-grams	Milli-grams	Milli-grams	Inter-national units	Retinol equiva-lents	Milli-grams	Milli-grams	Milli-grams	Milli-grams	
0	10	5	31	0.2	260	94	0	0	0.03	Tr	0.8	8	849
0	12	37	74	1.4	564	2	2,650	265	0.08	0.19	1.0	12	850
0	20	64	86	3.4	505	12	54,040	5,404	0.06	0.13	0.9	10	851
0	1	4	3	0.1	42	4	Tr	Tr	Tr	0.01	0.1	4	852
0	10	71	47	3.5	401	1,560	40	4	0.05	0.05	0.3	35	853
0	3	48	12	0.8	25	66	30	3	0.01	0.04	0.1	(^{1})	854
0	7	34	33	8.1	386	297	160	16	0.67	1.04	3.6	3	855
0	2	54	27	1.5	307	43	3,690	369	0.04	0.10	0.4	15	856
0	7	245	101	6.4	839	126	14,740	1,474	0.17	0.42	0.9	18	857
0	10	277	91	2.9	566	163	14,790	1,479	0.11	0.32	0.8	23	858
0	7	272	94	4.9	740	[72]683	18,780	1,878	0.03	0.30	0.8	31	859
184	3	230	231	1.3	201	763	3,460	675	0.09	0.30	0.5	3	860
0	8	49	70	0.6	346	2	520	52	0.08	0.07	0.9	10	861
0	18	29	41	0.7	896	2	7,290	729	0.17	0.05	1.4	20	862
0	28	32	63	0.5	397	11	24,880	2,488	0.08	0.14	0.7	28	863
0	37	32	41	0.8	278	20	25,750	2,575	0.08	0.21	1.0	26	864
8	29	27	27	1.2	198	74	4,400	440	0.02	0.04	0.4	7	865
0	59	77	133	3.4	536	191	38,570	3,857	0.07	0.23	2.4	13	866
0	8	9	20	0.4	125	21	3,190	319	0.01	0.02	0.3	11	867
0	5	9	28	0.6	255	10	1,390	139	0.07	0.06	0.7	22	868
0	10	62	46	1.5	530	[73]391	1,450	145	0.11	0.07	1.8	36	869
0	10	22	46	1.4	537	[74]881	1,360	136	0.11	0.08	1.6	45	870
0	49	92	207	7.8	2,442	[75]170	6,470	647	0.41	0.50	8.4	111	871
0	25	38	100	2.3	1,050	[76]50	3,400	340	0.18	0.14	4.3	88	872
0	18	34	78	1.9	909	[77]1,482	2,400	240	0.16	0.14	2.8	32	873
0	8	34	30	0.3	211	78	0	0	0.04	0.04	0.5	18	874
0	6	197	42	1.2	292	42	7,920	792	0.06	0.10	0.6	39	875
0	8	249	56	3.2	367	25	13,080	1,308	0.09	0.12	0.8	36	876
0	11	27	41	1.0	467	883	2,830	283	0.10	0.07	1.8	67	877
0	15	44	68	1.7	474	243	18,990	1,899	0.08	0.08	0.9	8	878
0	24	46	93	1.5	308	64	7,780	778	0.13	0.22	1.5	6	879
0	17	6	27	1.2	165	11	10	1	0.02	0.03	0.5	2	880

[75] With no added salt; if salt is added, sodium content is 2,070 mg.
[76] With no added salt; if salt is added, sodium content is 998 mg.
[77] With salt added.

Nutritive Value of the Edible Part of Food (Continued)

(Tr indicates nutrient present in trace amount.)

Item No.	Foods, approximate measures, units, and weight (weight of edible portion only)		Water	Food energy	Pro-tein	Fat	Fatty acids		
							Satu-rated	Mono-unsatu-rated	Poly-unsatu-rated
	Miscellaneous Items	Grams	Per-cent	Cal-ories	Grams	Grams	Grams	Grams	Grams
	Baking powders for home use:								
	Sodium aluminum sulfate:								
881	With monocalcium phosphate monohydrate----------------	1 tsp-----------	3	2	5	Tr	0	0.0	0.0	0.0
882	With monocalcium phosphate monohydrate, calcium sulfate--------------------	1 tsp-----------	2.9	1	5	Tr	0	0.0	0.0	0.0
883	Straight phosphate-------------	1 tsp-----------	3.8	2	5	Tr	0	0.0	0.0	0.0
884	Low sodium--------------------	1 tsp-----------	4.3	1	5	Tr	0	0.0	0.0	0.0
885	Catsup------------------------	1 cup-----------	273	69	290	5	1	0.2	0.2	0.4
886		1 tbsp----------	15	69	15	Tr	Tr	Tr	Tr	Tr
887	Celery seed----------------------	1 tsp-----------	2	6	10	Tr	1	Tr	0.3	0.1
888	Chili powder--------------------	1 tsp-----------	2.6	8	10	Tr	Tr	0.1	0.1	0.2
	Chocolate:								
889	Bitter or baking---------------	1 oz------------	28	2	145	3	15	9.0	4.9	0.5
	Semisweet, see Candy, (item 715).								
890	Cinnamon-----------------------	1 tsp-----------	2.3	10	5	Tr	Tr	Tr	Tr	Tr
891	Curry powder--------------------	1 tsp-----------	2	10	5	Tr	Tr	([1])	([1])	([1])
892	Garlic powder-------------------	1 tsp-----------	2.8	6	10	Tr	Tr	Tr	Tr	Tr
893	Gelatin, dry--------------------	1 envelope------	7	13	25	6	Tr	Tr	Tr	Tr
894	Mustard, prepared, yellow--------	1 tsp or indivi-dual packet---	5	80	5	Tr	Tr	Tr	0.2	Tr
	Olives, canned:								
895	Green-------------------------	4 medium or 3 extra large	13	78	15	Tr	2	0.2	1.2	0.1
896	Ripe, Mission, pitted----------	3 small or 2 large-------	9	73	15	Tr	2	0.3	1.3	0.2
897	Onion powder--------------------	1 tsp-----------	2.1	5	5	Tr	Tr	Tr	Tr	Tr
898	Oregano------------------------	1 tsp-----------	1.5	7	5	Tr	Tr	Tr	Tr	0.1
899	Paprika------------------------	1 tsp-----------	2.1	10	5	Tr	Tr	Tr	Tr	0.2
900	Pepper, black-------------------	1 tsp-----------	2.1	11	5	Tr	Tr	Tr	Tr	Tr
	Pickles, cucumber:								
901	Dill, medium, whole, 3-3/4 in long, 1-1/4-in diam.---------	1 pickle--------	65	93	5	Tr	Tr	Tr	Tr	0.1
902	Fresh-pack, slices 1-1/2-in diam., 1/4 in thick----------	2 slices--------	15	79	10	Tr	Tr	Tr	Tr	Tr
903	Sweet, gherkin, small, whole, about 2-1/2 in long, 3/4-in diam.	1 pickle--------	15	61	20	Tr	Tr	Tr	Tr	Tr
	Popcorn. See Grain Products, (items 497-499).								
904	Relish, finely chopped, sweet----	1 tbsp----------	15	63	20	Tr	Tr	Tr	Tr	Tr
905	Salt------------------------------	1 tsp-----------	5.5	0	0	0	0	0.0	0.0	0.0
906	Vinegar, cider------------------	1 tbsp----------	15	94	Tr	Tr	0	0.0	0.0	0.0
	Yeast:								
907	Baker's, dry, active-----------	1 pkg-----------	7	5	20	3	Tr	Tr	0.1	Tr
908	Brewer's, dry------------------	1 tbsp----------	8	5	25	3	Tr	Tr	Tr	0.0

[1]Value not determined.

Nutrients in Indicated Quantity

Cholesterol	Carbohydrate	Calcium	Phosphorus	Iron	Potassium	Sodium	Vitamin A value		Thiamin	Riboflavin	Niacin	Ascorbic acid	Item No.
							(IU)	(RE)					
Milligrams	Grams	Milligrams	Milligrams	Milligrams	Milligrams	Milligrams	International units	Retinol equivalents	Milligrams	Milligrams	Milligrams	Milligrams	
0	1	58	87	0.0	5	329	0	0	0.00	0.00	0.0	0	881
0	1	183	45	0.0	4	290	0	0	0.00	0.00	0.0	0	882
0	1	239	359	0.0	6	312	0	0	0.00	0.00	0.0	0	883
0	1	207	314	0.0	891	Tr	0	0	0.00	0.00	0.0	0	884
0	69	60	137	2.2	991	2,845	3,820	382	0.25	0.19	4.4	41	885
0	4	3	8	0.1	54	156	210	21	0.01	0.01	0.2	2	886
0	1	35	11	0.9	28	3	Tr	Tr	0.01	0.01	0.1	Tr	887
0	1	7	8	0.4	50	26	910	91	0.01	0.02	0.2	2	888
0	8	22	109	1.9	235	1	10	1	0.01	0.07	0.4	0	889
0	2	28	1	0.9	12	1	10	1	Tr	Tr	Tr	1	890
0	1	10	7	0.6	31	1	20	2	0.01	0.01	0.1	Tr	891
0	2	2	12	0.1	31	1	0	0	0.01	Tr	Tr	Tr	892
0	0	1	0	0.0	2	6	0	0	0.00	0.00	0.0	0	893
0	Tr	4	4	0.1	7	63	0	0	Tr	0.01	Tr	Tr	894
0	Tr	8	2	0.2	7	312	40	4	Tr	Tr	Tr	0	895
0	Tr	10	2	0.2	2	68	10	1	Tr	Tr	Tr	0	896
0	2	8	7	0.1	20	1	Tr	Tr	0.01	Tr	Tr	Tr	897
0	1	24	3	0.7	25	Tr	100	10	0.01	Tr	0.1	1	898
0	1	4	7	0.5	49	1	1,270	127	0.01	0.04	0.3	1	899
0	1	9	4	0.6	26	1	Tr	Tr	Tr	0.01	Tr	0	900
0	1	17	14	0.7	130	928	70	7	Tr	0.01	Tr	4	901
0	3	5	4	0.3	30	101	20	2	Tr	Tr	Tr	1	902
0	5	2	2	0.2	30	107	10	1	Tr	Tr	Tr	1	903
0	5	3	2	0.1	30	107	20	2	Tr	Tr	0.0	1	904
0	0	14	3	Tr	Tr	2,132	0	0	0.00	0.00	0.0	0	905
0	1	1	1	0.1	15	Tr	0	0	0.00	0.00	0.0	0	906
0	3	3	90	1.1	140	4	Tr	Tr	0.16	0.38	2.6	Tr	907
0	3	[78]17	140	1.4	152	10	Tr	Tr	1.25	0.34	3.0	Tr	908

[78]Value may vary from 6 to 60 mg.

*From Nutritive Value of Foods, United States Department of Agriculture, Home and Garden Bulletin Number 72. Prepared by Agricultural Research Service, Washington, DC. Revised 1989.

Appendix 6 Nutritive Value of Selected Ethnic Foods

FOOD	QUANTITY	GRAMS PER SERVING	Kcal	PRO (g)	FAT (g)	CHO (g)	Na (mg)	K (mg)	CHOL (mg)	SAT. FATTY ACIDS (g)	MONO. FATTY ACIDS (g)	POLY. FATTY ACIDS (g)	TOTAL DIETARY FIBER (g)
Navajo													
Starch/bread													
Blue corn mush with ash*	¾ c.	180	94	2.5	0.5	21.2	32	288	0	—	—	—	—
Flour tortilla, 8 in. diameter†‡	½	34	87	2.5	0.2	19.3	211	29	0	—	—	—	—
Steamed corn hominy, ck†	½ c.	115	70	1.8	1.0	13.3	18	108	0	—	—	—	—
Lean meat													
Mutton, flesh, lean only, ck without added fat§	1 oz	28	58	7.9	2.7¶	0	21	96	26	1.0	1.2	0.2	0
High-fat meat													
Mutton, flesh, lean and fat, ck without added fat§	1 oz	28	82	6.7	5.9¶	0	20	87	27	2.5	2.5	0.4	0
Fat													
Piñon nuts in shell	1 tbsp (25 nuts)	9	60	1.3	5.8	0.7	7	67	0	0.8	2.1	2.3	0.4
Alaskan Native													
Starch/bread													
Pilot bread, 4 in. diameter	1	25	104	2.1	2.0	18.2	142	57	—	—	—	—	—
Lean meats													
Caribou, ck	1 oz	28	47	8.3	1.2	0	17	87	31	0.5	0.4	0.2	—
Gumboots (leathery chiton)	2 oz	56	46	9.6	0.9	0	—	—	—	—	—	—	—
Halibut, ck	1 oz	28	39	7.5	0.8	0	20	164	12	0.1	0.3	0.3	—
Herring eggs, plain	0.5 c.	85	48	8.2	0.8	3.7	52	94	22	0.1	0.1	0.1	—
Moose, ck	1 oz	28	38	8.2	0.3	0	19	93	14	0.04	0.1	0.1	—
Pike, ck	1 oz	28	33	6.9	0.2	0	13	—	—	0.1	0.1	—	—
Seal meat, raw	1 oz	28	41	8.9	0.6	0	—	—	31	0.1	0.1	—	—
Venison, ck	1 oz	28	44	8.5	0.9	0	15	94	31	0.4	0.3	0.2	—
Walrus, raw	1 oz	28	56	5.4	3.9	0	—	—	22	0.7	2.4	0.7	—
Whale, bowhead, raw	1 oz	28	37	7.3	0.7	0	17	—	—	0.2	0.4	0.1	—
Medium-fat meats													
Dried fish (king salmon)	0.5 oz	14	60	7.1	5.3	0	—	—	—	—	—	—	—
Muskrat, ck	1 oz	28	67	8.5	3.3	0	27	91	—	—	—	—	—
Salmon, sockeye, ck	1 oz	28	60	7.6	3.1	0	18	105	24	0.5	1.5	0.7	—
High-fat meat													
Hooligan (eulachon), smoked	1 oz	28	86	5.7	6.9	0	—	—	—	—	—	—	—
Muktuk, skin and fat	1 × 1 × 2 in.	38	138	8	12	0	—	—	—	—	—	—	—
Vegetables													
Fiddlehead fern, raw	1 c.	180	34	3.2	0.2	5.0	84	—	—	—	—	—	—
Seaweed, dried black	1 c.	13	39	3.7	0.3	5.3	40	—	—	—	—	—	—
Willow greens, ck	0.5 c.	28	28	1.7	0.4	5.8	—	—	—	—	—	—	—
Sour dock, ck	0.5 c.	55	19	1.3	0.4	3.6	—	—	—	—	—	—	—
Fruits													
Highbush cranberries	1.25 c.	119	58	0.5	0.2	15	1	8	0	—	—	—	—
Huckleberries	1 c.	150	56	0.6	0.2	13	15	—	—	—	—	—	—
Salmonberries	1.25 c.	181	55	1.3	0.1	13	52	—	—	—	—	—	—
Fat													
Seal oil	1 tsp	5	45	0	5	0	—	0	8	0.6	3.0	1.4	—
Free													
Beach asparagus	1 c.	55	15	1	0.2	2.4	23	—	—	—	—	—	—

				Mexican American									
Starch/bread													
Bolillo, large, 4.5–5 in. long	¼	30	87	2.8	0.9	16.6	174	27	0	—	—	—	0.8
Frijoles cocidos	⅓ c.	56	77	4.6	0.3	14.4	1	262	0	0.1	0.1	0.1	3.5
Frijoles refritos, cn	⅓ c.	83	89	5.2	0.9	15.9	365	338	0	0.4	0.4	0.1	3.5
Tortilla, corn, 7.5 in. across, ready to bake/fry	1	30	69	1.7	0.8	12.8	7	46	0	0.1	0.2	0.5	0.9
Tortilla, flour, 7 in. across, ready to bake/fry (Starch/bread 1½)	1	40	118	3.5	2.7	22	164	52	0	0.8	1.3	0.8	0.9
Tortilla, flour, 9 in. across, ready to bake/fry	⅓	22	65	1.9	1.5	12	90	28.7	0	0.4	0.7	0.4	0.5
Starch/bread prepared with fat													
Taco shell, 5 in. across (corn tortilla, ready to use)	2	24	109	2.0	4.7	15.8	42	58	0	0.7	2.6	1.0	1.2
Lean meat													
Menudo	½ c.	—	55	8	1.5	1.8	431	24.5	25	—	—	—	—
Medium-fat meat													
Queso fresco	2 oz or ¼ c.	57	80	6.4	4.6	3.0	72	72	18	2.8	1.3	0.1	0
High-fat meat													
Chorizo (High-fat meat 1 + Fat 1)	1 oz	28.5	132	7.2	11.5	—	(367)	(58)	(30)	4.3	5.7	1.0	0
Vegetable													
Chayote, boiled, drained	½ c.	80	19	0.5	0.4	4.1	1	138	0	(0)	(0)	(0.2)	(0.6)
Jícama, ck	½ c.	(50)	23	0.6	0	5.2	3	90	0	0	0	0	—
Jícama, raw	½ c.	60	23	0.8	0.1	5.2	4	105	0	0	0	0	0.4
Nopales, raw	½ c.	59	24	0.4	0.3	5.6	3	130	0	0.1	0.1	0.1	2.1
Fruit													
Mango, raw	½ small	104	68	0.5	0.3	17.6	2	161	0	0	0	0	1.5
Papaya, raw	1 c.	140	54	0.9	0.2	13.7	4	359	0	0	0	0	1.7
Fat													
Avocado	⅛ medium	25	40	0.5	3.8	1.9	3	150	0	0.6	2.4	0.5	0.5
Free													
Cilantro	¼ c.	4	1	0	0	0	1	22	0	0	0	0	—
Jalapeño chili, cn, s + l, chopped	½ c.	68	17	0.5	0.4	3.3	995	92	0	(0)	(0)	(0.2)	(1.2)
Salsa de chile	2 tbsp	34	13	0.3	0	3.1	167	46	0	0	0	0	0.7
Verdolagas, ck	½ c.	58	10	0.9	0.1	2.1	26	283	0	0	0	0	(1.2)
Occasional													
Pan dulce, 4.5 in. across (no frosting or fruit) (Starch/bread 4 + Fat 1)	1	100	384	9.1	11.6	60.8	389	124	?	?	?	?	?
				Chinese American									
Starch/bread													
Cellophane or mung bean noodles, ck	¾ c.	93	73	—	—	18	—	—	—	—	—	—	—
Ginkgo seeds, cn	½ c.	76	86	1.8	1.2	17.1	238	139	—	0.24	0.46	0.46	—
Lotus root, ¼ in. thick, 2½ in. diameter, raw	10 slices	81	45	2.1	0.1	14	33	450	—	—	—	—	—
Mung beans or green gram beans, ck	⅓ c.	67	71	4.7	0.3	12.7	1	177	—	0.08	0.36	0.08	—
Red beans, ck	⅓ c.	58	61	4.1	0.3	11.0	0.9	153	—	0.08	0.36	0.08	—
Rice congee or soup	¾ c.	180	69	1.5	—	15	—	20	—	—	—	—	—
Rice noodles, fresh	½ c.	49	99	1.3	0.1	23	—	—	—	—	—	—	—
Rice vermicelli, ck	½ c.	64	56	1	0	13	—	—	—	—	—	—	—
Taro, ck	⅓ c.	44	62	0.2	0.1	15	7	210	—	—	—	—	—
Lean meat or substitute													
Beef jerky, 3½ in. × 1 in. piece	½ oz	14	44	6.98	1.3	0.7	(610)	—	—	—	—	—	—
Dried scallop, large	1	13	44	8.6	0.3	1.1	—	205	—	—	—	—	—
Dried shrimp, medium	1 tbsp or 10 shrimp	11	40	6.9	0.4	1.7	—	—	—	—	—	—	—
Soybeans, ck	3 tbsp	32	56	5.4	3	3.2	0	166	0	0.42	0.64	1.62	—
Squid, raw	2 oz	57	52	8.8	0.8	1.8	26	140	132	0.20	0.06	0.24	—
Tripe, beef, raw	2 oz	57	56	8.2	2.2	0	26	154	54	1.16	0.74	0.04	—

Table continued on following page

Chinese American

FOOD	QUANTITY	GRAMS PER SERVING	Kcal	PRO (g)	FAT (g)	CHO (g)	Na (mg)	K (mg)	CHOL (mg)	SAT. FATTY ACIDS (g)	MONO. FATTY ACIDS (g)	POLY. FATTY ACIDS (g)	TOTAL DIETARY FIBER (g)
Medium-fat meat or substitute													
Beef tongue	1 oz	28	81	6.3	5.9	0.1	17	51	30	2.54	2.70	0.22	—
Tofu or soybean curd, 2½ × 2¾ × 1 in.	4 oz or ½ cup	124	94	10	5.9	2.3	9	150	0	0.86	1.31	3.35	1.5
High-fat meat or substitute													
Salted duck egg	1 whole	68	137	9.8	10.3	0.5	—	171	—	—	—	—	—
Thousand-year-old or preserved limed duck egg	1 whole	63	114	8.8	7.3	2.6	—	323	—	—	—	—	—
High-fat meat + 1 fat													
Chinese sausage (pork and spices)	1 (2 oz)	56	199	11.9	16.4	3.7	493	—	—	6.1	7.5	1.8	—
Chinese sausage (pork, liver, and spices)	1 (2 oz)	56	205	14.9	15.7	—	560	—	—	5.8	7.2	1.7	—
Vegetable													
Amaranth or Chinese spinach, ck	½ c.	61	14	1.4	0.1	2.7	14	423	—	—	—	—	—
Arrowheads, or fresh corms, large, 3½ in. diameter, raw	1	25	25	1.2	0.2	5.0	6	470	—	—	—	—	—
Baby corn, cn	½ c.	64	13	1.9	0.3	1.9	730	117	—	—	—	—	—
Bamboo shoots, cn	½ c.	66	25	2.3	0.5	4.2	9	104	—	—	—	—	—
Bitter melon or bitter gourd, raw	1 c.	146	28	1.2	0.2	6.6	6	394	—	—	—	—	—
Chayote, raw	1 c.	124	32	1.2	0.4	7.2	4	198	—	—	—	—	—
Chinese celery, raw	1 c.	120	26	1.6	0.4	5.0	116	392	—	—	—	—	—
Chinese eggplant, white, ck	½ c.	87	20	0.9	0.1	4.9	—	—	—	—	—	—	—
Chinese eggplant, purple, ck	½ c.	72	17	0.7	0.1	4.0	—	—	—	—	—	—	—
Chinese or black mushrooms, medium, dried	2	8	22	0.7	0.1	5.6	1	115	—	—	—	—	—
Hairy melon or hairy cucumber, raw	1 c.	156	22	1.0	—	5.4	—	—	—	—	—	—	—
Leeks, ck	½ c.	52	16	0.4	0.1	4.0	6	46	—	—	—	—	—
Luffa, angled, raw	1 c.	178	30	1.2	0.2	7.2	2	252	—	—	—	—	—
Luffa, smooth or sponge, raw	1 c.	178	34	2.0	0.4	8.0	6	274	—	—	—	—	—
Mung bean sprouts, seed attached, raw	1 c.	104	32	3.2	0.2	6.2	6	144	—	—	—	—	—
Mung bean sprouts, seed attached, ck	½ c.	62	13	1.3	0.1	2.6	6	63	—	—	—	—	—
Mustard greens, ck	½ c.	70	11	1.6	0.2	1.5	11	141	—	—	—	—	—
Peapods or sugar peas, ck	½ c.	80	34	2.6	0.2	5.6	3	192	—	—	—	—	—
Soybean sprouts, seed attached, raw	½ c.	35	45	4.6	2.4	3.9	5	169	—	0.25	0.26	1.30	—
Soybean sprouts, seed attached, ck	½ c.	47	38	4.0	2.1	3.1	10	334	—	0.45	0.47	2.32	—
Straw mushrooms, cn	½ c.	66	20	1.5	0.1	3.8	172	47	—	—	—	—	—
Turnip, raw	1 c.	110	36	1.2	0.2	8.0	88	248	—	—	—	—	—
Water chestnuts, 1¼–2 in. diameter, raw	4 whole	36	38	0.5	0	8.6	5	210	—	—	—	—	—
Water chestnuts, cn (s + l)	½ c.	70	35	0.6	0.0	8.7	6	82	—	—	—	—	(1.3)
Winter melon or wax gourd, raw	1 c.	132	17	0.5	0.3	4.0	8	14.7	—	—	—	—	—
Yard-long beans, raw	1 c.	90	44	2.6	0.4	7.6	4	218	—	—	—	—	—
Yard-long beans, ck	½ c.	52	24	1.3	—	4.8	2	151	—	—	—	—	—
Fruit													
Carambola or star fruit, medium, raw	1½	191	63	1.0	0.6	14.8	2.5	230	—	—	—	—	—
Chinese banana, dwarf, raw	1	100	72	1.8	0.2	18.0	18	435	—	—	—	—	—
Guava, medium, raw	1½	135	69	1.2	0.9	15.9	3	384	—	—	—	—	—
Kumquat, medium, raw	5	100	60	1.0	—	16.0	5	220	—	—	—	—	—
Litchi or lychee, raw	10	96	60	0.7	0.4	16.0	0	144	—	—	—	—	—
Litchi or lychee, cn	½ c.	77	57	0.2	0.3	14.9	27	52	—	—	—	—	—
Longan, raw	30	96	60	1.2	0	14.4	0	27	—	—	—	—	—
Longan, cn	¾ c.	100	68	0.4	0.3	17.6	54	41	—	—	—	—	—
Mango, small, raw	½	104	68	0.5	0.3	17.6	2	161	—	—	—	—	—

Papaya, ripe, 3½ in. diameter, 5⅛ in. high, raw	½	152	59	0.9	0.2	14.9	4	389	—	—	—	—	—
Persimmon, Japanese (soft type), raw	½	84	59	0.5	0.2	15.6	2.0	135	—	—	—	—	—
Pummelo, raw	¾ c.	142	58	1.0	0.4	14.2	1	352	—	—	—	—	—
Milk													
Soybean milk, unsweetened	1 c.	240	78	6.6	4.6	4.4	30	338	0	0.52	0.78	2.0	—
Fat													
Coconut milk*	1 tbsp	15	35	0.3	3.6	0.8	2	39	0	3.17	0.15	0.04	—
Sesame paste	1½ tsp	8	48	1.4	4.0	2.0	1	46	0	0.57	1.54	1.78	
0.8													
Sesame seeds, whole, dried	1 tbsp	9	52	1.6	4.5	2.1	1	42	0	0.63	1.69	1.96	—
Free													
Amaranth or Chinese spinach, raw	1 c.	28	7	0.7	0.1	1.1	5	171	—	—	—	—	—
Bok choy, raw	1 c.	70	10	1.1	0.1	1.5	46	176	—	—	—	—	—
Bok choy, ck	½ c.	85	10	1.3	0.1	1.5	29	315	—	—	—	—	—
Chili pepper, raw	1	45	18	0.9	0.1	4.3	3	153	—	—	—	—	—
Chinese or Peking cabbage, raw	1 c.	76	12	0.9	0.2	2.5	7	181	—	—	—	—	—
Chinese or Peking cabbage, ck	½ c.	60	8	0.9	0.1	1.4	6	134	—	—	—	—	—
Choy sum or Chinese flowering cabbage, raw	1 c.	56	9	1.2	—	1.6	—	—	—	—	—	—	—
Coriander, raw	½ c.	8	2	—	—	0.2	2	44	—	—	—	—	—
Garland chrysanthemum, raw	1 c.	25	4	0.4	0	1.1	13	143	—	—	—	—	—
Gingerroot, raw	¼ c.	24	17	0.4	0.2	3.6	3	100	—	—	—	—	—
Mustard greens, salted and soured	2 tbsp	23	14	0.5	0.1	4.0	—	—	—	—	—	—	—
Oriental radish or daikon, raw	1 c.	88	16	0.6	0	1.8	9	—	—	—	—	—	—
Watercress, raw	1 c.	34	4	0.8	0	0.4	14	112	—	—	—	—	—
Combination													
Mock duck or wheat gluten, cn	½ c.	74	88	14	—	10	—	28	—	—	—	—	—
			Hmong American										
Starch/bread													
Cellophane or mung bean noodles, ck	¾ c.	93	73	—	—	18	—	—	—	—	—	—	—
Rice noodles, fresh	½ c.	49	99	1.3	0.1	23	—	—	—	—	—	—	—
Rice soup	¾ c.	180	69	1.5	—	15	—	20	—	—	—	—	—
Yard-long beans, pod and seeds, ck	½ c.	86	102	7.1	0.4	18.1	4	271	0	0.10	0.03	0.17	—
Medium-fat meat or substitute													
Pig's feet	2½ oz (= 2 exchanges)	71	138	13.6	8.8	0	—	—	71	3.04	4.13	0.96	0
Tofu or soybean curd, 2½ × 2¾ × 1 in.	4 oz or ½ cup	124	94	10	5.9	2.3	9	150	0	0.86	1.31	3.35	1.5
Vegetables													
Bamboo shoots, cn, drained	½ c.	66	13	1.1	0.3	2.1	4	52	0	0.06	0.01	0.11	0.43
Bitter melon, raw	1 c.	146	28	1.2	0.2	6.6	6	394	—	—	—	—	—
Cucuzzi squash (spaghetti squash), ck	½ c.	78	23	0.5	0.2	5.0	14	91	0	0.05	0.02	0.10	1.09
Luffa gourd/squash, angled, raw	1 c.	178	30	1.2	0.2	7.2	2	252	—	—	—	—	—
Luffa gourd/smooth or sponge, raw	1 c.	178	34	2	0.4	8	6	274	—	—	—	—	—
Mung bean sprouts, seeds attached, ck	½ c.	62	13	1.3	0.1	2.6	6	63	—	—	—	—	—
Pumpkin, ck	½ c.	122	24	0.9	0.1	6.0	2	281	0	0.04	0.01	0.00	1.01
Fruits													
Apple pear, raw, 2¼ in. high, 2½ in. diameter	1	122	51	0.6	0.3	13	0	148	0	0	0	0	—
Guava, medium, raw	1½	135	69	1.2	0.8	15.9	3	384	—	—	—	—	—
Jackfruit	½ c.	90	85	1	0.3	22	3	273	0	—	—	—	—
Fats													
Beef tallow	1 tsp	4.3	39	0	4.3	0	0	0	5	2.13	1.77	0.17	0
Chicken fat	1 tsp	4.3	38	0	4.3	0	—	—	4	1.27	1.9	0.9	0
Coconut cream	1 tbsp	19	36	0.5	3.4	1.6	10	19	0	2.99	0.14	0.04	—
Coconut milk, raw	1 tbsp	15	35	0.3	3.6	0.8	2	39	0	3.17	0.15	0.04	—

Table continued on following page

FOOD	QUANTITY	GRAMS PER SERVING	Kcal	PRO (g)	FAT (g)	CHO (g)	Na (mg)	K (mg)	CHOL (mg)	SAT. FATTY ACIDS (g)	MONO. FATTY ACIDS (g)	POLY. FATTY ACIDS (g)	TOTAL DIETARY FIBER (g)
Hmong American													
Coconut milk, cn	1 tbsp	15	30	0.3	3.2	0.9	2	33	0	2.89	0.14	0.04	—
Pork lard	1 tsp	4.2	39	0	4.3	0	0	0	4	1.67	1.93	0.47	0
Free													
Coriander (Chinese parsley), raw	1 c.	16	4	0.3	0.1	0.4	4	88	—	—	—	—	—
Fish sauce	1 tbsp	16	4	0.8	0.1	0	1088	—	—	—	—	—	0
Pumpkin blossom, ck	1 c.	134	20	1.5	0.1	4.4	8	142	0	0.05	0.02	0.01	—
Tender vines and leaves of pumpkin, squash, luffa gourd, and pea plant, ck	1 c.	70	14	2	0	2	6	306	0	0	0	0	—
Vinespinach, raw	1 c.	56	11	1	0.2	1.9	—	—	0	—	—	—	—
Occasional													
Condensed milk, sweetened	1 fl oz	38.2	123	3.0	3.3	20.8	49	142	13	2.10	0.93	0.13	0

* The addition of ash significantly increases the potassium content.

† Although data for flour tortillas and hominy are available from USDA sources, they reflect preparation techniques from other parts of the country. This data base contains information from a Navajo-specific study.

‡ The 8-inch diameter of the tortilla was chosen to represent the size that is commonly eaten.

§ Because of the lack of published data on mutton, the National Live Stock and Meat Board and the New Mexico Cooperative Extension Service recommend substituting lamb nutrient values for mutton, as has been done in this data base. However, everyday observation on the Navajo reservation suggests that the untrimmed mutton eaten by many clients is considerably higher in fat than the published data for lean and fat lamb. Thus, trimming mutton might reduce fat and kilocalories beyond the estimates given here.

¶ Total fat value includes fatty acids and glycerol.

** Raw liquid expressed from mixture of grated coconut meat and water.

KEY: CHO = carbohydrate; Chol = cholesterol; ck = cooked; cn = canned; K = potassium; Mono. = monounsaturated; Na = sodium; Poly. = polyunsaturated; Pro = protein; Sat. = saturated; s + l = small and large.

From Ethnic and Regional Food Practices, A Series. Navaho (1991), Alaskan Native (1993), Mexican American (1989), Chinese American (1990), and Hmong American (1992) Food Practices, Customs, and Holidays. The American Dietetic Association and American Diabetes Association, Inc.

Appendix 7 Dietary Fiber Content and Composition as Percentage of Sample Fresh Weight of 117 Frequently Consumed Foods

FOOD GROUP AND SAMPLE	MOISTURE[a]	SOLUBLE FIBER			INSOLUBLE FIBER					Total Dietary Fiber
		Hemicelluloses	Pectin	Total	Hemicelluloses	Cellulose	Pectin	Klason Lignin	Total	
Fruits										
Apple, Red Delicious, unpeeled	83.6*	tr[b]	0.2	0.2	0.5	0.6	0.5	0.2	1.8	2.0
Apple, Red Delicious, peeled	84.6*	tr	0.2	0.2	0.4	0.5	0.3	0.1	1.3	1.5
Apple, Granny Smith, unpeeled	83.8*	tr	0.3	0.3	0.8	1.0	0.5	0.1	2.4	2.7
Apricots, canned in syrup	73.4*	0.1	0.4	0.5	0.4	0.6	0.2	0.1	1.3	1.8
Banana	75.7*	0.2	0.3	0.5	0.2	0.3	0.1	0.6	1.2	1.7
Blueberries, fresh	85.4	0.1	0.2	0.3	0.7	0.4	0.4	0.9	2.4	2.7
Cantaloupe	88.7*	tr	0.1	0.1	0.1	0.3	0.2	tr	0.6	0.7
Cherries, tart, canned	90.9*	0.1	0.1	0.2	0.1	0.2	0.2	0.2	0.7	0.9
Grapefruit (Fla), pink, with membrane	86.9*	0.1	0.2	0.3	0.3	0.3	0.5	tr	1.1	1.4
Grapefruit (Fla), pink, without membrane	88.4*	tr	0.1	0.1	0.1	0.1	0.2	tr	0.4	0.5
Grapefruit (Tex), pink, without membrane	87.9*	0.1	tr	0.1	0.1	0.1	0.1	tr	0.3	0.4
Grapefruit (Fla), white, without membrane	88.2*	tr	0.1	0.1	0.1	tr	0.2	tr	0.3	0.4
Grapes, Thompson green	80.0*	tr	0.1	0.1	0.2	0.3	0.1	0.2	0.9	1.0
Nectarine, unpeeled	89.7*	0.2	0.2	0.4	0.3	0.3	0.1	0.1	0.8	1.2
Orange, navel	85.5*	0.1	0.2	0.3	0.5	0.4	0.5	tr	1.4	1.7
Orange (Fla)	86.8*	0.2	0.4	0.6	0.4	0.4	0.5	tr	1.3	1.9
Pear, canned in extra light syrup	89.7*	0.1	0.2	0.3	0.6	0.5	0.1	0.2	1.4	1.7
Pear, Bartlett, fresh, unpeeled	85.0*	0.1	0.3	0.4	0.9	0.7	0.4	0.4	2.4	2.8
Pineapple, canned in unsweetened juice	83.4*	0.1	tr	0.1	0.3	0.3	tr	tr	0.6	0.7
Plum, Friar, fresh, unpeeled	87.1*	0.1	0.3	0.4	0.2	0.2	0.2	0.2	0.8	1.2
Strawberries, fresh	90.2*	0.1	0.3	0.4	0.3	0.4	0.2	0.5	1.4	1.8
Tangerine	85.1*	0.1	0.3	0.4	0.4	0.4	0.5	0.1	1.4	1.8
Watermelon	90.1*	0.1	tr	0.1	0.1	0.1	0.1	tr	0.3	0.4
Vegetables										
Asparagus, whole spears, canned	93.3*	0.2	0.2	0.4	0.6	0.4	tr	0.2	1.2	1.6
Asparagus, fresh, cooked	91.4*	0.1	0.2	0.3	0.4	0.7	0.4	0.1	1.6	1.9
Bamboo shoots, canned	97.4*	0.1	tr	0.1	0.5	0.7	0.1	0.1	1.4	1.5
Bean sprouts, canned	96.2*	0.1	tr	0.1	0.5	0.3	0.2	0.1	1.1	1.2
Green beans, whole cut, canned	94.2*	0.3	0.2	0.5	0.5	0.5	0.2	0.2	1.4	1.9
Green beans, french cut, canned	93.2*	0.3	0.3	0.6	0.5	0.7	0.2	0.1	1.5	2.1
Beets, cut, canned	92.4*	0.1	0.3	0.4	0.4	0.7	0.2	tr	1.3	1.7
Broccoli, raw	88.5*	0.2	0.1	0.3	1.0	1.1	0.6	0.3	3.0	3.3
Broccoli, fresh, cooked	90.2*	0.2	0.2	0.4	0.9	1.2	0.7	0.3	3.1	3.5
Brussels sprouts, frozen, cooked	87.2*	0.2	0.3	0.5	1.5	1.3	0.7	0.1	3.6	4.1
Cabbage, raw	92.7*	tr	0.1	0.1	0.5	0.6	0.5	tr	1.6	1.7
Carrots, raw, peeled	87.2*	0.1	0.1	0.2	0.7	0.8	0.7	0.1	2.3	2.5
Cauliflower, raw	92.5*	0.1	0.2	0.3	0.7	0.8	0.4	0.1	2.0	2.3
Cauliflower, fresh, cooked	94.1*	0.1	0.2	0.3	0.7	0.7	0.4	tr	1.8	2.1
Celery, raw	94.5*	tr	tr	0.1	0.4	0.7	0.6	tr	1.7	1.8
Celery, fresh, cooked	95.2*	tr	0.1	0.1	0.8	0.4	0.5	tr	1.7	1.8
Corn, whole kernel, frozen	75.8*	0.1	tr	0.1	0.9	0.7	0.1	0.3	2.0	2.1

Table continued on following page

563

FOOD GROUP AND SAMPLE	MOISTURE[a]	SOLUBLE FIBER			INSOLUBLE FIBER					Total Dietary Fiber
		Hemicelluloses	Pectin	Total	Hemicelluloses	Cellulose	Pectin	Klason Lignin	Total	
Vegetables										
Corn, whole kernel, canned	76.7*	0.1	tr	0.1	0.5	0.7	0.1	0.5	1.8	1.9
Cucumber, peeled	96.2*	tr	tr	0.1	0.2	0.2	0.1	tr	0.5	0.6
Cucumber, unpeeled	95.8*	tr	tr	0.1	0.2	0.3	0.2	0.1	0.8	0.9
Mushrooms, canned	91.1‡	0.2	tr	0.2	0.3	1.8	0.1	0.1	2.3	2.5
Onion, green, raw	92.7*	tr	tr	tr	0.6	0.6	0.8	0.2	2.2	2.2
Onion, yellow, raw	90.3*	tr	tr	0.1	0.5	0.6	0.5	tr	1.6	1.7
Green pepper, raw	93.9*	tr	0.1	0.2	0.4	0.5	0.3	0.3	1.5	1.7
Potato, baked, with skin	73.3*	0.4	0.2	0.6	0.5	1.0	0.1	0.3	1.9	2.5
Potato, boiled, without skin	79.5*	0.2	0.1	0.3	0.4	0.5	0.1	tr	1.0	1.3
Potato, french fries	68.3*	0.2	0.2	0.4	0.7	0.9	0.2	0.1	1.8	2.3
Pumpkin, canned	90.2‡	0.1	0.4	0.5	0.4	1.4	0.4	0.2	2.4	2.9
Radish, red, raw	94.2*	tr	tr	0.1	0.3	0.6	0.4	tr	1.3	1.4
Squash, zucchini, raw	94.5*	0.1	tr	0.1	0.3	0.3	0.2	tr	0.8	0.9
Sweet potato, cut, canned in light syrup	75.6*	0.2	0.2	0.4	0.3	0.8	0.1	0.1	1.3	1.7
Tomatoes, canned	93.4*	tr	0.1	0.1	0.2	0.2	0.1	0.1	0.6	0.7
Turnip greens, frozen	92.9*	tr	0.1	0.1	0.6	0.9	0.8	0.1	2.4	2.5
Refined grain products[c]										
Biscuits, baking powder	16.7†	0.5	tr	0.5	0.9	0.6	tr	0.1	1.6	2.1
Bread, French	29.2†	0.7	tr	0.8	0.8	0.9	tr	0.1	1.9	2.7
Bread, Italian	26.9†	0.9	tr	0.9	1.2	0.9	0.1	0.7	2.9	3.8
Bread, Italian with sesame seeds	34.6†	0.9	tr	0.9	0.7	0.7	0.1	1.0	2.5	3.4
Bread, white wheat	33.1†	0.6	tr	0.6	0.8	0.6	0.1	0.5	2.0	2.6
Bun, hamburger	31.4‡	0.6	tr	0.7	0.9	0.7	tr	0.2	1.8	2.5
Cake, yellow	26.9*	0.3	tr	0.3	0.4	0.6	tr	0.1	1.1	1.4
Cereal, Total[d]	4.0‡	0.1	—	0.1	0.4	0.9	0.1	1.6	3.0	3.1
Cereal, cornflakes	10.9*	0.5	tr	0.5	0.9	2.1	0.1	0.7	3.8	4.3
Cereal, Cream of Wheat,[e] quick, cooked	87.9*	0.1	tr	0.1	0.2	0.3	tr	0.1	0.6	0.7
Cereal, Honey Smacks[f]	25.5*	0.5	tr	0.6	0.7	0.8	0.1	0.1	1.7	2.3
Cereal, oatmeal, old fashioned, cooked	84.2*	0.1	tr	0.7	0.4	0.1	0.1	0.5	1.2	1.9[g]
Cereal, Rice Krispies[f]	7.8*	0.5	tr	0.5	0.3	0.4	0.1	0.6	1.4	1.9
Cereal, Special K[f]	12.7*	0.2	tr	0.2	0.8	0.7	0.1	0.9	2.5	2.7
Cookies, ginger snaps	4.8†	0.6	tr	0.6	0.5	0.3	tr	0.4	1.2	1.8
Cookies, plain sugar	3.3*	0.4	tr	0.4	0.5	0.2	tr	tr	0.7	1.1
Corn bread	36.1*	0.2	tr	0.2	1.0	1.3	0.1	0.4	2.8	3.0
Hominy, white, cooked	85.0*	tr	tr	tr	0.1	0.5	tr	tr	0.6	0.6
Cracker, graham	4.4‡	0.8	tr	0.8	0.9	0.5	0.1	0.4	1.9	2.7
Cracker, saltine	4.3‡	1.2	tr	1.2	0.7	0.7	tr	0.5	1.9	3.1
Flour, all-purpose white wheat	9.2‡	0.9	0.1	1.0	1.2	0.5	0	0.2	1.9	2.9
Ice cream cone, Comet cup[e]	4.7†	1.0	tr	1.0	1.0	0.6	tr	0.5	2.1	3.1
Macaroni, cooked	69.6*	0.3	tr	0.3	0.6	0.4	tr	0.7	1.7	2.0
Muffin, English	38.0‡	0.6	tr	0.6	0.8	0.8	0.1	0.7	2.4	3.0
Muffin, plain	27.1*	0.4	tr	0.4	0.4	0.3	tr	0.4	1.1	1.5
Noodles, egg, Creamette,[h] cooked	67.2*	0.3	tr	0.3	0.5	0.5	tr	0.4	1.4	1.7

Food										
Pancake mix	8.3‡	1.0	tr	1.0	0.9	1.9	0.1	0.6	3.5	4.5
Pie crust	14.9†	0.5	tr	0.5	0.8	0.4	0	0.6	1.8	2.3
Rice, medium grain, regular, cooked	70.6*	0.1	tr	0.1	0.1	0.1	tr	0.1	0.3	0.4
Spaghetti, cooked	60.7*	0.4	tr	0.4	0.5	0.5	tr	tr	1.1	1.5
Roll, cinnamon	26.4*	0.6	tr	0.6	0.6	0.5	0.1	0.4	1.6	2.2
Tortilla, flour	33.0‡	0.5	tr	0.5	0.5	0.2	tr	0.3	1.0	1.5
Higher-fiber grain products										
Cereal, 40% bran flakes	3.2†	1.8	0.2	2.0	10.7	4.8	0.5	1.5	17.5	19.5
Cereal, All Bran[f]	5.7*	2.0	0.1	2.1	15.3	7.5	0.9	4.3	28.0	30.1
Cereal, Frosted Miniwheats[f]	15.0*	0.7	tr	0.7	3.8	2.5	0.2	1.0	7.5	8.2
Cereal, oat bran, uncooked	7.4†	1.5	0.1	6.5	3.7	1.0	0.3	3.5	10.5	17.0[i]
Cereal, Product 19[f]	3.4†	0.4	tr	0.5	1.6	1.7	0.2	1.5	5.0	5.5
Cereal, shredded wheat	7.6†	1.0	0.1	1.1	5.9	3.2	0.2	0.9	10.2	11.3
Cereal, Wheaties[d]	2.4†	1.7	0.1	1.8	4.9	2.8	0.5	1.4	9.6	11.4
Taco shell	7.7*	0.4	tr	0.4	2.5	2.7	0.3	0.9	6.4	6.8
Wheat germ	4.2‡	1.0	0.1	1.1	7.4	3.6	0.7	1.2	12.9	14.0
Legumes										
Kidney beans, canned	77.1*	0.9	0.2	1.1	1.2	2.2	0.4	0.3	4.1	5.2
Lima beans, green, canned	74.5*	0.3	0.1	0.4	1.2	2.2	0.3	0.1	3.8	4.2
Pork and beans, canned	75.0*	1.1	0.3	1.4	0.9	1.6	0.3	0.2	3.0	4.4
Peas, black-eyed, canned	78.6*	0.3	0.1	0.4	0.8	1.2	0.2	0.5	2.7	3.1
Peas, green, canned, Freshlike[j]	85.7*	0.2	0.2	0.4	0.4	2.1	0.3	0.1	2.9	3.3
Peas, green, canned, Del Monte[k]	81.5*	0.2	0.1	0.3	0.8	2.8	0.3	0.1	4.0	4.3
Peas, green, frozen	82.3*	0.1	0.2	0.3	0.7	2.0	0.5	tr	3.2	3.5
Nuts										
Almonds, with skin	4.7†	0.2	tr	0.2	1.8	3.3	1.6	1.9	8.6	8.8
Peanuts	1.6*	0.1	0.1	0.2	2.8	2.0	1.1	0.7	6.6	6.8
Peanut butter	1.7‡	0.2	0.1	0.3	2.7	1.6	0.9	0.8	6.0	6.3
Walnuts, English	3.5‡	0.1	tr	0.1	0.9	1.2	0.7	0.9	3.7	3.8
Miscellaneous foods										
Avocado (Calif)	77.3*	0.5	0.8	1.3	0.9	1.4	0.2	0.1	2.6	3.9
Catsup	66.7*	0.1	0.2	0.3	0.2	0.4	0.1	0.2	0.9	1.2
Coconut, shredded	18.5*	0.3	0.1	0.4	5.2	0.8	0.2	0	6.2	6.6
Olives, green, with pimento	76.5*	0.2	tr	0.2	0.5	0.6	0.3	0.4	1.8	2.0
Olives, black	80.5*	0.1	tr	0.1	0.6	0.6	0.3	0.6	2.1	2.2
Pickle, dill	94.9*	tr	tr	tr	0.3	0.4	0.3	0.1	1.1	1.1
Raisins	9.9*	0.3	0.3	0.6	0.4	0.8	0.6	1.8	3.6	4.2
Soup, cream of mushroom, canned	84.1*	0.1	tr	0.1	0.2	tr	tr	0	0.3	0.4
Soup, vegetarian vegetable, canned	82.3*	0.3	0.2	0.5	0.3	0.8	0.1	0.1	1.3	1.8

a Determined by lyophilization (*) or oven drying (†) or obtained from U.S. Dept. of Agriculture handbook no. 456 (‡).
b Tr = trace, less than 0.05%.
c Refined grain products are defined as those containing less than 5.0% total dietary fiber.
d General Mills, Minneapolis, Minn.
e Nabisco Brands, East Hanover, NJ.
f Kellogg Company, Battlecreek, Mich.
g Contains 0.7% β-glucan, 0.6% in the soluble and 0.1% in the insoluble fraction.
h Borden, Columbus, Ohio.
i Contains 6.9% β-glucan, 4.9% in the soluble and 2.0% in the insoluble fraction.
j The Larson Co, Green Bay, Wisc.
k Del Monte, San Francisco, Calif.

From Marlett JA: Content and composition of dietary fiber in 117 frequently consumed foods. © The American Dietetic Association. Reprinted by permission from Journal of the American Dietetic Association, 1992; 92: 175.

Appendix 8 Selected Enteral Liquid Supplements*

Product	Manufacturer	Form	NUTRIENT SOURCE		
			Major Protein Source	Major Fat Source	Major Carbohydrate Source
Citrisource	Sandoz Nutrition	Liquid	Whey protein concentrate	None added	Sugar, hydrolyzed cornstarch
Citrotein	Sandoz Nutrition	Powder	Egg white solids	Partially hydrogenated soybean oil	Sugar, hydrolyzed cornstarch
Compleat Regular	Sandoz Nutrition	Liquid	Beef, nonfat milk	Corn oil, beef	Maltodextrin, vegetables, fruits, lactose
Compleat Modified	Sandoz Nutrition	Liquid	Beef, calcium caseinate	Canola oil, beef	Maltodextrin, vegetables, fruits
Fibersource	Sandoz Nutrition	Liquid	Sodium and calcium caseinate	MCT, canola oil	Hydrolyzed cornstarch, soy fiber
Fibersource HN	Sandoz Nutrition	Liquid	Sodium and calcium caseinate	MCT, canola oil	Hydrolyzed cornstarch, soy fiber
Impact	Sandoz Nutrition	Liquid	Sodium and calcium caseinate, L-arginine	Structured lipid, menhaden oil	Hydrolyzed cornstarch
Impact with Fiber	Sandoz Nutrition	Liquid	Sodium and calcium caseinate, L-arginine	Structured lipid, menhaden oil	Hydrolyzed cornstarch, soy fiber, enzymatically modified guar
Isosource	Sandoz Nutrition	Liquid	Sodium and calcium caseinate, soy protein isolate	MCT, canola oil	Hydrolyzed cornstarch
Isosource HN	Sandoz Nutrition	Liquid	Sodium and calcium caseinate, soy protein isolate	MCT, canola oil	Hydrolyzed cornstarch
Isotein HN	Sandoz Nutrition	Powder	Delactosed lactalbumin	Partially hydrogenated soybean oil, MCT	Hydrolyzed cornstarch, fructose
Meritene Powder (Prepared with whole milk)	Sandoz Nutrition	Powder	Nonfat milk, whole milk	Milk fat	Lactose, sugar, hydrolyzed cornstarch
Resource Liquid	Sandoz Nutrition	Liquid	Sodium and calcium caseinate, soy protein isolate	Corn oil	Hydrolyzed cornstarch, sugar
Resource Plus Liquid	Sandoz Nutrition	Liquid	Sodium and calcium caseinate, soy protein isolate	Corn oil	Hydrolyzed cornstarch, sugar
Tolerex	Sandoz Nutrition	Powder	Free amino acids	Safflower oil	Glucose oligosaccharides
Vivonex Plus	Sandoz Nutrition	Powder	Free amino acids (30% BCAA)	Soybean oil	Maltodextrin, modified starch
Vivonex T.E.N.	Sandoz Nutrition	Powder	Free amino acids (33% BCAA)	Safflower oil	Maltodextrin
AlitraQ	Ross Laboratories	Powder	Peptides from soy hydrolysate, free amino acids, whey protein concentrate	MCT, safflower oil	Hydrolyzed cornstarch, sucrose
Criticare HN	Mead Johnson	Liquid	Enzymatically hydrolyzed casein, free amino acids	Safflower oil	Maltodextrin, modified cornstarch
Ensure with Fiber	Ross Laboratories	Liquid	Sodium and calcium caseinate, soy protein isolate	Corn oil	Hydrolyzed cornstarch, sucrose, soy polysaccharide
Ensure	Ross Laboratories	Liquid	Sodium and calcium caseinate, soy protein isolate	Corn oil	Corn syrup, sucrose
Ensure Plus	Ross Laboratories	Liquid	Sodium and calcium caseinate, soy protein isolate	Corn oil	Corn syrup, sucrose
Entrition RDA	Clintec	Liquid	Sodium and calcium caseinate	Corn oil	Maltodextrin
Entrition HN	Clintec	Liquid	Sodium and calcium caseinate	Corn oil	Maltodextrin
Glucerna	Ross Laboratories	Liquid	Sodium and calcium caseinate	High-oleic safflower oil, soy oil	Glucose polymers, soy fiber, fructose
Isocal	Mead Johnson	Liquid	Calcium and sodium caseinate, soy protein isolate	Soy oil, MCT	Maltodextrin
Isocal HN	Mead Johnson	Liquid	Calcium and sodium caseinate, soy protein isolate	Soy oil, MCT	Maltodextrin
Jevity	Ross Laboratories	Liquid	Sodium and calcium caseinate	MCT, corn oil, soy oil	Hydrolyzed cornstarch, soy polysaccharide
Osmolite	Ross Laboratories	Liquid	Sodium and calcium caseinate, soy protein isolate	MCT, corn oil, soy oil	Glucose polymers

													NUTRIENT ANALYSIS PER 1000 mL.								
Closed System	Protein (g/1000 mL)	Carbohydrate (g/1000 mL)	Fat (g/1000 mL)	% Cal from Protein	% Cal from Carbohydrate	% Cal from Fat	Calories/mL	N:Nonprotein Calorie Ratio	N:Calorie Ratio	mOsm/kg Water	Volume (mL) to meet 100% U.S. RDA	Water content (mL) per liter	Sodium mg (mEq)	Potassium mg (mEq)	Chloride mg (mEq)	Calcium mg (mEq)	Phosphorus mg (mMol)	Magnesium mg (mEq)	Iron (mg)	Fiber (g)	Trace Elements Added (Selenium, Chromium, Molybdenum)
No	37	150	0	20	80	0	0.76	1:105	1:131	700	*	876	210 (9)	85 (2)	930 (26)	570 (28)	680 (22)	210 (17)	9.5	—	No
No	41	120	1.6	25	73	2	0.67	1:76	1:101	480	1100	949	670 (29)	550 (14)	790 (22)	1100 (55)	1100 (35)	420 (35)	38	—	No
Yes	43	130	43	16	48	36	1.07	1:131	1:156	450	1500	843	1300 (57)	1400 (36)	1100 (31)	670 (33)	1200 (39)	270 (22)	12	4.2	Yes
Yes	43	140	37	16	53	31	1.07	1:131	1:156	300	1500	838	1000 (43)	1400 (36)	1100 (31)	670 (33)	870 (28)	270 (22)	12	4.2	Yes
Yes	43	170	41	14	56	30	1.2	1:151	1:177	390	1500	823	1100 (48)	1800 (46)	1100 (31)	670 (33)	670 (22)	270 (22)	12	10	Yes
Yes	53	160	41	18	52	30	1.2	1:118	1:144	390	1500	821	1100 (48)	1800 (46)	1100 (31)	670 (33)	670 (22)	270 (22)	12	6.7	Yes
Yes	56	130	28	22	53	25	1.0	1:71	1:91	375	1500	853	1100 (48)	1300 (33)	1300 (37)	800 (40)	800 (26)	270 (22)	12	—	Yes
No	56	140	28	22	53	25	1.0	1:71	1:91	375	1500	868	1100 (48)	1300 (33)	1300 (37)	800 (40)	800 (26)	270 (22)	12	10	Yes
Yes	43	170	41	14	56	30	1.2	1:148	1:173	360	1500	819	1200 (52)	1700 (43)	1100 (31)	670 (33)	670 (22)	270 (22)	12	—	Yes
Yes	53	160	41	18	52	30	1.2	1:116	1:141	330	1500	819	1100 (48)	1700 (43)	1100 (31)	670 (33)	670 (22)	270 (22)	12	—	Yes
No	68	160	34	23	52	25	1.19	1:86	1:111	300	1770	859	620 (27)	1100 (28)	960 (27)	560 (28)	560 (18)	230 (19)	10	—	Yes
No	69	120	34	26	45	29	1.06	1:71	1:96	690	1040	819	1100 (48)	2800 (72)	2200 (62)	2200 (110)	1900 (61)	380 (31)	17	—	No
No	37	140	37	14	54	32	1.06	1:154	1:179	430	1890	842	890 (39)	1600 (41)	1000 (28)	530 (27)	530 (17)	210 (17)	9.5	—	No
No	55	200	53	15	53	32	1.5	1:146	1:171	600	1400	764	1300 (57)	2100 (54)	1600 (45)	700 (35)	700 (23)	310 (26)	14	—	No
No	21	230	1.5	8	91	1.0	1.0	1:282	1:307	550	3160	864	470 (20)	1200 (31)	950 (27)	560 (28)	560 (18)	220 (18)	10	—	Yes
No	45	190	6.7	18	76	6	1.0	1:115	1:140	650	1800	850	610 (27)	1057 (27)	943 (27)	557 (28)	557 (18)	222 (19)	10	—	Yes
No	38	210	2.8	15	82	3	1.0	1:149	1:175	630	2000	853	460 (20)	780 (20)	820 (23)	500 (25)	500 (16)	200 (16)	9	—	Yes
No	53	165	16	21	66	13	1.0	1:94	1:120	575	1500	846	1000 (43)	1200 (31)	1300 (37)	733 (37)	733 (24)	267 (22)	15	—	Yes
No	38	220	5	14	82	5	1.06	1:149	1:174	650	1890	830	630 (27)	1320 (34)	1060 (30)	530 (27)	530 (17)	210 (17)	9.5	—	No
No	40	162	37	14	55	31	1.1	1:148	1:173	480	1391	829	845 (37)	1564 (40)	1440 (41)	719 (36)	719 (23)	288 (24)	13	14	Yes
No	37	145	37	14	54	32	1.06	1:153	1:178	470	1887	845	854 (37)	1564 (40)	1437 (41)	530 (27)	530 (17)	212 (17)	9.6	—	Yes
Yes	55	200	53	15	53	32	1.5	1:146	1:171	690	1420	769	1050 (46)	1940 (50)	1900 (54)	705 (35)	704 (23)	282 (23)	12.7	—	Yes
Yes	35	136	35	14	54	32	1.0	1:148	1:172	300	1500	844	800 (35)	1340 (34)	1340 (38)	670 (34)	670 (22)	268 (22)	12	—	Yes
Yes	44	114	41	18	45	37	1.0	1:117	1:142	300	1300	840	920 (40)	1579 (40)	1540 (44)	770 (39)	770 (25)	308 (25)	14	—	No
No	42	94	56	17	33	50	1.0	1:125	1:150	375	1422	874	928 (40)	1561 (40)	1435 (41)	704 (35)	704 (23)	282 (23)	12.7	14	Yes
No	34	133	44	13	50	37	1.06	1:167	1:192	270	1890	840	530 (23)	1320 (34)	1060 (30)	630 (32)	530 (17)	210 (17)	9.5	—	Yes
No	44	124	45	17	46	37	1.06	1:125	1:150	270	1180	840	930 (40)	1600 (41)	1430 (40)	840 (42)	840 (27)	340 (28)	15	—	Yes
Yes	44	152	37	17	53	30	1.06	1:125	1:150	310	1321	833	930 (40)	1564 (40)	1437 (41)	909 (45)	756 (24)	303 (25)	13.7	14	Yes
Yes	37	145	39	14	55	31	1.06	1:153	1:178	300	1887	841	640 (28)	1020 (26)	856 (24)	530 (27)	530 (17)	212 (17)	9.6	—	Yes

Table continued on following page

			NUTRIENT SOURCE		
Product	Manufacturer	Form	Major Protein Source	Major Fat Source	Major Carbohydrate Source
Osmolite HN	Ross Laboratories	Liquid	Sodium and calcium caseinate, soy protein isolate	MCT, corn oil, soy oil	Glucose polymers
Peptamen	Clintec	Liquid	Peptides from enzymatically hydrolyzed whey protein	MCT, sunflower oil	Maltodextrin, starch
Pulmocare	Ross Laboratories	Liquid	Sodium and calcium caseinate	Corn oil	Sucrose, hydrolyzed cornstarch
Reabilan HN	Elan Pharma	Liquid	Whey and casein peptides, nonphosphorylated casein peptides	MCT, primrose oil, soy oil	Maltodextrin, tapioca starch
Replete Unflavored	Clintec	Liquid	Calcium-potassium caseinate	Canola oil, MCT	Maltodextrin, corn syrup solids
Sustacal	Mead Johnson	Liquid	Calcium caseinate, soy protein isolate, sodium caseinate	Partially hydrogenated soy oil	Sucrose, corn syrup
Sustacal HC	Mead Johnson	Liquid	Calcium and sodium caseinate	Corn oil	Corn syrup solids, sugar
Sustacal with Fiber	Mead Johnson	Liquid	Calcium and sodium caseinate, soy protein isolate	Corn oil	Maltodextrin, sugar, soy fiber
Traumacal	Mead Johnson	Liquid	Calcium and sodium caseinate	Soybean oil, MCT	Corn syrup, sugar
Ultracal	Mead Johnson	Liquid	Sodium and calcium caseinate	Soy oil, MCT	Maltodextrin, soy fiber, oat fiber
Vital HN	Ross Laboratories	Powder	Partially hydrolyzed whey, meat and soy, free amino acids	Safflower oil, MCT	Hydrolyzed cornstarch, sucrose

* Based on manufacturer's available literature.

† Lack of fat precludes use as a total feeding.

‡ Contains selenium and chromium only.

Telephone numbers for leading manufacturers of liquid supplements: Clintec Nutrition Company 1-800-422-ASK2; Mead Johnson Nutritional Group 1-812-429-5000; Ross Laboratories 1-800-FOR-ROSS; Sandoz Nutrition 1-800-821-3559; Sherwood Medical 1-800-428-4400.

From Sandoz Nutrition, Your Source Chart. 1992 Clinical Products Division, Sandoz Nutrition Corporation, 5320 West 23rd Street, PO Box 370, Minneapolis, MN 55440.

NUTRITIONAL PROFILE / **NUTRIENT ANALYSIS PER 1000 mL.**

Closed System	Protein (g/1000 mL)	Carbohydrate (g/1000 mL)	Fat (g/1000 mL)	% Cal from Protein	% Cal from Carbohydrate	% Cal from Fat	Calories/mL	N:Nonprotein Calorie Ratio	N:Calorie Ratio	mOsm/kg Water	Volume (mL) to meet 100% U.S. RDA	Water content per liter (mL)	Sodium mg (mEq)	Potassium mg (mEq)	Chloride mg (mEq)	Calcium mg (mEq)	Phosphorous mg (mEq)	Magnesium mg (mMol)	Iron (mg)	Fiber (g)	Trace Elements Added (Selenium, Chromium, Molybdenum)
Yes	44	141	37	17	53	30	1.06	1:125	1:150	300	1321	841	930 (40)	1570 (40)	1440 (41)	758 (38)	758 (24)	303 (25)	13.7	—	Yes
No	40	127	39	16	51	33	1.0	1:131	1:156	270	1500	840	1000 (22)	1250 (32)	1000 (28)	800 (40)	700 (23)	400 (33)	12	—	Yes
No	63	106	92	17	28	55	1.5	1:125	1:150	520	947	786	1310 (57)	1902 (49)	1691 (48)	1056 (53)	1056 (34)	423 (35)	19	—	Yes
No	58	158	52	17	48	35	1.3	1:125	1:160	490	1875	800	1000 (43)	1661 (43)	2492 (70)	451 (23)	499 (16)	331 (27)	13	—	Yes
No	63	113	34	25	45	30	1.0	1:75	1:100	290	1000	844	500 (22)	1560 (40)	1000 (28)	1000 (50)	1000 (32)	400 (33)	18	—	Yes
No	61	140	23	24	55	21	1.01	1:79	1:104	650	1080	840	930 (40)	2100 (54)	1480 (42)	1010 (51)	930 (30)	380 (31)	17	—	No
No	61	190	58	16	50	34	1.5	1:134	1:160	650	1180	780	850 (37)	1480 (38)	1270 (36)	850 (43)	850 (27)	340 (28)	15	—	No
No	46	139	35	17	53	30	1.06	1:120	1:145	480	1390	840	720 (31)	1390 (36)	1390 (39)	850 (43)	710 (23)	280 (23)	12.7	6	No
No	82	142	68	22	38	40	1.5	1:91	1:116	490	2000	780	1180 (51)	1390 (36)	1600 (45)	750 (38)	750 (24)	200 (16)	9	—	No
No	44	123	45	17	46	37	1.06	1:130	1:152	310	1250	850	930 (40)	1610 (41)	1440 (41)	850 (43)	850 (27)	340 (28)	15	14	Yes
No	42	185	11	17	74	9	1.0	1:125	1:150	500	1500	867	467 (20)	1334 (34)	900 (25)	667 (33)	667 (22)	267 (22)	12	—	Yes

Appendix 9 The Exchange System

"This material has been modified from Exchange Lists for Meal Planning, which is the basis of a meal planning system designed by a committee of the American Diabetes Association and the American Dietetic Association. While designed primarily for people with diabetes and others who must follow special diets, the Exchange Lists are based on principles of good nutrition that apply to everyone." ©1986 American Diabetes Association, The American Dietetic Association.

AMOUNT OF NUTRIENTS IN ONE SERVING FROM EACH EXCHANGE LIST

EXCHANGE LIST	CARBOHYDRATE (g)	PROTEIN (g)	FAT (g)	KILOCALORIES
Starch/Bread	15	3	trace	80
Meat				
Lean	—	7	3	55
Medium-fat	—	7	5	75
High-fat	—	7	8	100
Vegetable	5	2	—	25
Fruit	15	—	—	60
Milk				
Skim	12	8	trace	90
Low-fat	12	8	5	120
Whole	12	8	8	150
Fat	—	—	5	45

STARCH/BREAD LIST

FOOD	PORTION	FOOD	PORTION
Cereals/Grains/Pasta		**Dried Beans/Peas/Lentils**	
Bran cereals, concentrated*	⅓ cup	Beans and peas (cooked) (such as kidney, white, split, blackeye)*	⅓ cup
Bran cereals, flaked* (such as Bran Buds, All Bran)	½ cup	Lentils (cooked)*	⅓ cup
Bulgar (cooked)	½ cup	Baked beans*	¼ cup
Cooked cereals	½ cup	**Starchy Vegetables**	
Cornmeal (dry)	2½ tbsp	Corn*	½ cup
Grapenuts	3 tbsp	Corn on cob, 6 in long*	1
Grits (cooked)	½ cup	Lima beans*	½ cup
Other ready-to-eat unsweetened cereals	¾ cup	Peas, green (canned or frozen)*	½ cup
Pasta (cooked)	½ cup	Plaintain*	½ cup
Puffed cereal	1½ cup	Potato, baked	1 small (3 oz)
Rice, white or brown (cooked)	⅓ cup	Potato, mashed	½ cup
Shredded wheat	½ cup	Squash, winter (acorn, butternut)	¾ cup
Wheat germ*	3 tbsp	Yam, sweet potato, plain	⅓ cup
Bread		**Crackers/Snacks**	
Bagel	½ (1 oz)	Animal crackers	8
Bread sticks, crisp, 4 in. long × ½ in.	2 (⅔ oz)	Graham crackers, 2½ in. square	3
Croutons, low fat	1 cup	Matzoh	¾ oz
English muffin	½	Melba toast	5 slices
Frankfurter or hamburger bun	½ (1 oz)	Oyster crackers	24
Pita, 6 in across	½	Popcorn (popped, no fat added)	3 cups
Plain roll, small	1 (1 oz)	Pretzels	¾ oz
Raisin, unfrosted	1 slice (1 oz)	Rye crisp, 2 in. × 3½ in.	4
Rye, pumpernickel*	1 slice (1 oz)	Saltine-type crackers	6
Tortilla, 6 in across	1	Whole wheat crackers, no fat added (crisp breads, such as Finn, Kavli, Wasa)	2–4 slices (¾ oz)
White (including French, Italian)	1 slice (1 oz)		
Whole wheat	1 slice (1 oz)		
Starch Foods Prepared with Fat†			
Biscuit, 2½ in across	1		
Chow mein noodles	½ cup		
Corn bread, 2 in cube	1 (2 oz)		
Cracker, round butter type	6		
French fried potatoes, 2 in to 3½ in long	10 (1½ oz)		
Muffin, plain small	1		
Pancake, 4 in across	2		
Stuffing, bread (prepared)	¼ cup		
Taco shell, 6 in across	2		
Waffle, 4½ in square	1		
Whole wheat crackers, fat added (such as Triscuits)	4–6 (1 oz)		

* Contains 3 grams or more of fiber (whole-grain products average about 2 grams of fiber per serving).
† Count as one starch/bread serving plus one fat serving.

MEAT LIST

FOOD		PORTION
Lean Meat and Substitutes		
Beef:	USDA Good or Choice grades of lean beef, such as round, sirloin, and flank steak; tenderloin; and chipped beef*	1 oz
Pork:	Lean pork, such as fresh ham; canned, cured or boiled ham*; Canadian bacon,* tenderloin	1 oz
Veal:	All cuts are lean except for veal cutlets (ground or cubed). Examples of lean veal are chops and roasts.	1 oz
Poultry:	Chicken, turkey, Cornish hen (without skin)	1 oz
Fish:	All fresh and frozen fish	1 oz
	Crab, lobster, scallops, shrimp, clams (fresh or canned in water*)	2 oz
	Oysters	6 medium
	Tuna* (canned in water)	¼ cup
	Herring (uncreamed or smoked)	1 oz
	Sardines (canned)	2 medium
Wild Game:	Venison, rabbit, squirrel	1 oz
	Pheasant, duck, goose (without skin)	1 oz
Cheese:	Any cottage cheese	¼ cup
	Grated parmesan	2 tbsp
	Diet cheeses* (with less than 55 kilocalories per ounce)	1 oz
Other:	95% fat-free luncheon meat	1 oz
	Egg whites	3 whites
	Egg substitutes with less than 55 kilocalories per ¼ cup.	¼ cup
Medium-fat Meat and Substitutes		
Beef:	Most beef products fall into this category. Examples are all ground beef, roast (rib, chuck, rump), steak (cubed, Porterhouse, T-bone), and meatloaf.	1 oz
Pork:	Most pork products fall into this category. Examples are chops, loin roast, Boston butt, cutlets.	1 oz
Lamb:	Most lamb products fall into this category. Examples are chops, leg, and roast.	1 oz
Veal:	Cutlet (ground or cubed, unbreaded)	1 oz
Poultry:	Chicken (with skin), domestic duck or goose (well-drained of fat), ground turkey	1 oz
Fish:	Tuna* (canned in oil and drained)	¼ cup
	Salmon* (canned)	¼ cup
Cheese:	Skim- or part–skim-milk cheeses, such as:	
	Ricotta	¼ cup
	Mozzarella	1 oz
	Diet cheeses* (with 56–80 kilocalories per ounce)	1 oz
Other:	86% fat-free luncheon meat*	1 oz
	Egg (high in cholesterol, limit to 3 per week)	1
	Egg substitutes with 56–80 kilocalories per ¼ cup	¼ cup
	Tofu (2½ in × 2¾ in × 1 in)	4 oz
	Liver, heart, kidney, sweetbreads (high in cholesterol)	1 oz
High-fat Meat and Substitutes†		
Beef:	Most USDA Prime cuts of beef, such as ribs, corned beef*	1 oz
Pork:	Spareribs, ground pork, pork sausage* (patty or link)	1 oz
Lamb:	Patties (ground lamb)	1 oz
Fish:	Any fried fish product	1 oz

MEAT LIST

FOOD		PORTION
High-fat Meat and Substitutes†		
Cheese:	All regular cheeses,* such as American, Blue, Cheddar, Monterey, Swiss	1 oz
Other:	Luncheon meat,* such as bologna, salami, pimento loaf	1 oz
	Sausage,* such as Polish, Italian	1 oz
	Knockwurst, smoked	1 oz
	Bratwurst*	1 oz
	Frankfurter* (turkey or chicken)	1 (10/lb)
	Peanut butter (contains unsaturated fat)	1 tbsp
High-fat Meat Plus Fat‡		
	Frankfurter* (beef, pork, or combination)	1 (10/lb)

* Contains 400 mg or more of sodium.
† High in saturated fat, cholesterol, and kilocalories; should be used only 3 times per week.
‡ Count as one meat serving plus one fat serving.

VEGETABLE LIST*

FOOD	PORTION†	FOOD	PORTION
Artichoke	½ medium	Mushrooms, cooked	½ cup
Asparagus	1 cup	Okra	1 cup
Beans (green, wax, Italian)	1 cup	Onions	1 cup
Bean sprouts	1 cup	Pea pods	1 cup
Beets	1 cup	Peppers (green)	1 cup
Broccoli	1 cup	Rutabaga	1 cup
Brussels sprouts	1 cup	Sauerkraut‡	½ cup
Cabbage, cooked	½ cup	Spinach, cooked	½ cup
Carrots	1 cup	Summer squash (crookneck)	1 cup
Cauliflower	1 cup	Tomato	1 large
Eggplant	1 cup	Tomato/vegetable juice‡	½ cup
Greens (collard, mustard, turnip)	1 cup	Turnips	1 cup
Kohlrabi	1 cup	Water chestnuts	1 cup
Leeks	1 cup	Zucchini, cooked	½ cup

* Starchy vegetables such as corn, peas, and potatoes are found on the Starch/Bread List. For free vegetables, see the Free Food List. Vegetables contain 2 to 3 g of fiber.
† Unless otherwise indicated, portion size is for raw vegetables.
‡ Contains 400 mg or more of sodium.

FRUIT LIST

FOOD	PORTION	FOOD	PORTION
Fresh, Frozen, and Unsweetened Canned Fruit			
Apple (raw, 2 in across)	1	Pears (canned)	½ cup or 2 halves
Applesauce (unsweetened)	½ cup	Persimmon (medium, native)	2
		Pineapple (raw)	¾ cup
Apricots (medium, raw)	4	Pineapple (canned)	⅓ cup
Apricots (canned)	½ cup or 4 halves	Plum (raw, 2 in across)	2
Banana (9 in long)	½	Pomegranate*	½
Blackberries (raw)*	¾ cup	Raspberries (raw)*	1 cup
Blueberries (raw)*	¾ cup	Strawberries (raw, whole)*	1¼ cup
Cantaloupe (5 in across)	⅓	Tangerine (2½ in across)	2
(cubes)	1 cup	Watermelon (cubes)	1¼ cup
Cherries (large, raw)	12		
Cherries (canned)	½ cup	**Dried Fruit**	
Figs (raw, 2 in across)	2	Apples*	4 rings
Fruit cocktail (canned)	½ cup	Apricots*	7 halves
Grapefruit (medium)	½	Dates	2½ medium
Grapefruit (segments)	¾ cup	Figs*	1½
Grapes (small)	15	Prunes*	3 medium
Honeydew melon (medium)	⅛	Raisins	2 tbsp
(cubes)	1 cup		
Kiwi (large)	1	**Fruit Juice**	
Mandarin oranges	¾ cup	Apple juice/cider	½ cup
Mango (small)	½	Cranberry juice cocktail	⅓ cup
Nectarine (1½ in across)*	1	Grapefruit juice	½ cup
Orange (2½ in across)	1	Grape juice	⅓ cup
Papaya	1 cup	Orange juice	½ cup
Peach (2¾ in across)	1 or ¾ cup	Pineapple juice	½ cup
Peaches (canned)	½ cup or 2 halves	Prune juice	⅓ cup
Pear	½ large or 1 small		

* Contains 3 or more g of fiber (fresh, frozen, and dry fruits have about 2 g fiber per serving).

MILK LIST

FOOD	PORTION	FOOD	PORTION
Skim and Very Lowfat Milk		**Lowfat Milk**	
Skim milk	1 cup	2% milk	1 cup
½% milk	1 cup	Plain lowfat yogurt (with added nonfat milk solids)	8 oz
1% milk	1 cup		
Lowfat buttermilk	1 cup	**Whole Milk**	
Evaporated skim milk	½ cup	Whole milk	1 cup
Dry nonfat milk	⅓ cup	Evaporated whole milk	½ cup
Plain nonfat yogurt	8 oz	Whole plain yogurt	8 oz

FAT LIST

FOOD	PORTION	FOOD	PORTION
		Unsaturated Fats	
Avocado	⅛ medium	Salad dressing, mayonnaise-type	2 tsp
Margarine	1 tsp	Salad dressing, mayonnaise-type, reduced-calorie	1 tbsp
Margarine, diet*	1 tbsp		
Mayonnaise	1 tsp	Salad dressing (all varieties)*	1 tbsp
Mayonnaise, reduced-calorie*	1 tbsp	Salad dressing, reduced-calorie†	2 tbsp
Nuts and Seeds:			
Almonds, dry roasted	6 whole	**Saturated Fats**	
Cashews, dry roasted	1 tbsp	Butter	1 tsp
Pecans	2 whole	Bacon*	1 slice
Peanuts	20 small or 10 large	Chitterlings	½ oz
Walnuts	2 whole	Coconut, shredded	2 tbsp
Other nuts	1 tbsp	Coffee whitener, liquid	2 tbsp
Seeds, pine nuts, sunflower (without shells)	1 tbsp	Coffee whitener, powder	4 tsp
		Cream (light, coffee, table)	2 tbsp
Pumpkin seeds	2 tsp	Cream, sour	2 tbsp
Oil (corn, cottonseed, safflower, soybean, sunflower, olive, peanut)	1 tsp	Cream (heavy, whipping)	1 tbsp
		Cream cheese	1 tbsp
		Salt pork*	¼ oz
Olives*	10 small or 5 large		

* If more than 2 servings are eaten, these foods have 400 mg or more of sodium.
† Contains 400 mg or more of sodium.

FREE FOODS*

Drinks
Bouillon† or broth without fat
Bouillon, low-sodium
Carbonated drinks, sugar-free
Carbonated water
Club soda
Cocoa powder, unsweetened
    (1 tbsp)
Coffee/Tea
Drink mixes, sugar-free
Tonic water, sugar-free

Nonstick pan spray

Fruit
Cranberries, unsweetened (½
    cup)
Rhubarb, unsweetened (½ cup)

Vegetables (raw, 1 cup)
Cabbage
Celery
Chinese cabbage‡
Cucumber
Green onion
Hot peppers
Mushrooms
Radishes
Zucchini‡

Salad Greens
Endive
Escarole
Lettuce
Romaine
Spinach

Sweet substitutes
Candy, hard, sugar-free
Gelatin, sugar-free
Gum, sugar-free
Jam/Jelly, sugar-free (2 tsp)
Pancake syrup, sugar-free
    (1–2 tbsp)
Sugar substitutes (saccharin,
    aspartame)
Whipped topping
    (2 tbsp)

Condiments
Catsup (1 tbsp)
Horseradish
Mustard
Pickles,† dill, unsweetened
Salad dressing, low-calorie
    (2 tbsp)
Taco sauce (1 tbsp)
Vinegar

Seasonings§
Basil (fresh)
Celery seeds
Cinnamon
Chili powder
Chives
Curry
Dill
Flavoring extracts (vanilla, al-
    mond, walnut, peppermint,
    butter, lemon, etc.)
Garlic
Garlic powder
Herbs
Hot pepper sauce
Lemon
Lemon juice
Lime
Lime juice
Mint
Onion powder
Oregano
Paprika
Pepper
Pimento
Spices
Soy sauce†
Soy sauce, low sodium ("lite")
Wine, used in cooking (¼ cup)
Worcestershire sauce

* Contain less than 20 kilocalories per serving. If no serving size is indicated, these foods can be eaten freely. If serving size is indicated, 2 or 3 servings can be eaten per day.
    † Contain 400 mg or more of sodium.
    ‡ Contain 3 g or more of fiber.
    § Read labels carefully to choose seasonings without salt or sodium.

COMBINATION FOODS

FOOD	AMOUNT	EXCHANGES
Casseroles, homemade	1 cup (8 oz)	2 starch, 2 medium-fat meat, 1 fat
Cheese pizza,* thin crust	¼ of 15 oz or ¼ of 10"	2 starch, 1 medium-fat meat, 1 fat
Chili with beans (commercial)*†	1 cup (8 oz)	2 starch, 2 medium-fat meat, 2 fat
Chow mein (without noodles or rice)	2 cups (16 oz)	1 starch, 2 vegetable, 2 lean meat
Macaroni and cheese*	1 cup (8 oz)	2 starch, 1 medium-fat meat, 2 fat
Soup		
Bean*†	1 cup (8 oz)	1 starch, 1 vegetable, 1 lean meat
Chunky, all varieties*	10-¾ oz can	1 starch, 1 vegetable, 1 medium-fat meat
Cream* (made with water)	1 cup (8 oz)	1 starch, 1 fat
Vegetable* or broth*	1 cup (8 oz)	1 starch
Spaghetti and meatballs* (canned)	1 cup (8 oz)	2 starch, 1 medium-fat meat, 1 fat
Sugar-free pudding (made with skim milk)	½ cup	1 starch
If beans are used as a meat substitute:		
Dried beans,† peas,† lentils†	1 cup (cooked)	2 starch, 1 lean meat

* Contains 400 mg or more of sodium.
† Contains 3 grams or more of fiber.

FOODS FOR OCCASIONAL USE

FOOD	AMOUNT	EXCHANGES
Angel food cake	1/12 cake	2 starch
Cake, no icing	1/12 cake, or a 3" square	2 starch, 2 fat
Cookies	2 small (1¾" across)	1 starch, 1 fat
Frozen fruit yogurt	⅓ cup	1 starch
Gingersnaps	3	1 starch
Granola	¼ cup	1 starch, 1 fat
Granola bars	1 small	1 starch, 1 fat
Ice cream, any flavor	½ cup	1 starch, 2 fat
Ice milk, any flavor	½ cup	1 starch, 1 fat
Sherbet, any flavor	¼ cup	1 starch
Snack chips,* all varieties	1 oz	1 starch, 2 fat
Vanilla wafers	6 small	1 starch, 1 fat

* Contains 400 mg or more of sodium.

Appendix 10 Sample Tube-feeding Administration Schedule

Continuous Drip Schedule

Day	Time (h)	Strength	Rate (mL/h)	Volume (mL)	Kilocalories
1	1st 8	Full	50	400	400
	2nd 8	Full	75	600	600
	3rd 8	Full	100	800	800
					1800
					Total Calories
2	24	Full	100–125	2400–3000	2400–3000
					Total Kilocalories

Intermittent Drip Schedule

Day	Time (h)	Strength	Rate (5–10 mL/min)	Volume (mL)	Kilocalories
1	7AM–11PM	Full	100 mL q 2h (7AM, 9AM)	200	200
		Full	150 mL q 2h (11AM, 1PM, 3PM)	450	450
		Full	200 mL q 2h (5PM, 7PM, 9PM, 11PM)	800	800
					1450
					Total Calories
2	7AM–11PM	Full	250 mL q 2h (8 feedings)	2000	2000
					Total Calories
			up to 400 mL q 3h (5 feedings)	2000	2000
					Total Calories

From Consultant Dietitians in Health Care Facilities, A Practice Group of the American Dietetic Association, Pocket Resource for Nutrition Assessment, 1990.

Appendix II Total Parenteral Nutrition Administration Schedule

RATE (mL/h)	TOTAL VOLUME PER 24 h (mL)	D50W+ 5.5%AA*	D70W+ 5.5%AA	D50W+ 8.5%AA	D70W+ 8.5%AA	D50W+ 10%AA	D70W+ 10%AA
50	1200	1162 kcal† 33 g pro 5.3 g N$_2$	1569 kcal 33 g pro 5.3 g N$_2$	1239 kcal 51 g pro 8 g N$_2$	1648 kcal 51 g pro 8 g N$_2$	1278 kcal 60 g pro 9.5 g N$_2$	1686 kcal 60 g pro 9.5 g N$_2$
75	1800	1745 kcal 50 g pro 8 g N$_2$	2357 kcal 50 g pro 8 g N$_2$	1861 kcal 77 g pro 12.3 g N$_2$	2473 kcal 77 g pro 12.3 g N$_2$	1971 kcal 90 g pro 14.4 g N$_2$	2529 kcal 90 g pro 14.4 g N$_2$
85	2040	1974 kcal 56 g pro 9 g N$_2$	2668 kcal 56 g pro 9 g N$_2$	2108 kcal 87 g pro 14 g N$_2$	2802 kcal 87 g pro 14 g N$_2$	2173 kcal 102 g pro 16.3 g N$_2$	2866 kcal 102 g pro 16.3 g N$_2$
100	2400	2325 kcal 66 g pro 10.6 g N$_2$	3139 kcal 66 g pro 10.6 g N$_2$	2478 kcal 102 g pro 16.3 g N$_2$	3295 kcal 102 g pro 16.3 g N$_2$	2556 kcal 120 g pro 19.2 g N$_2$	3372 kcal 120 g pro 19.2 g N$_2$
125	3000	2907 kcal 83 g pro 13.3 g N$_2$	3926 kcal 83 g pro 13.3 g N$_2$	3100 kcal 128 g pro 20.4 g N$_2$	4120 kcal 128 g pro 20.4 g N$_2$	3195 kcal 150 g pro 24 g N$_2$	4215 kcal 150 g pro 24 g N$_2$
150	3600	3486 kcal 99 g pro 15.8 g N$_2$	4709 kcal 99 g pro 15.8 g N$_2$	3718 kcal 153 g pro 24.5 g N$_2$	4941 kcal 153 g pro 24.5 g N$_2$	3834 kcal 180 g pro 28.8 g N$_2$	5058 kcal 180 g pro 28.8 g N$_2$

* For reference: D5W is 0.17 kcal/mL; D10W is 0.34 kcal/mL; D20W is 0.68 kcal/mL; D50W is 1.70 kcal/mL; D70W is 2.38 kcal/mL; 1 L 10% AA is 100 g pro; 1 L 8.5% AA is 85 g pro; 1 L 5.5% AA is 55 g pro; 20% fat is 2.0 kcal/mL; 10% fat is 1.1 kcal/mL; Standard AA (g) ÷ 6.25 = g N$_2$.

† Kilocalorie levels are based on total (carbohydrate and protein) kilocalories; generally nonprotein kilocalories are used.

Key: AA = amino acids; N$_2$ = nitrogen; pro = protein.

From Consultant Dietitians in Health Care Facilities, A Practice Group of the American Dietetic Association, Pocket Resource for Nutrition Assessment, 1990.

Appendix 12 Harris-Benedict Estimated Basal Energy Expenditure (BEE)

MALES*

Weight

lbs	kg	kcal	lbs	kg	kcal
88.0	40	616	187.0	85	1235
90.2	41	630	189.2	86	1249
92.4	42	644	191.4	87	1263
94.6	43	658	193.6	88	1276
96.8	44	671	195.8	89	1290
99.0	45	685	198.0	90	1304
101.2	46	699	200.2	91	1318
103.4	47	713	202.4	92	1331
105.6	48	726	204.6	93	1345
107.8	49	740	206.8	94	1359
110.0	50	754	209.0	95	1373
112.2	51	768	211.2	96	1386
114.4	52	781	213.4	97	1400
116.6	53	795	215.6	98	1414
118.8	54	809	217.8	99	1428
121.0	55	823	220.0	100	1441
123.2	56	836	222.2	101	1455
125.4	57	850	224.4	102	1469
127.6	58	864	226.6	103	1483
129.8	59	878	228.8	104	1496
132.0	60	891	231.0	105	1510
134.2	61	905	233.2	106	1524
136.4	62	919	235.4	107	1538
138.6	63	933	237.6	108	1551
140.8	64	946	239.8	109	1565
143.0	65	960	242.0	110	1579
145.2	66	974	244.2	111	1593
147.4	67	988	246.4	112	1606
149.6	68	1001	248.6	113	1620
151.8	69	1015	250.8	114	1634
154.0	70	1029	253.0	115	1648
156.2	71	1043	255.2	116	1661
158.4	72	1056	257.4	117	1675
160.6	73	1070	259.6	118	1689
162.8	74	1084	261.8	119	1703
165.0	75	1098	264.0	120	1716
167.2	76	1111	266.2	121	1730
169.4	77	1125	268.4	122	1744
171.6	78	1139	270.6	123	1758
173.8	79	1153	272.8	124	1771
176.0	80	1166			
178.2	81	1180			
180.4	82	1194			
182.6	83	1208			
184.8	84	1221			

Height

ft in	in	cm	kcal
4' 7"	55	139.7	699
8	56	142.2	711
9	57	144.8	724
10	58	147.3	737
11	59	149.9	749
5' 0"	60	152.4	762
1	61	154.9	775
2	62	157.5	787
3	63	160.0	800
4	64	162.6	813
5' 5"	65	165.1	825
6	66	167.6	838
7	67	170.2	851
8	68	172.7	864
9	69	175.3	876
5'10"	70	177.8	889
11	71	180.3	902
6' 0"	72	182.9	914
1	73	185.4	927
2	74	188.0	940
6' 3"	75	190.5	953
4	76	193.0	965
5	77	195.6	978
6	78	198.1	991
7	79	200.7	1003
6' 8"	80	203.2	1016
9	81	205.7	1029
10	82	208.3	1041
11	83	210.8	1054
7 0	84	213.4	1067

Age

yr	kcal	yr	kcal	yr	kcal
18	122	48	324	73	493
19	128	49	331	74	500
20	135	50	338	75	507
21	142	51	345	76	514
22	149	52	352	77	521
23	155	53	358	78	527
24	162	54	365	79	534
25	169	55	372	80	541
26	176	56	379	81	548
27	183	57	385	82	554
28	189	58	392	83	561
29	196	59	399	84	568
30	203	60	406	85	575
31	210	61	412	86	581
32	216	62	419	87	588
33	223	63	426	88	595
34	230	64	433	89	602
35	237	65	439	90	608
36	243	66	446	91	615
37	250	67	453	92	622
38	257	68	460	93	629
39	264	69	466	94	635
40	270	70	473	95	642
41	277	71	480	96	649
42	284	72	487	97	656
43	291				
44	297				
45	304				
46	311				
47	318				

How to use this table:

STEP 1 Obtain weight, height, and age of subject.

STEP 2 BEE = weight kcal + height kcal — age kcal

Example: 70-kilogram, 178-centimeter, 45-year-old male

BEE = 1029 + 889 — 304

BEE = 1614‡

FEMALES†

Weight

lbs	kg	kcal	lbs	kg	kcal
77.0	35	990	176.0	80	1420
79.2	36	999	178.2	81	1429
81.4	37	1009	180.4	82	1439
83.6	38	1018	182.6	83	1449
85.8	39	1028	184.8	84	1458
88.0	40	1038	187.0	85	1468
90.2	41	1047	189.2	86	1477
92.4	42	1057	191.4	87	1487
94.6	43	1066	193.6	88	1496
96.8	44	1076	195.8	89	1506
99.0	45	1085	198.0	90	1516
101.2	46	1095	200.2	91	1525
103.4	47	1104	202.4	92	1535
105.6	48	1114	204.6	93	1544
107.8	49	1124	206.8	94	1554
110.0	50	1133	209.0	95	1563
112.2	51	1143	211.2	96	1573
114.4	52	1152	213.4	97	1582
116.6	53	1162	215.6	98	1592
118.8	54	1171	217.8	99	1602
121.0	55	1181	220.0	100	1611
123.2	56	1190	222.2	101	1621
125.4	57	1200	224.4	102	1630
127.6	58	1210	226.6	103	1640
129.8	59	1219	228.8	104	1649
132.0	60	1229	231.0	105	1659
134.2	61	1238	233.2	106	1668
136.4	62	1248	235.4	107	1678
138.6	63	1257	237.6	108	1688
140.8	64	1267	239.8	109	1697
143.0	65	1277	242.0	110	1707
145.2	66	1286	244.2	111	1716
147.4	67	1296	246.4	112	1726
149.6	68	1305	248.6	113	1735
151.8	69	1315	250.8	114	1745
154.0	70	1324	253.0	115	1755
156.2	71	1334	255.2	116	1764
158.4	72	1343	257.4	117	1774
160.6	73	1353	259.6	118	1783
162.8	74	1363	261.8	119	1793
165.0	75	1372			
167.2	76	1382			
169.4	77	1391			
171.6	78	1401			
173.8	79	1410			

Height

ft in	in	cm	kcal
4' 0"	48	121.9	226
1	49	124.5	230
2	50	127.0	235
3	51	129.5	240
4	52	132.1	244
4' 5"	53	134.6	249
6	54	137.2	254
7	55	139.7	258
8	56	142.2	263
9	57	144.8	268
4'10"	58	147.3	273
11	59	149.9	277
5' 0"	60	152.4	282
1	61	154.9	287
2	62	157.5	291
5' 3"	63	160.0	296
4	64	162.6	301
5	65	165.1	305
6	66	167.6	310
7	67	170.2	315
5' 8"	68	172.7	320
9	69	175.3	324
10	70	177.8	329
11	71	180.3	334
6 0	72	182.9	338

Age

yr	kcal	yr	kcal	yr	kcal
18	84	48	225	78	365
19	89	49	229	79	370
20	94	50	234	80	374
21	98	51	239	81	379
22	103	52	243	82	384
23	108	53	248	83	388
24	112	54	253	84	393
25	117	55	257	85	398
26	122	56	262	86	402
27	126	57	267	87	407
28	131	58	271	88	412
29	136	59	276	89	417
30	140	60	281	90	421
31	145	61	285	91	426
32	150	62	290	92	431
33	154	63	295	93	435
34	159	64	300	94	440
35	164	65	304	95	445
36	168	66	309	96	449
37	173	67	314	97	454
38	178	68	318	98	459
39	183	69	323	99	463
40	187	70	328	100	468
41	192	71	332	101	473
42	197	72	337	102	477
43	201	73	342		
44	206	74	346		
45	211	75	351		
46	215	76	356		
47	220	77	360		

Example: 55-kilogram, 163-centimeter, 45-year-old female

BEE = 1181 + 301 — 211

BEE = 1271‡

* Based on the Harris-Benedict equation: BEE = $66.47 + (13.75 \times \text{weight in kg}) + (5.0 \times \text{height in cm}) - (6.76 \times \text{age in yrs.})$

† Based on the Harris-Benedict equation: BEE = $655.10 + (9.56 \times \text{weight in kg}) + (1.85 \times \text{height in cm}) - (4.68 \times \text{age in yrs.})$

‡ Multiply BEE by 1.2 to 2.1 to allow for activity and stress levels.

From Harris J, Benedict F: *A Biometric Study of Basal Metabolism in Man.* Publication 279. Washington, DC: Carnegie Institution, 1919, pp. 40–44. Chart published by Consultant Dietitians in Health Care Facilities, A Practice Group of the American Dietetic Association, Pocket Resource for Nutrition Assessment, 1990.

Appendix 13 Growth Charts for Boys and Girls from Birth to 18 Years of Age

Take all measurements with the child nude or with minimal clothing and without shoes. Measure length with the infant (under 3 years; use "Birth to 36 months" chart) lying on his or her back fully extended. Two people are needed to measure recumbent length properly. Measure stature with the child (at least 2 years of age; use "2 to 18 years" chart) standing. Use a beam balance to measure weight.

From the Department of Health, Education, and Welfare, Public Health Service, Health Resource Administration, National Center for Health Statistics, and Centers for Disease Control and Prevention.

BOYS FROM BIRTH TO 36 MONTHS

LENGTH FOR AGE

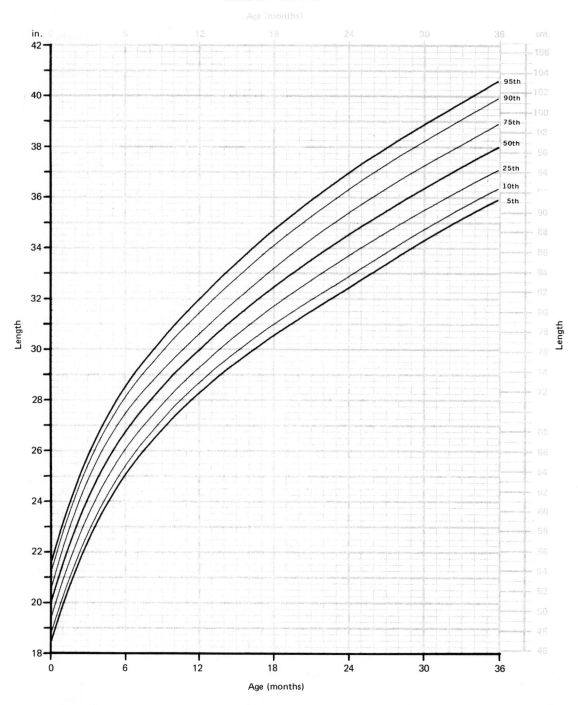

BOYS FROM BIRTH TO 36 MONTHS

WEIGHT FOR AGE

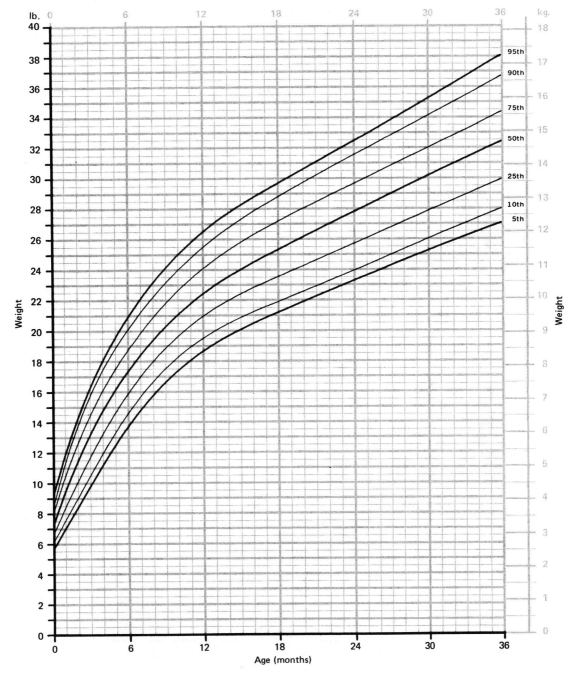

BOYS FROM BIRTH TO 36 MONTHS

HEAD CIRCUMFERENCE FOR AGE

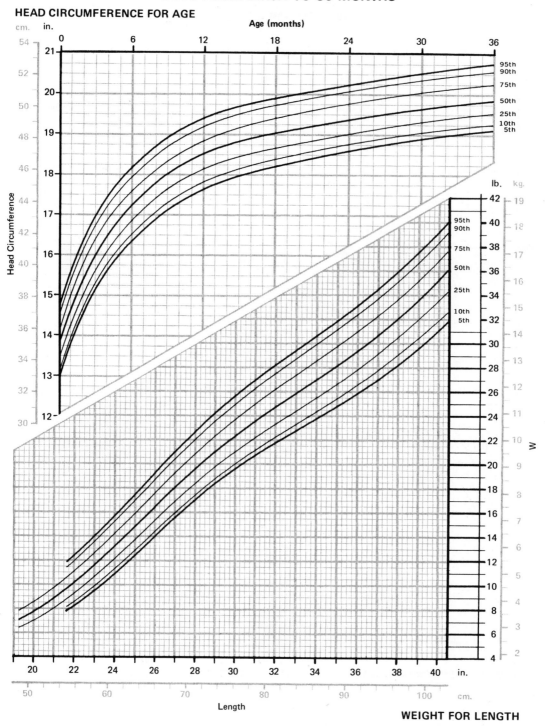

WEIGHT FOR LENGTH

GIRLS FROM BIRTH TO 36 MONTHS

LENGTH FOR AGE

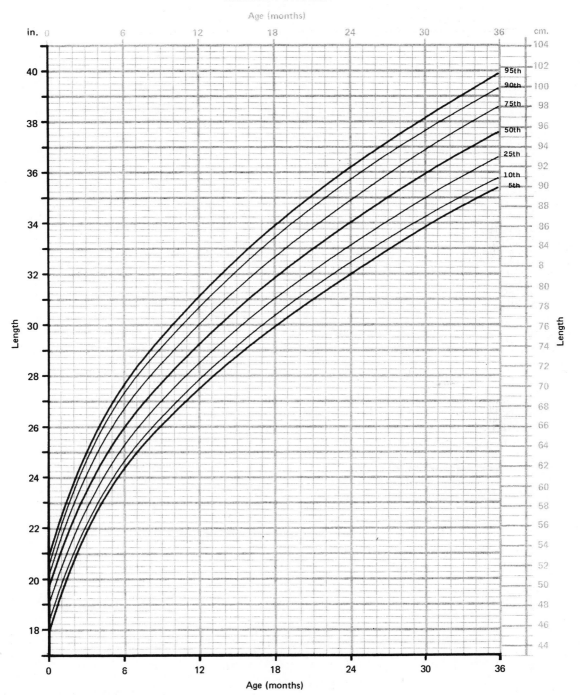

GIRLS FROM BIRTH TO 36 MONTHS

WEIGHT FOR AGE

Age (months)

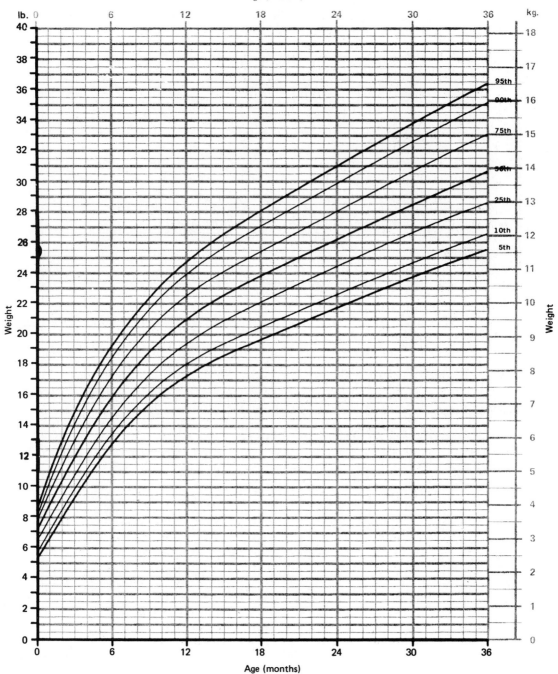

GIRLS FROM BIRTH TO 36 MONTHS

HEAD CIRCUMFERENCE FOR AGE

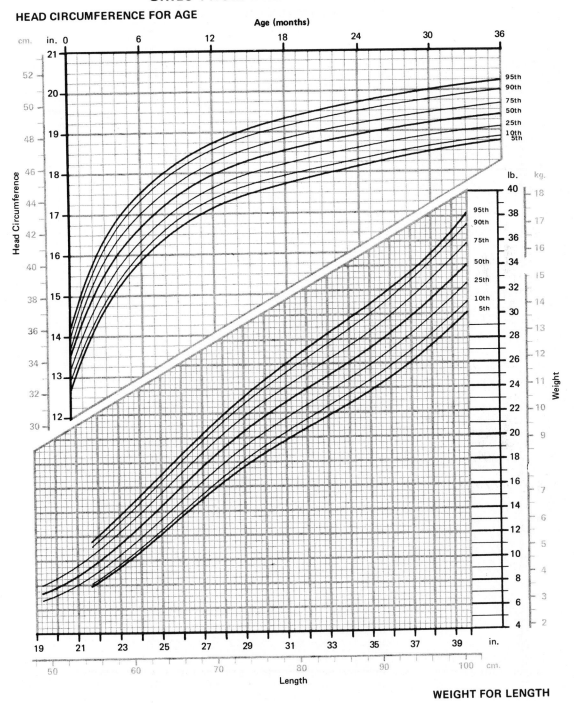

WEIGHT FOR LENGTH

BOYS FROM 2 TO 18 YEARS

STATURE FOR AGE

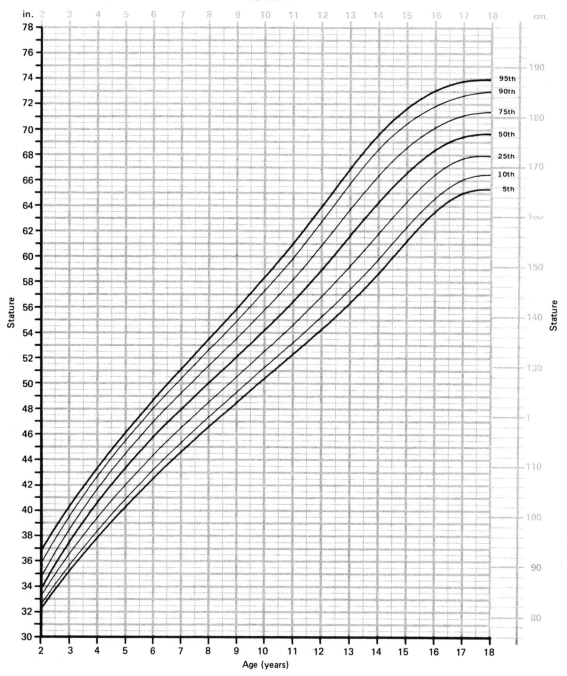

BOYS FROM 2 TO 18 YEARS

WEIGHT FOR AGE

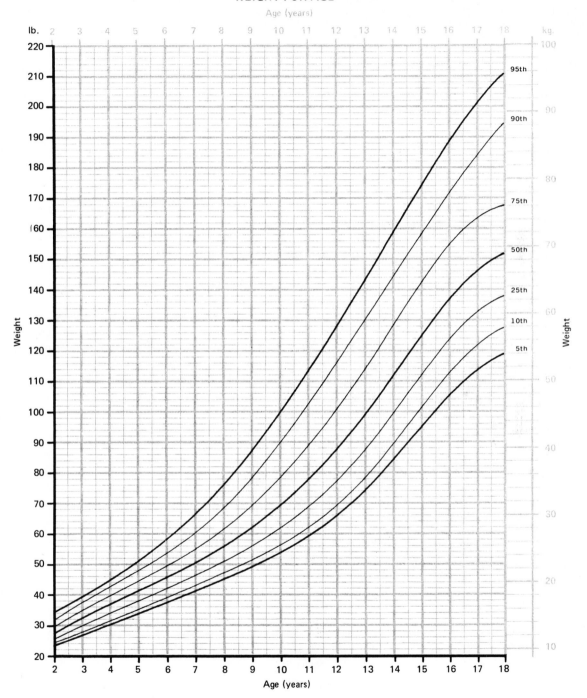

PRE-PUBERTAL BOYS FROM 2 TO 11½ YEARS

WEIGHT FOR STATURE

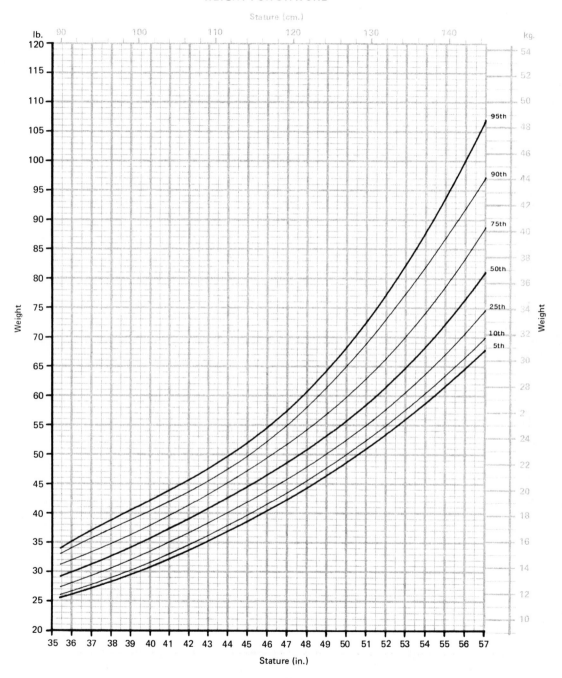

GIRLS FROM 2 TO 18 YEARS

STATURE FOR AGE

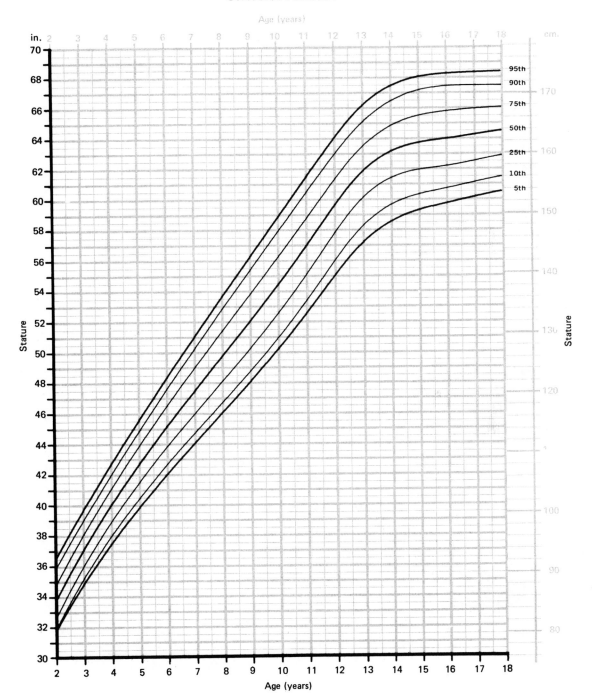

GIRLS FROM 2 TO 18 YEARS
WEIGHT FOR AGE

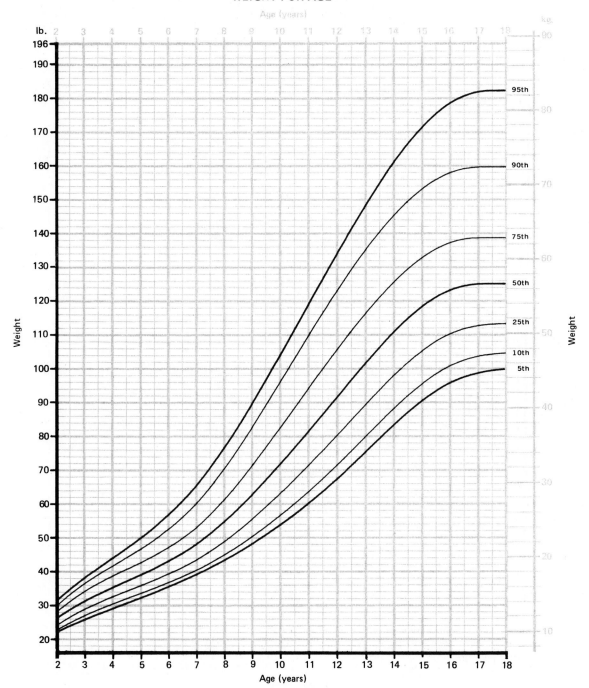

PRE-PUBERTAL GIRLS FROM 2 TO 10 YEARS

WEIGHT FOR STATURE

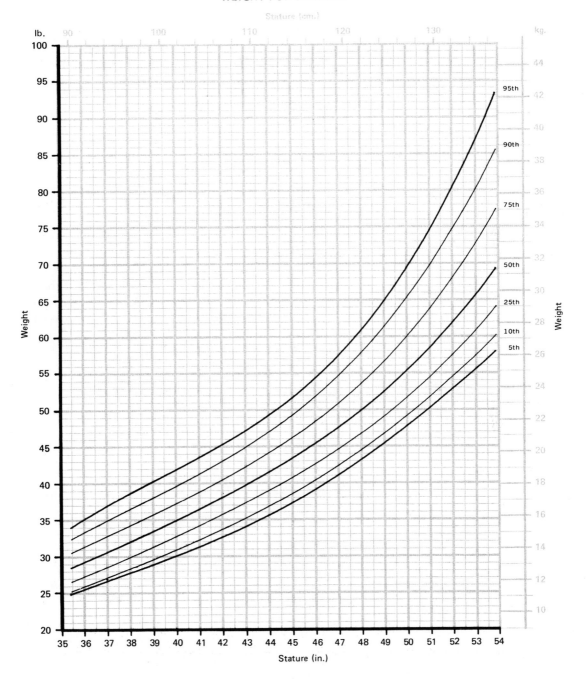

Appendix 14 Estimating Body Frame Size

1. Frame size may be determined by wrist circumference. Values are affected by variability of soft tissue. Wrist circumference is determined by measuring the smallest part of the wrist distal to the styloid process of the ulna and radius. The "r" value is then determined by this formula:

$$\frac{\text{height in centimeters}}{\text{wrist circumference in centimeters}}$$

Then refer to the following r value table to determine frame size:

Men r value	frame size	Women r value
10.4 or greater	small	11.0 or greater
9.6 to 10.4	medium	10.1 to 11.0
9.6 or less	large	10.1 or less

2. Elbow breadth is measured with the forearm upward at a 90-degree angle. The distance between the outer aspects of the two prominent bones on either side of the elbow is considered to be the elbow breadth. Elbow breadth less than that listed for medium frame indicates a small frame. Elbow breadth greater than that listed for medium frame indicates a large frame.

Frame Size for Women

Height in 1-inch heels	Elbow breadth for medium frames
4'10" to 4'11"	2-¼" to 2-½"
5'0" to 5'3"	2-¼" to 2-½"
5'4" to 5'7"	2-⅜" to 2-⅝"
5'8" to 5'11"	2-⅜" to 2-⅝"
6'0"	2-½" to 2-¾"

Frame Size for Men

Height in 1-inch heels	Elbow breadth for medium frames
5'2" to 5'3"	2-½" to 2-⅞"
5'4" to 5'7"	2-⅝" to 2-⅞"
5'8" to 5'11"	2-¾" to 3"
6'0" to 6'3"	2-¾" to 3-⅛"
6'4"	2-⅞" to 3-¼"

From Manual for Clinical Dietetics, The American Dietetic Association, 1988, found in Consultant Dietitians in Health Care Facilities, A Practice Group of the American Dietetic Association: Pocket Resource for Nutrition Assessment, 1990.

Appendix 15 Metropolitan Life Height and Weight Tables

The Metropolitan Life Insurance Company has published height and weight tables as a public service. The weights are associated with greatest longevity for people aged 25 to 59, and the revised charts of 1983 are guidelines based on a mortality study of 4.2 million policy holders over the preceding 22 years. The study found that the average man is heavier than he was 20 years ago and that deaths associated with hypertension and overweight were noted to be fewer since then. It was also found that mildly elevated blood pressure can be treated effectively so that normal life expectancy results. Longer life is still apparently associated with weighing somewhat less than what is average for one's height.

The tables, which reflect the findings of the study, have created controversy in the medical community, since the weights are from 1 to 13 per cent higher than those published in 1959. Heart specialists are concerned that these new figures will foster a misconception that overweight or obesity may not be as detrimental to one's health after all. From the dietitian's point of view, also, it is still best to set personalized weight goals according to the needs of the individual and not based on population samples. The height and weight tables are not intended to give ideal weights.

Men (Ages 25–59)*					Women (Ages 25–59)*				
Height		**Small**	**Medium**	**Large**	**Height**		**Small**	**Medium**	**Large**
Feet	**Inches**	**Frame**	**Frame**	**Frame**	**Feet**	**Inches**	**Frame**	**Frame**	**Frame**
5	2	128–134	131–141	138–150	4	10	102–111	109–121	118–131
5	3	130–136	133–143	140–153	4	11	103–113	111–123	120–134
5	4	132–138	135–145	142–156	5	0	104–115	113–126	122–137
5	5	134–140	137–148	144–160	5	1	106–118	115–129	125–140
5	6	136–142	139–151	146–164	5	2	108–121	118–132	128–143
5	7	138–145	142–154	149–168	5	3	111–124	121–135	131–147
5	8	140–148	145–157	152–172	5	4	114–127	124–138	134–151
5	9	142–151	148–160	155–176	5	5	117–130	127–141	137–155
5	10	144–154	151–163	158–180	5	6	120–133	130–144	140–159
5	11	146–157	154–166	161–184	5	7	123–136	133–147	143–163
6	0	149–160	157–170	164–188	5	8	126–139	136–150	146–167
6	1	152–164	160–174	168–192	5	9	129–142	139–153	149–170
6	2	155–168	164–178	172–197	5	10	132–145	142–156	152–173
6	3	158–172	167–182	176–202	5	11	135–148	145–159	155–176
6	4	162–176	171–187	181–207	6	0	138–151	148–162	158–179

Based on lowest mortality. Weight is given in pounds according to frame (in indoor clothing weighing 5 lbs [men] or 3 lbs [women], shoes with 1" heels). Source of basic data: 1979 Build Study, Society of Actuaries and Association of Life Insurance Medical Directors of America, 1980. Copyright 1983, Metropolitan Life Insurance Company.

Appendix 16 Body Mass Index

Measure height to the nearest inch and weight to the nearest pound. Mark them on the body mass index (BMI) nomogram. Then use a straight edge (paper, ruler) to connect the two points and circle the spot where this straight line crosses the center line to obtain the BMI value. Note: When computing BMI with the equation weight $\div$ height^2, kilograms and meters should be used.

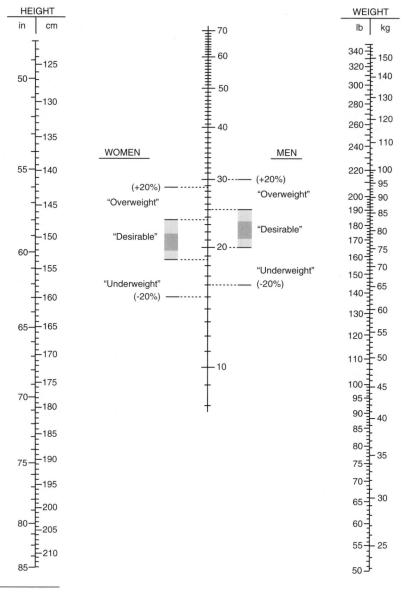

Redrawn from Thomas E, McKay DA, Cutlin MB: Nomograph for body mass index (kg/m^2). Am J Clin Nutr. 1976;29:302–304; with permission.

Appendix 17 Nomogram to Estimate Stature from Knee Height in Persons Aged 60 to 90 Years

An elderly person's stature can be estimated from the nomogram below. To use this nomogram, locate the person's age on the left column and knee height on the middle column, and connect these two points. Mark where the connecting line crosses the stature column for the appropriate sex to find the estimated stature.

A knee-height caliper can be obtained from Ross Laboratory, 1-800-848-2607. In OH, PA, and WV, call 1-800-367-7677 or contact your local Ross representative.

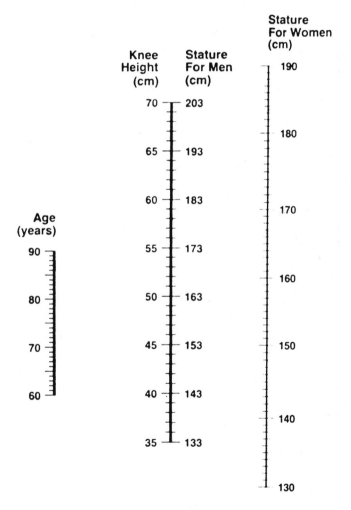

From Consultant Dietitians in Health Care Facilities, A Practice Group of the American Dietetic Association, Pocket Resource for Nutrition Assessment, 1990.

Appendix 18 1994 Federal Poverty Levels*

FAMILY SIZE†	1994 FEDERAL POVERTY LEVEL	175% OF FEDERAL POVERTY LEVEL	200% OF FEDERAL POVERTY LEVEL
1	7,696	13,468	15,392
2	10,064	17,612	20,128
3	12,432	21,756	24,864
4	14,800	25,900	29,600
5	17,168	30,044	34,336
6	19,536	34,188	39,072

* As per 93-INF-47 (to be used for Title XX eligibility determinations). Many community nutrition programs use 185% of Federal Poverty Level for eligibility.
† For each additional member, add $750.

Appendix 19 School Lunch Patterns for Various Age/Grade Groups

COMPONENTS	MINIMUM QUANTITIES*				RECOMMENDED QUANTITIES†	SPECIFIC REQUIREMENTS
	PRESCHOOL		GRADES K–3	GRADES 4–12	GRADES 7–12	
	Ages 1–2 (Group I)	Ages 3–4 (Group II)	Ages 5–8 (Group III)	Age 9 & Over (Group IV)	Age 12 & Over (Group V)	
MEAT OR MEAT ALTERNATE A serving of one of the following or a combination to give an equivalent quantity:						• Must be served in the main dish or the main dish and one other menu item. • Vegetable protein products, cheese alternate products, and enriched macaroni with fortified protein may be used to meet part of the meat/meat alternate requirement. Fact sheets on each of these alternate foods give detailed instructions for use. • No more than one-half of the total requirement may be met with full-strength fruit or vegetable juice. • Cooked dry beans or peas may be used as a meat alternate or as a vegetable but not as both in the same meal.
Lean meat, poultry, or fish (edible portion as served)	1 oz	1½ oz	1½ oz	2 oz	3 oz	
Cheese	1 oz	1½ oz	1½ oz	2 oz	3 oz	
Large egg(s)	½	¾	¾	1	1½	
Cooked dry beans or peas	¼ cup	3/8 cup	3/8 cup	½ cup	¾ cup	
Peanut butter	2 Tbsp	3 Tbsp	3 Tbsp	4 Tbsp	6 Tbsp	
VEGETABLE AND/OR FRUIT Two or more servings of vegetable or fruit or both to total	½ cup	½ cup	½ cup	¾ cup	¾ cup	
BREAD OR BREAD ALTERNATE Servings of bread or bread alternate A serving is: • 1 slice of whole-grain or enriched bread • A whole-grain or enriched biscuit, roll, muffin, etc. • ½ cup of cooked whole-grain or enriched rice, macaroni, noodles, whole grain or enriched pasta products, or other cereal grains such as bulgur or corn grits • A combination of any of the above	5 per week	8 per week	8 per week	8 per week	10 per week	• At least ½ serving of bread or an equivalent quantity of bread alternate for Group I, and 1 serving for Groups II–V, must be served daily. • Enriched macaroni with fortified protein may be used as a meat alternate or as a bread alternate but not as both in the same meal. NOTE: *Food Buying Guide for Child Nutrition Programs, PA-1331 (1983)* provides the information for the minimum weight of a serving.
MILK A serving of fluid milk	¾ cup (6 fl oz)	¾ cup (6 fl oz)	½ pint (8 fl oz)	½ pint (8 fl oz)	½ pint (8 fl oz)	At least one of the following forms of milk must be offered: • Unflavored lowfat milk • Unflavored skim milk • Unflavored buttermilk NOTE: This requirement does not prohibit offering other milks, such as whole milk or flavored milk, along with one or more of the above.

* USDA recommends, but does not require, that you adjust portions by age/grade group to better meet the food and nutritional needs of children according to their ages if you adjust portions. Groups I–IV are minimum requirements for the age/grade groups specified. If you do *not* adjust portions, the Group IV portions are the portions to serve all children.

† Group V specifies recommended, not required, quantities for students 12 years and older. These students may request smaller portions, but not smaller than those specified in Group IV.

From the U.S. Dept. of Agriculture, National School Lunch Program, Food Buying Guide, January, 1984.

Appendix 20 Celiac and Other Allergy Resources

Celiac Support Groups

Celiac Sprue Association/United States of America (CSA/USA), PO Box 31700, Omaha, NE 68131-0700; 402/558-0600.

Gluten Intolerance Group of North America (GIG), PO Box 23053, Broadway Station, Seattle, WA 98102-0353; 206/325-6980.

Canadian Celiac Association, 6519-B Mississauga Road, Mississauga, Ontario L5N1A6, Canada; 416/567-7195.

Gluten-Free Special Products List

AlpineAire Foods
PO Box 926
Nevada City, CA 95959
(916) 272-1971

Excellent source for freeze-dried foods for backpacking and camping. All foods are vacuum-packed. They contain no preservatives, no added sugar, no artificial flavors or colors. Note: Their "vegetable pasta" listed in Pasta Roma and Vegetable Pasta Stew CONTAINS WHEAT FLOUR as its major ingredient. Mail orders accepted.

Dietary Specialties
PO Box 227
Rochester, NY 14601
1-800-544-0099

Dietary Specialties, Wel-plan, and Aproten brands. Gluten-free bread, crackers, cookies, and pasta. Mixes for bread, cakes, muffins, and brownies. Mail orders accepted.

El Molino Mills
345 N. Baldwin Park Blvd.
City of Industry, CA 91746
(213) 962-7167

Produce a variety of gluten-free cereals and flours. Available through local distributors only. No retail mail sales. Will forward name and address of distributor in your area and product ingredient information.

Ener-G Foods, Inc.
PO Box 84487
Seattle, WA 98124-5787
(206) 767-6660
1-800-331-5222

Jolly Joan brand gluten-free flours and flour mixes available. Will ship gluten-free flours in bulk also. Variety of baked products including breads, cinnamon rolls, cookies, and pizza crusts. Gluten-free pasta and crackers available. Mail orders accepted. Write for complete product information.

Fearn Soya Foods
Div. of Richard Foods Corp.
Melrose Park, IL 60160
(312) 345-2335

Variety of gluten-free flours, baking mixes, and other baking ingredients (Fearn brand). Mail orders accepted.

NuVita Foods, Inc.
7524 SW Macadam
Portland, OR 97219
(503) 246-5433

Produce Lange's "Mello Gold" brand gluten-free flours. Mail orders accepted.

Red Mill Farms, Inc.
Gluten-Free Products Division
290 S. 5th Street
Brooklyn, NY 11211
(718) 384-2150

Gluten-free, lactose-free Dutch Chocolate Cake, Banana-Nut Cake, and Coconut Macaroons. All vacuum-packed. Excellent products! Mail order only.

Allergy Cookbooks

Hagman B: *The Gluten-Free Gourmet, Living Well Without Wheat.* New York, NY: Henry Holt & Company, 1990.
Hartsook E: *Gluten Intolerance Group Cookbook,* 2nd ed. GIG, PO Box 23053, Seattle, WA 98102-0353, 1990.
USDA, U.S. Department of Health and Human Services. *Cooking for People with Food Allergies.* USDA Home and Garden Bulletin No. 246, 1988.
Yoder ER: *Allergy-Free Cooking.* Reading, Mass: Addison-Wesley Publishing Co, 1987.
Zukin Jane: *Dairy-Free Cookbook.* Rocklin, CA: Prima Publishing & Communications, 1989.

GLOSSARY

Absorption—the passage of liquids and end products of digestion into the villi of the intestine

Achalasia—a condition in which the esophagus and gastrointestinal tract fail to relax, causing a feeling of fullness, vomiting, and possible aspiration of esophagael contents into the respiratory passages

Acid-base balance—a state of equilibrium between acidity and alkalinity of body fluids; problems with acidosis or alkalosis are determined by pH and blood gas analysis

Activities of daily living (ADL)—activities that the average person performs routinely during a day

Adipose tissue—body fat

Adrenaline—a hormone that works to raise blood sugar levels; also causes increased heart rate

Aerobic exercise—any form of exercise that requires an increased intake of oxygen, such as brisk walking or running

AIDS enteropathy—a condition related to AIDS that causes malabsorption and resultant diarrhea

Albumin—a plasma protein responsible for regulating the osmotic force of blood

Alimentary enzymes—enzymes in the digestive tract, such as sucrase, lactase, maltase, and lipase

Alkali—a chemical substance with a pH greater than 7

Allergen—a substance that induces hypersensitivity

Amino acids—the substances that make protein: essential amino acids must be supplied by the diet; non-essential amino acids can be synthesized by the body

Amylase—an enzyme that hastens the hydrolysis of starch into sugar

Anabolism—the constructive phase of metabolism resulting in growth and repair; adj., anabolic

Anaerobic exercise—any exercise that does not increase the intake of oxygen, such as weight lifting

Analog—a fabricated food resembling another food in texture and flavor

Anemia—a reduction in the number of red blood cells or hemoglobin

Antagonist—a substance that renders another substance inactive

Anorexia—loss of appetite

Anorexia nervosa—a serious chronic condition with severe restriction of food intake unrelated to appetite and refusal to accept a normal weight as desirable; often associated with adolescent girls but also occurs with boys and athletes who require a low body weight

Anthropometry—the science of body measurements, such as size, weight, and proportion

Arteriosclerosis—the hardening and thickening of the walls of the arteries

Ascites—an accumulation of excess fluids in the abdomen

Aspiration—inhaling food or liquid into the lungs; can cause pneumonia

Atherosclerosis—a build-up of plaque inside the arteries and blood vessels that leads to heart disease

Azotemia—abnormally increased levels of nitrogen in the blood

Basal metabolism—the lowest level of metabolism to support life; does not take into account physical activity

Behavior modification—techniques used to change learned behavior

Beta cells—the cells of the pancreas where insulin is produced

Bile—a yellow fluid produced by the liver and stored in the gallbladder until needed in the small intestine for digestion of dietary fat

Biological value of protein—refers to the amount of essential amino acids in relation to the total quantity of protein; animal protein sources (meat, eggs, milk) have a high biological value of protein

Body mass index (BMI)—originally called the Quetelet Index, weight in kilograms divided by the square of the height in meters; felt to be a better indicator for appropriate height and weight measures than Metropolitan Life charts

Botulism—an often fatal form of food poisoning caused by a poisonous endotoxin, *Clostridium botulinum*

Bulimarexia—a condition vacillating between anorexic and bulimic eating patterns

Bulimia—a condition of overeating coupled with purging or laxative abuse

Cancer cachexia—malnutrition associated with cancer

Carbohydrate loading—a strategy used by athletes to increase the amount of stored glycogen available to the muscles

Carbohydrates—substances found in food that provide 4 kilocalories per gram; made up of the elements carbon, hydrogen, and oxygen

Cariogenic—contributing to dental caries

Carnitine—a molecule primarily synthesized in the kidneys with a role in fatty acid oxidation in tissue cells, especially those of cardiac and skeletal muscles

Catabolism—a destructive process that releases energy; adj., catabolic

Catalyst—a substance that causes or accelerates a chemical reaction

Catheter—a tubular instrument inserted into a body channel for administering or withdrawing fluids

Cellulose—structural fiber in fruits, vegetables, and grains

Cerebrovascular accident (CVA)—an embolus or blood clot in the brain; often called a "stroke"

Cheilosis—a condition characterized by dry, scaly lips and cracks at the corners of the mouth; a symptom of riboflavin deficiency

Cholesterol—a fat-related compound produced in the livers of animals; found in animal fats but does not provide kilocalories

Chyme—the semiliquid form of digested food that passes from the stomach into the duodenum after undergoing the action of gastric juice

Cleft palate—an opening or hole in the roof of the mouth, sometimes extending to the lip, that needs to be surgically repaired

Clostridium perfringens—a type of bacterium that causes food poisoning

Colostrum—the nutritious substance that precedes breast milk production in the first few days after delivery

Constipation—defecation of bowel matter less than three times per week with hard stools; objective signs include a palpable mass and decreased bowel sounds

Cortisol—a hormone produced in the adrenal glands that works in the opposite manner to insulin to raise blood sugar levels

Counter regulatory hormones—hormones that work in the opposite manner to insulin; raise blood sugar levels principally through the release of stored glycogen in the liver or through the inhibition of insulin action

Custodial approach—a method of health care, usually in an institutional setting, in which patients are not asked to take responsibility for their own needs; results in a form of dependency

D50W/D70W—dextrose in water solutions with 50 or 70 per cent concentrations

Daily Reference Values (DRV)—a system developed for use on food labels to indicate recommended nutrient intakes for 2000 and 2500 kilocalorie diets

Deficiency disease—a condition resulting from the lack of one or more essential nutrients in the diet; may be related to inadequate dietary intake, digestive problems, or malabsorption

Dental enamel—the outside hard protective covering of teeth

Dental plaque—a calcified coating on teeth that offers a perfect growing medium for bacteria; plaque needs to be removed regularly to prevent dental decay

Denver Developmental Screening Test—an observational test based on infant developmental progress according to age-related tasks such as sitting, crawling, walking, and looking for objects

Depapillation—the smooth appearance of the papilla (elevations on the surface of the tongue containing taste buds) resulting from B-vitamin deficiency

Desirable weight—a body mass index (BMI) between 20 and 25; or a realistic weight that allows for good health for an individual

DETERMINE check list—a tool to identify elderly persons who are at nutritional risk; developed by the American Academy of Family Physicians, the American Dietetic Association, and the National Council on the Aging

Diabetes mellitus—a condition of inadequate insulin production and/or use

Diagnosis related groups (DRGs)—a system in which similar illnesses are grouped together and the estimated duration of health care is predetermined for purposes of financial reimbursement to the health institution

Diarrhea—rapid movement of fecal matter through the intestinal system resulting in poor absorption of water and food nutrients

Dietitian—a person with a minimum of 4 years college training in the science of nutrition; registered dietitians (R.D.s) have additional training and have passed an exam by the American Dietetic Association

Digestion—the mechanical and chemical process of breaking food material down to allow for absorbtion in the intestinal tract

Digestive enzymes—chemicals produced in the body to help in the digestive process; terms ending in "ase" indicate enzymes, such as lactase and sucrase

Disaccharides—double sugars such as sucrose and lactose

Diuresis—excess urination

Diuretic—a substance promoting urine secretion

Dumping syndrome—a condition characterized by nausea, weakness, sweating, palpitation, fainting, often a warm feeling, sometimes diarrhea; symptoms occur after eating in people who have had a partial gastrectomy

Dysgeusia—impaired sense of taste

Dyspepsia—impaired digestion related to epigastric discomfort after meals

Dysphagia—difficulty in swallowing

Edema—an abnormal accumulation of extracellular fluid

Edentulous—without teeth

Efficient body weight—the weight at which fat reserves will allow best performance in a sport

Elbow breadth—a measurement used in anthropometry to determine frame size

Electrolyte—a substance that disassociates into ions when fused or in solution so that electricity can be conducted

Elemental feeding—a complete liquid nutrition supplement that does not require digestion

Elimination diets—diets used to diagnose food allergies; common allergens are eliminated from the diet and reintroduced in an attempt to identify foods that cause individual allergy reactions

Empty kilocalorie foods—foods that provide sugar or fat but few vitamins, minerals, or protein

Emulsify—to mix one liquid that is dispersed in another liquid (e.g., fat droplets in bile)

Energy balance—the level of energy taken in (kilocalories) that equals that amount of energy expended (basal metabolism plus activity needs)

Enrichment—the replacement of nutrients lost in processing foods

Enteral—by way of the small intestine

Enteral nutrition—a form of nutritional support usually with liquid nutrition supplements

Enzyme—a protein that can hasten or produce a change in a substance; names of enzymes usually end in -ase

Fad diet—a weight loss diet that is usually deficient in nutrients and often promises a "quick-fix" and an easy solution to weight control

Fats—substances found in food that provide at least 9 kilocalories per gram; fats, like carbohydrates, contain the elements carbon, hydrogen, and oxygen but in a more concentrated form

Fat-soluble—a substance that dissolves in fat; generally ascribed to a type of vitamin

Fatty acid—an organic compound of carbon, hydrogen, and oxygen that combines with glycerol to form fat

Fiber—the most complex form of carbohydrate; resists digestion; generally referred to as dietary fiber and includes two broad types: soluble and insoluble (related to the ability to dissolve in water)

Fifteen:fifteen (15:15) rule—treatment and re-evaluation of hypoglycemia; treatment with 15 grams of carbohydrate for someone who is still conscious with a recheck of blood sugar levels in 15 minutes (procedure to continue if blood sugar remains low)

Fluoride—a mineral that promotes uptake of calcium by teeth and bones; currently used as a preventive measure against dental caries

Food additives—substances added for stabilization or to increase shelf-life and safety of food

Food allergens—protein material found in food that induces an allergic reaction

Food allergy—an abnormal hypersensitive reaction to foods containing allergens

Food and Drug Administration (FDA)—a federal agency that helps to ensure safety of food and drug products

Food distribution system—the process from food production to consumer use; generally based on monetary exchange

Food exchange lists—a food guide that groups food based on equivalent amounts of carbohydrate, protein, and fat

Food Guide Pyramid—a food guide that combines the old Basic Four Food Groups with the US Dietary Guidelines; portrays both minimum and maximum amounts of food necessary for good health

Food intolerance—a nonimmune intolerance to certain foods related to poor digestion or another factor

Food jags—a term applied to childhood eating habits in which a few foods are eaten for days and weeks at a time

Food resource management—strategies to use efficiently limited resources pertaining to food, such as budgeting, storage, and preparation techniques

Fore milk—breast milk that is released from the front of the breasts and has a lower fat content than hind milk

Fortification—the addition of nutrients to greater than the natural level found in a food

Gastric—pertaining to the stomach

Gavage feeding—forced feeding

Gestational diabetes—a form of diabetes occurring during pregnancy beginning usually between the 24th to 28th weeks of gestation

Gingivitis—an inflammation of the gums

Glomerular filtration rate (GFR)—amount of glomerular filtrate in milliliters cleared through the kidneys in 1 minute; rates less than 30 mL/minute indicate kidney disease; the presence of lower rates calls for aggressive management

Glucagon—a counter regulatory hormone that is given by injection during severe bouts of hypoglycemia in an unconscious diabetic person

Gluconeogenesis—the formation of glucose from protein

Glucose—the form of sugar found in the blood; the end product of carbohydrate digestion

Gluten—the protein portion of wheat, oats, rye, barley, and triticale (a hybrid grain); complete avoidance is often necessary in the control of celiac disease

Glycemia—blood glucose level

Glycemic index—a means of rating food based on predictive impact on blood sugar levels; fats have the lowest and sugars have the highest glycemic index

Glycerol—a component of fats

Glycogen—the storage form of carbohydrate found in the liver and muscle tissues; released in the form of sugar as needed for energy or during times of physiological stress

Glycogen loading—a process by which the glycogen stores in the liver are increased beyond normal levels to allow for the demands for endurance in athletic competition

Glycogenolysis—the breakdown of stored carbohydrate in the liver from glycogen to glucose

Goiter—a swelling of the thyroid gland on the neck caused by iodine deficiency

GRAS list—Generally Recognized As Safe; standards for acceptable levels of food additives

Grazing—a term applied to a manner of continuous eating as opposed to three distinct meals

Growth hormone—a substance that stimulates growth; works opposite to insulin to raise blood sugar levels

Growth spurts—bouts of increased growth such as during adolescence; found commonly at 3 and 6 weeks of age and again at 3 months

Gustatory—pertaining to taste

Hematocrit—the volume percentage of red blood cells in whole blood

Hematuria—blood in the urine

Heme iron—the form of iron found in meat which is readily absorbed

Hemicellulose—a carbohydrate that is more soluble and more easily decomposed than cellulose

Hemodialysis—a procedure used to remove toxic wastes from the blood of a patient with acute or chronic renal failure

Hemoglobin—the oxygen-carrying pigment of the blood; the principal protein in the red blood cell

Hemoglobin A_{1C} (HbA_{1C})—a portion of the hemoglobin which when found in elevated amounts indicates possible diabetes; a test of the HbA_{1C} levels is used to determine long-term diabetes management

Hiatal hernia—protrusion of part of the stomach through the opening of the esophageal hiatus of the diaphragm

Hind milk—breast milk released from upper parts of the breast in response to the hormone oxytocin; very rich in fat

HIV—human immunodeficiency virus; the infectious agent that causes AIDS

Holistic health—having to do with the whole; considering all factors affecting one's state of health

Homogenize—the process by which fat particles become so finely dispersed that they do not rise in a liquid

Honeymoon period—usually the first year after diagnosis of insulin-dependent diabetes mellitus; before the complete destruction of the beta cells

Hormone—chemical produced by cells of the body to stimulate certain life processes such as growth and reproduction

Host—a human, animal, or plant that provides sustenance for another organism or tumor

Hydrogenated fat—a liquid vegetable oil that has the element hydrogen added to make a solid fat

Hydrolysis—the addition of water to a molecule; an important process related to energy release

Hyperalimentation—also referred to as total parenteral nutrition (TPN); administration of all nutrients directly into the blood system

Hyperchlorhydria—an excess of hydrochloric acid in gastric juice

Hyperemesis—excessive vomiting

Hyperglycemia—an elevation of glucose in the blood; two fasting blood sugar measurements over 140 mg/dL are diagnostic of diabetes

Hyperglycemic Hyperosmolar Nonketotic Coma (HHNK)—a condition often associated with diabetes in an older person; indicated by blood sugars in the 500 mg/dL range or higher with severe dehydration and confusion evident

Hyperplasty—a term related to the fat cell theory that describes a situation in which a person has an excess number of fat cells

Hypertension—high blood pressure

Hypochlorhydria—a deficiency of hydrochloric acid in gastric juice

Hypocupremia—low copper levels in the blood

IgE antibody—the immune factor related to food and other allergies

Ileum—the lower part of the small intestine

Immune—resistant to a disease

Ingestion—eating; taking food into the digestive tract

Inorganic—not containing carbon

Insoluble fiber—a form of dietary fiber that does not dissolve in water; referred to as roughage; whole wheat contains this type of fiber

Insulin—a protein hormone formed in the pancreas and secreted into the blood for the purpose of regulating carbohydrate, lipid, and amino acid metabolism

Insulin-dependent diabetes mellitus (IDDM)—a form of diabetes that usually develops in children and young adults; once known as juvenile on-set diabetes

Insulin resistance—a condition in which the body cells resist the action of insulin; often found in conjunction with obesity and with a high-fat diet; often a genetic predisposition exists

Insulin shock—excess amounts of injected insulin result in profound hypoglycemia; glucose needed to treat either orally in a conscious state or via a venous route (IV dextrose).

Intrinsic factor—a substance produced in the stomach that helps absorb vitamin B_{12}.

Iron overload—a rare disease of unknown origin and characterized by widespread iron deposits in the body that can lead to pancreatic cirrhosis and other problems

IU—International Unit, a unit of measure in the International System of Units, or Système International d'Unites (SI Units)

Jejunum—the middle portion of the small intestine connecting the duodenum and the ileum

Ketoacidosis—an accumulation of excess ketones (acid) that changes the pH of the blood; seen in uncontrolled diabetes mellitus

Ketogenic diet—a diet containing large amounts of fat and minimal amounts of protein and carbohydrate; sometimes used in treating certain types of epilepsy in children

Ketosis—the accumulation in the blood and tissues of large quantities of ketone bodies as a result of oxidation of fats

Kilocalorie (kcal)—a unit of measure applied to food energy; one pound of body fat is equivalent to 3500 kilocalories of food

Krebs cycle—the chemical process found at the cell level that converts food matter into energy

Kwashiorkor—protein deficiency disease

La Leche League—a private volunteer agency that has local meetings nationwide to support women in their attempt to breast-feed successfully

Lactation—the secretion of milk for breast-feeding; the period during which this takes place

Lactose—the form of carbohydrate found in milk; referred to as "milk sugar"

Lactose intolerance—inability to digest lactose due to inadequate amounts of the lactase enzyme; common symptoms are bloating of the abdomen with flatus and diarrhea

Legume—the fruit or seed of pod-bearing plants such as peas, beans, lentils, and peanuts

Let-down reflex—phenomenon of the hormone oxytocin allowing the hind milk to flow during breast-feeding; characterized by a gentle "pins and needles" sensation

Linoleic acid—an essential fatty acid

Lipase—an enzyme that hastens the splitting of fats into glycerol and fatty acids

Lipids—a term relating to all forms of fat

Lipogenic—related to substances that induce the promotion of body fat; insulin is a lipogenic hormone

Lipolysis—the breakdown of body fat

Malnutrition—a state of inadequate nutrient intake (such as marasmus) or an excess (such as obesity)

Marasmus—protein-kilocalorie (or protein-energy) malnutrition

Mastication—chewing of food

Meals on Wheels—a community-sponsored program that provides meals to elderly, homebound individuals

Medium chain triglyceride (MCT)—a type of fat that does not require digestion; often used as a form of enteral nutritional support in conditions of fat malabsorption

Megadose—a large dose; generally used to describe supplements of vitamins and minerals that are greater than 10 times the RDA

Metabolism—the process that includes the buildup phase of cell growth (anabolic phase) and the breakdown phase such as with weight loss (catabolic phase)

Metabolite—a substance produced during metabolism

Micronutrient—a substance in food needed in small amounts, such as vitamins and minerals

Mid-arm circumference—a measurement used in anthropometry to help determine body fat percentage

Milk anemia—a form of iron deficiency anemia attributable to an excess intake of milk, which replaces other iron sources such as meat

Minerals—naturally found nonorganic substances needed for health

Modified skim milk—skim milk to which extra protein has been added

Monosaccharide—the simplest form of carbohydrate; one-unit sugar molecules; glucose and fructose

Nasogastric—used to describe the placement of a feeding tube from the nose to the stomach

Nasojejunal—used to describe the placement of a feeding tube from the nose to the jejunum

National Academy of Sciences—a federal advisory group that is involved with setting the Recommended Dietary Allowances (RDAs)

Nitrogen balance—a state in which nitrogen intake through protein ingestion equals the amount being excreted through the kidneys

Non–insulin-dependent diabetes mellitus (NIDDM)—a form of diabetes that typically is found in overweight adults; insulin injection is sometimes necessary for good blood sugar control but is not required for survival

Nutrient—substance found in food needed for health

Nutrient density—the ratio of nutrients to kilocalories; high nutrient density means a large amount of nutrients per serving of food

Nutrition—the sum of the processes by which the body uses food to support health

Nutrition labeling—a description of nutrition analysis found on food labels

Nutrition Program for the Elderly—a federal food assistance program for older persons that emphasizes meals in a congregate setting or delivery of food to homebound persons

Nutrition Screening Initiative—a national attempt to improve the nutritional status of older Americans; includes the DETERMINE checklist.

Nutritional support—provision of enteral and parenteral nutrition; also used to describe the provision of liquid supplements for weight gain

Nutritionist—no legal definition; registered dietitians are nutritionists in the sense that they are trained in the science of nutrition; qualified nutritionists include persons with a minimum of a 4-year degree in the science of nutrition

Obesity—a weight greater than 20 per cent ideal body weight; a body mass index greater than 30

Oliguria—decreased urinary output

Omega-3 fatty acids—the type of fat found in fish oil and some plant products

Optimal nutrition—the level of nutrient intake as appropriate for an individual without excess or inadequacy

Osmolality—the number of particles dissolved in a solution

Overweight—an excess of 10 per cent body weight over an ideal weight

Oxidation—a chemical process of energy metabolism in which oxygen removes electrons from atoms

Oxytocin—a hormone that causes uterine contraction and promotes the let-down reflex in breast-feeding

Palliative care—treatment to relieve or lessen pain or other uncomfortable symptoms but not to effect a cure

Palmar grasp—hand grasp characterized by use of the palm

Pancreas—a gland behind the stomach that releases insulin, glucagon, and some enzymes of digestion for fats and proteins

Pancreatitis—inflammation of the pancreas often associated with alcoholism and fat malabsorption

Parenteral—not through the gastrointestinal tract

Parenteral nutrition—provision of a liquid nutrition formula directly into the blood system via the subclavian vein or other site

Pasteurization—the heating of milk or other liquid to a temperature of 60° C (140° F) for 30 minutes, killing pathogenic bacteria and considerably delaying the development of other bacteria

Pectin—a form of soluble fiber

Pellagra—a nutritional deficiency disease caused by long-term lack of niacin, resulting in a number of nervous, digestive, and skin symptoms

Periodontal—around or near a tooth

Peripheral parenteral nutrition (PPN)—administration of nutrients through peripheral veins

Peristalsis—the waves of contraction by which the digestive tract propels its contents

Pernicious anemia—a form of anemia caused by a lack of the intrinsic factor normally produced by the stomach mucosa, leading to a deficiency in vitamin B_{12}

Phenylalanine—an amino acid found in the sugar substitute Nutrasweet and naturally occurring in protein foods

Physiological stress—physical conditions that disturb the body's homeostasis; examples include injury, infection, and surgery

Pica—an abnormal craving for nonfood substances

Pincer grasp—hand grasp characterized by use of the thumb and index finger

Polydipsia—excess thirst

Polyphagia—excess appetite

Polysaccharides—the most complex form of carbohydrates; many units of sugar linked together

Polyunsaturated fatty acids (PUFA)—found in liquid oils

Postprandial—after meals

Pre-term milk—breast milk from a mother who has given birth to a premature baby

Protein—large organic substances in food that contain nitrogen for building purposes related to growth; provides 4 kilocalories per gram

Protein-energy malnutrition—also known as marasmus

Prudent diet—a diet that is very low in fat

P:S ratio—the ratio of polyunsaturated to saturated fats found in the diet

Purging—describes bulimic actions such as intentional vomiting and laxative abuse

Purine—a compound found in meat and meat extracts; sometimes avoided as a treatment for gout

Reactive hypoglycemia—a form of low blood sugar that may be a precursor to diabetes; characterized by excess but delayed insulin production in response to simple carbohydrate intake

Rebound scurvy—a type of vitamin C deficiency disease caused by rapid withdrawal from chronic ingestion of megadoses of vitamin C

Recommended Dietary Allowances (RDAs)—the amount of nutrients recommended to achieve health; felt to easily meet the nutritional needs of 95 per cent of the population

Refined cereal—cereal that has had its nutritional value reduced by removal of the bran layer and germ from the grain

Residue—the undigested material found in food

Restoration—the process by which the nutrients that have been lost in refining foods are replaced (see also **Enrichment**)

Restorative approach—health care approach with a goal of restoring a person's independence; opposite of the custodial approach

Retinol equivalents (REs)—a means of measuring vitamin A content of food

Rickets—a bone disease that begins in childhood, is caused by lack of vitamin D, and results in bowing of legs

Salmonella—rod-shaped bacteria often associated with dairy products, eggs, and chicken that cause a form of gastroenteritis

Saturated fat—solid fats; found in most animal fats in association with cholesterol and in hydrogenated fats

Self monitoring blood glucose (SMBG)—monitoring of blood glucose levels at home with a blood glucose meter for improved diabetes management

Set point theory—a theory related to the phenomenon of regaining weight lost in dieting, which states that individuals have a set weight that their body seems to return to

Soluble fiber—forms of dietary fiber that dissolve in water and the digestive tract; oat bran and legumes are high in soluble fiber

Specific dynamic action—the increase in metabolism related to the process of digesting food

Sports anemia—anemia in athletes unrelated to iron intake

Steatorrhea—a condition characterized by excess fat in the stool

Steroids—an important group of body compounds that includes sex and adrenal hormones, vitamin D, and cholesterol

Sugar alcohols—a form of sugar found in sugar substitutes that does not promote dental caries (mannitol and sorbitol)

Sulfonylureas—oral compounds that stimulate insulin secretion

Therapeutic diet—a diet modified in nutrients and used as therapy for diabetes, renal and cardiovascular disease, and other diseases and conditions (also Medical Nutrition Therapy)

Total parenteral nutrition (TPN)—administration of nutrients through the superior vena cava

Trans fatty acids—the form of fat found in hydrogenated fats

Transferase—an enzyme that hastens a transfer from one molecule to another

Transferrin—a serum globulin or protein that binds and transports iron

Triceps skinfold—an anthropometric measurement in which calipers measure the fat on the back of the arm; requires training for accuracy

Triglycerides—the form of food fat found in the blood and body tissues

Trypsin—an enzyme produced in the intestine that hastens the hydrolysis of protein

Tube feeding—the provision of a liquid supplement through a tube which extends to either the stomach or the jejunum

Underweight—a body mass index less than 19

Unsaturated fat—fat with low levels of hydrogen; liquid or soft form of fat

US Dietary Guidelines—guidelines aimed at reducing the mortality and morbidity rates of several diseases such as cardiovascular disease, hypertension, cancer, and diabetes mellitus; recommend increased intake of complex carbohydrates and dietary fiber, with reduced intake of fat, sugar, salt, and alcohol; recommend maintaining or achieving desirable weight and including a variety of foods in the diet

US Recommended Dietary Allowances (US RDAs)—a percentage system used in the past for food labels based on the maximum amount of nutrient needs

Vegan—a person who does not eat animal products; protein is derived from plant sources such as legumes, nuts, and seeds

Vegetarian—a person who avoids eating meat for health or spiritual reasons; some vegetarians avoid red meat only

Videofluoroscopy—a test to determine a person's swallowing ability

Villi—the hairlike projections inside the intestinal tract; involved in absorption of digested food matter

Vitamins—substances found in food needed for health; compounds made genetically within plant products and also found in animal products

Water-soluble—a substance that dissolves in water; generally refers to a type of vitamin or certain forms of dietary fiber

Weaning—substituting other forms of feeding for breast-feeding; may also be used to describe gradually discontinuing nutrition support or other life support measures

WIC—the acronym used for the Women, Infants, and Children Supplemental Nutrition Program, a federal food assistance and nutritional education program

Xerostomia—diminished or absent production of saliva

COMMON PREFIXES

cardio—referring to the heart
chemo—chemical, chemistry
dys—abnormal, disordered
extra—outside
hyper—greater than normal
hypo—less than normal
naso—referring to the nose
peri—around, near
poly—many, much
pre—preceding, before

COMMON SUFFIXES

-emia—found in the blood
-genic—producing, forming
-itis—inflammation
-lysis—destruction, decomposition of
-ostomy—an artificial opening formed by surgery (e.g., gastrostomy, ileostomy)
-uria—found in the urine

INDEX

Note: page numbers in *italics* refer to illustrations;
page numbers followed by t refer to tables.

A

Absorption, 84
Achalasia, 258–260
Acid-base balance, 126
Acquired immunodeficiency
　syndrome (AIDS), 297–305
　definition of, 299
　kilocalorie needs in, 302–303
　nutrition in management of, 299–
　　303
　nutritional management of,
　　nurse's and health care
　　professional's role in, 304
　nutritional support in manage-
　　ment of, 310
　pediatric, 303–304
Active listening, 46
Acute renal failure (ARF),
　nutritional treatment of,
　246–249
Addiction, drug, in pregnancy, 354
Additives, food, 475, 476t
Adipose tissue, growth of,
　nutritional factors affecting, 374
Adolescent(s), eating patterns of,
　387–388
　good nutrition for, nurse's and
　　health care professional's role
　　in, 389, 391
　nutritional requirements of, 389
　pregnancy in, 354
Adrenaline, in nutrient metabolism
　and absorption, 92
Aerobic exercise, for weight
　management, 430–431
Affective realm, in nutritional
　assessment, 46
African American food patterns, 25t
Aging. See also *Elderly.*
　definition of, 452
　nutritional status and, 452–456
AIDS (acquired immunodeficiency
　syndrome), 297–305. See also
　*Acquired immunodeficiency
　syndrome (AIDS).*
AIDS enteropathy, 303
AIDS related complex (ARC), 298
　nutrition concerns in, 300
Albumin, low serum levels of, high-
　protein diet for, 162

Albumin *(Continued)*
　in nutritional assessment, 40
　screening for, in diabetes manage-
　　ment, 233
Albuminuria, 243
Alcohol, nutritional status and, 35
　sugar, 65
　use of, by diabetic patient, 229
　in pregnancy, 354
Allergens, food, 330–331
Allergy(ies), cookbooks for, 612
　food, 329–334
　　definition of, 330
　　diagnosis of, 331
　　treatment of, 332–334
Alzheimer's disease, in elderly,
　460–461
Ambulatory care, definition of, 473
Ambulatory care services, offering
　nutrition guidance, 473–475
Amenorrhea, calcium intake and,
　435
America, hunger in, 469–470
American Heart Association (AHA),
　50
　dietary guidelines of, 194, 197
Amino acids, 67–68
　essential, 55, 67
Anabolic phase, of healing, 310
Anabolism, 84
Anaerobic exercise, for weight
　management, 431
Anaphylactic shock, from food
　allergies, 330
Anemia, hemoglobin levels and, 121
　high-iron diet for, 164
　iron-deficiency, in children, 378–
　　381
　　diagnosis and treatment of,
　　　380–381
　　prevention of, 379
　megaloblastic, drugs causing, 179
　milk, 361
　pernicious, 114
　　in elderly, 460
　　high-protein diet for, 162
　in pregnancy, 351
　in renal disease, 250
　sports, 435
Anorexia, cancer and, 288
Anorexia nervosa, 335–336

Anthropometry, in nutritional status
　assessment, 169–172
Anticonvulsants, nutrient
　interactions with, 403
Antidiuretic hormone, release of,
　with excess fluid intake, 359
Antigens, food, 330–331
Antioxidants, 203
　in cancer prevention, 288
Anuria, 243
Appetite, loss of, as drug side effect,
　184
　stimulation of, as drug side effect,
　185
Arachidonic acid, 74
Arsenic, 124
Arteriosclerosis, 192
Arthralgias, in iron overload, 121
Arthritis, in elderly, 458–459
Ascites, 279
　restricted-sodium diet for, 163
Ascorbic acid, 103t, 115–117
Assessment strategies, in nutrition
　care planning process, 40–41
Assistive devices, for eating
　problems, *413*
Atonic constipation, 269
Attention deficit hyperactivity
　disorder (ADHD), 337
Autism, 395
Autonomic neuropathy, complicating
　diabetes, 236
Azotemia, 243

B

Baby-bottle tooth decay, 422–423
Bacterial foodborne illness,
　480t–481t
Balance, 133
Basal energy expenditure, Harris-
　Benedict estimated, 592
Basal metabolism, 85–86
Behavior, malnutrition and,
　375–378
Behavior modification, in obesity
　treatment, 443, 446–447
Behavioral problems, eating
　problems from, 400
Beriberi, 111

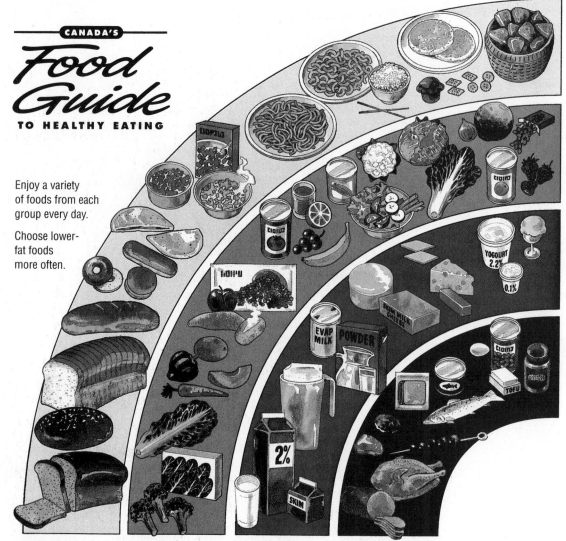

Health and Welfare Canada

Santé et Bien-être social Canada

Canada's Food Guide

TO HEALTHY EATING

Enjoy a variety of foods from each group every day.

Choose lower-fat foods more often.

Grain Products
Choose whole grain and enriched products more often.

Vegetables & Fruit
Choose dark green and orange vegetables and orange fruit more often.

Milk Products
Choose lower-fat milk products more often.

Meat & Alternatives
Choose leaner meats, poultry and fish, as well as dried peas, beans and lentils more often.

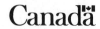